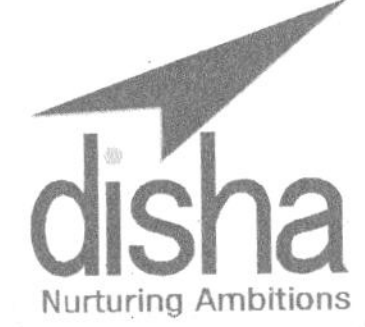

43 JEE MAIN MATHEMATICS

ONLINE & OFFLINE

2019 - 2012 | 2018 - 2002

CHAPTER-WISE + TOPIC-WISE
SOLVED PAPERS

• **Corporate Office :** 45, 2nd Floor, Maharishi Dayanand Marg, Corner Market,
Malviya Nagar, New Delhi-110017
Tel. : 011-49842349 / 49842350

By
D.P. GUPTA
WASIM HUSSAIN BABA

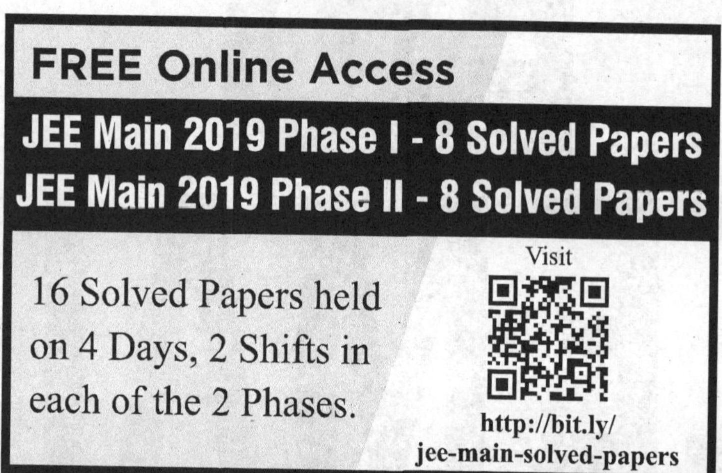

Typeset by Disha DTP Team

DISHA PUBLICATION

For further information about the books from DISHA,
Log on to **www.dishapublication.com** or email to **info@dishapublication.com**

Contents

JEE Main Solved Papers 2019

(Refer to the Main Chapters for Topics)

CHAPTER-1 : Sets

TOPIC-2

1. In a class of 140 students numbered 1 to 140, all even numbered students opted Mathematics course, those whose number is divisible by 3 opted Physics course and those whose number is divisible by 5 opted Chemistry course. Then the number of students who did not opt for any of the three courses is: **[Set II, Jan 2019]**

(a) 102 (b) 42 (c) 1 (d) 38

CHAPTER-2 : Relations and Functions

TOPIC-2

2. If $f(x) = \log_e\left(\frac{1-x}{1+x}\right)$, $|x| < 1$, then $f\left(\frac{2x}{1+x^2}\right)$ is equal to : **[Set I, April 2019]**

(a) $2f(x)$ (b) $2f(x^2)$

(c) $(f(x))^2$ (d) $-2f(x)$

CHAPTER-3 : Trigonometric Functions

TOPIC-1

3. For any $\theta \in \left(\frac{\pi}{4}, \frac{\pi}{2}\right)$ the expression

$3(\sin\theta - \cos\theta)^4 + 6(\sin\theta + \cos\theta)^2 + 4\sin^6\theta$ equals: **[Set I, Jan 2019]**

(a) $13 - 4\cos^2\theta + 6\sin^2\theta\cos^2\theta$

(b) $13 - 4\cos^6\theta$

(c) $13 - 4\cos^2\theta + 6\cos^4\theta$

(d) $13 - 4\cos^4\theta + 2\sin^2\theta\cos^2\theta$

TOPIC-2

4. If $\cos(\alpha + \beta) = \frac{3}{5}$, $\sin(\alpha - \beta) = \frac{5}{13}$ and $0 < \alpha, \beta < \frac{\pi}{4}$, then $\tan(2\alpha)$ is equal to : **[Set I, April 2019]**

(a) $\frac{63}{52}$ (b) $\frac{63}{16}$ (c) $\frac{21}{16}$ (d) $\frac{33}{52}$

5. The value of **[Set II, April 2019]**
$\cos^2 10° - \cos 10° \cos 50° + \cos^2 50°$ is :

(a) $\frac{3}{4} + \cos 20°$ (b) 3/4

(c) $\frac{3}{2}(1 + \cos 20°)$ (d) 3/2

TOPIC-3

6. Let $S = \{\theta \in [-2\pi, 2\pi] : 2\cos^2\theta + 3\sin\theta = 0\}$.
Then the sum of the elements of S is: **[Set II, April 2019]**

(a) $\frac{13\pi}{6}$ (b) $\frac{5\pi}{3}$

(c) 2π (d) π

CHAPTER-4 : Principle of Mathematical Induction

TOPIC-1

7. Consider the statement: "P(n) : $n^2 - n + 41$ is prime." Then which one of the following is true? **[Set II, Jan 2019]**

(a) Both P(3) and P(5) are true.

(b) P(3) is false but P(5) is true.

(c) Both P(3) and P(5) are false.

(d) P(5) is false but P(3) is true.

CHAPTER-5 : Complex Numbers and Quadratic Equations

TOPIC-1

8. Let $A = \left\{\theta \in \left(-\frac{\pi}{2}, \pi\right) : \frac{3 + 2i\sin\theta}{1 - 2i\sin\theta} \text{ is purely imaginary}\right\}$.
Then the sum of the elements in A is: **[Set I, Jan 2019]**

(a) $\frac{5\pi}{6}$ (b) π

(c) $\frac{3\pi}{4}$ (d) $\frac{2\pi}{3}$

9. Let z_1 and z_2 be any two non-zero complex numbers such that $3|z_1| = 4|z_2|$. If $z = \frac{3z_1}{2z_2} + \frac{2z_2}{3z_1}$ then: **[Set II, Jan 2019]**

(a) $\text{Re}(z) = 0$ (b) $|z| = \sqrt{\frac{5}{2}}$

(c) $|z| = \frac{1}{2}\sqrt{\frac{17}{2}}$ (d) $\text{Im}(z) = 0$

TOPIC-3

10. If α and β be the roots of the equation $x^2 - 2x + 2 = 0$, then the least value of n for which $\left(\frac{\alpha}{\beta}\right)^n = 1$ is : **[Set I, April 2019]**
(a) 2 (b) 5
(c) 4 (d) 3

11. The sum of the solutions of the equation $\left|\sqrt{x}-2\right| + \sqrt{x}\left(\sqrt{x}-4\right) + 2 = 0, (x > 0)$ is equal to: **[Set I, April 2019]**
(a) 9 (b) 12
(c) 4 (d) 10

12. Let p, q ϵ R. If $2 - \sqrt{3}$ is a root of the quadratic equation, $x^2 + px + q = 0$, then: **[Set II, April 2019]**
(a) $p^2 - 4q + 12 = 0$ (b) $q^2 - 4p - 16 = 0$
(c) $q^2 + 4p + 14 = 0$ (d) $p^2 - 4q - 12 = 0$

13. Let α and β be two roots of the equation $x^2 + 2x + 2 = 0$, then $\alpha^{15} + \beta^{15}$ is equal to: **[Set I, Jan 2019]**
(a) – 256 (b) 512
(c) –512 (d) 256

TOPIC-4

14. If 5, 5r, $5r^2$ are the lengths of the sides of a triangle, then r cannot be equal to: **[Set II, Jan 2019]**
(a) $\frac{3}{4}$ (b) $\frac{5}{4}$ (c) $\frac{7}{4}$ (d) $\frac{3}{2}$

15. Consider the quadratic equation $(c - 5)x^2 - 2cx + (c - 4) = 0$, $c \neq 5$. Let S be the set of all integral values of c for which one root of the equation lies in the interval (0, 2) and its other root lies in the interval (2, 3). Then the number of elements in S is: **[Set II, Jan 2019]**
(a) 18 (b) 12 (c) 10 (d) 11

CHAPTER-7 : Permutations and Combinations

TOPIC-2

16. All possible numbers are formed using the digits 1, 1, 2, 2, 2, 2, 3, 4, 4 taken all at a time. The number of such numbers in which the odd digits occupy even places is : **[Set I, April 2019]**
(a) 180 (b) 175
(c) 160 (d) 162

17. A committee of 11 members is to be formed from 8 males and 5 females. If m is the number of ways the committee is formed with at least 6 males and n is the number of ways the committee is formed with at least 3 females, then: **[Set II, April 2019]**
(a) m + n = 68 (b) m = n = 78
(c) n = m – 8 (d) m = n = 68

18. Consider a class of 5 girls and 7 boys. The number of different teams consisting of 2 girls and 3 boys that can be formed from this class, if there are two specific boys A and B, who refuse to be the members of the same team, is: **[Set I, Jan 2019]**
(a) 500 (b) 200 (c) 300 (d) 350

19. If $\sum_{i=1}^{20}\left(\frac{{}^{20}C_{i-1}}{{}^{20}C_i + {}^{20}C_{i-1}}\right)^3 = \frac{k}{21}$, then k equals: **[Set II, Jan 2019]**
(a) 400 (b) 50 (c) 200 (d) 100

CHAPTER-8 : Binomial Theorem

TOPIC-1

20. The sum of the co-efficients of all even degree terms in x in the expansion of $\left(x+\sqrt{x^3-1}\right)^6 + \left(x-\sqrt{x^3-1}\right)^6$, $(x > 1)$ is equal to : **[Set I, April 2019]**
(a) 29 (b) 32
(c) 26 (d) 24

21. If the fourth term in the Binomial expansion of $\left(\frac{2}{x} + x^{\log_8 x}\right)^6$ (x > 0) is 20×8^7, then a value of x is: **[Set II, April 2019]**
(a) 8^3 (b) 8^2
(c) 8 (d) 8^{-2}

22. If the fractional part of the number $\frac{2^{403}}{15}$ is $\frac{k}{15}$, then k is equal to: **[Set I, Jan 2019]**
(a) 6 (b) 8 (c) 4 (d) 14

23. If the third term in the binomial expansion of $\left(1 + x^{\log_2 x}\right)^5$ equals 2560, then a possible value of x is: **[Set II, Jan 2019]**
(a) $\frac{1}{4}$ (b) $4\sqrt{2}$
(c) $\frac{1}{8}$ (d) $2\sqrt{2}$

TOPIC-3

24. The sum of the series $2 \cdot {}^{20}C_0 + 5 \cdot {}^{20}C_1 + 8 \cdot {}^{20}C_2 + 11 \cdot {}^{20}C_3 + \ldots + 62 \cdot {}^{20}C_{20}$ is equal to : **[Set I, April 2019]**
(a) 2^{26} (b) 2^{25}
(c) 2^{23} (d) 2^{24}

CHAPTER-9 : Sequences and Series

TOPIC-1

25. The sum of all natural numbers 'n' such that $100 < n < 200$ and H.C.F. $(91, n) > 1$ is : **[Set I, April 2019]**
(a) 3203 (b) 3303
(c) 3221 (d) 3121

26. Let the sum of the first n terms of a non-constant A.P., $a_1, a_2, a_3, \ldots\ldots$ be $50n + \frac{n(n-7)}{2}A$, where A is a constant. If d is the common difference of this A.P., then the ordered pair (d, a_{50}) is equal to: **[Set II, April 2019]**
(a) (50, 50 + 46A) (b) (50, 50 + 45A)
(c) (A, 50 + 45A) (d) (A, 50 + 46A)

27. Let $a_1, a_2, \ldots, a_{30}$ be an A.P., $S = \sum_{i=1}^{30} a_i$ and $T = \sum_{i=1}^{15} a_{(2i-1)}$. If $a_5 = 27$ and $S - 2T = 75$, then a_{10} is equal to: **[Set I, Jan 2019]**
(a) 52 (b) 57
(c) 47 (d) 42

28. The sum of all two digit positive numbers which when divided by 7 yield 2 or 5 as remainder is: **[Set II, Jan 2019]**
(a) 1256 (b) 1465
(c) 1365 (d) 1356

TOPIC-2

29. Let $\sum_{k=1}^{10} f(a+k) = 16(2^{10}-1)$, where the function f satisfies $f(x + y) = f(x) f(y)$ for all natural numbers x, y and f(1) = 2. Then the natural number 'a' is: **[Set II, April 2019]**
(a) 2 (b) 16
(c) 4 (d) 3

30. If a, b and c be three distinct real numbers in G.P. and $a + b + c = xb$, then x cannot be: **[Set I, Jan 2019]**
(a) –2 (b) –3 (c) 4 (d) 2

TOPIC-3

31. The sum of all values of $\theta \in \left(0, \frac{\pi}{2}\right)$ satisfying $\sin^2 2\theta + \cos^4 2\theta = \frac{3}{4}$ is: **[Set II, Jan 2019]**
(a) π (b) $\frac{5\pi}{4}$ (c) $\frac{\pi}{2}$ (d) $\frac{3\pi}{8}$

CHAPTER-10 : Straight Lines and Pair of Straight Lines

TOPIC-1

32. Let O(0, 0) and A(0, 1) be two fixed points. Then the locus of a point P such that the perimeter of ΔAOP is 4, is : **[Set I, April 2019]**
(a) $8x^2 - 9y^2 + 9y = 18$
(b) $9x^2 - 8y^2 + 8y = 16$
(c) $9x^2 + 8y^2 - 8y = 16$
(d) $8x^2 + 9y^2 - 9y = 18$

TOPIC-2

33. A point on the straight line, $3x + 5y = 15$ which is equidistant from the coordinate axes will lie only in : **[Set I, April 2019]**
(a) 4th quadrant (b) 1st quadrant
(c) 1st and 2nd quadrants (d) 1st, 2nd and 4th quadrants

34. Slope of a line passing through P(2, 3) and intersecting the line x + y = 7 at a distance of 4 units from P, is: **[Set II, April 2019]**
(a) $\frac{1-\sqrt{5}}{1+\sqrt{5}}$ (b) $\frac{1-\sqrt{7}}{1+\sqrt{7}}$
(c) $\frac{\sqrt{7}-1}{\sqrt{7}+1}$ (d) $\frac{\sqrt{5}-1}{\sqrt{5}+1}$

35. A point P moves on the line $2x - 3y + 4 = 0$. If Q(1, 4) and R(3, –2) are fixed points, then the locus of the centroid of ΔPQR is a line: **[Set II, Jan 2019]**
(a) with slope $\frac{3}{2}$ (b) parallel to x-axis
(c) with slope $\frac{2}{3}$ (d) parallel to y-axis

36. If the line 3x + 4y – 24 = 0 intersects the x-axis at the point A and the y-axis at the point B, then the incentre of the triangle OAB, where O is the origin, is: **[Set II, Jan 2019]**
(a) (3, 4) (b) (2, 2) (c) (4, 3) (d) (4, 4)

TOPIC-3

37. Consider the set of all lines $px + qy + r = 0$ such that $3p + 2q + 4r = 0$. Which one of the following statements is true? **[Set I, Jan 2019]**
(a) The lines are concurrent at the point $\left(\frac{3}{4}, \frac{1}{2}\right)$.
(b) Each line passes through the origin.
(c) The lines are all parallel.
(d) The lines are not concurrent.

CHAPTER-11 : Conic Sections

TOPIC-1

38. The sum of the squares of the lengths of the chords intercepted on the circle, $x^2 + y^2 = 16$, by the lines, $x + y = n$, $n \in N$, where N is the set of all natural numbers, is : **[Set I, April 2019]**
(a) 320 (b) 105 (c) 160 (d) 210

39. All the points in the set $S = \left\{\frac{\alpha+i}{\alpha-1} : \alpha \in R\right\} (i = \sqrt{-1})$ lie on a: **[Set II, April 2019]**
(a) straight line whose slope is 1.
(b) circle whose radius is 1.
(c) circle whose radius is $\sqrt{2}$.
(d) straight line whose slope is –1.

40. If a tangent to the circle $x^2 + y^2 = 1$ intersects the coordinate axes at distinct points P and Q, then the locus of the mid-point of PQ is: **[Set II, April 2019]**

(a) $x^2 + y^2 - 4x^2y^2 = 0$ (b) $x^2 + y^2 - 2xy = 0$

(c) $x^2 + y^2 - 16x^2y^2 = 0$ (d) $x^2 + y^2 - 2x^2y^2 = 0$

41. Three circles of radii a, b, c (a < b < c) touch each other externally. If they have *x*-axis as a common tangent, then: **[Set I, Jan 2019]**

(a) $\frac{1}{\sqrt{a}} = \frac{1}{\sqrt{b}} + \frac{1}{\sqrt{c}}$

(b) $\frac{1}{\sqrt{b}} = \frac{1}{\sqrt{a}} + \frac{1}{\sqrt{c}}$

(c) a, b, c are in A.P

(d) $\sqrt{a}, \sqrt{b}, \sqrt{c}$ are in A.P.

42. If a circle C passing through the point (4, 0) touches the circle $x^2 + y^2 + 4x - 6y = 12$ externally at the point (1, – 1), then the radius of C is: **[Set II, Jan 2019]**

(a) $2\sqrt{5}$ (b) 4

(c) 5 (d) $\sqrt{57}$

TOPIC-2

43. The shortest distance between the line $y = x$ and the curve $y^2 = x - 2$ is : **[Set I, April 2019]**

(a) 2 (b) $\frac{7}{8}$ (c) $\frac{7}{4\sqrt{2}}$ (d) $\frac{11}{4\sqrt{2}}$

44. If one end of a focal chord of the parabola, $y^2 = 16x$ is at (1, 4), then the length of this focal chord is: **[Set II, April 2019]**

(a) 25 (b) 22 (c) 24 (d) 20

45. Axis of a parabola lies along x-axis. If its vertex and focus are at distance 2 and 4 respectively from the origin, on the positive *x*-axis then which of the following points does not lie on it? **[Set I, Jan 2019]**

(a) $(5, 2\sqrt{6})$ (b) (8, 6)

(c) $(6, 4\sqrt{2})$ (d) (4, – 4)

46. Equation of a common tangent to the circle, $x^2 + y^2 - 6x = 0$ and the parabola, $y^2 = 4x$, is : **[Set I, Jan 2019]**

(a) $2\sqrt{3}y = 12x + 1$ (b) $\sqrt{3}y = x + 3$

(c) $2\sqrt{3}y = -x - 12$ (d) $\sqrt{3}y = 3x + 1$

47. If the parabolas $y^2 = 4b(x - c)$ and $y^2 = 8ax$ have a common normal, then which one of the following is a valid choice for the ordered triad (a, b, c)? **[Set II, Jan 2019]**

(a) $\left(\frac{1}{2}, 2, 3\right)$ (b) (1, 1, 3)

(c) $\left(\frac{1}{2}, 2, 0\right)$ (d) (1, 1, 0)

TOPIC-3

48. If the tangents on the ellipse $4x^2 + y^2 = 8$ at the points (1, 2) and (*a*, *b*) are perpendicular to each other, then a^2 is equal to : **[Set I, April 2019]**

(a) $\frac{128}{17}$ (b) $\frac{64}{17}$ (c) $\frac{4}{17}$ (d) $\frac{2}{17}$

TOPIC-4

49. If the line $y = mx + 7\sqrt{3}$ is normal to the hyperbola $\frac{x^2}{24} - \frac{y^2}{18} = 1$, then a value of m is : **[Set II, April 2019]**

(a) $\frac{\sqrt{5}}{2}$ (b) $\frac{\sqrt{15}}{2}$ (c) $\frac{2}{\sqrt{5}}$ (d) $\frac{3}{\sqrt{5}}$

50. Let $0 < \theta < \frac{\pi}{2}$. If the eccentricity of the hyperbola $\frac{x^2}{\cos^2\theta} - \frac{y^2}{\sin^2\theta} = 1$ is greater than 2, then the length of its latus rectum lies in the interval: **[Set I, Jan 2019]**

(a) $(3, \infty)$ (b) (3/2, 2]

(c) (2, 3] (d) (1, 3/2]

51. The equation of a tangent to the hyperbola $4x^2 - 5y^2 = 20$ parallel to the line $x - y = 2$ is: **[Set II, Jan 2019]**

(a) $x - y + 1 = 0$ (b) $x - y + 7 = 0$

(c) $x - y + 9 = 0$ (d) $x - y - 3 = 0$

CHAPTER-12 : Limits and Derivatives

TOPIC-1

52. $\lim_{x\to 0} \frac{\sin^2 x}{\sqrt{2} - \sqrt{1+\cos x}}$ equals : **[Set I, April 2019]**

(a) $4\sqrt{2}$ (b) $\sqrt{2}$ (c) $2\sqrt{2}$ (d) 4

53. $\lim_{y\to 0} \frac{\sqrt{1+\sqrt{1+y^4}} - \sqrt{2}}{y^4}$ **[Set I, Jan 2019]**

(a) exists and equals $\frac{1}{4\sqrt{2}}$

(b) exists and equals $\frac{1}{2\sqrt{2}(\sqrt{2}+1)}$

(c) exists and equals $\frac{1}{2\sqrt{2}}$

(d) does not exist

54. For each $t \in \mathbf{R}$, let [t] be the greatest integer less than or equal to t. Then, **[Set II, Jan 2019]**

$$\lim_{x\to 1+} \frac{(1 - |x| + \sin|1 - x|)\sin\left(\frac{\pi}{2}[1 - x]\right)}{|1 - x|[1 - x]}$$

(a) equals 1 (b) equals 0

(c) equals – 1 (d) does not exist

CHAPTER-13 : Mathematical Reasoning

TOPIC-1

55. If the Boolean expression $(p \oplus q) \wedge (\sim p \odot q)$ is equivalent to $p \wedge q$, where $\oplus, \odot \in \{\wedge, \vee\}$ then the ordered pair $(\oplus, \odot)$ is: **[Set I, Jan 2019]**

(a) $(\vee, \wedge)$ (b) $(\vee, \vee)$

(c) $(\wedge, \vee)$ (d) $(\wedge, \wedge)$

TOPIC-2

56. The contrapositive of the statement "If you are born in India, then you are a citizen of India", is : **[Set I, April 2019]**

(a) If you are not a citizen of India, then you are not born in India.
(b) If you are a citizen of India, then you are born in India.
(c) If you are born in India, then you are not a citizen of India.
(d) If you are not born in India, then you are not a citizen of India.

57. For any two statements p and q, the negation of the expression $p \vee (\sim p \wedge q)$ is: **[Set II, April 2019]**

(a) $\sim p \wedge \sim q$ (b) $p \wedge q$

(c) $p \leftrightarrow q$ (d) $\sim p \vee \sim q$

CHAPTER-14 : Statistics

TOPIC-2

58. The mean and variance of seven observations are 8 and 16, respectively. If 5 of the observations are 2, 4, 10, 12, 14, then the product of the remaining two observations is : **[Set I, April 2019]**

(a) 45 (b) 49

(c) 48 (d) 40

59. If the standard deviation of the numbers –1, 0, 1, k is $\sqrt{5}$ where $k > 0$, then k is equal to: **[Set II, April 2019]**

(a) $2\sqrt{6}$ (b) $2\sqrt{\frac{10}{3}}$

(c) $4\sqrt{\frac{5}{3}}$ (d) $\sqrt{6}$

60. 5 students of a class have an average height 150 cm and variance 18 cm^2. A new student, whose height is 156 cm, joined them. The variance (in cm^2) of the height of these six students is: **[Set I, Jan 2019]**

(a) 16 (b) 22 (c) 20 (d) 18

61. The mean of five observations is 5 and their variance is 9.20. If three of the given five observations are 1, 3 and 8, then a ratio of other two observations is: **[Set II, Jan 2019]**

(a) 10 : 3 (b) 4 : 9

(c) 5 : 8 (d) 6 : 7

CHAPTER-16 : Relations and Functions

TOPIC-2

62. For $x \in \mathbf{R} - \{0, 1\}$, let $f_1(x) = \frac{1}{x}$, $f_2(x) = 1 - x$ and $f_3(x) = \frac{1}{1-x}$ be three given functions. If a function, J(x) satisfies $(f_2 o J o f_1)(x) = f_3(x)$ then J(x) is equal to: **[Set I, Jan 2019]**

(a) $f_3(x)$ (b) $\frac{1}{x} f_3(x)$

(c) $f_2(x)$ (d) $f_1(x)$

CHAPTER-17 : Inverse Trigonometric Functions

TOPIC-2

63. If $\alpha = \cos^{-1}\left(\frac{3}{5}\right)$, $\beta = \tan^{-1}\left(\frac{1}{3}\right)$, where $0 < \alpha, \beta < \frac{\pi}{2}$, then $\alpha - \beta$ is equal to : **[Set I, April 2019]**

(a) $\tan^{-1}\left(\frac{9}{5\sqrt{10}}\right)$ (b) $\cos^{-1}\left(\frac{9}{5\sqrt{10}}\right)$

(c) $\tan^{-1}\left(\frac{9}{14}\right)$ (d) $\sin^{-1}\left(\frac{9}{5\sqrt{10}}\right)$

64. If $\cos^{-1}\left(\frac{2}{3x}\right) + \cos^{-1}\left(\frac{3}{4x}\right) = \frac{\pi}{2}\left(x > \frac{3}{4}\right)$, then x is equal to: **[Set I, Jan 2019]**

(a) $\frac{\sqrt{145}}{12}$ (b) $\frac{\sqrt{145}}{10}$

(c) $\frac{\sqrt{146}}{12}$ (d) $\frac{\sqrt{145}}{11}$

CHAPTER-18 : Matrices

TOPIC-1

65. Let $A = \begin{bmatrix} \cos\alpha & -\sin\alpha \\ \sin\alpha & \cos\alpha \end{bmatrix}$, $(\alpha \in R)$ such that $A^{32} = \begin{bmatrix} 0 & -1 \\ 1 & 0 \end{bmatrix}$. Then a value of α is : **[Set I, April 2019]**

(a) $\frac{\pi}{32}$ (b) 0 (c) $\frac{\pi}{64}$ (d) $\frac{\pi}{16}$

CHAPTER-19 : Determinants

TOPIC-2

66. Let α and β be the roots of the equation $x^2 + x + 1 = 0$. Then for $y \neq 0$ in R, $\begin{vmatrix} y+1 & \alpha & \beta \\ \alpha & y+\beta & 1 \\ \beta & 1 & y+\alpha \end{vmatrix}$ is equal to: **[Set II, April 2019]**

(a) $y(y^2 - 1)$ (b) $y(y^2 - 3)$

(c) y^3 (d) $y^3 - 1$

67. Let d∈**R**, and

$$A = \begin{bmatrix} -2 & 4+d & (\sin\theta)^{-2} \\ 1 & (\sin\theta)+2 & d \\ 5 & (2\sin\theta)-d & (-\sin\theta)+2+2d \end{bmatrix},$$

$\theta \in [0, 2\pi]$. If the minimum value of det (A) is 8, then a value of d is: **[Set II, Jan 2019]**

(a) -5 (b) -7
(c) $2\left(\sqrt{2}+1\right)$ (d) $2\left(\sqrt{2}+2\right)$

TOPIC-3

68. If

$$\begin{bmatrix}1 & 1\\0 & 1\end{bmatrix}\cdot\begin{bmatrix}1 & 2\\0 & 1\end{bmatrix}\cdot\begin{bmatrix}1 & 3\\0 & 1\end{bmatrix}\cdots\cdots\begin{bmatrix}1 & n-1\\0 & 1\end{bmatrix}=\begin{bmatrix}1 & 78\\0 & 1\end{bmatrix},$$

then the inverse of $\begin{bmatrix}1 & n\\0 & 1\end{bmatrix}$ is: **[Set II, April 2019]**

(a) $\begin{bmatrix}1 & 0\\12 & 1\end{bmatrix}$ (b) $\begin{bmatrix}1 & -13\\0 & 1\end{bmatrix}$
(c) $\begin{bmatrix}1 & -12\\0 & 1\end{bmatrix}$ (d) $\begin{bmatrix}1 & 0\\13 & 1\end{bmatrix}$

69. If $A = \begin{bmatrix}\cos\theta & -\sin\theta\\ \sin\theta & \cos\theta\end{bmatrix}$, then the matrix A^{-50} when

$\theta = \dfrac{\pi}{12}$, is equal to: **[Set I, Jan 2019]**

(a) $\begin{bmatrix}\frac{1}{2} & -\frac{\sqrt{3}}{2}\\ \frac{\sqrt{3}}{2} & \frac{1}{2}\end{bmatrix}$ (b) $\begin{bmatrix}\frac{\sqrt{3}}{2} & -\frac{1}{2}\\ \frac{1}{2} & \frac{\sqrt{3}}{2}\end{bmatrix}$
(c) $\begin{bmatrix}\frac{\sqrt{3}}{2} & \frac{1}{2}\\ -\frac{1}{2} & \frac{\sqrt{3}}{2}\end{bmatrix}$ (d) $\begin{bmatrix}\frac{1}{2} & \frac{\sqrt{3}}{2}\\ -\frac{\sqrt{3}}{2} & \frac{1}{2}\end{bmatrix}$

TOPIC-4

70. The greatest value of $c \in R$ for which the system of linear equations

$x - cy - cz = 0;\ cx - y + cz = 0;\ cx + cy - z = 0$

has a non-trivial solution, is : **[Set I, April 2019]**

(a) -1 (b) $\dfrac{1}{2}$ (c) 2 (d) 0

71. If the system of equations **[Set II, Jan 2019]**

$x + y + z = 5$
$x + 2y + 3z = 9$
$x + 3y + \alpha z = \beta$

has infinitely many solutions, then $\beta - \alpha$ equals:

(a) 21 (b) 8
(c) 18 (d) 5

CHAPTER-20 : Continuity and Differentiability

TOPIC-1

72. If the function f defined on $\left(\dfrac{\pi}{6}, \dfrac{\pi}{3}\right)$ by

$$f(x) = \begin{cases} \dfrac{\sqrt{2}\cos x - 1}{\cot x - 1}, & x \neq \dfrac{\pi}{4} \\ k, & x = \dfrac{\pi}{4} \end{cases}$$

is continuous, then k is equal to: **[Set II, April 2019]**

(a) 2 (b) $\dfrac{1}{2}$
(c) 1 (d) $\dfrac{1}{\sqrt{2}}$

73. Let $f : \mathbf{R} \to \mathbf{R}$ be a function defined as

$$f(x) = \begin{cases} 5, & \text{if } x \le 1 \\ a + bx, & \text{if } 1 < x < 3 \\ b + 5x, & \text{if } 3 \le x < 5 \\ 30, & \text{if } x \ge 5 \end{cases}$$

Then, f is : **[Set I, Jan 2019]**

(a) continuous if a = 5 and b = 5
(b) continuous if a = – 5 and b = 10
(c) continous if a = 0 and b = 5
(d) not continuous for any values of a and b

TOPIC-2

74. Let $f(x) = 15 - |x - 10|$; $x \in R$. Then the set of all values of x, at which the function, $g(x) = f(f(x))$ is not differentiable, is: **[Set II, April 2019]**

(a) {5, 10, 15} (b) {10, 15}
(c) {5, 10, 15, 20} (d) {10}

75. Let $f(x) = \begin{cases} \max\{|x|, x^2\} & |x| \le 2 \\ 8 - 2|x|, & 2 < |x| \le 4 \end{cases}$

Let S be the set of points in the interval (– 4, 4) at which f is not differentiable. Then S: **[Set II, Jan 2019]**

(a) is an empty set
(b) equals {– 2, – 1, 0, 1, 2}
(c) equals {– 2, – 1, 1, 2}
(d) equals {– 2, 2}

TOPIC-3

76. If $2y = \left(\cot^{-1}\left(\dfrac{\sqrt{3}\cos x + \sin x}{\cos x - \sqrt{3}\sin x}\right)\right)^2$, $x \in \left(0, \dfrac{\pi}{2}\right)$ then $\dfrac{dy}{dx}$ is equal to : **[Set I, April 2019]**

(a) $\dfrac{\pi}{6} - x$ (b) $x - \dfrac{\pi}{6}$
(c) $\dfrac{\pi}{3} - x$ (d) $2x - \dfrac{\pi}{3}$

TOPIC-4

77. Let $f : \mathbf{R} \to \mathbf{R}$ be a function such that $f(x) = x^3 + x^2 f'(1) + xf''(2) + f'''(3)$, $x \in \mathbf{R}$. Then $f(2)$ equals: **[Set II, Jan 2019]**

(a) -4 (b) 30

(c) -2 (d) 8

CHAPTER-21 : Applications of Derivatives

TOPIC-2

78. Let $f: [0 : 2] \to R$ be a twice differentiable function such that $f''(x) > 0$, for all $x \in (0, 2)$. If $\phi(x) = f(x) + f(2-x)$, then ϕ is : **[Set I, April 2019]**

(a) increasing on (0, 1) and decreasing on (1, 2).
(b) decreasing on (0, 2)
(c) decreasing on (0, 1) and increasing on (1, 2).
(d) increasing on (0, 2)

79. If the function $f : R - \{1, -1\} \to A$ defined by $f(x) = \frac{x^2}{1-x^2}$, is surjective, then A is equal to: **[Set II, April 2019]**

(a) $R - \{-1\}$ (b) $[0, \infty)$

(c) $R - [-1, 0)$ (d) $R - (-1, 0)$

TOPIC-3

80. If the tangent to the curve, $y = x^3 + ax - b$ at the point $(1, -5)$ is perpendicular to the line, $-x + y + 4 = 0$, then which one of the following points lies on the curve? **[Set II, April 2019]**

(a) $(-2, 1)$ (b) $(-2, 2)$
(c) $(2, -1)$ (d) $(2, -2)$

81. Let S be the set of all values of x for which the tangent to the curve $y = f(x) = x^3 - x^2 - 2x$ at (x, y) is parallel to the line segment joining the points $(1, f(1))$ and $(-1, f(-1))$, then S is equal to: **[Set II, April 2019]**

(a) $\left\{\frac{1}{3}, 1\right\}$ (b) $\left\{-\frac{1}{3}, -1\right\}$

(c) $\left\{\frac{1}{3}, -1\right\}$ (d) $\left\{-\frac{1}{3}, 1\right\}$

82. If θ denotes the acute angle between the curves, $y = 10 - x^2$ and $y = 2 + x^2$ at a point of their intersection, then $|\tan\theta|$ is equal to: **[Set I, Jan 2019]**

(a) $\frac{4}{9}$ (b) $\frac{8}{15}$

(c) $\frac{7}{17}$ (d) $\frac{8}{17}$

83. The shortest distance between the point $\left(\frac{3}{2}, 0\right)$ and the curve $y = \sqrt{x}$, $(x > 0)$, is: **[Set II, Jan 2019]**

(a) $\frac{\sqrt{5}}{2}$ (b) $\frac{\sqrt{3}}{2}$ (c) $\frac{3}{2}$ (d) $\frac{5}{4}$

TOPIC-4

84. If S_1 and S_2 are respectively the sets of local minimum and local maximum points of the function, $f(x) = 9x^4 + 12x^3 - 36x^2 + 25$, $x \in R$, then : **[Set I, April 2019]**

(a) $S_1 = \{-2\}$; $S_2 = \{0, 1\}$ (b) $S_1 = \{-2, 0\}$; $S_2 = \{1\}$
(c) $S_1 = \{-2, 1\}$; $S_2 = \{0\}$ (d) $S_1 = \{-1\}$; $S_2 = \{0, 2\}$

85. The maximum volume (in cu.m) of the right circular cone having slant height 3 m is: **[Set I, Jan 2019]**

(a) 6π (b) $3\sqrt{3}\pi$ (c) $\frac{4}{3}\pi$ (d) $2\sqrt{3}\pi$

CHAPTER-22 : Integrals

TOPIC-1

86. $\int \frac{\sin\frac{5x}{2}}{\sin\frac{x}{2}} dx$ is equal to :

(where c is a constant of integration.) **[Set I, April 2019]**

(a) $2x + \sin x + 2\sin 2x + c$ (b) $x + 2\sin x + 2\sin 2x + c$
(c) $x + 2\sin x + \sin 2x + c$ (d) $2x + \sin x + \sin 2x + c$

87. If f(x) is a non-zero polynomial of degree four, having local extreme points at $x = -1, 0, 1$; then the set $S = \{x \in R : f(x) = f(0)\}$ contains exactly: **[Set II, April 2019]**

(a) four irrational numbers.
(b) four rational numbers.
(c) two irrational and two rational numbers.
(d) two irrational and one rational number.

88. The integral $\int \sec^{2/3} x \operatorname{cosec}^{4/3} x \, dx$ is equal to: **[Set II, April 2019]**

(a) $-3\tan^{-1/3} x + C$ (b) $-\frac{3}{4}\tan^{-4/3} x + C$

(c) $-3\cot^{-1/3} x + C$ (d) $3\tan^{-1/3} x + C$

(Here C is a constant of integration)

89. For $x^2 \neq n\pi + 1$, $n \in N$ (the set of natural numbers), the integral **[Set I, Jan 2019]**

$$\int x\sqrt{\frac{2\sin(x^2-1) - \sin 2(x^2-1)}{2\sin(x^2-1) + \sin 2(x^2-1)}}\, dx$$ is equal to:

(a) $\log_e\left|\frac{1}{2}\sec^2(x^2-1)\right| + c$

(b) $\frac{1}{2}\log_e|\sec(x^2-1)| + c$

(c) $\frac{1}{2}\log_e\left|\sec^2\left(\frac{x^2-1}{2}\right)\right| + c$

(d) $\log_e\left|\sec\left(\frac{x^2-1}{2}\right)\right| + c$

(where c is a constant of integration)

90. Let $I=\int_a^b (x^4-2x^2)dx$. If I is minimum then the ordered pair (a, b) is: **[Set II, Jan 2019]**

(a) $\left(0,\sqrt{2}\right)$ (b) $\left(-\sqrt{2},0\right)$

(c) $\left(\sqrt{2},-\sqrt{2}\right)$ (d) $\left(-\sqrt{2},\sqrt{2}\right)$

TOPIC-3

91. If $f(x)=\dfrac{2-x\cos x}{2+x\cos x}$ and $g(x)=\log_e x$, (x > 0) then the value of the integral $\int_{-\frac{\pi}{4}}^{\frac{\pi}{4}} g(f(x))dx$ is: **[Set I, April 2019]**

(a) $\log_e 3$ (b) $\log_e e$
(c) $\log_e 2$ (d) $\log_e 1$

92. The value of $\int_0^{\pi/2}\dfrac{\sin^3 x}{\sin x+\cos x}dx$ is: **[Set II, April 2019]**

(a) $\dfrac{\pi-2}{8}$ (b) $\dfrac{\pi-1}{4}$

(c) $\dfrac{\pi-2}{4}$ (d) $\dfrac{\pi-1}{2}$

93. The value of $\int_0^{\pi}|\cos x|^3\,dx$ is: **[Set I, Jan 2019]**

(a) 0 (b) $\dfrac{4}{3}$

(c) $\dfrac{2}{3}$ (d) $-\dfrac{4}{3}$

94. Let n ≥ 2 be a natural number and $0<\theta<\dfrac{\pi}{2}$

Then $\int\dfrac{(\sin^n\theta+\sin\theta)^{\frac{1}{n}}\cos\theta}{\sin^{n+1}\theta}d\theta$ is equal to: **[Set II, Jan 2019]**

(a) $\dfrac{n}{n^2-1}\left(1-\dfrac{1}{\sin^{n-1}\theta}\right)^{\frac{n+1}{n}}+C$

(b) $\dfrac{n}{n^2+1}\left(1-\dfrac{1}{\sin^{n-1}\theta}\right)^{\frac{n+1}{n}}+C$

(c) $\dfrac{n}{n^2-1}\left(1+\dfrac{1}{\sin^{n-1}\theta}\right)^{\frac{n+1}{n}}+C$

(d) $\dfrac{n}{n^2-1}\left(1-\dfrac{1}{\sin^{n+1}\theta}\right)^{\frac{n+1}{n}}+C$

(where C is a constant of integration)

CHAPTER-23 : Applications of Integrals

TOPIC-1

95. The area (in sq. units) of the region $A=\{(x,y)\in R\times R|0\le x\le 3, 0\le y\le 4, y\le x^2+3x\}$ is: **[Set I, April 2019]**

(a) $\dfrac{53}{6}$ (b) 8

(c) $\dfrac{59}{6}$ (d) $\dfrac{26}{3}$

TOPIC-2

96. The area (in sq. units) of the region $A=\{(x,y):x^2\le y\le x+2\}$ is: **[Set II, April 2019]**

(a) $\dfrac{10}{3}$ (b) $\dfrac{9}{2}$

(c) $\dfrac{31}{6}$ (d) $\dfrac{13}{6}$

97. The area (in sq. units) bounded by the parabola $y=x^2-1$, the tangent at the point (2, 3) to it and the y-axis is: **[Set I, Jan 2019]**

(a) $\dfrac{8}{3}$ (b) $\dfrac{32}{3}$

(c) $\dfrac{56}{3}$ (d) $\dfrac{14}{3}$

98. If the area enclosed between the curves $y=kx^2$ and $x=ky^2$, (k > 0), is 1 square unit. Then k is: **[Set II, Jan 2019]**

(a) $\dfrac{\sqrt{3}}{2}$ (b) $\dfrac{1}{\sqrt{3}}$

(c) $\sqrt{3}$ (d) $\dfrac{2}{\sqrt{3}}$

CHAPTER-24 : Differential Equations

TOPIC-2

99. If $\dfrac{dy}{dx}+\dfrac{3}{\cos^2 x}y=\dfrac{1}{\cos^2 x}, x\in\left(\dfrac{-\pi}{3},\dfrac{\pi}{3}\right)$, and $y\left(\dfrac{\pi}{4}\right)=\dfrac{4}{3}$, then $y\left(-\dfrac{\pi}{4}\right)$ equals: **[Set II, Jan 2019]**

(a) $\dfrac{1}{3}+e^6$ (b) $\dfrac{1}{3}$ (c) $-\dfrac{4}{3}$ (d) $\dfrac{1}{3}+e^3$

TOPIC-3

100. Let $y=y(x)$ be the solution of the differential equation, $(x^2+1)^2\dfrac{dy}{dx}+2x(x^2+1)y=1$ such that $y(0)=0$. If $\sqrt{a}\,y(1)=\dfrac{\pi}{32}$, then the value of 'a' is: **[Set I, April 2019]**

(a) $\dfrac{1}{4}$ (b) $\dfrac{1}{2}$ (c) 1 (d) $\dfrac{1}{16}$

101. The solution of the differential equation $x\frac{dy}{dx} + 2y = x^2$ $(x \neq 0)$ with $y(1) = 1$, is: **[Set II, April 2019]**

(a) $y = \frac{4}{5}x^3 + \frac{1}{5x^2}$ (b) $y = \frac{x^3}{5} + \frac{1}{5x^2}$

(c) $y = \frac{x^2}{4} + \frac{3}{4x^2}$ (d) $y = \frac{3}{4}x^2 + \frac{1}{4x^2}$

102. If $y = y(x)$ is the solution of the differential equation, $x\frac{dy}{dx} + 2y = x^2$ satisfying $y(1) = 1$, then $\left(-\right)$ is equal to: **[Set I, Jan 2019]**

(a) $\frac{7}{64}$ (b) $\frac{1}{4}$ (c) $\frac{49}{16}$ (d) $\frac{13}{16}$

CHAPTER-25 : Vector Algebra

TOPIC-2

103. Let $\vec{a} = 2\hat{i} + \lambda_1\hat{j} + 3\hat{k}, \vec{b} = 4\hat{i} + (3 - \lambda_2)\hat{j} + 6\hat{k}$ and $\vec{c} = 3\hat{i} + 6\hat{j} + (\lambda_3 - 1)\hat{k}$ be three vectors such that $\vec{b} = 2\vec{a}$ and $\vec{a}$ is perpendicular to $\vec{c}$ Then a possible value of $(\lambda_1, \lambda_2, \lambda_3)$ is: **[Set II, Jan 2019]**

(a) (1, 3, 1) (b) $\left(-\frac{1}{2}, 4, 0\right)$

(c) $\left(\frac{1}{2}, 4, -2\right)$ (d) (1, 5, 1)

TOPIC-3

104. The magnitude of the projection of the vector $2\hat{i} + 3\hat{j} + \hat{k}$ on the vector perpendicular to the plane containing the vectors $\hat{i} + \hat{j} + \hat{k}$ and $\hat{i} + 2\hat{j} + 3\hat{k}$, is : **[Set I, April 2019]**

(a) $\frac{\sqrt{3}}{2}$ (b) $\sqrt{6}$

(c) $3\sqrt{6}$ (d) $\sqrt{\frac{3}{2}}$

105. Let $\vec{\alpha} = 3\hat{i} + \hat{j}$ and $\vec{\beta} = 2\hat{i} - \hat{j} + 3\hat{k}$. If $\vec{\beta} = \vec{\beta}_1 - \vec{\beta}_2$, where $\vec{\beta}_1$ is parallel to $\vec{\alpha}$ and $\vec{\beta}_2$ is perpendicular to $\vec{\alpha}$, then $\vec{\beta}_1 \times \vec{\beta}_2$ is equal to: **[Set II, April 2019]**

(a) $-3\hat{i} + 9\hat{j} + 5\hat{k}$ (b) $3\hat{i} - 9\hat{j} - 5\hat{k}$

(c) $\frac{1}{2}\left(-3\hat{i} + 9\hat{j} + 5\hat{k}\right)$ (d) $\frac{1}{2}\left(3\hat{i} - 9\hat{j} + 5\hat{k}\right)$

106. Let $\vec{a} = \hat{i} - \hat{j}, \vec{b} = \hat{i} + \hat{j} + \hat{k}$ and $\vec{c}$ be a vector such that $\vec{a} \times \vec{c} + \vec{b} = \vec{0}$ and $\vec{a}.\vec{c} = 4$, then $|\vec{c}|^2$ is equal to: **[Set I, Jan 2019]**

(a) $\frac{19}{2}$ (b) 9 (c) 8 (d) $\frac{17}{2}$

CHAPTER-26 : Three Dimensional Geometry

TOPIC-2

107. The length of the perpendicular from the point (2, –1, 4) on the straight line, $\frac{x+3}{10} = \frac{y-2}{-7} = \frac{z}{1}$ is : **[Set I, April 2019]**

(a) greater than 3 but less than 4

(b) less than 2

(c) greater than 2 but less than 3

(d) greater than 4

TOPIC-3

108. The equation of a plane containing the line of intersection of the planes $2x - y - 4 = 0$ and $y + 2z - 4 = 0$ and passing through the point (1, 1, 0) is : **[Set I, April 2019]**

(a) $x - 3y - 2z = -2$ (b) $2x - z = 2$

(c) $x - y - z = 0$ (d) $x + 3y + z = 4$

109. If the line, $\frac{x-1}{2} = \frac{y+1}{3} = \frac{z-2}{4}$ meets the plane, $x + 2y + 3z = 15$ at a point P, then the distance of P from the origin is: **[Set II, April 2019]**

(a) $\sqrt{5}/2$ (b) $2\sqrt{5}$

(c) 9/2 (d) 7/2

110. A plane passing through the points (0, –1, 0) and (0, 0, 1) and making an angle $\frac{\pi}{4}$ with the plane $y - z + 5 = 0$, also passes through the point: **[Set II, April 2019]**

(a) $(-\sqrt{2}, 1, -4)$ (b) $(\sqrt{2}, -1, 4)$

(c) $(-\sqrt{2}, -1, -4)$ (d) $(\sqrt{2}, 1, 4)$

111. The system of linear equations

$x + y + z = 2$

$2x + 3y + 2z = 5$

$2x + 3y + (a^2 - 1)z = a + 1$ **[Set I, Jan 2019]**

(a) is inconsistent when a = 4

(b) has a unique solution for $|a| = \sqrt{3}$

(c) has infinitely many solutions for a = 4

(d) is inconsistent when $|a| = \sqrt{3}$

112. The equation of the line passing through (–4, 3, 1), parallel to the plane $x + 2y - z - 5 = 0$ and intersecting the line $\frac{x+1}{-3} = \frac{y-3}{2} = \frac{z-2}{-1}$ is: **[Set I, Jan 2019]**

(a) $\frac{x-4}{2} = \frac{y+3}{1} = \frac{z+1}{4}$

(b) $\frac{x+4}{1} = \frac{y-3}{1} = \frac{z-1}{3}$

(c) $\frac{x+4}{3} = \frac{y-3}{-1} = \frac{z-1}{1}$

(d) $\frac{x+4}{-1} = \frac{y-3}{1} = \frac{z-1}{1}$

113. The plane through the intersection of the planes $x + y + z = 1$ and $2x + 3y - z + 4 = 0$ and parallel to y-axis also passes through the point: **[Set I, Jan 2019]**

(a) $(-3, 0, -1)$ (b) $(-3, 1, 1)$

(c) $(3, 3, -1)$ (d) $(3, 2, 1)$

114. The plane passing through the point $(4, -1, 2)$ and parallel to the lines $\frac{x+2}{3} = \frac{y-2}{-1} = \frac{z+1}{2}$ and $\frac{x-2}{1} = \frac{y-3}{2} = \frac{z-4}{3}$ also passes through the point: **[Set II, Jan 2019]**

(a) $(1, 1, -1)$ (b) $(1, 1, 1)$

(c) $(-1, -1, -1)$ (d) $(-1, -1, 1)$

115. Let A be a point on the line $\vec{r} = (1 - 3\mu)\hat{i} + (\mu - 1)\hat{j} + (2 + 5\mu)\hat{k}$ and B(3, 2, 6) be a point in the space. Then the value of μ for which the vector $\overrightarrow{AB}$ is parallel to the plane $x - 4y + 3z = 1$ is: **[Set II, Jan 2019]**

(a) $\frac{1}{4}$ (b) $\frac{1}{8}$

(c) $\frac{1}{2}$ (d) $-\frac{1}{4}$

CHAPTER-27 : Probability

TOPIC-1

116. Let A and B be two non-null events such that $A \subset B$. Then, which of the following statements is always correct? **[Set I, April 2019]**

(a) $P(A|B) = P(B) - P(A)$ (b) $P(A|B) \geq P(A)$

(c) $P(A|B) \leq P(A)$ (d) $P(A|B) = 1$

117. Four persons can hit a target correctly with probabilities $\frac{1}{2}, \frac{1}{3}, \frac{1}{4}$ and $\frac{1}{8}$ respectively. If all hit at the target independently, then the probability that the target would be hit, is: **[Set II, April 2019]**

(a) $\frac{25}{192}$ (b) $\frac{7}{32}$

(c) $\frac{1}{192}$ (d) $\frac{25}{32}$

118. An unbiased coin is tossed. If the outcome is a head then a pair of unbiased dice is rolled and the sum of the numbers obtained on them is noted. If the toss of the coin results in tail then a card from a well-shuffled pack of nine cards numbered 1, 2, 3, ..., 9 is randomly picked and the number on the card is noted. The probability that the noted number is either 7 or 8 is: **[Set II, Jan 2019]**

(a) $\frac{13}{36}$ (b) $\frac{15}{72}$

(c) $\frac{19}{72}$ (d) $\frac{19}{36}$

TOPIC-2

119. Two cards are drawn successively with replacement from a well-shuffled deck of 52 cards. Let X denote the random variable of number of aces obtained in the two drawn cards. Then $P(X = 1) + P(X = 2)$ equals: **[Set I, Jan 2019]**

(a) 49/169 (b) 52/169

(c) 24/169 (d) 25/169

CHAPTER-28 : Properties of Triangles

TOPIC-2

120. Consider a triangular plot ABC with sides AB = 7 m, BC = 5 m and CA = 6 m. A vertical lamp-post at the mid point D of AC subtends an angle 30° at B. The height (in m) of the lamp-post is: **[Set II, Jan 2019]**

(a) $\frac{3}{2}\sqrt{21}$ (b) $\frac{2}{3}\sqrt{21}$

(c) $2\sqrt{21}$ (d) $7\sqrt{3}$

Hints & Solutions

Chapter 1
Topic-2

1. **(d)**

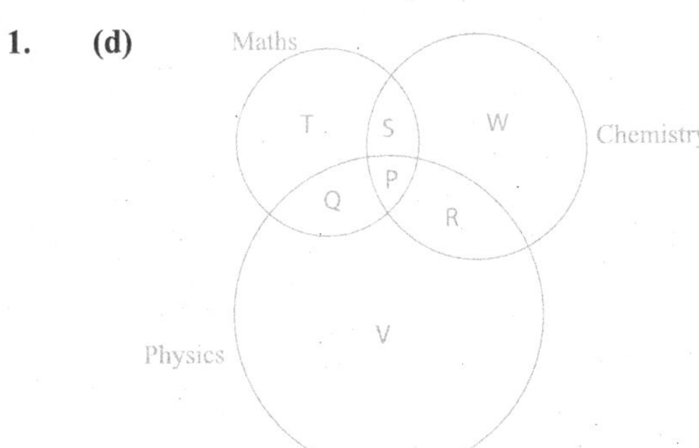

$P = \{30, 60, 90, 120\}$

$\Rightarrow n(P) = 4$

$Q = \{6n: n \in N, 1 \le n \le 23\} - P$

$\Rightarrow n(Q) = 19$

$R = \{15n: n \in N, 1 \le n \le 9\} - P$

$\Rightarrow n(R) = 5$

$S = \{10n: n \in N, 1 \le n \le 14\} - P$

$\Rightarrow n(S) = 10$

$n(T) = 70 - n(P) - n(Q) - n(S) = 70 - 33 = 37$

$n(V) = 46 - n(P) - n(Q) - n(R) = 46 - 28 = 18$

$n(W) = 28 - n(P) - n(R) - n(S) = 28 - 19 = 9$

$\Rightarrow$ Number of required students

$= 140 - (4 + 19 + 5 + 10 + 37 + 18 + 9)$

$= 140 - 102 = 38$

Chapter 2
Topic-2

2. **(a)** $f(x) = \log\left(\frac{1-x}{1+x}\right), |x| < |$

$$f\left(\frac{2x}{1+x^2}\right) = \log\left(\frac{1-\frac{2x}{1+x^2}}{1+\frac{2x}{1+2x^2}}\right)$$

$$= \log\left(\frac{1+x^2-2x}{1+x^2+2x}\right) = \log\left(\frac{1-x}{1+x}\right)^2$$

$$= 2\log\left(\frac{1-x}{1+x}\right) = 2f(x)$$

Chapter 3
Topic-1

3. **(b)** $3(\sin\theta - \cos\theta)^4 + 6(\sin\theta + \cos\theta)^2 + 4\sin^6\theta$

$= 3(1 - 2\sin\theta\cos\theta)^2 + 6(1 + 2\sin\theta\cos\theta) + 4\sin^6\theta$

$= 3(1 + 4\sin^2\theta\cos^2\theta - 4\sin\theta\cos\theta) + 6 + 12\sin\theta\cos\theta + 4\sin^6\theta$

$= 9 + 12\sin^2\theta\cos^2\theta + 4\sin^6\theta$

$= 9 + 12\cos^2\theta(1 - \cos^2\theta) + 4(1 - \cos^2\theta)^3$

$= 9 + 12\cos^2\theta - 12\cos^4\theta + 4(1 - \cos^6\theta - 3\cos^2\theta + 3\cos^4\theta)$

$= 9 + 4 - 4\cos^6\theta$

$= 13 - 4\cos^6\theta$

Topic-2

4. **(b)** $\because$ $\alpha + \beta$ and $\alpha - \beta$ both are acute angles.

$\cos(\alpha + \beta) = \frac{3}{5}$, then $\sin(\alpha + \beta) = \sqrt{1-\left(\frac{3}{5}\right)^2} = \frac{4}{5}$

$\Rightarrow \tan(\alpha + \beta) = \frac{4}{3}$

And $\sin(\alpha - \beta) = \frac{5}{13}$, then

$\cos(\alpha - \beta) = \sqrt{1-\left(\frac{5}{13}\right)^2} = \frac{12}{13}$

$\Rightarrow \tan(\alpha - \beta) = \frac{5}{12}$

Now, $\tan 2\alpha = \tan((\alpha + \beta) + (\alpha - \beta))$

$$= \frac{\tan(\alpha+\beta) + \tan(\alpha-\beta)}{1 - \tan(\alpha+\beta).\tan(\alpha-\beta)} = \frac{\frac{4}{3}+\frac{5}{12}}{1-\frac{4}{3}.\frac{5}{12}} = \frac{63}{16}$$

5. **(b)** $\cos^2 10° - \cos 10° \cos 50° + \cos^2 50°$

$$= \left(\frac{1+\cos 20°}{2}\right) + \left(\frac{1+\cos 100°}{2}\right) - \frac{1}{2}(2\cos 10°\cos 50°)$$

$$= 1 + \frac{1}{2}(\cos 20° + \cos 100°) - \frac{1}{2}[\cos 60° + \cos 40°]$$

$$= \left(1 - \frac{1}{4}\right) + \frac{1}{2}[\cos 20° + \cos 100° - \cos 40°]$$

$$= \frac{3}{4} + \frac{1}{2}[2\cos 60° \times \cos 40° - \cos 40°]$$

$$= \frac{3}{4}$$

Topic-3

6. **(c)** $2\cos^2\theta + 3\sin\theta = 0$

$\Rightarrow (2\sin\theta + 1)(\sin\theta - 2) = 0$

$\Rightarrow \sin\theta = -\frac{1}{2}$ or $\sin\theta = 2 \rightarrow$ Not possibe

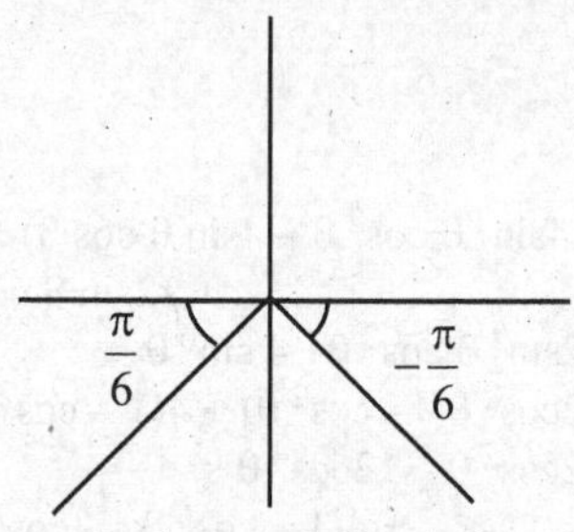

The required sum of all solutions in $[-2\pi, 2\pi]$ is

$$=\left(\pi+\frac{\pi}{6}\right)+\left(2\pi-\frac{\pi}{6}\right)+\left(-\frac{\pi}{6}\right)+\left(-\pi+\frac{\pi}{6}\right)=2\pi$$

Chapter 4

Topic-1

7. (a) $P(n) = n^2 - n + 41$

$\Rightarrow P(3) = 9 - 3 + 41 = 47$ (prime)

& $P(5) = 25 - 5 + 41 = 61$ (prime)

$\therefore$ $P(3)$ and $P(5)$ are both prime i.e., true.

Chapter 5

Topic-1

8. (d) Suppose $z = \dfrac{3+2i\sin\theta}{1-2i\sin\theta}$

Since, z is purely imaginary, then $z + \bar{z} = 0$

$$\Rightarrow \frac{3+2i\sin\theta}{1-2i\sin\theta}+\frac{3-2i\sin\theta}{1+2i\sin\theta}=0$$

$$\Rightarrow \frac{(3+2i\sin\theta)(1+2i\sin\theta)+(3-2i\sin\theta)(1-2i\sin\theta)}{1+4\sin^2\theta}=0$$

$$\Rightarrow \sin^2\theta = \frac{3}{4} \Rightarrow \sin\theta = \frac{\sqrt{3}}{2}$$

$$\Rightarrow \theta = -\frac{\pi}{3}, \frac{\pi}{3}, \frac{2\pi}{3}$$

Now, the sum of elements in $A = -\dfrac{\pi}{3}+\dfrac{\pi}{3}+\dfrac{2\pi}{3}=\dfrac{2\pi}{3}$

9. (none) Let $z_1 = r_1 e^{i\theta}$ and $z_2 = r_2 e^{i\phi}$

$$3|z_1| = 4|z_2| \Rightarrow 3r_1 = 4r_2$$

$$z=\frac{3z_1}{2z_2}+\frac{2z_2}{3z_1}=\frac{3r_1}{2r_2}e^{i(\theta-\phi)}+\frac{2}{3}\frac{r_2}{r_1}e^{i(\phi-\theta)}$$

$$=\frac{3}{2}\times\frac{4}{3}(\cos(\theta-\phi)+i\sin(\theta-\phi))+$$

$$\frac{2}{3}\times\frac{3}{4}[\cos(\theta-\phi)-i\sin(\theta-\phi)]$$

$$z=\left(2+\frac{1}{2}\right)\cos(\theta-\phi)+i\left(2-\frac{1}{2}\right)\sin(\theta-\phi)$$

$$\therefore \quad |z|=\sqrt{\frac{25}{4}\cos^2(\theta-\phi)+\frac{9}{4}\sin^2(\theta-\phi)}$$

$$=\sqrt{\frac{16}{4}\cos^2(\theta-\phi)+\frac{9}{4}} \Rightarrow \frac{3}{2}\le|z|\le\frac{5}{2}$$

Topic-3

10. (c) The given quadratic equation is $x^2 - 2x + 2 = 0$

Then, the roots of the this equation are $\dfrac{2\pm\sqrt{-4}}{2}=1\pm i$

Now, $\dfrac{\alpha}{\beta}=\dfrac{1-i}{1+i}=\dfrac{(1-i)^2}{1-i^2}=i$

or $\dfrac{\alpha}{\beta}=\dfrac{1-i}{1+i}=\dfrac{(1-i)^2}{1-i^2}=-i$ So, $\dfrac{\alpha}{\beta}=\pm i$

Now, $\left(\dfrac{\alpha}{\beta}\right)^n = 1 \Rightarrow (\pm i)^n = 1$

$\Rightarrow$ n must be a multiple of 4.

Hence, the required least value of $n = 4$.

11. (d) Let $\sqrt{x} = a$

$\therefore$ given equation will become:

$|a-2| + a(a-4) + 2 = 0$

$\Rightarrow |a-2| + a^2 - 4a + 4 - 2 = 0$

$\Rightarrow |a-2| + (a-2)^2 - 2 = 0$

Let $|a-2| = y$ (Clearly $y \ge 0$)

$\Rightarrow y + y^2 - 2 = 0$

$\Rightarrow y = 1$ or -2 (rejected)

$\Rightarrow |a-2| = 1 \Rightarrow a = 1, 3$

When $\sqrt{x} = 1 \Rightarrow x = 1$

When $\sqrt{x} = 3 \Rightarrow x = 9$

Hence, the required sum of solutions of the equation $= 10$

12. (d) Since $2-\sqrt{3}$ is a root of the quadratic equation $x^2 + px + q = 0$

$\therefore 2+\sqrt{3}$ is the other root

$$\Rightarrow x^2+px+q=[x-(2-\sqrt{3})][x-(2+\sqrt{3})]$$

$$=x^2-(2+\sqrt{3})x-(2-\sqrt{3})x+(2^2-(\sqrt{3})^2)$$

$$=x^2-4x+1$$

Now, by comparing $p = -4, q = 1$

$\Rightarrow p^2 - 4q - 12 = 16 - 4 - 12 = 0$

13. (a) Consider the equation

$$x^2 + 2x + 2 = 0$$

$$x=\frac{-2\pm\sqrt{4-8}}{2}=-1\pm i$$

Let $\alpha = -1 + i, \beta = -1 - i$

$$\alpha^{15} + \beta^{15} = (-1+i)^{15} + (-1-i)^{15}$$

$$=\left(\sqrt{2}e^{i\frac{3\pi}{4}}\right)^{15}+\left(\sqrt{2}e^{-i\frac{3\pi}{4}}\right)^{15}$$

$$=\left(\sqrt{2}\right)^{15}\left[e^{\frac{i45\pi}{4}}+e^{\frac{-i45\pi}{4}}\right]$$

$$=\left(\sqrt{2}\right)^{15}.2\cos\frac{45\pi}{4}=\left(\sqrt{2}\right)^{15}.2\cos\frac{3\pi}{4}$$

$$==\frac{-2}{\sqrt{2}}\left(\sqrt{2}\right)^{15}$$

$$=-2\left(\sqrt{2}\right)^{14}=-256$$

Topic-4

14. (c)

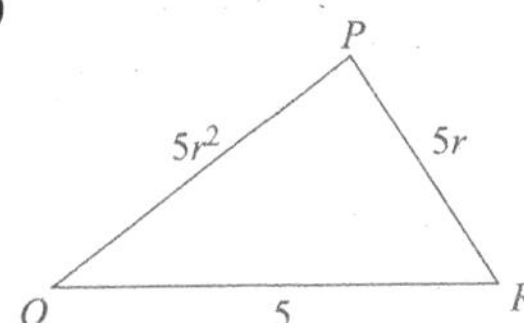

ΔPQR is possible if

$$5+5r>5r^2$$

$$\Rightarrow \quad 1+r>r^2$$

$$\Rightarrow \quad r^2-r-1<0$$

$$\Rightarrow \quad \left(r-\frac{1}{2}+\frac{\sqrt{5}}{2}\right)\left(r-\frac{1}{2}-\frac{\sqrt{5}}{2}\right)<0$$

$$\Rightarrow \quad r\in\left(\frac{-\sqrt{5}+1}{2},\frac{\sqrt{5}+1}{2}\right)$$

$$\because \quad \frac{7}{4}\notin\left(\frac{-\sqrt{5}+1}{2},\frac{\sqrt{5}+1}{2}\right) \quad \therefore \quad r\neq\frac{7}{4}$$

15. (d) Consider the quadratic equation

$$(c-5)x^2-2cx+(c-4)=0$$

Now, $f(0).f(3)>0$ and $f(0).f(2)<0$

$$\Rightarrow \quad (c-4)(4c-49)>0 \text{ and } (c-4)(c-24)<0$$

$$\Rightarrow \quad c\in(-\infty,4)\cup\left(\frac{49}{4},\infty\right) \text{ and } c\in(4,24)$$

$$\Rightarrow \quad c\in\left(\frac{49}{4},24\right)$$

Integral values in the interval $\left(\frac{49}{4},24\right)$ are 13, 14, ..., 23.

$\therefore \quad S=\{13, 14, ..., 23\}$

Chapter 7

Topic-2

16. (a) $\because$ There are total 9 digits and out of which only 3 digits are odd.

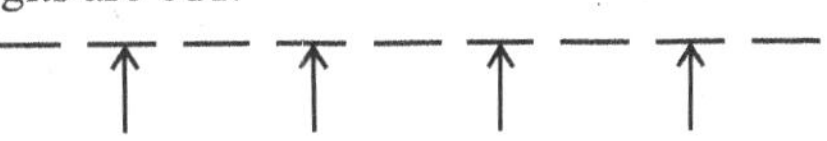

$\therefore$ Number of ways to arrange odd digits first

$$={}^4C_3.\frac{3!}{2!}$$

Hence, total number of 9 digit numbers

$$=\left({}^4C_3.\frac{3!}{2!}\right).\frac{6!}{2!\,4!}$$

$$=180$$

17. (b) Since, m = number of ways the committee is formed with at least 6 males
$={}^8C_6\,.\,{}^5C_5+{}^8C_7\,.\,{}^5C_4+{}^8C_8\,.\,{}^5C_3=78$
and n = number of ways the committee is formed with at least 3 females
$={}^5C_3\,.\,{}^8C_8+{}^5C_4\,.\,{}^8C_7+{}^5C_5\,.\,{}^8C_6=78$
Hence, m = n = 78

18. (c) Since, the number of ways to select 2 girls is ${}^5C_2$.
Now, 3 boys can be selected in 3 ways.

(a) Selection of A and selection of any 2 other boys (except B) in ${}^5C_2$ ways
(b) Selection of B and selection of any 2 two other boys (except A) in ${}^5C_2$ ways
(c) Selection of 3 boys (except A and B) in ${}^5C_3$ ways

Hence, required number of different teams
$={}^5C_2\,({}^5C_2+{}^5C_2+{}^5C_3)=300$

19. (d) Consider the expression,

$$\frac{{}^{20}C_{i-1}}{{}^{20}C_i+{}^{20}C_{i-1}}=\frac{{}^{20}C_{i-1}}{{}^{21}C_1}$$

$$=\frac{20!}{(i-1)!(21-i)!}\times\frac{i!(21-i)!}{21!}=\frac{i}{21}$$

$$\therefore \quad \sum_{i=1}^{20}\left(\frac{{}^{20}C_{i-1}}{{}^{20}C_i+{}^{20}C_{i-1}}\right)^3=\sum_{i=1}^{20}\left(\frac{i}{21}\right)^3=\frac{(1)}{(21)^3}\sum_{i=1}^{20}i^3$$

$$=\frac{1}{(21)^3}\times\left(\frac{20\times21}{2}\right)^2=\frac{100}{21}$$

$$\because \quad \sum_{i=1}^{20}\left(\frac{{}^{20}C_{i-1}}{{}^{20}C_i+{}^{20}C_{i-1}}\right)^3=\frac{k}{21}$$

$$\therefore \quad k=100$$

Chapter 8

Topic-1

20. (d) $(x+\sqrt{x^3-1})^6+(x-\sqrt{x^3-1})^6$

$= 2[{}^6C_0x^6 + {}^6C_2x^4(x^3-1) + {}^6C_4x^2(x^3-1)^2 + {}^6C_6(x^3-1)^3]$

$= 2[x^6 + 15x^7 - 15x^4 + 15x^8 - 30x^5 + 15x^2 + x^9 - 3x^6 + 3x^3 - 1]$

Hence, the sum of coefficients of even powers of

$x = 2[1 - 15 + 15 + 15 - 3 - 1] = 24$

21. (b) $\because T_4 = 20 \times 8^7$

$\Rightarrow {}^6C_3\left(\frac{2}{x}\right)^3 \times (x^{\log_8 x})^3 = 20\times 8^7$

$\Rightarrow 8\times 20\times\left(\frac{x^{\log_8 x}}{x}\right)^3 = 20\times 8^7 \quad \Rightarrow \frac{x^{\log_8 x}}{x} = 64$

Now, take $\log_8$ on both sides, then

$(\log_8 x)^2 - (\log_8 x) = 2$

$\Rightarrow \log_8 x = -1$ or $\log_8 x = 2$

$\Rightarrow x = \frac{1}{8}$ or $x = 8^2$

22. (b) $2^{403} = 2^{400}\cdot 2^3$

$= 2^{4\times 100}\cdot 2^3$

$= (2^4)^{100}\cdot 8$

$= 8(2^4)^{100} = 8(16)^{100}$

$= 8(1+15)^{100}$

$= 8 + 15\mu$

When 2^{403} is divided by 15, then remainder is 8.

Hence, fractional part of the number is $\frac{8}{15}$

Therefore value of k is 8

23. (a) Third term of $(1+x^{\log_2 x})^5 = {}^5C_2(x^{\log_2 x})^{5-3}$

$= {}^5C_2(x^{\log_2 x})^2$

Given, ${}^5C_2\,(x^{\log_2 x})^2 = 2560$

$\Rightarrow \quad (x^{\log_2 x})^2 = 256 = (\pm 16)^2$

$\Rightarrow \quad x^{\log_2 x} = 16$ or $x^{\log_2 x} = -16$ (rejected)

$\Rightarrow \quad x^{\log_2 x} = 16 \Rightarrow \log_2 x \log_2 x = \log_2 16 = 4$

$\Rightarrow \quad \log_2 x = \pm 2 \Rightarrow x = 2^2$ or 2^{-2}

$\Rightarrow \quad x = 4$ or $\frac{1}{4}$

Topic-3

24. (b) $2.{}^{20}C_0 + 5.{}^{20}C_1 + 8.{}^{20}C_2 + ... + 62.{}^{20}C_{20}$

$= \sum_{r=0}^{20}(3r+2)\,{}^{20}C_r = 3\sum_{r=0}^{20} r.\,{}^{20}C_r + 2\sum_{r=0}^{20}{}^{20}C_r$

$= 60\sum_{r=1}^{20}{}^{19}C_{n-1} + 2\sum_{r=0}^{20}{}^{20}C_r$

$= 60\times 2^{19} + 2\times 2^{20} = 2^{21}[15+1] = 2^{25}$

Chapter 9

Topic-1

25. (d) $\because \quad 91 = 13\times 7$

Then, the required numbers are either divisible by 7 or 13.

$\therefore$ Sum of such numbers = Sum of no. divisible by 7 + sum of the no. divisible by 13 – Sum of the numbers divisible by 91

$= (105 + 112 + ... + 196) + (104 + 117 + ... + 195) - 182$

$= 2107 + 1196 - 182$

$= 3121$

26. (d) $\because S_n = \left(50 - \frac{7A}{2}\right)n + n^2\times\frac{A}{2} \quad \Rightarrow a_1 = 50 - 3S$

$\therefore d = a_2 - a_1 = S_{n_2} - S_{n_1} - S_{n_1} \Rightarrow d = \frac{A}{2}\times 2 = A$

Now, $a_{50} = a_1 + 49\times d$

$= (50 - 3A) + 49A$

$= 50 + 46A$

So, $(d, a_{50}) = (A, 50 + 46A)$

27. (a) $S = \sum_{i=1}^{30} a_i = \frac{30}{2}[2a_1 + 29d]$

$T = \sum_{i=1}^{15} a_{(2i-1)} = \frac{15}{2}[2a_1 + 28d]$

Since, $S - 2T = 75$

$\Rightarrow 30a_1 + 435d - 30a_1 - 420d = 75$

$\Rightarrow d = 5$

Also, $a_5 = 27 \quad \Rightarrow \quad a_1 + 4d = 27$

$\Rightarrow a_1 = 7,$

Hence, $a_{10} = a_1 + 9d = 7 + 9\times 5 = 52$

28. **(d)** Two digit positive numbers which when divided by 7 yield 2 as remainder are 12 terms i.e,16, 23, 30, ..., 93

Two digit positive numbers which when divided by 7 yield 5 as remainder are 13 terms i.e,12, 19, 26, ..., 96

By using AP sum of 16, 23, ..., 93, we get

$S_1 = 16 + 23 + 30 + ... + 93 = 654$

By using AP sum of 12, 19, 26, ..., 96, we get

$S_1 = 12 + 19 + 26 + ... + 96 = 702$

$\therefore$ required Sum $= S_1 + S_2 = 654 + 702 = 1356$

Topic-2

29. (d) $\because$ f(x + y) = f(x) . f(y)

$\Rightarrow$ Let $f(x) = t^x$

f(1) = 2

$\therefore$ t' = 2

$\Rightarrow f(x) = 2^x$

Since, $\sum_{k=1}^{10} f(a+k) = 16(2^{10}-1)$

Then, $\sum_{k=1}^{10} 2^{a+k} = 16(2^{10}-1)$

$\Rightarrow 2^a \sum_{k=1}^{10} 2^k = 16(2^{10}-1)$

$\Rightarrow 2^a \times \frac{((2^{10})-1)\times 2}{(2-1)} = 16\times(2^{10}-1) \Rightarrow 2.2^a = 16$

$\Rightarrow$ a = 3

30. (d) $\because$ a, b, c, are in G.P.

$\Rightarrow \quad b^2 = ac$

Since, $a + b + c = xb$

$\Rightarrow \quad a + c = (x-1)b$

Take square on both sides, we get

$a^2 + c^2 + 2ac = (x-1)^2 b^2$

$\Rightarrow \quad a^2 + c^2 = (x-1)^2 ac - 2ac \quad [\because b^2 = ac]$

$\Rightarrow \quad a^2 + c^2 = ac[(x-1)^2 - 2]$

$\Rightarrow \quad a^2 + c^2 = ac[x^2 - 2x - 1]$

$\because a^2 + c^2$ are positive and $b^2 = ac$ which is also positive.

Then, $x^2 - 2x - 1$ would be positive but for $x = 2$, $x^2 - 2x - 1$ is negative.

Hence, x cannot be taken as 2.

Topic-3

31. **(c)** $\sin^2 2\theta + \cos^4 2\theta = \frac{3}{4}$

$\Rightarrow \quad 1 - \cos^2 2\theta + \cos^4 2\theta = \frac{3}{4}$

$\Rightarrow \quad \cos^2 2\theta(1 - \cos^2 2\theta) = \frac{1}{4}$ ...(1)

$\because \quad$ G.M. $\le$ A.M.

$\therefore \quad (\cos^2 2\theta)(1 - \cos^2 2\theta) \le \left(\frac{\cos^2 2\theta + (1 - \cos^2 2\theta}{2}\right)^2$

$= \frac{1}{4}$ ...(2)

So, from equation (1) and (2) we get.

G.M. = A.M.

It is possible only if,

$\cos^2 2\theta = 1 - \cos^2 2\theta$

$\Rightarrow \quad \cos^2 2\theta = \frac{1}{2} \Rightarrow \cos 2\theta = \pm\frac{1}{\sqrt{2}}$

$\Rightarrow \quad \theta = \frac{\pi}{8}, \frac{3\pi}{8} \quad \therefore$ Sum $= \frac{\pi}{8} + \frac{3\pi}{8} = \frac{\pi}{2}$

Chapter 10

Topic-1

32. (c) Let point $P(h, k)$

$\because \quad OA = 1$

So, $OP + AP = 3$

$\Rightarrow \quad \sqrt{h^2 + k^2} + \sqrt{h^2 + (k-1)^2} = 3$

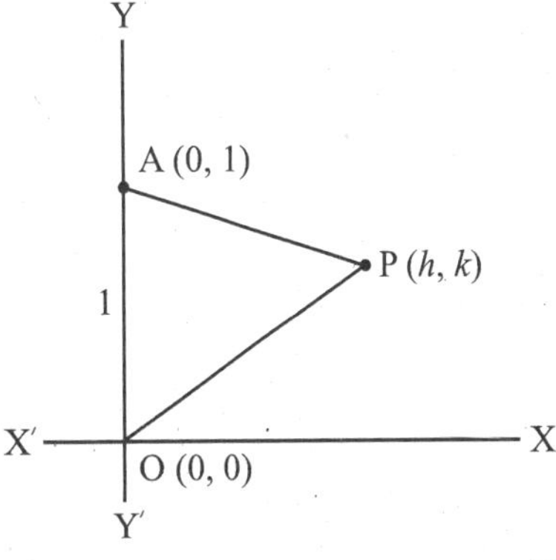

$\Rightarrow h^2 + (k-1)^2 = 9 + h^2 + k^2 - 6\sqrt{h^2 + k^2}$

$\Rightarrow 6\sqrt{h^2 + k^2} = 2k + 8$

$\Rightarrow 9h^2 + 8k^2 - 8k - 16 = 0$

Hence, locus of point P is

$9x^2 + 8y^2 - 8y - 16 = 0$

Topic-2

33. (c) A point which is equidistant from both the axes lies on either $y = x$ and $y = -x$.

Since, point lies on the line $3x + 5y = 15$

Then the required point

$3x + 5y = 15$

$x + y = 0$

$x = -\frac{15}{2}$

$y = \frac{15}{2} \Rightarrow (x, y) = \left(-\frac{15}{2}, \frac{15}{2}\right)$ {2nd quadrant}

or $3x + 5y = 15$

$x - y = 0$

$x = \frac{15}{8}$

$y = \frac{15}{8} \Rightarrow (x, y) = \left(\frac{15}{8}, \frac{15}{8}\right)$ {1st quadrant}

Hence, the required point lies in 1st and 2nd quadrant.

34. (b)

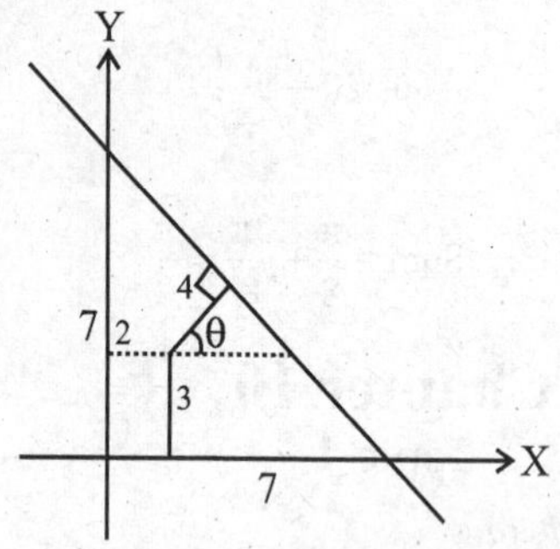

Since point at 4 units from P (2, 3) will be A (4 cosθ + 2, 4 sinθ + 3) and this point will satisfy the equation of line x + y = 7

$\Rightarrow \cos\theta + \sin\theta = \frac{1}{2}$

On squaring

$\Rightarrow \sin 2\theta - \frac{3}{4} \Rightarrow \frac{2\tan\theta}{1+\tan^2\theta} = -\frac{3}{4}$

$\Rightarrow 3\tan^2\theta + 8\tan\theta + 3 = 0$

$\Rightarrow \tan\theta = \frac{-8 \pm 2\sqrt{7}}{6}$ (ignoring –ve sign)

$\Rightarrow \tan\theta = \frac{-8 \pm 2\sqrt{7}}{6} = \frac{1-\sqrt{7}}{1+\sqrt{7}}$

35. (c)

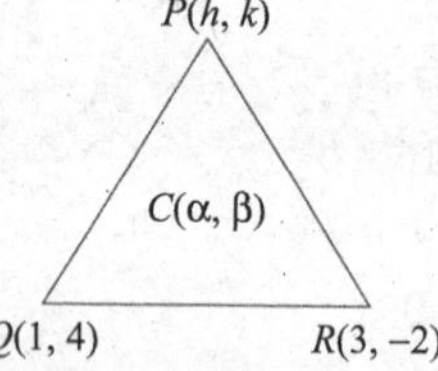

Let centroid C be (α, β)

we have $\alpha = \frac{1+3+h}{3} \Rightarrow h = 3\alpha - 4$

$\beta = \frac{4-2+k}{3} \Rightarrow k = 3\beta - 2$

but $P(h, k)$ lies on $2x - 3y + 4 = 0$

$\Rightarrow \quad 2(3\alpha - 4) - 3(3\beta - 2) + 4 = 0$

$\Rightarrow \quad 6\alpha - 9\beta - 8 + 6 + 4 = 0$

$\Rightarrow \quad 6\alpha - 9\beta + 2 = 0$

Locus: $6x - 9y + 2 = 0$

$\Rightarrow \quad y = \frac{6}{9}x + \frac{2}{9} \quad \therefore$ its slope $= \frac{6}{9} = \frac{2}{3}$

36. **(b)** Equation of the line is:

$3x + 4y = 24$

or $\frac{x}{8} + \frac{y}{6} = 1$

$\therefore$ coordinates of A, B & O are (8, 0), (0, 6) & (0, 0) respectively.

$\Rightarrow \quad OA = 8, OB = 6 \;\&\; AB = 10.$

$\therefore$ Incentre of ΔOAB is given as:

$$I \equiv \left(\frac{8\times0+6\times8+10\times0}{8+6+10}, \frac{8\times6+6\times0+10\times0}{8+6+10}\right) \equiv (2,2).$$

Topic-3

37. (a) The given equations of the set of all lines

$$px + qy + r = 0 \quad ...(1)$$

and given condition is :

$3p + 2q + 4r = 0$

$$\Rightarrow \quad \frac{3}{4}p + \frac{2}{4}q + r = 0 \quad ...(2)$$

From (1) & (2) we get :

$\therefore \quad x = \frac{3}{4}, y = \frac{1}{2}$

Hence the set of lines are concurrent and passing through the fixed point $\left(\frac{3}{4}, \frac{1}{2}\right)$

Chapter 11

Topic-1

38. (d) Let the chord $x + y = n$ cuts the circle $x^2 + y^2 = 16$ at P and Q Length of perpendicular from O on PQ

$= \left|\frac{0+0-n}{\sqrt{1^2+1^2}}\right| = \frac{n}{\sqrt{2}}$

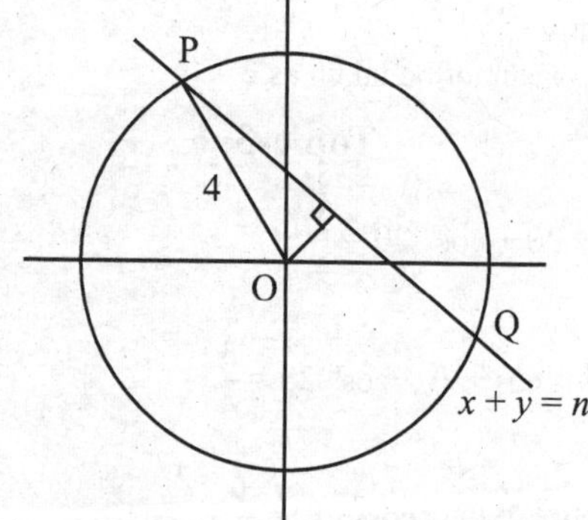

Then, length of chord $PQ = 2\sqrt{4^2 - \left(\frac{n}{\sqrt{2}}\right)^2}$

$= 2\sqrt{16 - \frac{n^2}{2}}$

Thus only possible values of n are 1, 2, 3, 4, 5.
Hence, the sum of squares of lengths of chords

$= \sum_{n=1}^{5} 4\left(16 - \frac{n^2}{2}\right) = 64 \times 5 - 2.\frac{5\times6\times11}{6} = 210$

39. (b) Let $z \in S$ then $z = \dfrac{\alpha + i}{\alpha - i}$

Since, z is a complex number and let $z = x + iy$

Then, $x + iy = \dfrac{(\alpha + i)^2}{\alpha^2 + 1}$ (by rationalisation)

$\Rightarrow x + iy = \dfrac{(\alpha^2 - 1)}{\alpha^2 + 1} + \dfrac{i(2\alpha)}{\alpha^2 + 1}$

Then compare both sides

$$x = \frac{\alpha^2 - 1}{\alpha^2 + 1} \quad ...(1)$$

$$y = \frac{2\alpha}{\alpha^2 + 1} \quad ...(2)$$

Now squaring and adding equations (1) and (2)

$$\Rightarrow x^2 + y^2 = \frac{(\alpha^2 - 1)^2}{(\alpha^2 + 1)^2} + \frac{4\alpha^2}{(\alpha^2 + 1)^2} = 1$$

40. (a) Let any tangent to circle $x^2 + y^2 = 1$ is $x\cos\theta + y\sin\theta = 1$

Since, P and Q are the point of intersection on the co-ordinate axes.

Then $P \equiv \left(\dfrac{1}{\cos\theta}, 0\right)$ & $Q \equiv \left(0, \dfrac{1}{\sin\theta}\right)$

$\therefore$ mid-point of PQ be $M \equiv \left(\dfrac{1}{2\cos\theta}, \dfrac{1}{2\sin\theta}\right) \equiv (h, k)$

$$\Rightarrow \cos\theta = \frac{1}{2h} \quad ...(1)$$

$$\sin\theta = \frac{1}{2k} \quad ...(2)$$

Now squaring and adding equation (1) and (2)

$$\frac{1}{h^2} + \frac{1}{k^2} = 4$$

$\therefore$ locus of M is : $x^2 + y^2 = 4x^2y^2$

$\Rightarrow h^2 + k^2 = 4h^2k^2$

41. (a)

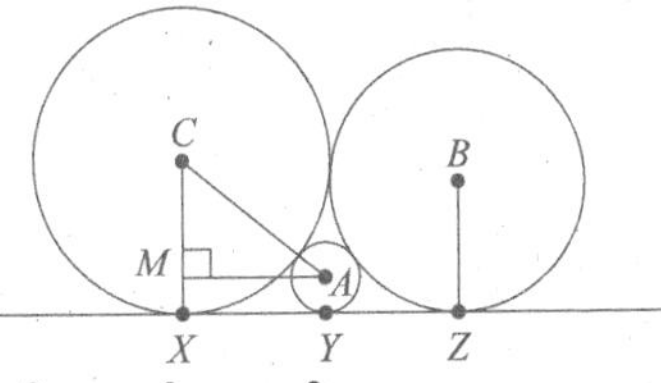

$AM^2 = AC^2 - MC^2$

$= (a + c)^2 - (a - c)^2 = 4ac$

$\Rightarrow AM^2 = XY^2 = 4ac$

$\Rightarrow XY = 2\sqrt{ac}$

Similarly, $YZ = 2\sqrt{ba}$ and $XZ = 2\sqrt{bc}$

Then, $XZ = XY + YZ$

$\Rightarrow 2\sqrt{bc} = 2\sqrt{ac} + 2\sqrt{ba}$

$\Rightarrow \dfrac{1}{\sqrt{a}} = \dfrac{1}{\sqrt{b}} + \dfrac{1}{\sqrt{c}}$

42. (c) The equation of circle $x^2 + y^2 + 4x - 6y = 12$ can be written as $(x + 2)^2 + (y - 3)^2 = 25$

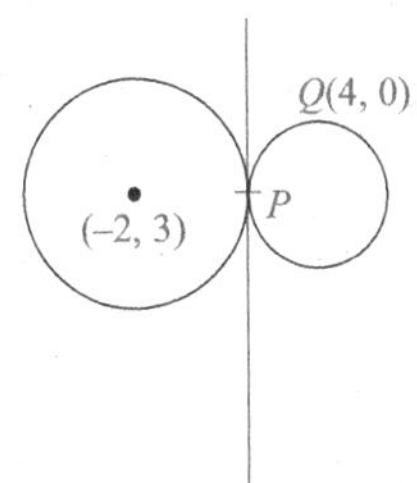

Let $P = (1, -1)$ & $Q = (4, 0)$

Equation of tangent at $P(1, -1)$ to the given circle :

$x(1) + y(-1) + 2(x + 1) - 3(y - 1) - 12 = 0$

$$3x - 4y - 7 = 0 \quad ...(1)$$

The required circle is tangent to (1) at $(1, -1)$.

$$\therefore \quad (x - 1)^2 + (y + 1)^2 + \lambda(3x - 4y - 7) = 0 \quad ...(2)$$

Equation (2) passes through $Q(4, 0)$

$\Rightarrow \quad 3^2 + 1^2 + \lambda(12 - 7) = 0 \Rightarrow 5\lambda + 10 = 0 \Rightarrow \lambda = -2$

Equation (2) becomes $x^2 + y^2 - 8x + 10y + 16 = 0$

radius $= \sqrt{(-4)^2 + (5)^2 - 16} = 5$

Topic-2

43. (c) The shortest distance between line $y = x$ and parabola = the distance LM between line $y = x$ and tangent of parabola having slope 1.

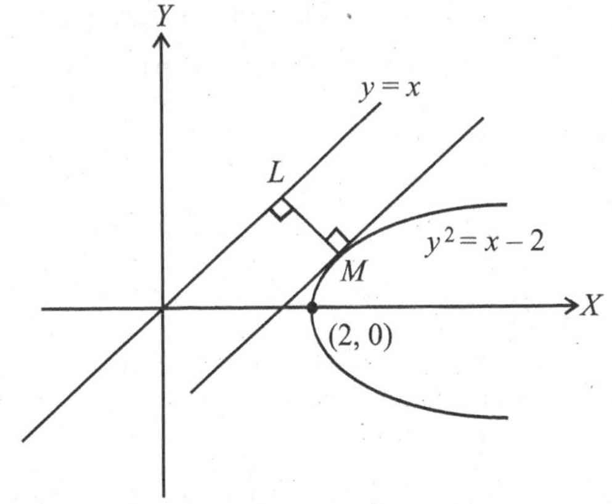

Let equation of tangent of parabola having slope 1 is,

$y = m(x-2) + \frac{a}{m}$

Here $m = 1$ and $a = \frac{1}{4}$

$\therefore$ equation of tangent is: $y = x - \frac{7}{4}$

Distance between the line $y - x = 0$ and $y - x + \frac{7}{4} = 0$

$= \left|\frac{\frac{7}{4} - 0}{\sqrt{1^2+1^2}}\right| = \frac{7}{4\sqrt{2}}$

44. (a) $\because y^2 = 16x$

$\Rightarrow a = 4$

One end of focal chord of the parabola is at (1, 4)

y – coordinate of focal chord is 2at

$\therefore 2at = 4$

$\Rightarrow t = \frac{1}{2}$

Hence, the required length of focal chord

$= a\left(t + \frac{1}{t}\right)^2 = 4 \times \left(2 + \frac{1}{2}\right)^2 = 25$

45. (b) Since, vertex and focus of given parabola is (2, 0) and (4, 0) respectively

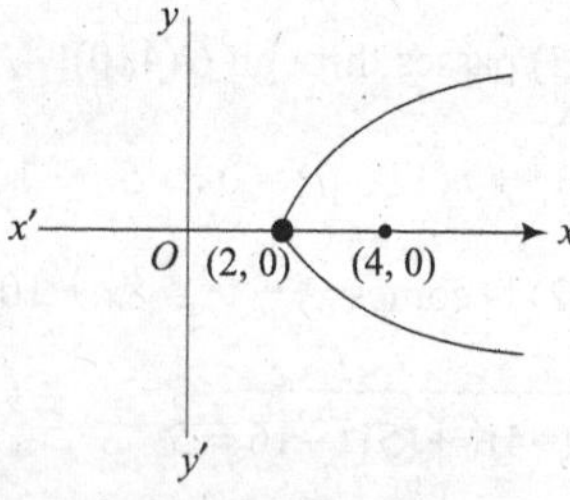

Then, equation of parabola is

$(y-0)^2 = 4 \times 2(x-2)$

$\Rightarrow \quad y^2 = 8x - 16$

Hence, the point (8, 6) does not lie on given parabola.

46. (b) Since, the equation of tangent to parabola $y^2 = 4x$ is

$y = mx + \frac{1}{m}$ ...(1)

The line (1) is also the tangent to circle

$x^2 + y^2 - 6x = 0$

Then centre of circle = (3, 0)

radius of circle = 3

The perpendicular distance from centre to tangent is equal to the radius of circle

$\therefore \quad \frac{\left|3m + \frac{1}{m}\right|}{\sqrt{1+m^2}} = 3 \Rightarrow \left(3m + \frac{1}{m}\right)^2 = 9(1+m^2)$

$\Rightarrow \quad m = \pm\frac{1}{\sqrt{3}}$

Then, from equation (1): $y = \pm\frac{1}{\sqrt{3}}x \pm \sqrt{3}$

Hence, $\sqrt{3}y = x + 3$ is one of the required common tangent.

47. (a, b, c, d)

Normal to $y^2 = 8ax$ is

$y = mx - 4am - 2am^3$ ...(1)

and normal to $y^2 = 4b(x-c)$ with slope m is

$y = m(x-c) - 2bm - bm^3$ ...(2)

Since, both parabolas have a common normal.

$\therefore \quad 4am + 2am^3 = cm + 2bm + bm^3$

$\Rightarrow \quad 4a + 2am^2 = c + 2b + bm^2$ or $m = 0$

$\Rightarrow \quad (4a - c - 2b) = (b - 2a)m^2$

or (X-axis is common normal always)

Since, x-axis is a common normal. Hence all the options are correct for $m = 0$.

Topic-3

48. (d) Since (a, b) touches the given ellipse $4x^2 + y^2 = 8$

$\therefore \quad 4a^2 + b^2 = 8$ ...(1)

Equation of tangent on the ellipse at the point A (1, 2) is:

$4x + 2y = 8 \Rightarrow 2x + y = 4 \Rightarrow y = -2x + 4$

But, also equation of tangent at $P(a, b)$ is:

$4ax + by = 8 \Rightarrow y = \frac{-4a}{b} + \frac{8}{b}$.

Since, tangents are perpendicular to each other.

$\Rightarrow \quad \frac{-4a}{b} = \frac{-1}{2} \quad \Rightarrow b = 8a$ ...(2)

from (1) & (2) we get:

$\Rightarrow a = \pm\frac{2}{\sqrt{34}} \Rightarrow a^2 = \frac{2}{17}$

Topic-4

49. (c) Since, lx + my + n = 0 is a normal to $\frac{x^2}{a^2} - \frac{y^2}{b^2} = 1$,

then $\frac{a^2}{l^2} - \frac{b^2}{m^2} = \frac{(a^2+b^2)^2}{n^2}$

but it is given that $mx - y + 7\sqrt{3}$ is normal to hyperbola

$\frac{x^2}{24} - \frac{y^2}{18} = 1$

then $\frac{24}{m^2} - \frac{18}{(-1)^2} = \frac{(24+18)^2}{(7\sqrt{3})^2} \Rightarrow m = \frac{2}{\sqrt{5}}$

50. (a) $\because a^2 = \cos^2\theta, b^2 = \sin^2\theta$

and $e > 2 \Rightarrow e^2 > 4 \Rightarrow 1 + b^2/a^2 > 4$

$\Rightarrow \quad 1 + \tan^2\theta > 4$

$\Rightarrow \quad \sec^2\theta > 4 \quad \Rightarrow \quad \theta \in \left(\frac{\pi}{3}, \frac{\pi}{2}\right)$

Latus rectum,

$$LR = \frac{2b^2}{a} = \frac{2\sin^2\theta}{\cos\theta} = 2(\sec\theta - \cos\theta)$$

$$\Rightarrow \quad \frac{d(LR)}{d\theta} = 2(\sec\theta\tan\theta + \sin\theta) > 0 \ \forall\ \theta \in \left(\frac{\pi}{3}, \frac{\pi}{2}\right)$$

$$\therefore \quad \min(LR) = 2\left(\sec\frac{\pi}{3} - \cos\frac{\pi}{3}\right) = 2\left(2 - \frac{1}{2}\right) = 3$$

max (LR) tends to infinity as $\theta \to \frac{\pi}{2}$

Hence, length of latus rectum lies in the interval $(3, \infty)$

51. **(a)** Given, the equation of line,

$x - y = 2 \Rightarrow y = x - 2$

$\therefore$ its slope $= m = 1$

Equation of hyperbola is:

$$\frac{x^2}{5} - \frac{y^2}{4} = 1 \Rightarrow a^2 = 5, b^2 = 4$$

The equation of tangent to the hyperbola is,

$$y = mx \pm \sqrt{a^2m^2 - b^2}$$

$$= x \pm \sqrt{5-4}$$

$$\Rightarrow \quad y = x \pm 1$$

Chapter 12

Topic-1

52. **(a)** $\lim\limits_{x\to 0} \frac{\sin^2 x}{\sqrt{2} - \sqrt{1+\cos x}}$

$$= \lim_{x\to 0} \frac{\sin^2 x}{\sqrt{2} - \sqrt{2\cos^2\frac{x}{2}}} \qquad \left[\frac{0}{0}\right]$$

$$= \lim_{x\to 0} \frac{\sin^2 x}{\sqrt{2}\left[1-\cos\frac{x}{2}\right]} = \lim_{x\to 0} \frac{\sin^2 x}{2\sqrt{2}\sin^2\frac{x}{4}}$$

$$= \lim_{x\to 0} \frac{\left(\frac{\sin x}{x}\right)^2 .16}{2\sqrt{2}\left(\frac{\sin\frac{x}{4}}{\frac{x}{4}}\right)^2} = \frac{16}{2\sqrt{2}} = 4\sqrt{2}$$

53. **(a)** $L = \lim\limits_{y\to 0} \frac{\sqrt{1+\sqrt{1+y^4}} - \sqrt{2}}{y^4}$

$$= \lim_{y\to 0} \frac{\left(\sqrt{1+\sqrt{1+y^4}} - \sqrt{2}\right)\left(\sqrt{1+\sqrt{1+y^4}} + \sqrt{2}\right)}{y^4\left(\sqrt{1+\sqrt{1+y^4}} + \sqrt{2}\right)}$$

$$= \lim_{y\to 0} \frac{1+\sqrt{1+y^4} - 2}{y^4\left(\sqrt{1+\sqrt{1+y^4}} + \sqrt{2}\right)}$$

$$= \lim_{y\to 0} \frac{\left(\sqrt{1+y^4} - 1\right)\left(\sqrt{1+y^4} + 1\right)}{y^4\left(\sqrt{1+\sqrt{1+y^4}} + \sqrt{2}\right)\left(\sqrt{1+y^4} + 1\right)}$$

$$= \lim_{y\to 0} \frac{1+y^4 - 1}{y^4\left(\sqrt{1+\sqrt{1+y^4}} + \sqrt{2}\right)\left(\sqrt{1+y^4} + 1\right)}$$

$$= \frac{1}{2\sqrt{2}\times 2} = \frac{1}{4\sqrt{2}}$$

54. **(b)** $\lim\limits_{\to} \frac{(1-|x| + \sin(|1-x|))\sin\left(-[1-x]\right)}{|1-x|[1-x]}$

$$= \lim_{h\to 0} \frac{(1-|1+h| + \sin(|1-1-h|))\sin\left(\frac{\pi}{2}[1-1-h]\right)}{|1-1-h|[1-1-h]}$$

$$= \lim_{h\to 0} \frac{(1-1-h+\sinh)\sin\left(\frac{\pi}{2}(-1)\right)}{h([0-h])}$$

$$= \lim_{h\to 0} \frac{(-h+\sin h)\sin\left(-\frac{\pi}{2}\right)}{h(-1)} = 0$$

Chapter 13

Topic-1

55. **(c)** Check each option

(a) $(p \vee q) \wedge (\sim p \wedge q) = (\sim p \wedge q)$

(b) $(p \vee q) \wedge (\sim p \vee q) = q$

(c) $(p \wedge q) \wedge (\sim p \vee q) = p \wedge q$

(d) $(p \wedge q) \wedge (\sim p \wedge q) = F$

Topic-2

56. **(a)** S: "If you are born in India, then you are a citizen of India."

Contrapositive of $p \to q$ is $\sim q \to \sim p$

So contrapositive of statement S will be :

"If you are not a citizen of India, then you are not born in India."

57. **(d)** $\sim(p \vee (\sim p \wedge q)) = \sim(\sim p \wedge q) \wedge \sim p$

$= (\sim q \vee p) \wedge \sim p$

$= \sim p \wedge (p \vee \sim q)$

$= (\sim q \wedge \sim p) \vee (p \wedge \sim p)$

$= (\sim p \wedge \sim q)$

Chapter 14

Topic-2

58. (c) Let the remaining numbers are a and b.

Mean ( ) $= \frac{\sum x_i}{N} = \frac{2+4+10+12+14+a+b}{7} = 8$

$\Rightarrow a + b = 14$ ...(i)

Variance $(\sigma^2) = \frac{\sum x_i^2}{N} - (\bar{x})^2 = 16$

$\Rightarrow \frac{2^2+4^2+10^2+12^2+14^2+a^2+b^2}{7} - (8)^2 = 16$

$\Rightarrow a^2 + b^2 = 100$ ...(ii)

From (i) and (ii), $(14 - b)^2 + b^2 = 100$

$\Rightarrow 196 + b^2 - 28b + b^2 = 100$

$\Rightarrow b^2 - 14b + 48 = 0$

$\Rightarrow b = 6, 8$

$\therefore$ $a = 8, 6.$

$\therefore$ $(a, b) = (6, 8)$ or $(8, 6)$

Hence, the product of the remaining two observations $= ab = 48$

59. (a) Mean of given observation $= \frac{k}{4}$

$\because$ Standard deviation = 5

$\therefore \sigma^2 = 5$

$\Rightarrow \sigma^2 = \frac{1}{n}\Sigma(x_i - \bar{x})^2 = \frac{\left(\frac{k}{4}+1\right)^2 + \left(\frac{k}{4}\right)^2 + \left(\frac{k}{4}-1\right)^2 + \left(\frac{3k}{4}\right)^2}{4} = 5$

$\Rightarrow \frac{\frac{12k^2}{16}+2}{4} = 5 \Rightarrow k = 2\sqrt{6}$

60. (c) $\because$ Variance $= \sigma^2 = \frac{\Sigma x_i^2}{N} - (\bar{x})^2$

$\Rightarrow \quad 18 = \frac{\Sigma x_i^2}{5} - (150)^2$

$\Rightarrow \quad \Sigma x_i^2 = 90 + 112590 = 112590$

Then, variance of the height of six students

$V' = \frac{112590 + (156)^2}{6} - \left(\frac{750+156}{6}\right)^2$

$= 22821 - 22801$

$= 20$

61. (b) Since mean of x_1, x_2, x_3, x_4 and x_5 is 5

$\Rightarrow \quad x_1 + x_2 + x_3 + x_4 + x_5 = 25$

$\Rightarrow \quad 1 + 3 + 8 + x_4 + x_5 = 25$

$\Rightarrow \quad x_4 + x_5 = 13$ ...(1)

$\because \quad \frac{\sum_{i=1}^{5} x_i^2}{5} - (5)^2 = 9.2 \Rightarrow \sum_{i=1}^{5} x_i^2 = 5(25 + 9.2)$

$= 125 + 46 = 171$

$\Rightarrow \quad (1)^2 + (3)^2 + (8)^2 + x_4^2 + x_5^2 = 171$

$\Rightarrow \quad x_4^2 + x_5^2 = 97$ ...(2)

$\Rightarrow \quad (x_4 + x_5)^2 - 2x_4 x_5 = 97$

$\Rightarrow \quad 2x_4 x_5 = 13^2 - 97 = 72 \Rightarrow x_4 x_5 = 36$ ...(3)

(1) and (3) $\Rightarrow x_4 : x_5 = \frac{4}{9}$ or $\frac{9}{4}$

Chapter 16

Topic-2

62. (a) The given relation is

$(f_2 o J o f_1)(x) = f_3(x) = \frac{1}{1-x}$

$\Rightarrow (f_2 o J)(f_1(x)) = \frac{1}{1-x}$

$\Rightarrow (f_2 o J)\left(\frac{1}{x}\right) = \frac{1}{1-\frac{1}{\frac{1}{x}}} = \frac{\frac{1}{x}}{\frac{1}{x}-1}$ $\left[\because f_1(x) = \frac{1}{x}\right]$

$\Rightarrow (f_2 o J)(x) = \frac{x}{x-1}$ $\left[\frac{1}{x} \text{ is replaced by } x\right]$

$\Rightarrow f_2(J(x)) = \frac{x}{x-1}$

$\Rightarrow 1 - J(x) = \frac{x}{x-1}$ $[\because f_2(x) = 1 - x]$

$\therefore J(x) = 1 - \frac{x}{x-1} = \frac{1}{1-x} = f_3(x)$

Chapter 17

Topic-2

63. (d) $\because$ $\cos\alpha = \frac{3}{5}$, then $\sin\alpha = \frac{4}{5}$

$\Rightarrow \tan\alpha = \frac{4}{3}$

and $\tan\beta = \frac{1}{3}$

$\because \tan(\alpha-\beta) = \frac{\tan\alpha - \tan\beta}{1+\tan\alpha.\tan\beta}$

$= \frac{\frac{4}{3}-\frac{1}{3}}{1+\frac{4}{9}} = \frac{1}{\frac{13}{9}} = \frac{9}{13}$

$\therefore\ \alpha-\beta = \tan^{-1}\left(\frac{9}{13}\right) = \sin^{-1}\left(\frac{9}{5\sqrt{10}}\right)$

$= \cos^{-1}\left(\frac{13}{5\sqrt{10}}\right)$

64. (a) $\cos^{-1}\left(\frac{2}{3x}\right)+\cos^{-1}\left(\frac{3}{4x}\right) = \frac{\pi}{2}; \left(x>\frac{3}{4}\right)$

$\Rightarrow\ \cos^{-1}\left(\frac{2}{3x}\right) = \frac{\pi}{2}-\cos^{-1}\left(\frac{3}{4x}\right)$

$\Rightarrow\ \cos^{-1}\left(\frac{2}{3x}\right) = \sin^{-1}\left(\frac{3}{4x}\right)\ \left[\because \sin^{-1}x+\cos^{-1}x = \frac{\pi}{2}\right]$

Put $\sin^{-1}\left(\frac{3}{4x}\right) = \theta \qquad \Rightarrow \sin\theta = \frac{3}{4x}$

$\Rightarrow\ \cos\theta = \sqrt{1-\sin^2\theta} = \sqrt{1-\frac{9}{16x^2}}$

$\Rightarrow\ \theta = \cos^{-1}\left(\frac{\sqrt{16x^2-9}}{4x}\right)$

$\therefore\ \cos^{-1}\left(\frac{2}{3x}\right) = \cos^{-1}\left(\frac{\sqrt{16x^2-9}}{4x}\right)$

$\Rightarrow\ \frac{2}{3x} = \frac{\sqrt{16x^2-9}}{4x} \Rightarrow x^2 = \frac{64+81}{9\times16} \quad \Rightarrow\ x = \pm\sqrt{\frac{145}{144}}$

$\Rightarrow\ x = \frac{\sqrt{145}}{12} \qquad \left(\because x>\frac{3}{4}\right)$

Chapter 18

Topic-1

65. (c) $A = \begin{bmatrix}\cos\alpha & -\sin\alpha\\ \sin\alpha & \cos\alpha\end{bmatrix}$

$A^2 = \begin{bmatrix}\cos\alpha & -\sin\alpha\\ \sin\alpha & \cos\alpha\end{bmatrix}\begin{bmatrix}\cos\alpha & -\sin\alpha\\ \sin\alpha & \cos\alpha\end{bmatrix}$

$= \begin{bmatrix}\cos2\alpha & -\sin2\alpha\\ \sin2\alpha & \cos2\alpha\end{bmatrix}$

Similarly, $A^4 = A^2 . A^2 = \begin{bmatrix}\cos4\alpha & -\sin4\alpha\\ \sin4\alpha & \cos4\alpha\end{bmatrix}$

and so on $A^{32} = \begin{bmatrix}\cos32\alpha & -\sin32\alpha\\ \sin32\alpha & \cos32\alpha\end{bmatrix} = \begin{bmatrix}0 & -1\\ 1 & 0\end{bmatrix}$

Then $\sin32\alpha = 1$ and $\cos32\alpha = 0$

$\Rightarrow\ 32\alpha = n\pi + (-1)^n\frac{\pi}{2}$ and $32\alpha = 2n\pi + \frac{\pi}{2}$

$\Rightarrow\ \alpha = \frac{n\pi}{32}+(-1)^n\frac{\pi}{64}$ and $\alpha = \frac{n\pi}{16}+\frac{\pi}{64}$ where $n\in z$

Put $n = 0$, $\alpha = \frac{\pi}{64}$

Hence, required value of α is $\frac{\pi}{64}$.

Chapter 19

Topic-2

66. (c) Let $\alpha = \omega$ and $\beta = \omega^2$ are roots of $x^2+x+1 = 0$

& *Let* $\Delta = \begin{vmatrix}y+1 & \omega & \omega^2\\ \omega & y+\omega^2 & 1\\ \omega^2 & 1 & y+\omega\end{vmatrix} = \Delta$

Applying $C_1 \to C_1+C_2+C_3$

$\Delta = \begin{vmatrix}y+1+\omega+\omega^2 & \omega & \omega^2\\ y+1+\omega+\omega^2 & y+\omega^2 & 1\\ 1+\omega+\omega^2+y & 1 & y+\omega\end{vmatrix}$

$\Delta = \begin{vmatrix}y & \omega & \omega^2\\ y & y+\omega^2 & 1\\ y & 1 & y+\omega\end{vmatrix} (\because 1+\omega+\omega^2 = 0)$

$\Delta = y\begin{vmatrix}1 & \omega & \omega^2\\ 1 & y+\omega^2 & 1\\ 1 & 1 & y+\omega\end{vmatrix}$

Applying $R_2 \to R_2 - R_1\ \&\ R_3 \to R_3 - R_1$

$\Delta = y\begin{vmatrix}y+\omega^2-\omega & 1-\omega^2\\ 1-\omega & y+\omega-\omega^2\end{vmatrix}$

$\Rightarrow \Delta = y\left[y-(\omega-\omega^2)(y+(\omega-\omega^2)-(1-\omega)(1-\omega^2)\right]$

$\Rightarrow \Delta = y\left[y^2-(\omega-\omega^2)^2-1+\omega^2+\omega-\omega^3\right]$

$\Rightarrow \Delta = y\left[y^2-\omega^2-\omega^4+2\omega^3-1+\omega^2+\omega^4-\omega^3\right](\because \omega^4 = \omega)$

$\Rightarrow\ \Delta = y(y^2) = y^3$

67. (a) $\det(A)=\begin{vmatrix}-2 & 4+d & \sin\theta-2\\ 1 & \sin\theta+2 & d\\ 5 & 2\sin\theta-d & -\sin\theta+2+2d\end{vmatrix}$

Applying $R_3 \to R_3-2R_2+R_1$ we get

$$\det(A)=\begin{vmatrix}-2 & 4+d & \sin\theta-2\\ 1 & \sin\theta+2 & d\\ 1 & 0 & 0\end{vmatrix}$$

$= d(4+d)-(\sin^2\theta-4)$

$\Rightarrow$ $\det(A)=d^2+4d+4-\sin^2\theta=(d+2)^2-\sin^2\theta$

Minimum value of det (A) is attained when $\sin^2\theta = 1$

$\therefore$ $(d+2)^2-1=8 \Rightarrow (d+2)^2=9 \Rightarrow d+2=\pm 3$

$\Rightarrow$ $d=-5$ or 1

Topic-3

68. (b) $\begin{bmatrix}1 & 1\\ 0 & 1\end{bmatrix}\begin{bmatrix}1 & 2\\ 0 & 1\end{bmatrix}\begin{bmatrix}1 & 3\\ 0 & 1\end{bmatrix}\begin{bmatrix}1 & 4\\ 0 & 1\end{bmatrix}\cdots\begin{bmatrix}1 & n-1\\ 0 & 1\end{bmatrix}=\begin{bmatrix}1 & 78\\ 0 & 1\end{bmatrix}$

$\Rightarrow \begin{bmatrix}1 & 1+2+3+\ldots+(n-1)\\ 0 & 1\end{bmatrix}=\begin{bmatrix}1 & 78\\ 0 & 1\end{bmatrix}$

$\Rightarrow \dfrac{(n-1)n}{2}=78 \Rightarrow n^2-n-15=0$

$\Rightarrow n=13$

Now, the matrix $\begin{bmatrix}1 & n\\ 0 & 1\end{bmatrix}=\begin{bmatrix}1 & 13\\ 0 & 1\end{bmatrix}$

Then, the required inverse of $\begin{bmatrix}1 & 13\\ 0 & 1\end{bmatrix}=\begin{bmatrix}1 & -13\\ 0 & 1\end{bmatrix}$

69. (c) $A=\begin{bmatrix}\cos\theta & -\sin\theta\\ \sin\theta & \cos\theta\end{bmatrix} \Rightarrow |A|=1$

$$\text{adj}(A)=\begin{bmatrix}+\cos\theta & -\sin\theta\\ +\sin\theta & +\cos\theta\end{bmatrix}^T=\begin{bmatrix}\cos\theta & \sin\theta\\ -\sin\theta & \cos\theta\end{bmatrix}$$

$$\Rightarrow \quad A^{-1}=\begin{bmatrix}\cos\theta & \sin\theta\\ -\sin\theta & \cos\theta\end{bmatrix}=B$$

$$B^2=\begin{bmatrix}\cos\theta & \sin\theta\\ -\sin\theta & \cos\theta\end{bmatrix}\begin{bmatrix}\cos\theta & \sin\theta\\ -\sin\theta & \cos\theta\end{bmatrix}$$

$$=\begin{bmatrix}\cos 2\theta & \sin 2\theta\\ -\sin 2\theta & \cos 2\theta\end{bmatrix}$$

$$\Rightarrow \quad B^3=\begin{bmatrix}\cos 3\theta & \sin 3\theta\\ -\sin 3\theta & \cos 3\theta\end{bmatrix}$$

$$\Rightarrow \quad A^{-50}=B^{50}=\begin{bmatrix}\cos(50\theta) & \sin(50\theta)\\ -\sin(50\theta) & \cos(50\theta)\end{bmatrix}$$

$$(A^{-50})_{\theta=\frac{\pi}{12}}=\begin{bmatrix}\frac{\sqrt{3}}{2} & \frac{1}{2}\\ -\frac{1}{2} & \frac{\sqrt{3}}{2}\end{bmatrix}$$

$$\left[\because \cos\left(\frac{50\pi}{12}\right)=\cos\left(4\pi+\frac{\pi}{6}\right)=\cos\frac{\pi}{6}=\frac{\sqrt{3}}{2}\right]$$

Topic-4

70. (b) If the system of equations has non-trivial solutions, then the determinant of coefficient matrix is zero

$$\begin{vmatrix}1 & -c & -c\\ c & -1 & c\\ c & c & -1\end{vmatrix}=0$$

$\Rightarrow (1-c^2)+c(-c-c^2)-c(c^2+c)=0$

$\Rightarrow (1+c)(1-c)-2c^2(1+c)=0$

$\Rightarrow (1+c)(1-c-2c^2)=0$

$\Rightarrow (1+c)^2(1-2c)=0$

$\Rightarrow c=-1$ or $\dfrac{1}{2}$

Hence, the greatest value of c is $\frac{1}{2}$ for which the system of linear equations has non-trivial solution.

71. (b) $\Delta=\begin{vmatrix}1 & 1 & 1\\ 1 & 2 & 3\\ 1 & 3 & \alpha\end{vmatrix}=2\alpha-9-\alpha+3+1=\alpha-5$

$$\Delta_1=\begin{vmatrix}5 & 1 & 1\\ 9 & 2 & 3\\ \beta & 3 & \alpha\end{vmatrix}=5(2\alpha-9)-1(9\alpha-3\beta)+(27-2\beta)$$

$= 10\alpha-45-9\alpha+3\beta+27-2\beta$

$=\alpha+\beta-18$

$$\Delta_2=\begin{vmatrix}1 & 5 & 1\\ 1 & 9 & 3\\ 1 & \beta & \alpha\end{vmatrix}=9\alpha-3\beta-5(\alpha-3)+1(\beta-9)$$

$=9\alpha-3\beta-5\alpha+15+\beta-9=4\alpha-2\beta+6$

$$\Delta_3=\begin{vmatrix}1 & 1 & 5\\ 1 & 2 & 9\\ 1 & 3 & \beta\end{vmatrix}=2\beta-27-\beta+9+5=\beta-13$$

Since, the system of equations has infinite many solutions. Hence,

$\Delta_1=\Delta_2=\Delta_3=\Delta=0$

$\Rightarrow$ $\alpha=5, \beta=13 \Rightarrow \beta-\alpha=8$

Chapter 20

Topic-1

72. **(b)** Since, f(x) is continuous, then

$$\lim_{x\to\frac{\pi}{4}} f(x) = f\left(\frac{\pi}{4}\right)$$

$$\lim_{x\to\frac{\pi}{4}} \frac{\sqrt{2}\cos x-1}{\cot x-1} = k$$

Now by L- hospital's rule

$$\lim_{x\to\frac{\pi}{4}} \frac{\sqrt{2}\sin x}{\operatorname{cosec}^2 x} = k \Rightarrow \frac{\sqrt{2}\left(\frac{1}{\sqrt{2}}\right)}{(\sqrt{2})^2} = k \quad \Rightarrow k = \frac{1}{2}$$

73. **(d)** Let $f(x)$ is continuous at $x = 1$, then

$f(1^-) = f(1) = f(1^+)$

$\Rightarrow \quad 5 = a + b$ ...(1)

Let $f(x)$ is continuous at $x = 3$, then

$f(3^-) = f(3) = f(3^+)$

$\Rightarrow \quad a + 3b = b + 15$ ...(2)

Let $f(x)$ is continuous at $x = 5$, then

$f(5^-) = f(5) = f(5^+)$

$\Rightarrow \quad b + 25 = 30$

$\Rightarrow \quad b = 30 - 25 = 5$

From (1), $a = 0$

But $a = 0$, $b = 5$ do not satisfy equation (2)

Hence, $f(x)$ is not continuous for any values of a and b

Topic-2

74. **(a)** Since, f(x) = 15 – |(10 – x)|

$\therefore$ g(x) = f(f(x)) = 15 – |10 – [15 – |10 – x|]|

= 15 – ||10 – x| – 5|

$\therefore$ Then, the points where function g(x) is Non-differentiable are

10 – x = 0 and |10 – x| = 5

$\Rightarrow$ x = 10 and x – 10 = ± 5

$\Rightarrow$ x = 10 and x = 15, 5

75. **(b)** Given $f(x) = \begin{cases} \max\{|x|, x^2\} & |x| \le 2 \\ 8-2|x| & 2<|x|\le 4 \end{cases}$

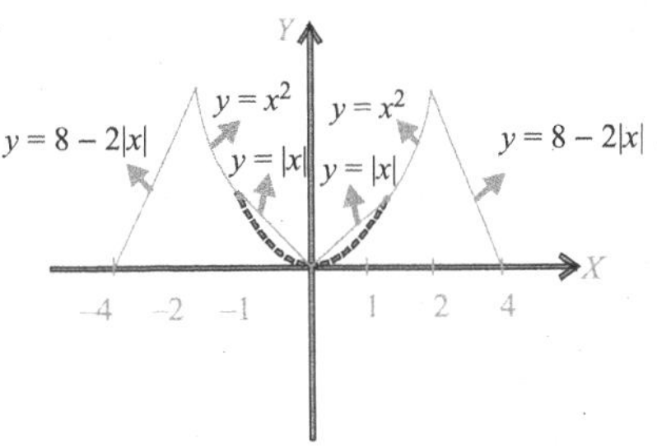

$\because f(x)$ is not differentiable at –2, –1, 0, 1 and 2.

$\therefore S = \{-2, -1, 0, 1, 2\}$

Topic-3

76. **(none)** $2y = \left[\cot^{-1}\left(\frac{\frac{\sqrt{3}}{2}\cos x + \frac{1}{2}\sin x}{\frac{1}{2}\cos x - \frac{\sqrt{3}}{2}\sin x}\right)\right]^2$

$$\Rightarrow 2y = \left[\cot^{-1}\left(\frac{\cos\left(\frac{\pi}{6}-x\right)}{\sin\left(\frac{\pi}{6}-x\right)}\right)\right]^2$$

$$\Rightarrow 2y = \left[\cot^{-1}\left(\cot\left(\frac{\pi}{6}-x\right)\right)\right]^2 \quad \because \frac{\pi}{6}-x \in \left(-\frac{\pi}{3},\frac{\pi}{6}\right)$$

$$\Rightarrow 2y = \begin{cases} \left(\frac{7\pi}{6}-x\right)^2, & \text{if } \frac{\pi}{6}-x \in \left(\frac{-\pi}{3},0\right) \\ \left(\frac{\pi}{6}-x\right)^2, & \text{if } \frac{\pi}{6}-x \in \left(0,\frac{\pi}{0}\right) \end{cases}$$

$$\Rightarrow \frac{dy}{dx} = \begin{cases} x-\frac{7\pi}{6} & \text{if } x \in \left(\frac{\pi}{6},\frac{\pi}{2}\right) \\ x-\frac{\pi}{6} & \text{if } x \in \left(0,\frac{\pi}{6}\right) \end{cases}$$

Topic-4

77. **(c)** Let $f(x) = x^3 + ax^2 + bx + c$

$f'(x) = 3x^2 + 2ax + b \Rightarrow f'(1) = 3 + 2a + b$

$f''(x) = 6x + 2a \Rightarrow f''(2) = 12 + 2a$

$f'''(x) = 6 \Rightarrow f'''(3) = 6$

$\because \quad f(x) = x^3 + f'(1)x^2 + f''(2)x + f'''(3)$

$\therefore \quad f'(1) = a \Rightarrow 3 + 2a + b = a \Rightarrow a + b = -3$ ...(1)

also $f''(2) = b \Rightarrow 12 + 2a = b \Rightarrow 2a - b = -12$ ...(2)

and $f''(3) = c \Rightarrow c = 6$

Add (1) and (2)

$3a = -15 \Rightarrow a = -5 \Rightarrow b = 2$

$\Rightarrow f(x) = x^3 - 5x^2 + 2x + 6$

$\Rightarrow f(2) = 8 - 20 + 4 + 6 = -2$

Chapter 21

Topic-2

78. (c) $\phi(x) = f(x) + f(2-x)$

Now, differentiate w.r.t. x,

$\phi'(x) = f'(x) - f'(2-x)$

For $\phi(x)$ to be increasing $\phi'(x) > 0$

$\Rightarrow f'(x) - f'(2-x) > 0$

$\Rightarrow f'(x) > f'(2-x)$

But $f''(x) > 0 \Rightarrow f'(x)$ is an increasing function

Then, $f'(x) > f'(2-x) > 0$

$\Rightarrow x > 2 - x$

$\Rightarrow x > 1$

Hence, $\phi(x)$ is increasing on (1, 2) and decreasing on (0, 1).

79. (c) $f(x) = \dfrac{x^2}{1-x^2}$

$$\Rightarrow f(-x) = \frac{x^2}{1-x^2} = f(x)$$

$$f'(-x) = \frac{2x}{(1-x^2)^2}$$

$\therefore$ f(x) increases in $x \in (10, \infty)$

Also f(0) = 0 and

$\lim_{x \to \pm\infty} f(x) = -1$ and f(x) is even function

$\therefore$ Set A = R – [–1, 0)

And the graph of function f(x) is

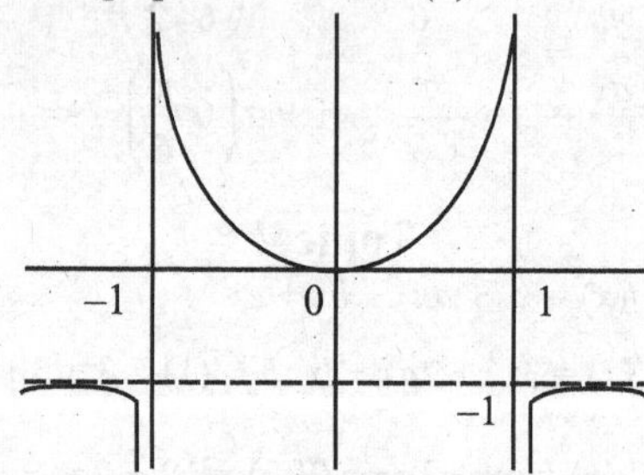

Topic-3

80. (d) $y = x^3 + ax - b$

Since, the point (1, –5) lies on the curve.

$\Rightarrow 1 + a - b = -5$

$\Rightarrow a - b = -6$ ...(1)

$\dfrac{dy}{dx} = 3x^2 + a$

$\left(\dfrac{dy}{dx}\right)_{at\ x=1} = 3 + a$

Since, required line is perpendicular to y = x – 4, then slope of tangent at the point P (1, –5) = –1

$\therefore 3 + a = -1$

$\Rightarrow a = -4$

$\Rightarrow b = 2$

$\therefore$ the equation of the curve is $y = x^3 - 4x - 2$

$\Rightarrow$ (2, –2) lies on the curve

81. (d) $y = f(x) = x^3 - x^2 - 2x$

$$\Rightarrow \frac{dy}{dx} - 3x^2 - 2x - 2$$

$f(1) = 1 - 1 - 2 = -2, \quad f(-1) = -1 - 1 + 2 = 0$

Since the tangent to the curve is parallel to the line segment joining the points (1, –2) (–1, 0)

Since their slopes are equal

$$\Rightarrow 3x^2 - 2x - 2 = \frac{-2-0}{2}$$

$$\Rightarrow x = 1, \frac{-1}{3}$$

Hence, the required set $S = \left\{\dfrac{-1}{3}, 1\right\}$

82. (b) Since, the equation of curves are

$y = 10 - x^2$ ...(1)

$y = 2 + x^2$ ...(2)

Adding eqn (1) and (2), we get

$2y = 12 \Rightarrow y = 6$

Then, from eqn (1)

$x = \pm 2$

Differentiate equation (1) with respect to x

$$\frac{dy}{dx} = -2x \Rightarrow \left(\frac{dy}{dx}\right)_{(2,6)} = -4 \text{ and } \left(\frac{dy}{dx}\right)_{(-2,6)} = 4$$

Differentiate equation (2) with respect to x

$$\frac{dy}{dx} = 2x \Rightarrow \left(\frac{dy}{dx}\right)_{(2,6)} = 4 \text{ and } \left(\frac{dy}{dx}\right)_{(-2,6)} = -4$$

$$\text{At (2, 6) } \tan\theta = \left(\frac{(-4)-(4)}{1+(-4)\times(4)}\right) = \frac{8}{15}$$

$$\text{At (–2, 6), } \tan\theta = \frac{(4)-(-4)}{1+(4)(-4)} = \frac{8}{-15} \Rightarrow |\tan\theta| = \frac{8}{15}$$

$$\therefore |\tan\theta| = \frac{8}{15}$$

83. (a)

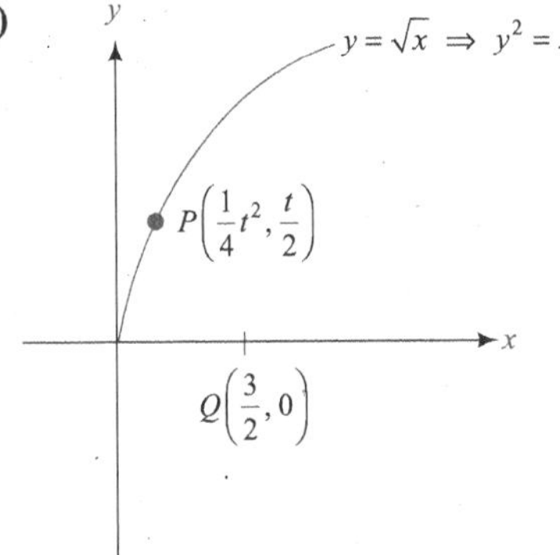

Here the curve is parabola with $a = \frac{1}{4}$.

Let P(at^2, 2at) or $P\left(\frac{t^2}{4}, \frac{t}{2}\right)$ be a point on the curve.

Now, $y^2 = x$

$\Rightarrow \quad 2y\frac{dy}{dx} = 1 = \frac{dy}{dx} = \frac{1}{2\sqrt{x}}$

$\Rightarrow \quad \left(\frac{dy}{dx}\right)_{at\ p} = \frac{1}{t}$

$\therefore$ equation of normal at P to $y^2 = x$ is,

$$\left(y - \frac{t}{2}\right) = -t\left(x - \frac{1}{4}t^2\right)$$

$\Rightarrow \quad y = -tx + \frac{1}{2}t + \frac{1}{4}t^3$ ...(1)

For minimum PQ, (1) passes through $Q\left(\frac{3}{2}, 0\right)$

$\Rightarrow \quad \frac{-3}{2}t + \frac{t}{2} + \frac{t^3}{4} = 0 \Rightarrow -4t + t^3 = 0$

$\Rightarrow \quad t(t^2 - 4) = 0 \Rightarrow t = -2, 0, 2$

$\because \quad t \geq 0 \Rightarrow t = 0, 2$

If $t = 0$, $P(0, 0) \Rightarrow AP = \frac{3}{2}$

If $t = 2$, $P(1, 1) \Rightarrow AP = \frac{\sqrt{5}}{2}$

$\Rightarrow$ Shortest distance $\left(\frac{3}{2}, 0\right)$ and $y = \sqrt{x}$ is $\frac{\sqrt{5}}{2}$

Topic-4

84. (c) $f(x) = 9x^4 + 12x^3 - 36x^2 + 25$

$f'(x) = 36[x^3 + x^2 - 2x] = 36x(x-1)(x+2)$

$$\begin{array}{cccccccc} - & & + & & - & & + \\ & -2 & & 0 & & 1 & \end{array}$$

Here at –2 & 1, $f'(x)$ changes from negative value to positive value.

$\Rightarrow$ –2 & 1 are local minimum points. At 0, $f'(x)$ changes from positive value to negative value.

$\Rightarrow$ 0 is the local maximum point.

Hence, $S_1 = \{-2, 1\}$ and $S_2 = \{0\}$

85. (d)

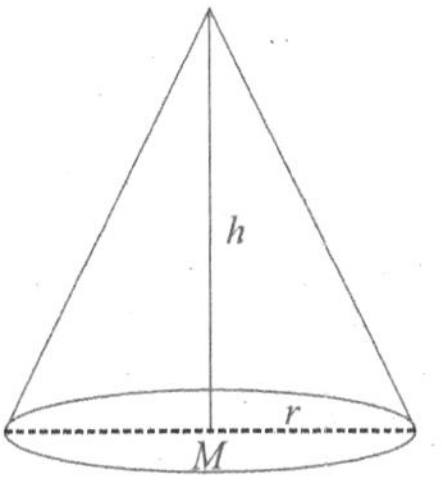

$h^2 + r^2 = \ell^2 = 9$ ...(1)

Volume of cone

$V = \frac{1}{3}\pi r^2 h$ ...(2)

From (1) and (2),

$\Rightarrow \quad V = \frac{1}{3}\pi(9 - h^2)h$

$\Rightarrow \quad V = \frac{1}{3}\pi(9h - h^3) \quad \Rightarrow \quad \frac{dv}{dh} = \frac{1}{3}\pi(9 - 3h^2)$

For maxima/minima,

$$\frac{dV}{dh} = 0 \Rightarrow \frac{1}{3}\pi(9 - 3h^2) = 0$$

$\Rightarrow \quad h = \pm\sqrt{3} \Rightarrow h = \sqrt{3}$

($\because h > 0$)

Now; $\frac{d^2V}{dh^2} = \frac{1}{3}\pi(-6h)$

Here, $\left(\frac{d^2V}{dh^2}\right)_{at\ h=\sqrt{3}} < 0$

Then, $h = \sqrt{3}$ is point of maxima

Hence, the required maximum volume is,

$$V = \frac{1}{3}\pi(9-3)\sqrt{3} = 2\sqrt{3}\pi$$

Chapter 22

Topic-1

86. (c) $\int \frac{\sin\left(\frac{5x}{2}\right)}{\sin\left(\frac{x}{2}\right)}dx = \int \frac{2\cos\frac{x}{2}.\sin\frac{5x}{2}}{2\cos\frac{x}{2}.\sin\frac{x}{2}}dx$

$= \int \frac{\sin 3x + \sin 2x}{\sin x}dx$

$= \int (3 - 4\sin^2 x + 2\cos x)dx$

$[\because \sin 2x = 2\sin x\cos x \text{ and } \sin 3x = 3\sin x - 4\sin^3 x]$

$= \int (3 - 2(1 - \cos 2x) + 2\cos x)dx$

$= \int (1 + 2\cos x + 2\cos 2x)dx$

$= x + 2\sin x + \sin 2x + c$

87. (d) Since, function f(x) have local extreem points at x = –1, 0, 1. Then

$f'(x) = K(x+1)x(x-1)$

$= K(x^3 - x)$

$\Rightarrow f(x) = K\left(\frac{x^4}{4} - \frac{x^2}{2}\right) + C$ (using integration)

$\Rightarrow f(0) = C$

$\because f(x) = f(0) \Rightarrow K\left(\frac{x^4}{4} - \frac{x^2}{2}\right) = 0$

$\Rightarrow \frac{x^2}{2}\left(\frac{x^2}{2} - 1\right) = 0$

$\Rightarrow x = 0, 0, \sqrt{2}, -\sqrt{2}$

$\therefore S = \{0, -\sqrt{2}, \sqrt{2}\}$

88. (a) $I = \int \sec^{\frac{2}{3}} x.\text{cosec}^{\frac{4}{3}} dx$

$I = \int \frac{\sec^2 x dx}{\tan^{\frac{4}{3}} x}$

Put tan x = z

$\Rightarrow \sec^2 x\, dx = dz$

$\Rightarrow I = \int z^{-\frac{4}{3}} \cdot dz = \frac{z^{\frac{-1}{3}}}{\left(\frac{-1}{3}\right)} + C \Rightarrow I = -3(\tan x)^{\frac{-1}{3}} + C$

89. (c, d) Consider the given integral

$I = \int x\sqrt{\frac{2\sin(x^2-1) - 2\sin(x^2-1)\cos(x^2-1)}{2\sin(x^2-1) + 2\sin(x^2-1)\cos(x^2-1)}}dx$

$(\because \sin 2\theta = 2\sin\theta\cos\theta)$

$\Rightarrow I = \int x\sqrt{\frac{1-\cos(x^2-1)}{1+\cos(x^2-1)}}dx$

$\Rightarrow I = \int x\left|\tan\left(\frac{x^2-1}{2}\right)\right|dx,$

Now let $\frac{x^2-1}{2} = t \Rightarrow \frac{2x}{2}dx = dt$

$\therefore I = \int |\tan(t)|\,dt = \ln|\sec t| + C$

or $I = \ln\left|\sec\left(\frac{x^2-1}{2}\right)\right| + c = \frac{1}{2}\ln\left|\sec^2\left(\frac{x^2-1}{2}\right)\right| + c$

90. (d) $I = \int_a^b (x^4 - 2x^2)dx$

$\Rightarrow \frac{dI}{dx} = x^4 - 2x^2 = 0$ (for minimum)

$\Rightarrow x = 0, \pm\sqrt{2}$

Also, $I = \left[\frac{x^5}{5} - \frac{2x^3}{3}\right]_a^b$

For a = 0, b = $\sqrt{2}$

$I = \frac{-8\sqrt{2}}{15}$

For a = $-\sqrt{2}$, b = 0

$I = \frac{-8\sqrt{2}}{15}.$

For a = $\sqrt{2}$, b = $-\sqrt{2}$

$I = \frac{16\sqrt{2}}{15}.$

For a = $-\sqrt{2}$, b = $\sqrt{2}$

$I = \frac{-16\sqrt{2}}{15}.$

$\therefore$ I is minimum when $(a, b) = (-\sqrt{2}, \sqrt{2})$

Topic-3

91. (d) $g(f(x)) = \log\left(\frac{2 - x\cos x}{2 + x\cos x}\right), x > 0$

Let $I = \int_{-\pi/4}^{\pi/4} \log\left(\frac{2 - x\cos x}{2 + x\cos x}\right)dx$ ...(1)

Use the property $\int_a^b f(x)dx = \int_a^b f(a+b-x)dx$

Then, equation (1) becomes,

$$I=\int_{-\pi/4}^{\pi/4}\log\left(\frac{2+x\cos x}{2-x\cos x}\right)dx \quad ...(2)$$

Adding (1) and (2)

$$2I=\int_{-\pi/4}^{\pi/4}\log\left(\frac{2-x\cos x}{2+x\cos x}\cdot\frac{2+x\cos x}{2-x\cos x}\right)dx$$

$$2I=\int_{-\pi/2}^{\pi/2}\log(1)dx=0$$

$\Rightarrow I=0=\log 1$

92. **(b)** Let $I=\int_0^{\pi/2}\frac{\sin^3 x dx}{\sin x+\cos x}$ ...(1)

Use the property $\int_0^a f(x)dx=\int_0^a f(a-x)dx$

$$I=\int_0^{\pi/2}\frac{\cos^3 x\,dx}{\sin x+\cos x} \quad ...(2)$$

Adding equation (1) and (2), we get

$$\Rightarrow 2I=\int_0^{\pi/2}\left(1-\frac{1}{2}\sin(2x)\right)dx$$

$$\Rightarrow I=\frac{1}{2}\left[x+\frac{1}{4}\cos 2x\right]_0^{\pi/2}$$

$$\Rightarrow I=\frac{\pi-1}{4}$$

93. **(b)** $I=\int_0^{\pi}|\cos x|^3\,dx$

$$=2\int_0^{\pi/2}\cos^3 x\,dx$$

$$=\frac{2}{4}\int_0^{\pi/2}(3\cos x+\cos 3x)dx$$

$[\because \cos 3\theta=4\cos^3\theta-3\cos\theta]$

$$=\frac{1}{2}\left[3\sin x+\frac{\sin 3x}{3}\right]_0^{\pi/2}$$

$$=\frac{1}{2}\left(3-\frac{1}{3}\right)=\frac{4}{3}$$

94. **(a)** Let, $I=\int\frac{(\sin^n\theta-\sin\theta)^{\frac{1}{n}}\cos\theta}{\sin^{n+1}\theta}d\theta$

Let $\sin\theta=u$

$\Rightarrow \cos\theta\,d\theta=du$

$$\therefore \quad I=\int\frac{(u^n-u)^{\frac{1}{n}}}{u^{n+1}}du$$

$$=\int\frac{\left(1-\frac{1}{u^{n-1}}\right)^{\frac{1}{n}}}{u^n}du=\int u^{-n}(1-u^{1-n})^{\frac{1}{n}}du$$

Let $1-u^{1-n}=v$

$\Rightarrow -(1-n)u^{-n}\,du=dv$

$$\Rightarrow u^{-n}\,du=\frac{dv}{n-1}$$

$$\therefore \quad I=\int v^{\frac{1}{n}}\cdot\frac{dv}{n-1}=\frac{1}{n-1}\cdot\frac{v^{\frac{1}{n}+1}}{\frac{1}{n}+1}$$

$$=\frac{n}{n^2-1}v^{\frac{n+1}{n}}+C=\frac{n}{n^2-1}\left(1-\frac{1}{u^{n-1}}\right)^{\frac{n+1}{n}}+C$$

$$=\frac{n}{n^2-1}\left(1-\frac{1}{\sin^{n-1}\theta}\right)^{\frac{n+1}{n}}+C$$

Chapter 23

Topic-1

95. **(c)** Since, the relation $y\le x^2+3x$ represents the region below the parabola in the 1st quadrant

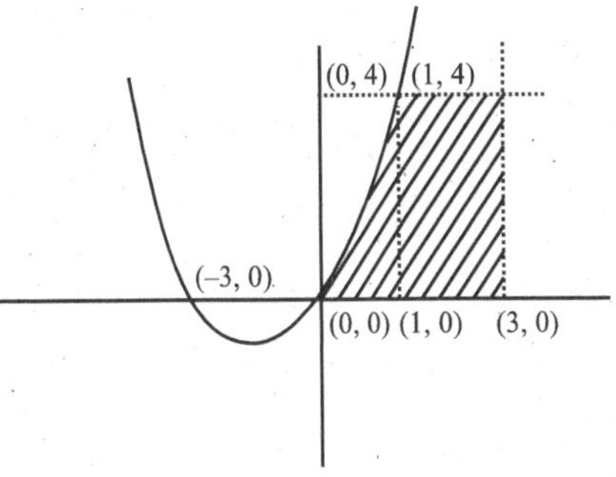

$\because y=4$

$\Rightarrow x^2+3x=4 \Rightarrow x=1,-4$

$\therefore$ the required area = area of shaded region

$$=\int_0^1(x^2+3x)dx+\int_1^3 4.dx=\left[\frac{x^3}{3}+\frac{3x^2}{2}\right]_0^1+[4x]_1^3$$

$$=\frac{1}{3}+\frac{3}{2}+8=\frac{59}{6}$$

Topic-2

96. (b)

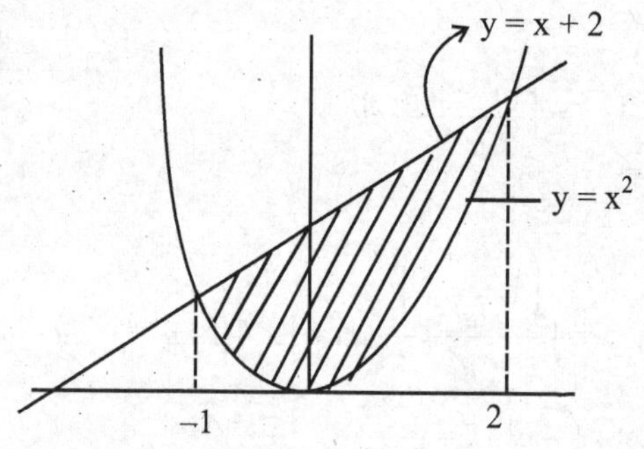

Required area is equal to the area under the curves $y \geq x^2$ and $y \leq x + 2$

$\therefore$ required area $\int_{-1}^{2} ((x+2)-x^2)dx$

$$=\left(\frac{x^2}{2}+2x-\frac{x^3}{3}\right)_{-1}^{2}$$

$$=\left(2+4-\frac{8}{3}\right)-\left(+\frac{1}{2}-2+\frac{1}{3}\right)=\frac{9}{2}$$

97. (a)

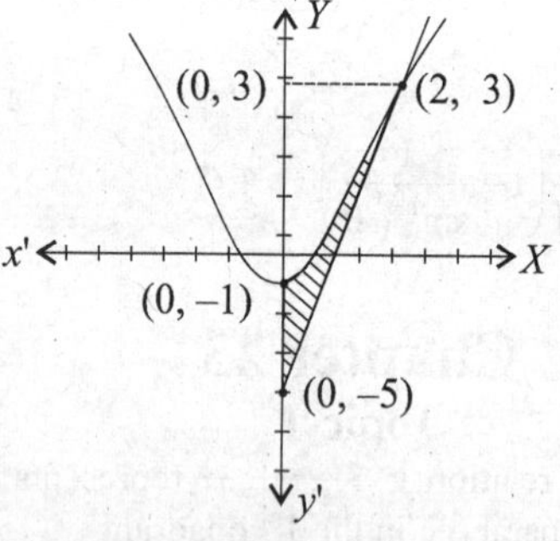

$\because$ Curve is given as :
$y = x^2 - 1$

$\Rightarrow \quad \frac{dy}{dx} = 2x$

$\Rightarrow \quad \left(\frac{dy}{dx}\right)_{(2,3)} = 4$

$\therefore$ equation of tangent at (2, 3)

$(y - 3) = 4 (x - 2)$

$\Rightarrow y = 4x - 5$

but $x = 0$

$\Rightarrow y = -5$

Here the curve cuts Y–axis

$\therefore$ required area

$$= \frac{1}{4}\int_{-5}^{3}(y+5)dy - \int_{-1}^{3}\sqrt{y+1}\,dy$$

$$= \frac{1}{4}\left[\frac{y^2}{2}+5y\right]_{-5}^{3} - \frac{2}{3}\left[(y+1)^{3/2}\right]_{-1}^{3}$$

$$= \frac{1}{4}\left[\frac{9}{2}+15-\frac{25}{2}+25\right]$$

$$= -\frac{2}{3}\left[4^{3/2}-0\right]$$

$$= \frac{32}{4}-\frac{16}{3}=\frac{8}{3} \text{ sq-units.}$$

98. (b)

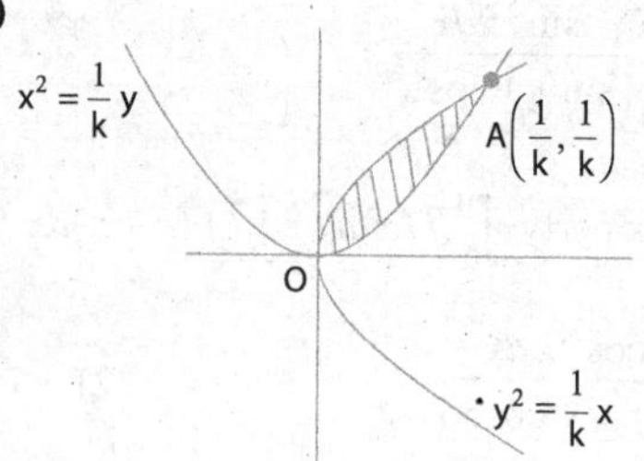

Two curves will intersect in the Ist quadrant at $A\left(\frac{1}{R},\frac{1}{R}\right)$

$\because$ area of shaded region = 1.

$$\therefore \quad \int_{0}^{\frac{1}{k}}\left(\frac{\sqrt{x}}{\sqrt{k}}-kx^2\right)dx = 1$$

$$\Rightarrow \quad \left(\frac{1}{\sqrt{k}}\cdot\frac{x^{\frac{3}{2}}}{\frac{3}{2}}\right)_{0}^{\frac{1}{k}} - \left(k\cdot\frac{x^3}{3}\right)_{0}^{\frac{1}{k}} = 1$$

$$\Rightarrow \quad \frac{2}{3\sqrt{k}}\cdot\frac{1}{k^{\frac{3}{2}}}-\frac{k}{3k^3}=1$$

$$\Rightarrow \quad \frac{2}{3k^2}-\frac{1}{3k^2}=1$$

$\Rightarrow \quad 3k^2 = 1$

$$\Rightarrow \quad k=\pm\frac{1}{\sqrt{3}}$$

$$\therefore \quad k=\frac{1}{\sqrt{3}} \quad (\because k > 0)$$

Chapter 24

Topic-2

99. **(a)** Given, $\frac{dy}{dx}+\frac{3}{\cos^2 x}y=\frac{1}{\cos^2 x}$

$$\frac{dy}{dx}=\sec^2 x(1-3y)$$

$$\Rightarrow \int\frac{dy}{(1-3y)}=\int\sec^2 x\,dx$$

$$\Rightarrow -\frac{1}{3}\ln|1-3y|=\tan x+C \quad ...(i)$$

$$\because y\left(\frac{\pi}{4}\right)=\frac{4}{3} \quad \text{(Given)}$$

$$\Rightarrow -\frac{1}{3}\ln|1-4|=\tan\frac{\pi}{4}+C$$

$$\Rightarrow -\frac{1}{3}\ln 3=C+1\Rightarrow C=-1-\frac{1}{3}\ln 3$$

$\therefore$ in eq. (i), we get

$$\frac{-1}{3}\ln|1-3y|=\tan x-1-\frac{1}{3}\ln 3$$

Put, $x=-\frac{\pi}{4}$

$$\Rightarrow -\frac{1}{3}\ln|1-3y|=\tan\left(-\frac{\pi}{4}\right)-1-\frac{1}{3}\ln 3$$

$$=-1-1-\frac{1}{3}\ln 3$$

$$\Rightarrow \ln|1-3y|=6+\ln 3$$

$$\Rightarrow \ln\left|\frac{1}{3}-y\right|=6\Rightarrow\left|\frac{1}{3}-y\right|=e^6\Rightarrow y=\frac{1}{3}\pm e^6$$

Topic-3

100. **(d)** $(1+x^2)^2\frac{dy}{dx}+2x(1+x^2)y=1$

$$\Rightarrow \frac{dy}{dx}+\left(\frac{2x}{1+x^2}\right)y=\frac{1}{(1+x^2)^2}$$

Since, the above differential equation is a linear differential equation

$$\therefore \text{ I.F.}=e^{\int\frac{2x}{1+x^2}dx}=e^{\log(1+x^2)}=1+x^2$$

Then, the solution of the differential equation

$$\Rightarrow y(1+x^2)=\int\frac{dx}{1+x^2}+c$$

$$\Rightarrow y(1+x^2)=\tan^{-1}x+c \quad ...(1)$$

If $x=0$ then $y=0$ (given)

$\Rightarrow 0=0+c$

$\Rightarrow c=0$

Then, equation (1) becomes,

$\Rightarrow y(1+x^2)=\tan^{-1}x$

Now put $x=1$ in above equation, then

$$2y=\frac{\pi}{4}$$

$$\Rightarrow 2\left(\frac{\pi}{32\sqrt{a}}\right)=\frac{\pi}{4} \qquad \left[\sqrt{a}\,y(1)=\frac{\pi}{32}\right]$$

$$\Rightarrow \sqrt{a}=\frac{1}{4}$$

$$\Rightarrow a=\frac{1}{16}$$

101. **(c)** $\frac{dy}{dx}+\frac{2}{x}y=x$ y(1) = 1 (given)

Since, the above differential equation is the linear differential equation, then $I.F=e^{\int\frac{2}{x}dx}=x^2$

Now, the solution of the linear differential equation

$$y\times x^2=\int x^3dx$$

$$\Rightarrow yx^2=\frac{x^4}{4}+C$$

$$\because y(1)=1$$

$$\therefore 1\times1=\frac{1}{4}+C\Rightarrow C=\frac{3}{4}$$

$\therefore$ Solution becomes.

$$y=\frac{x^2}{4}+\frac{3}{4x^2}$$

102. **(c)** Since, $x\frac{dy}{dx}+2y=x^2$

$$\Rightarrow \frac{dy}{dx}+\frac{2}{x}y=x$$

$$\text{I.F.}=e^{\int\frac{2}{x}dx}=e^{2\ln x}=e^{\ln x^2}=x^2.$$

Solution of differential equation is:

$$y \cdot x^2 = \int x \cdot x^2 dx$$

$$y \cdot x^2 = \frac{x^4}{4} + C \quad ...(1)$$

$\because \quad y(1) = 1$

$\therefore \quad C = \frac{3}{4}$

Then, from equation (1)

$$y \cdot x^2 = \frac{x^4}{4} + \frac{3}{4}$$

$$\therefore \quad y = \frac{x^2}{4} + \frac{3}{4x^2}$$

$$\therefore \quad y\left(\frac{1}{2}\right) = \frac{1}{16} + 3 = \frac{49}{16}$$

Chapter 25

Topic-2

103. **(b)** $\because \vec{b} = 2\vec{a}$

$\therefore \quad 4\hat{i} + (3 - \lambda_2)\hat{j} + 6\hat{k} = 4\hat{i} + 2\lambda_1\hat{j} + 6\hat{k}$

$\therefore \quad 3 - \lambda_2 = 2\lambda_1 \quad ...(1)$

$\because \vec{a}$ is perpendicular to $\vec{c}$

$\therefore \quad \vec{a} \cdot \vec{c} = 0$

$\Rightarrow \quad 6 + 6\lambda_1 + 3(\lambda_3 - 1) = 0$

$\Rightarrow \quad 2 + 2\lambda_1 + \lambda_3 - 1 = 0$

$\Rightarrow \quad \lambda_3 = -2\lambda_1 - 1 \quad ...(2)$

Since $\left(\frac{-1}{2}, 4, 0\right)$ satisfies equation (1) and (2). Hence, one of possible value of

$$\lambda_1 = -\frac{1}{2}, \lambda_2 = 4 \text{ and } \lambda_3 = 0$$

Topic-3

104. **(d)** Let $\vec{a} = \hat{i} + \hat{j} + \hat{k}$ and $\vec{b} = \hat{i} + 2\hat{j} + 3\hat{k}$

$\therefore$ vector perpendicular to $\vec{a}$ and $\vec{b}$ is $\vec{a} \times \vec{b}$

$$\therefore \quad \vec{a} \times \vec{b} = \begin{vmatrix} \hat{i} & \hat{j} & \hat{k} \\ 1 & 1 & 1 \\ 1 & 2 & 3 \end{vmatrix} = \hat{i} - 2\hat{j} + \hat{k}$$

Now, projection of vector $\vec{c} = 2\hat{i} + 3\hat{j} + \hat{k}$ on $\vec{a} \times \vec{b}$ is

$$= \left|\frac{\vec{c}.(\vec{a} \times \vec{b})}{|\vec{a} \times \vec{b}|}\right| = \left|\frac{2 - 6 + 1}{\sqrt{6}}\right| = \frac{3}{\sqrt{6}} = \sqrt{\frac{3}{2}}$$

105. **(c)** $\vec{\beta} = \vec{\beta_1} - \vec{\beta_2} \quad ...(1)$

Since, $\vec{\beta_2}$ is perpendicular to $\vec{\alpha}$.

$\therefore \vec{\beta_2}.\vec{\alpha} = 0$

Since, $\vec{\beta_1}$ is parallel to $\vec{a}$.

then $\vec{\beta_1} = \lambda\vec{\alpha}$ (say)

$\vec{a}.\vec{\beta} = \vec{a}.\vec{\beta_1} - \vec{\alpha}.\vec{\beta_2}$

$\Rightarrow 5 = \lambda\alpha^2 \Rightarrow 5 = \lambda \times 10 \quad (\because |\vec{\alpha}| = \sqrt{10}).$

$\Rightarrow \lambda = \frac{1}{2} \quad \therefore \vec{B_1} = \frac{\vec{\alpha}}{2}$

$\therefore \vec{\beta_1} = \frac{\vec{\alpha}}{2}$

Cross product with $\vec{B_1}$ in equation (1)

$\Rightarrow \vec{\beta} \times \vec{B_1} = -\vec{B_2} \times \vec{B_1}$

$\Rightarrow \vec{\beta} \times \vec{B_1} = \vec{B_1} \times \vec{B_2} \quad \Rightarrow \vec{\beta_1} \times \vec{\beta_2} = \frac{\vec{\beta} \times \vec{\alpha}}{2}$

$$\Rightarrow \vec{B_1} \times \vec{B2} = \frac{1}{2}\begin{vmatrix} \hat{i} & j & k \\ 2 & -1 & 3 \\ 3 & 1 & 0 \end{vmatrix}$$

$$= \frac{1}{2}\left[-3\hat{i} - \hat{j}(-9) + \hat{k}(5)\right] = \frac{1}{2}\left[-3\hat{i} + 9\hat{j} + 5\hat{k}\right]$$

106. **(a)** $\because |\vec{a} \times \vec{c}|^2 = |\vec{a}|^2 |\vec{c}|^2 - (\vec{a}.\vec{c})^2$

$\Rightarrow \quad |-\vec{b}|^2 = 2|\vec{c}|^2 - 16 \quad \Rightarrow 3 = 2|\vec{c}|^2 - 16$

$\Rightarrow \quad |\vec{c}|^2 = \frac{19}{2}$

Chapter 26

Topic-2

107. **(a)** Let P be the foot of perpendicular from point $T(2, -1, 4)$ on the given line. So P can be assumed as $P(10\lambda - 3, -7\lambda + 2, \lambda)$

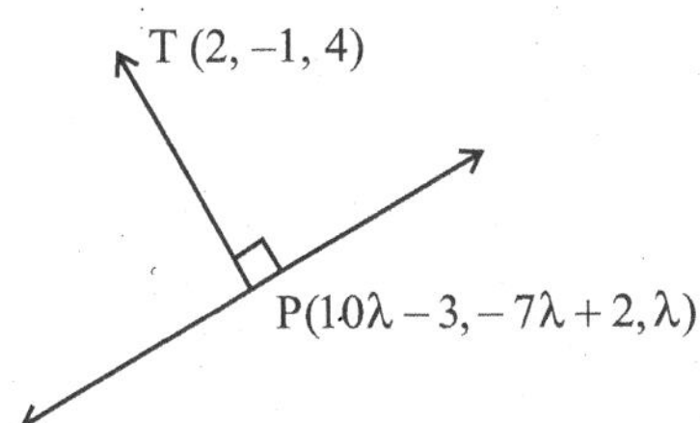

DR's of $TP \propto$ to $10\lambda - 5, -7\lambda + 3, \lambda - 4$

$\because$ TP and given line are perpendicular, so

$10(10\lambda - 5) - 7(-7\lambda + 3) + 1(\lambda - 4) = 0$

$\Rightarrow \lambda = \frac{1}{2}$

$\Rightarrow TP = \sqrt{(10\lambda - 5)^2 + (-7\lambda + 3)^2 + (\lambda - 4)^2}$

$= \sqrt{0 + \frac{1}{4} + \frac{49}{4}} = \sqrt{12.5} = 3.54$

Hence, the length of perpendicular is greater than 3 but less than 4.

Topic-3

108. (c) Let the equation of required plane be;

$(2x - y - 4) + \lambda(y + 2z - 4) = 0$

$\because$ This plane passes through the point (1, 1, 0) then

$(2 - 1 - 4) + \lambda(1 + 0 - 4) = 0$

$\Rightarrow \lambda = -1$

Then, equation of required plane is,

$(2x - y - 4) - (y + 2z - 4) = 0$

$\Rightarrow 2x - 2y - 2z = 0 \Rightarrow x - y - z = 0$

109. (c) Let point on line be P (2k + 1, 3k – 1, 4k + 2)

Since, point P lies on the plane x + 2y + 3z = 15

$\therefore$ 2k + 1 + 6k – 2 + 12k + 6 = 15

$\Rightarrow k = \frac{1}{2}$

$\therefore P \equiv \left(2, \frac{1}{2}, 4\right)$

Then the distance of the point P from the origin is

$OP = \sqrt{4 + \frac{1}{4} + 16} = \frac{9}{2}$

110. (d) Let the required plane passing through the points (0, –1, 0) and (0, 0, 1) be $\frac{x}{\lambda} + \frac{y}{-1} + \frac{z}{1} = 1$ and the given plane is y – z + 5 = 0

$\therefore \cos\frac{\pi}{4} = \frac{-1-1}{\sqrt{\left(\frac{1}{\lambda^2} + 1 + 1\right)}\sqrt{2}}$

$\Rightarrow \lambda^2 = \frac{1}{2} \Rightarrow \frac{1}{\lambda} = \pm\sqrt{2}$

Then, the equation of plane is

$\pm\sqrt{2}x - y + z = 1$

Then the point $(\sqrt{2}, 1, 4)$ satisfies the equation of plane

111. (d) Since the system of linear equations are

$$x + y + z = 2 \qquad ...(1)$$

$$2x + 3y + 2z = 5 \qquad ...(2)$$

$$2x + 3y + (a^2 - 1)z = a + 1 \qquad ...(3)$$

Now, $\Delta = \begin{vmatrix} 1 & 1 & 1 \\ 2 & 3 & 2 \\ 2 & 3 & a^2 - 1 \end{vmatrix}$

(Applying $R_3 \to R_3 - R_2$)

$\Rightarrow \Delta = \begin{vmatrix} 1 & 1 & 1 \\ 2 & 3 & 2 \\ 0 & 0 & a^2 - 3 \end{vmatrix}$

$= a^2 - 3$

When, $\Delta = 0 \Rightarrow a^2 - 3 = 0 \Rightarrow |a| = \sqrt{3}$

If $a^2 = 3$, then plane represented by eqn (2) and eqn (3) are parallel.

Hence, the given system of equation is inconsistent.

112. (c) Let any point on the intersecting line

$\frac{x+1}{-3} = \frac{y-3}{2} = \frac{z-2}{-1} = \lambda$ (say)

is $(-3\lambda - 1, 2\lambda + 3, -\lambda + 2)$

Since, the above point lies on a line which passes through the point (–4, 3, 1)

Then, direction ratio of the required line

$= \langle -3\lambda - 1 + 4, 2\lambda + 3 - 3, -\lambda + 2 - 1 \rangle$

or $\langle -3\lambda + 3, 2\lambda, -\lambda + 1 \rangle$

Since, line is parallel to the plane

$x + 2y - z - 5 = 0$

Then, perpendicular vector to the line is $\hat{i} + 2\hat{j} - \hat{k}$

Now $(-3\lambda + 3)(1) + (2\lambda)(2) + (-\lambda + 1)(-1) = 0$

$\Rightarrow \lambda = -1$

Now direction ratio of the required line = $\langle 6, -2, 2 \rangle$ or $\langle 3, -1, 1 \rangle$

Hence required equation of the line is

$\frac{x+4}{3} = \frac{y-3}{-1} = \frac{z-1}{1}$

113. (d) Since, equation of plane through intersection of planes

$x + y + z = 1$ and $2x + 3y - z + 4 = 0$ is

$(2x + 3y - z + 4) + \lambda(x + y + z - 1) = 0$

$(2 + \lambda)x + (3 + \lambda)y + (-1 + \lambda)z + (4 - \lambda) = 0 \quad ...(1)$

But, the above plane is parallel to y-axis then

$(2 + \lambda) \times 0 + (3 + \lambda) \times 1 + (-1 + \lambda) \times 0 = 0$

$\Rightarrow \lambda = -3$

Hence, the equation of required plane is

$-x - 4z + 7 = 0$

$\Rightarrow x + 4z - 7 = 0$

Therefore, (3, 2, 1) the passes through the point.

114. (b) Equation of required plane is

$$\begin{vmatrix} x-4 & y+1 & z-2 \\ 3 & -1 & 2 \\ 1 & 2 & 3 \end{vmatrix} = 0$$

$(x-4)(-3-4) - (y+1)(9-2) + (z-2)(6+1) = 0$

$\Rightarrow \quad -7(x-4) - 7(y+1) + 7(z-2) = 0$

$\Rightarrow \quad x - 4 + y + 1 - z + 2 = 0$

$\Rightarrow \quad x + y - z - 1 = 0$

$\because$ point (1, 1, 1) satisfies this equation

$\therefore$ point (1, 1, 1) lies on the plane

115. (a) $\because$ A be a point on given line.

$\therefore$ Position vector of A

$$\overrightarrow{OA} = \vec{r} = (1-3\mu)\hat{i} + (\mu-1)\hat{j} + (2+5\mu)\hat{k}$$

Position vector of $B = \overrightarrow{OB} = 3\hat{i} + 2\hat{j} + 6\hat{k}$

$\therefore \quad \overrightarrow{AB} = \overrightarrow{OB} - \overrightarrow{OA}$

$= (3\mu + 2)\hat{i} + (3-\mu)\hat{j} + (4 - 5\mu)\hat{k}$

Equation of plane is: $x - 4y + 3z = 1$

$\because \quad \overrightarrow{AB}$ is parallel to this plane.

$\therefore \quad 1(3\mu + 2) - 4(3 - \mu) + 3(4 - 5\mu) = 0$

$\Rightarrow \quad 3\mu + 2 - 12 + 4\mu + 12 - 15\mu = 0$

$\Rightarrow \quad 2 - 8\mu = 0$

$\Rightarrow \quad \mu = \frac{1}{4}$

Chapter 27

Topic-1

116. (b) $\because \quad A \subset B$; so $A \cap B = A$

Now, $P\left(\frac{A}{B}\right) = \frac{P(A \cap B)}{P(B)}$

$\Rightarrow \quad P\left(\frac{A}{B}\right) = \frac{P(A)}{P(B)}$

$\because \quad P(B) \leq 1$

$\Rightarrow \quad P\left(\frac{A}{B}\right) \geq P(A)$

117. (d) P (at least one hits the target)

= 1 – P (none of them hits the target)

$$= 1 - \left(1 - \frac{1}{2}\right)\left(1 - \frac{1}{3}\right)\left(1 - \frac{1}{4}\right)\left(1 - \frac{1}{8}\right)$$

$$= 1 - \frac{1}{2} \times \frac{2}{3} \times \frac{3}{4} \times \frac{7}{8} = 1 - \frac{7}{32} = \frac{25}{32}$$

118. (c) $P(\text{Outcome is head}) = \frac{1}{2}$

$P(\text{Outcome is tail}) = –$

$P(\text{7 or 8 is the sum of two dice}) = \frac{6}{36} + \frac{5}{36} = \frac{11}{36}$

$P(\text{7 or 8 is the number of card}) = \frac{1}{9} + \frac{1}{9} = \frac{2}{9}$

Required probability $= \frac{1}{2} \times \frac{11}{36} + \frac{1}{2} \times \frac{2}{9}$

$= \frac{1}{2}\left(\frac{11+8}{36}\right) = \frac{19}{72}$

Topic-2

119. (d) X = number of aces drawn

$\therefore \quad P(X = 1) + P(X = 2)$

$$= \left\{\frac{4}{52} \times \frac{48}{52} + \frac{48}{52} \times \frac{4}{52}\right\} + \left\{\frac{4}{52} \times \frac{4}{52}\right\}$$

$$= \frac{24}{169} + \frac{1}{169} = \frac{25}{169}$$

Chapter 28

Topic-2

120. (b) Let the height of the lamp-post is h.

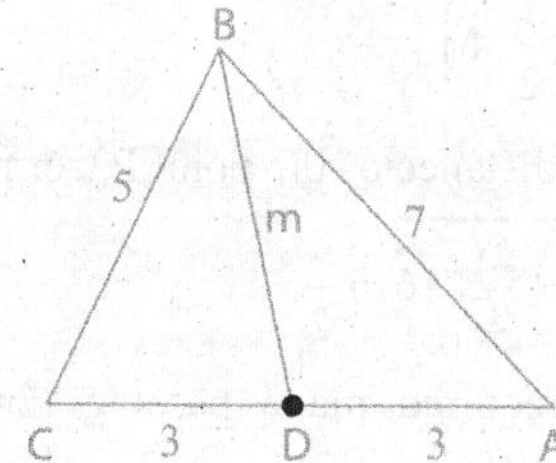

By Appolonius Theorem,

$$2\left(BD^2 + \left(\frac{AC}{2}\right)^2\right) = BC^2 + AB^2$$

$\Rightarrow \quad 2(m^2 + 3^2) = 25 + 49 \Rightarrow m = 2\sqrt{7}$

$\tan 30° = \frac{h}{BD}$

$\Rightarrow \quad h = 2\sqrt{7} \times \frac{1}{\sqrt{3}} = \frac{2\sqrt{21}}{3}$

JEE Main Solved Papers 2018
Offline + Online
(Refer to the Main Chapters for Topics)

CHAPTER-1 : Sets

TOPIC-1

1. Let $S = \{x \in R : x \geq 0$ and $2|\sqrt{x}-3|+\sqrt{x}(\sqrt{x}-6)+6=0$. Then S : **[2018]**
   (a) contains exactly one element.
   (b) contains exactly two elements.
   (c) contains exactly four elements.
   (d) is an empty set.

CHAPTER-3 : Trigonometric Functions

TOPIC-3

2. If sum of all the solutions of the equation $8\cos x \cdot \left(\cos\left(\frac{\pi}{6}+x\right)\cdot\cos\left(\frac{\pi}{6}-x\right)-\frac{1}{2}\right)-1$ in $[0, \pi]$ is $k\pi$, then k is equal to : **[2018]**
   (a) $\frac{13}{9}$ (b) $\frac{8}{9}$
   (c) $\frac{20}{9}$ (d) $\frac{2}{3}$

3. The number of solutions of $\sin 3x = \cos 2x$, in the interval $\left(\frac{\pi}{2}, \pi\right)$ is **[Online April 15, 2018]**
   (a) 3 (b) 4
   (c) 2 (d) 1

CHAPTER-5 : Complex Numbers and Quadratic Equations

TOPIC-1

4. The set of all $\alpha \in R$, for which $w = \frac{1+(1-8\alpha)z}{1-z}$ is a purely imaginary number, for all $z \in C$ satisfying $|z| = 1$ and $Re\, z \neq 1$, is **[Online April 15, 2018]**
   (a) $\{0\}$ (b) an empty set
   (c) $\left\{0, \frac{1}{4}, -\frac{1}{4}\right\}$ (d) equal to R

5. If $f(x)$ is a quadratic expression such that $f(1)+f(2)=0$, and -1 is a root of $f(x)=0$, then the other root of $f(x)=0$ is **[Online April 15, 2018]**
   (a) $-\frac{5}{8}$ (b) $-\frac{8}{5}$
   (c) $\frac{5}{8}$ (d) $\frac{8}{5}$

TOPIC-2

6. The least positive integer n for which $\left(\frac{1+i\sqrt{3}}{1-i\sqrt{3}}\right)^n = 1$, is **[Online April 16, 2018]**
   (a) 2 (b) 6
   (c) 5 (d) 3

7. If $|z-3+2i| \leq 4$ then the difference between the greatest value and the least value of $|z|$ is **[Online April 15, 2018]**
   (a) $\sqrt{13}$ (b) $2\sqrt{13}$
   (c) 8 (d) $4+\sqrt{13}$

TOPIC-3

8. If $\alpha, \beta \in C$ are the distinct roots, of the equation $x^2 - x + 1 = 0$, then $\alpha^{101} + \beta^{107}$ is equal to : **[2018]**
   (a) 0 (b) 1
   (c) 2 (d) -1

9. Let p, q and r be real numbers ($p \neq q$, $r \neq 0$), such that the roots of the equation $\frac{1}{x+p}+\frac{1}{x+q}=\frac{1}{r}$ are equal in magnitude but opposite in sign, then the sum of squares of these roots is equal to. **[Online April 16, 2018]**
   (a) $p^2+q^2+r^2$ (b) p^2+q^2
   (c) $2(p^2+q^2)$ (d) $\frac{p^2+q^2}{2}$

10. If an angle A of a Δ ABC satisfies 5 cos A + 3 = 0, then the roots of the quadratic equation, $9x^2+27x+20=0$ are. **[Online April 16, 2018]**

(a) $\sin A, \sec A$ (b) $\sec A, \tan A$
(c) $\tan A, \cos A$ (d) $\sec A, \cot A$

11. If $\lambda \in R$ is such that the sum of the cubes of the roots of the equation, $x^2+(2-\lambda)x+(10-\lambda)=0$ is minimum, then the magnitude of the difference of the roots of this equation is **[Online April 15, 2018]**

(a) 20 (b) $2\sqrt{5}$
(c) $2\sqrt{7}$ (d) $4\sqrt{2}$

12. If $\tan A$ and $\tan B$ are the roots of the quadratic equation, $3x^2-10x-25=0$ then the value of $3\sin^2(A+B)-10\sin(A+B).\cos(A+B)-25\cos^2(A+B)$ is **[Online April 15, 2018]**

(a) 25 (b) −25
(c) −10 (d) 10

CHAPTER-7 : Permutations and Combinations

TOPIC-1

13. The number of numbers between 2,000 and 5,000 that can be formed with the digits 0, 1, 2, 3, 4, (repetition of digits is not allowed) and are multiple of 3 is? **[Online April 16, 2018]**

(a) 30 (b) 48
(c) 24 (d) 36

14. n – digit numbers are formed using only three digits 2, 5 and 7. The smallest value of n for which 900 such distinct numbers can be formed, is **[Online April 15, 2018]**

(a) 6 (b) 8
(c) 9 (d) 7

TOPIC-2

15. From 6 different novels and 3 different dictionaries, 4 novels and 1 dictionary are to be selected and arranged in a row on a shelf so that the dictionary is always in the middle. The number of such arrangements is : **[2018]**

(a) less than 500
(b) at least 500 but less than 750
(c) at least 750 but less than 1000
(d) at least 1000

16. The number of four letter words that can be formed using the letters of the word BARRACK is **[Online April 15, 2018]**

(a) 144 (b) 120
(c) 264 (d) 270

CHAPTER-8 : Binomial Theorem

TOPIC-1

17. The sum of the co-efficients of all odd degree terms in the expansion of **[2018]**

$(x+\sqrt{x^3-1})^5+(x-\sqrt{x^3-1})^5, (x>1)$ is :

(a) 0 (b) 1
(c) 2 (d) −1

18. The coefficient of x^2 in the expansion of the product $(2-x^2).((1+2x+3x^2)^6+(1-4x^2)^6)$ is **[Online April 16, 2018]**

(a) 106 (b) 107
(c) 155 (d) 108

19. If n is the degree of the polynomial,

$$\left[\frac{1}{\sqrt{5x^3+1}-\sqrt{5x^3-1}}\right]^8+\left[\frac{1}{\sqrt{5x^3+1}+\sqrt{5x^3-1}}\right]^8$$ and

m is the coefficient of x^n in it, then the ordered pair (n, m) is equal to **[Online April 15, 2018]**

(a) $(12,(20)^4)$ (b) $(8,5(10)^4)$
(c) $(24,(10)^8)$ (d) $(12,8(10)^4)$

20. The coefficient of x^{10} in the expansion of $(1+x)^2(1+x^2)^3(1+x^3)^4$ is equal to **[Online April 15, 2018]**

(a) 52 (b) 44
(c) 50 (d) 56

CHAPTER-9 : Sequences and Series

TOPIC-1

21. Let $a_1, a_2, a_3, \ldots, a_{49}$ be in A.P. such that $\sum_{k=0}^{12} a_{4k+1}=416$ and $a_9+a_{43}=66$. If $a_1^2+a_2^2+\ldots+a_{17}^2=140m$, then m is equal to : **[2018]**

(a) 68 (b) 34
(c) 33 (d) 66

22. Let $\frac{1}{x_1}, \frac{1}{x_2}, \frac{1}{x_3}, \ldots\ldots, (x_i \neq 0$ for $i=1,2,\ldots, n)$ be in A.P. such that $x_1=4$ and $x_{21}=20$. If n is the least positive integer for which $x_n>50$, then $\sum_{i=1}^{n}\left(\frac{1}{x_i}\right)$ is equal to. **[Online April 16, 2018]**

(a) 3 (b) $\frac{13}{8}$
(c) $\frac{13}{4}$ (d) $\frac{1}{8}$

23. If $x_1, x_2, ..., x_n$ and $\frac{1}{h_1}, \frac{1}{h^2}, ... \frac{1}{h_n}$ are two A.P's such that $x_3 = h_2 = 8$ and $x_8 = h_7 = 20$, then $x_5 . h_{10}$ equals. **[Online April 15, 2018]**

(a) 2560 (b) 2650
(c) 3200 (d) 1600

TOPIC-2

24. If b is the first term of an infinite G. P whose sum is five, then b lies in the interval. **[Online April 15, 2018]**

(a) $(-\infty, -10)$ (b) $(10, \infty)$
(c) $(0, 10)$ (d) $(-10, 0)$

25. Let $A_n = \left(\frac{3}{4}\right) - \left(\frac{3}{4}\right)^2 + \left(\frac{3}{4}\right)^3 - ... + (-1)^{n-1}\left(\frac{3}{4}\right)^n$ and $B_n = 1 - A_n$. Then, the least odd natural number p, so that $B_n > A_n$, for all $n \geq p$ is **[Online April 15, 2018]**

(a) 5 (b) 7
(c) 11 (d) 9

26. If a, b, c are in A.P. and a^2, b^2, c^2 are in G.P. such that $a < b < c$ and $a + b + c = \frac{3}{4}$, then the value of a is **[Online April 15, 2018]**

(a) $\frac{1}{4} - \frac{1}{3\sqrt{2}}$ (b) $\frac{1}{4} - \frac{1}{4\sqrt{2}}$

(c) $\frac{1}{4} - \frac{1}{\sqrt{2}}$ (d) $\frac{1}{4} - \frac{1}{2\sqrt{2}}$

TOPIC-4

27. Let A be the sum of the first 20 terms and B be the sum of the first 40 terms of the series

$1^2 + 2 \cdot 2^2 + 3^2 + 2.4^2 + 5^2 + 2.6^2 + ...$

If $B - 2A = 100\lambda$, then λ is equal to : **[2018]**

(a) 248 (b) 464
(c) 496 (d) 232

28. The sum of the first 20 terms of the series

$1 + \frac{3}{2} + \frac{7}{4} + \frac{15}{8} + \frac{31}{16} + ...$ is? **[Online April 16, 2018]**

(a) $38 + \frac{1}{2^{20}}$ (b) $39 + \frac{1}{2^{19}}$

(c) $39 + \frac{1}{2^{20}}$ (d) $38 + \frac{1}{2^{19}}$

CHAPTER-10 : Straight Lines and Pair of Straight Lines

TOPIC-1

29. Let the orthocentre and centroid of a triangle be A(–3, 5) and B(3, 3) respectively. If C is the circumcentre of this triangle, then the radius of the circle having line segment AC as diameter, is : **[2018]**

(a) $2\sqrt{10}$ (b) $3\sqrt{\frac{5}{2}}$

(c) $\frac{3\sqrt{5}}{2}$ (d) $\sqrt{10}$

TOPIC-2

30. A straight line through a fixed point (2, 3) intersects the coordinate axes at distinct points P and Q. If O is the origin and the rectangle OPRQ is completed, then the locus of R is : **[2018]**

(a) $2x + 3y = xy$ (b) $3x + 2y = xy$
(c) $3x + 2y = 6xy$ (d) $3x + 2y = 6$

31. In a triangle ABC, coordianates of A are (1, 2) and the equations of the medians through B and C are $x + y = 5$ and $x = 4$ respectively. Then area of ΔABC (in sq. units) is **[Online April 15, 2018]**

(a) 5 (b) 9
(c) 12 (d) 4

TOPIC-3

32. The foot of the perpendicular drawn from the origin, on the line, $3x + y = \lambda(\lambda \neq 0)$ is P. If the line meets x-axis at A and y-axis at B, then the ratio $BP : PA$ is **[Online April 15, 2018]**

(a) $9:1$ (b) $1:3$
(c) $1:9$ (d) $3:1$

33. The sides of a rhombus $ABCD$ are parallel to the lines, $x - y + 2 = 0$ and $7x - y + 3 = 0$. If the diagonals of the rhombus intersect at $P(1, 2)$ and the vertex A (different from the origin) is on the y-axis, then the ordinate of A is **[Online April 15, 2018]**

(a) 2 (b) $\frac{7}{4}$

(c) $\frac{7}{2}$ (d) $\frac{5}{2}$

CHAPTER-11 : Conic Sections

TOPIC-1

34. If the tangent at (1, 7) to the curve $x^2 = y - 6$ touches the circle $x^2 + y^2 + 16x + 12y + c = 0$ then the value of c is : **[2018]**

(a) 185 (b) 85
(c) 95 (d) 195

35. If a circle C, whose radius is 3, touches externally the circle, $x^2 + y^2 + 2x - 4y - 4 = 0$ at the point (2, 2), then the length of the intercept cut by this circle c, on the x-axis is equal to **[Online April 16, 2018]**

(a) $\sqrt{5}$ (b) $2\sqrt{3}$
(c) $3\sqrt{2}$ (d) $2\sqrt{5}$

36. A circle passes through the points (2, 3) and (4, 5). If its centre lies on the line, $y - 4x + 3 = 0$, then its radius is equal to **[Online April 15, 2018]**

(a) $\sqrt{5}$ (b) 1
(c) $\sqrt{2}$ (d) 2

37. Two parabolas with a common vertex and with axes along x-axis and y-axis, respectively, intersect each other in the first quadrant. if the length of the latus rectum of each parabola is 3, then the equation of the common tangent to the two parabolas is? **[Online April 15, 2018]**

(a) $3(x+y)+4=0$ (b) $8(2x+y)+3=0$
(c) $4(x+y)+3=0$ (d) $x+2y+3=0$

38. The tangent to the circle $C_1 : x^2 + y^2 - 2x - 1 = 0$ at the point (2, 1) cuts off a chord of length 4 from a circle C_2 whose centre is (3, – 2). The radius of C_2 is **[Online April 15, 2018]**

(a) $\sqrt{6}$ (b) 2
(c) $\sqrt{2}$ (d) 3

TOPIC-2

39. Tangent and normal are drawn at P(16, 16) on the parabola $y^2 = 16x$, which intersect the axis of the parabola at A and B, respectively. If C is the centre of the circle through the points P, A and B and $\angle CPB = \theta$, then a value of $\tan\theta$ is : **[2018]**

(a) 2 (b) 3
(c) $\frac{4}{3}$ (d) $\frac{1}{2}$

40. Tangents drawn from the point (– 8, 0) to the parabola $y^2 = 8x$ touch the parabola at P and Q. If F is the focus of the parabola, then the area of the triangle PFQ (in sq. units) is equal to **[Online April 15, 2018]**

(a) 48 (b) 32
(c) 24 (d) 64

TOPIC-3

41. Two sets A and B are as under :

$A = \{(a, b) \in R \times R : |a - 5| < 1 \text{ and } |b - 5| < 1\}$;

$B = \{(a, b) \in R \times R : 4(a-6)^2 + 9(b-5)^2 \le 36\}$. Then : **[2018]**

(a) $A \subset B$
(b) $A \cap B = \phi$ (an empty set)
(c) neither $A \subset B$ nor $B \subset A$
(d) $B \subset A$

42. If the length of the latus rectum of an ellipse is 4 units and the distance between a focus and its nearest vertex on the major axis is $\frac{3}{2}$ units, then its eccentricity is? **[Online April 16, 2018]**

(a) $\frac{1}{2}$ (b) $\frac{2}{3}$
(c) $\frac{1}{9}$ (d) $\frac{1}{3}$

TOPIC-4

43. Tangents are drawn to the hyperbola $4x^2 - y^2 = 36$ at the points P and Q. If these tangents intersect at the point T(0, 3) then the area (in sq. units) of ΔPTQ is : **[2018]**

(a) $54\sqrt{3}$ (b) $60\sqrt{3}$
(c) $36\sqrt{5}$ (d) $45\sqrt{5}$

44. The locus of the point of intersection of the lines, $\sqrt{2}x - y + 4\sqrt{2}k = 0$ and $\sqrt{2}kx + ky - 4\sqrt{2} = 0$ (k is any non-zero real parameter) is. **[Online April 16, 2018]**

(a) A hyperbola with length of its transverse axis $8\sqrt{2}$
(b) An ellipse with length of its major axis $8\sqrt{2}$
(c) An ellipse whose eccentricity is $\frac{1}{\sqrt{3}}$
(d) A hyperbola whose eccentricity is $\sqrt{3}$

CHAPTER-12 : Limits and Derivatives

TOPIC-1

45. For each $t \in R$, let $[t]$ be the greatest integer less than or equal to t. Then **[2018]**

$$\lim_{x \to 0^+} x\left(\left[\frac{1}{x}\right] + \left[\frac{2}{x}\right] + \ldots + \left[\frac{15}{x}\right]\right)$$

(a) is equal to 15.
(b) is equal to 120.
(c) does not exist (in R).
(d) is equal to 0.

46. $\lim_{x\to 0}\frac{x\tan 2x - 2x\tan x}{(1-\cos 2x)^2}$ equals. **[Online April 15, 2018]**

(a) 1 (b) $-\frac{1}{2}$

(c) $\frac{1}{4}$ (d) $\frac{1}{2}$

TOPIC-2

47. $\lim_{x\to 0}\frac{(27+x)^{\frac{1}{3}}-3}{9-(27+x)^{\frac{2}{3}}}$ equals. **[Online April 16, 2018]**

(a) $-\frac{1}{3}$ (b) $\frac{1}{6}$

(c) $-\frac{1}{6}$ (d) $\frac{1}{3}$

TOPIC-3

48. Let $f(x)$ be a polynomial of degree 4 having extreme values at $x = 1$ and $x = 2$. If $\lim_{x\to 0}\left(\frac{f(x)}{x^2}+1\right) = 3$ then $f(-1)$ is equal to **[Online April 15, 2018]**

(a) $\frac{1}{2}$ (b) $\frac{3}{2}$

(c) $\frac{5}{2}$ (d) $\frac{9}{2}$

CHAPTER-13 : Mathematical Reasoning

TOPIC-1

49. The Boolean expression

$\sim(p\vee q)\vee(\sim p\wedge q)$ is equivalent to : **[2018]**

(a) p (b) q

(c) ~q (d) ~p

50. If $p\rightarrow(\sim p\vee\sim q)$ is false, then the truth values of p and q are respectively. **[Online April 16, 2018]**

(a) T, F (b) F, F

(c) F, T (d) T, T

51. If $(p\wedge\sim q)\wedge(p\wedge r)\rightarrow\sim p\vee q$ is false, then the truth values of p, q and r are respectively **[Online April 15, 2018]**

(a) F, T, F (b) T, F, T

(c) F, F, F (d) T, T, T

52. Consider the following two statements.

Statement *p*:

The value of sin 120° can be divided by taking $\theta = 240°$ in the equation $2\sin\frac{\theta}{2} = \sqrt{1+\sin\theta}-\sqrt{1-\sin\theta}$.

Statement *q*:

The angles A, B, C and D of any quadrilateral $ABCD$ satisfy the equation $\cos\left(\frac{1}{2}(A+C)\right)+\cos\left(\frac{1}{2}(B+D)\right)=0$

Then the truth values of p and q are respectively. **[Online April 15, 2018]**

(a) F, T (b) T, T

(c) F, F (d) T, F

CHAPTER-14 : Statistics

TOPIC-1

53. The mean of a set of 30 observations is 75. If each other observation is multiplied by a non-zero number λ and then each of them is decreased by 25, their mean remains the same. The λ is equal to **[Online April 15, 2018]**

(a) $\frac{10}{3}$ (b) $\frac{4}{3}$

(c) $\frac{1}{3}$ (d) $\frac{2}{3}$

TOPIC-2

54. If $\sum_{i=1}^{9}(x_i-5)=9$ and $\sum_{i=1}^{9}(x_i-5)^2=45$, then the standard deviation of the 9 items $x_1, x_2, ..., x_9$ is : **[2018]**

(a) 4 (b) 2

(c) 3 (d) 9

55. The mean and the standard deviation (s.d.) of five observations are 9 and 0, respectively.

If one of the observations is changed such that the mean of the new set of five observations becomes 10, then their s.d. is? **[Online April 16, 2018]**

(a) 0 (b) 4

(c) 2 (d) 1

56. If the mean of the data : 7, 8, 9, 7, 8, 7, λ, 8 is 8, then the variance of this data is **[Online April 15, 2018]**

(a) $\frac{9}{8}$ (b) 2

(c) $\frac{7}{8}$ (d) 1

CHAPTER-15 : Probability

TOPIC-1

57. Two different families A and B are blessed with equal number of children. There are 3 tickets to be distributed amongst the children of these families so that no child gets more than one ticket.

If the probability that all the tickets go to the children of the family B is $\frac{1}{12}$, then the number of children in each family is? **[Online April 16, 2018]**

(a) 4 (b) 6

(c) 3 (d) 5

58. A box $'A'$ contanis 2 white, 3 red and 2 black balls. Another box $'B'$ contains 4 white, 2 red and 3 black balls. If two balls are drawn at random, without replacement, from a randomly selected box and one ball turns out to be white while the other ball turns out to be red, then the probability that both balls are drawn from box $'B'$ is **[Online April 15, 2018]**

(a) $\frac{7}{16}$ (b) $\frac{9}{32}$

(c) $\frac{7}{8}$ (d) $\frac{9}{16}$

CHAPTER-16 : Relations and Functions

TOPIC-1

59. Let N denote the set of all natural numbers. Define two binary relations on N as $R_1 = \{(x, y) \in N \times N : 2x + y = 10\}$ and $R_2 = \{(x, y) \in N \times N : x + 2y = 10\}$. Then **[Online April 16, 2018]**

(a) Both R_1 and R_2 are transitive relations

(b) Both R_1 and R_2 are symmetric relations

(c) Range of R_2 is $\{1, 2, 3, 4\}$

(d) Range of R_1 is $\{2, 4, 8\}$

60. Consider the following two binary relations on the set $A = \{a, b, c\} : R_1 = \{(c, a) (b, b), (a, c), (c, c), (b, c), (a, a)\}$ and $R_2 = \{(a, b), (b, a), (c, c), (c, a), (a, a), (b, b), (a, c)$. Then **[Online April 15, 2018]**

(a) R_2 is symmetric but it is not transitive

(b) Both R_1 and R_2 are transitive

(c) Both R_1 and R_2 are not symmetric

(d) R_1 is not symmetric but it is transitive

TOPIC-2

61. Let $f: A \rightarrow B$ be a function defined as $f(x) = \frac{x-1}{x-2}$, where $A = R - \{2\}$ and $B = R - \{1\}$. Then f is **[Online April 15, 2018]**

(a) invertible and $f^{-1}(y) = \frac{2y+1}{y-1}$

(b) invertible and $f^{-1}(y) = \frac{3y-1}{y-1}$

(c) no invertible

(d) invertible and $f^{-1}(y) = \frac{2y-1}{y-1}$

CHAPTER-18 : Matrices

TOPIC-1

62. Let $A = \begin{bmatrix} 1 & 0 & 0 \\ 1 & 1 & 0 \\ 1 & 1 & 1 \end{bmatrix}$ and $B = A^{20}$. Then the sum of the elements of the first column of B is? **[Online April 16, 2018]**

(a) 211 (b) 210

(c) 231 (d) 251

CHAPTER-19 : Determinants

TOPIC-2

63. If $\begin{vmatrix} x-4 & 2x & 2x \\ 2x & x-4 & 2x \\ 2x & 2x & x-4 \end{vmatrix} = (A+Bx)(x-A)^2$, then the ordered pair (A, B) is equal to : **[2018]**

(a) $(-4, 3)$ (b) $(-4, 5)$

(c) $(4, 5)$ (d) $(-4, -5)$

TOPIC-3

64. Let A be a matrix such that $A \cdot \begin{bmatrix} 1 & 2 \\ 0 & 3 \end{bmatrix}$ is a scalar matrix and $|3A| = 108$. Then A^2 equals **[Online April 15, 2018]**

(a) $\begin{bmatrix} 4 & -32 \\ 0 & 36 \end{bmatrix}$ (b) $\begin{bmatrix} 4 & 0 \\ -32 & 36 \end{bmatrix}$

(c) $\begin{bmatrix} 36 & 0 \\ -32 & 4 \end{bmatrix}$ (d) $\begin{bmatrix} 36 & -32 \\ 0 & 4 \end{bmatrix}$

65. Suppose A is any 3×3 non-singular matrix and $(A-3I)(A-5I) = O$, where $I = I_3$ and $O = O_3$. If $\alpha A + \beta A^{-1} = 4I$, then $\alpha + \beta$ is equal to **[Online April 15, 2018]**

(a) 8 (b) 12

(c) 13 (d) 7

TOPIC-4

66. If the system of linear equations

$x + ky + 3z = 0$
$3x + ky - 2z = 0$
$2x + 4y - 3z = 0$

has a non-zero solution (x, y, z), then $\frac{xz}{y^2}$ is equal to : **[2018]**

(a) 10 (b) -30

(c) 30 (d) -10

67. The number of values of k for which the system of linear equations, $(k+2)x + 10y = k$, $kx + (k+3)y = k-1$ has no solution, is [Online April 16, 2018]
(a) Infinitely many (b) 3
(c) 1 (d) 2

68. Let S be the set of all real values of k for which the system of linear equations
$x + y + z = 2$
$2x + y - z = 3$
$3x + 2y + kz = 4$
has a unique solution. Then S is [Online April 15, 2018]
(a) an empty set (b) equal to $R - \{0\}$
(c) equal to $\{0\}$ (d) equal to R

69. If the system of linear equations
$x + ay + z = 3$
$x + 2y + 2z = 6$
$x + 5y + 3z = b$
has no solution, then [Online April 15, 2018]
(a) $a = 1, b \neq 9$ (b) $a \neq -1, b = 9$
(c) $a = -1, b = 9$ (d) $a = -1, b \neq 9$

CHAPTER-20 : Continuity and Differentiability

TOPIC-1

70. If the function f defined as

$$f(x) = \frac{1}{x} - \frac{k-1}{e^{2x}-1}$$

$x \neq 0$, is continuous at $x = 0$,
then the ordered pair $(k, f(0))$ is equal to? [Online April 16, 2018]
(a) (3, 1) (b) (3, 2)
(c) $\left(\frac{1}{3}, 2\right)$ (d) (2, 1)

71. Let $f(x) = \begin{cases} (x-1)^{\frac{1}{2-x}}, & x > 1, x \neq 2 \\ k, & x = 2 \end{cases}$

The value of k for which f is continuous at $x = 2$ is [Online April 15, 2018]
(a) e^{-2} (b) e
(c) e^{-1} (d) 1

TOPIC-2

72. Let S = $\{t \in R : f(x) = |x - \pi|(e^{|x|} - 1)\sin|x|$ is not differentiable at t$\}$. Then the set S is equal to : [2018]
(a) $\{0\}$ (b) $\{\pi\}$
(c) $\{0, \pi\}$ (d) ϕ (an empty set)

73. Let $S = \{(\lambda, \mu) \in R \times R : f(t) = (|\lambda|e^{|t|} - \mu) . \sin(2|t|), t \in R$, is a differentiable function$\}$. Then S is a subest of? [Online April 15, 2018]
(a) $R \times [0, \infty)$ (b) $(-\infty, 0) \times R$
(c) $[0, \infty) \times R$ (d) $R \times (-\infty, 0)$

TOPIC-3

74. If $x = \sqrt{2^{\text{cosec}^{-1} t}}$ and $y = \sqrt{2^{\sec^{-1} t}}$ $(|t| \geq 1)$, then $\frac{dy}{dx}$ is equal to. [Online April 16, 2018]
(a) $\frac{y}{x}$ (b) $-\frac{y}{x}$
(c) $-\frac{x}{y}$ (d) $\frac{x}{y}$

75. If $f(x) = \begin{vmatrix} \cos x & x & 1 \\ 2\sin x & x^2 & 2x \\ \tan x & x & 1 \end{vmatrix}$, then $\lim_{x \to 0} \frac{f'(x)}{x}$ [Online April 15, 2018]
(a) Exists and is equal to – 2
(b) Does not exist
(c) Exist and is equal to 0
(d) Exists and is equal to 2

76. If $f(x) = \sin^{-1}\left(\frac{2 \times 3^x}{1 + 9^x}\right)$, then $f'\left(-\frac{1}{2}\right)$ equals. [Online April 15, 2018]
(a) $\sqrt{3}\log_e\sqrt{3}$ (b) $-\sqrt{3}\log_e\sqrt{3}$
(c) $-\sqrt{3}\log_e 3$ (d) $\sqrt{3}\log_e 3$

TOPIC-4

77. If $x^2 + y^2 + \sin y = 4$, then the value of $\frac{d^2y}{dx^2}$ at the point $(-2, 0)$ is [Online April 15, 2018]
(a) -34 (b) -32
(c) -2 (d) 4

CHAPTER-21 : Applications of Derivatives

TOPIC-3

78. If the curves $y^2 = 6x, 9x^2 + by^2 = 16$ intersect each other at right angles, then the value of b is : [2018]
(a) $\frac{7}{2}$ (b) 4
(c) $\frac{9}{2}$ (d) 6

79. Let P be a point on the parabola, $x^2 = 4y$. If the distance of P from the centre of the circle, $x^2+y^2+6x+8=0$ is minimum, then the equation of the tangent to the parabola at P, is **[Online April 16, 2018]**

(a) $x+4y-2=0$ (b) $x+2y=0$

(c) $x+y+1=0$ (d) $x-y+3=0$

80. If the tangents drawn to the hyperbola $4y^2=x^2+1$ intersect the co-ordinate axes at the distinct points A and B, then the locus of the mid point of AB is **[Online April 15, 2018]**

(a) $x^2-4y^2+16x^2y^2=0$

(b) $4x^2-y^2+16x^2y^2=0$

(c) $4x^2-y^2-16x^2y^2=0$

(d) $x^2-4y^2-16x^2y^2=0$

81. If β is one of the angles between the normals to the ellipse, $x^2 + 3y^2 = 9$ at the points $(3\cos\theta, \sqrt{3}\sin\theta)$ and $(-3\sin\theta, \sqrt{3}\cos\theta)$; $\in\left(0,\frac{\pi}{2}\right)$; then $\frac{2\cot\beta}{\sin 2\theta}$ is equal to **[Online April 15, 2018]**

(a) $\sqrt{2}$ (b) $\frac{2}{\sqrt{3}}$

(c) $\frac{1}{\sqrt{3}}$ (d) $\frac{\sqrt{3}}{4}$

82. A normal to the hyperbola, $4x^2 - 9y^2 = 36$ meets the co-ordinate axes x and y at A and B, respectively. If the parallelogram $OABP$ (O being the origin) is formed, then the locus of P is **[Online April 15, 2018]**

(a) $4x^2-9y^2=121$ (b) $4x^2+9y^2=121$

(c) $9x^2-4y^2=169$ (d) $9x^2+4y^2=169$

TOPIC-4

83. Let $f(x)=x^2+\frac{1}{x^2}$ and $g(x)=x-\frac{1}{x}$, $x\in R-\{-1,0,1\}$.

If $h(x)=\frac{f(x)}{g(x)}$, then the local minimum value of h(x) is : **[2018]**

(a) -3 (b) $-2\sqrt{2}$

(c) $2\sqrt{2}$ (d) 3

84. Let M and m be respectively the absolute maximum and the absolute minimum values of the function, $f(x)=2x^3-9x^2+12x+5$ in the interval [0, 3]. Then $M-m$ is equal to **[Online April 16, 2018]**

(a) 1 (b) 5

(c) 4 (d) 9

85. If a right circular cone having maximum volume, is inscribed in a sphere of radius 3 cm, then the curved surface area (in cm^2) of this cone is **[Online April 15, 2018]**

(a) $8\sqrt{3}\pi$ (b) $6\sqrt{2}\pi$

(c) $6\sqrt{3}\pi$ (d) $8\sqrt{2}\pi$

CHAPTER-22 : Integrals

TOPIC-1

86. The integral

$$\int\frac{\sin^2 x\cos^2 x}{(\sin^5 x+\cos^3 x\sin^2 x+\sin^3 x\cos^2 x+\cos^5 x)^2}dx \text{ is equal to :}$$

[2018]

(a) $\frac{-1}{3(1+\tan^3 x)}+C$ (b) $\frac{1}{1+\cot^3 x}+C$

(c) $\frac{-1}{1+\cot^3 x}+C$ (d) $\frac{1}{3(1+\tan^3 x)}+C$

(where C is a constant of integration)

87. If $\int\frac{\tan x}{1+\tan x+\tan^2 x}dx = x-\frac{K}{\sqrt{A}}\tan^{-1}\left(\frac{K\tan x+1}{\sqrt{A}}\right)+C$, ($C$ is a constant of integration), then the ordered pair (K, A) is euqal to **[Online April 16, 2018]**

(a) (2, 3) (b) (2, 1)

(c) (−2, 1) (d) (−2, 3)

88. If $f\left(\frac{x-4}{x+2}\right)=2x+1$, $(x\in R=\{1,-2\})$, then $\int f(x)\,dx$ is equal to (where C is a constant of integration) **[Online April 15, 2018]**

(a) $12\log_e|1-x|-3x+c$ (b) $-12\log_e|1-x|-3x+c$

(c) $-12\log_e|1-x|+3x+c$ (d) $12\log_e|1-x|+3x+c$

89. $\int\frac{2x+5}{\sqrt{7-6x-x^2}}dx = A\sqrt{7-6x-x^2}+B\sin^{-1}\left(\frac{x+3}{4}\right)+C$ (where C is a constant of integration), then the ordered pair (A, B) is equal to **[Online April 15, 2018]**

(a) (−2, −1) (b) (2, −1)

(c) (−2, 1) (d) (2, 1)

TOPIC-3

90. The value of $\int_{-\frac{\pi}{2}}^{\frac{\pi}{2}}\frac{\sin^2 x}{1+2^x}dx$ is : **[2018]**

(a) $\frac{\pi}{2}$ (b) 4π

(c) $\frac{\pi}{4}$ (d) $\frac{\pi}{8}$

91. If $f(x)=\int_0^x t(\sin x-\sin t)\,dt$ then **[Online April 16, 2018]**

(a) $f'''(x)+f'(x)=\cos x-2x\sin x$

(b) $f'''(x)+f''(x)-f'(x)=\cos x$

(c) $f'''(x)-f''(x)=\cos x-2x\sin x$

(d) $f'''(x)+f''(x)=\sin x$

92. The value of integral $\int_{\frac{\pi}{4}}^{\frac{3\pi}{4}} \frac{x}{1+\sin x} dx$ is **[Online April 15, 2018]**

(a) $\frac{\pi}{2}(\sqrt{2}+1)$ (b) $\pi(\sqrt{2}-1)$

(c) $2\pi(\sqrt{2}-1)$ (d) $\pi\sqrt{2}$

93. If $I_1 = \int_0^1 e^{-x} \cos^2 x\, dx$; $I_2 = \int_0^1 e^{-x^2} \cos^2 x\, dx$ and $I_3 = \int_0^1 e^{-x^3} dx$; then **[Online April 15, 2018]**

(a) $I_2 > I_3 > I_1$ (b) $I_3 > I_1 > I_2$

(c) $I_2 > I_1 > I_3$ (d) $I_3 > I_2 > I_1$

TOPIC-4

94. The value of the integral $\int_{-\frac{\pi}{2}}^{\frac{\pi}{2}} \sin^4 x \left(1+\log\left(\frac{2+\sin x}{2-\sin x}\right)\right) dx$ is **[Online April 15, 2018]**

(a) $\frac{3}{16}\pi$ (b) 0

(c) $\frac{3}{8}\pi$ (d) $\frac{3}{4}$

CHAPTER-23 : Applications of Integrals

TOPIC-1

95. Let $g(x) = \cos x^2, f(x) = \sqrt{x}$, and $\alpha, \beta\ (\alpha < \beta)$ be the roots of the quadratic equation $18x^2 - 9\pi x + \pi^2 = 0$. Then the area (in sq. units) bounded by the curve $y = (gof)(x)$ and the lines $x = \alpha, x = \beta$ and $y = 0$, is : **[2018]**

(a) $\frac{1}{2}(\sqrt{3}+1)$ (b) $\frac{1}{2}(\sqrt{3}-\sqrt{2})$

(c) $\frac{1}{2}(\sqrt{2}-1)$ (d) $\frac{1}{2}(\sqrt{3}-1)$

TOPIC-2

96. If the area of the region bounded by the curves, $y = x^2$, $y = \frac{1}{x}$ and the lines $y = 0$ and $x = t\ (t > 1)$ is 1 sq. unit, then t is equal to **[Online April 16, 2018]**

(a) $\frac{4}{3}$ (b) $e^{2/3}$

(c) $\frac{3}{2}$ (d) $e^{3/2}$

97. The area (in sq. units) of the region

$\{x \in R : x \geq 0, y \geq 0, y \geq x-2 \text{ and } y \leq \sqrt{x}\}$, is

[Online April 15, 2018]

(a) $\frac{13}{3}$ (b) $\frac{10}{3}$

(c) $\frac{5}{3}$ (d) $\frac{8}{3}$

CHAPTER-24 : Differential Equations

TOPIC-1

98. The differential equation representing the family of ellipse having foci either on the x-axis or on the y-axis centre at the origin and passing through the point (0, 3) is: **[Online April 16, 2018]**

(a) $xyy' + y^2 - 9 = 0$ (b) $x + yy'' = 0$

(c) $xyy'' + x(y')^2 - yy' = 0$ (d) $xyy' - y^2 + 9 = 0$

TOPIC-2

99. Let $y - y(x)$ be the solution of the differential equation $\sin x \frac{dy}{dx} + y\cos x = 4x, x \in (0, \pi)$. If $y\left(\frac{\pi}{2}\right) = 0$, then $y\left(\frac{\pi}{6}\right)$ is equal to : **[2018]**

(a) $\frac{-8}{9\sqrt{3}}\pi^2$ (b) $-\frac{8}{9}\pi^2$

(c) $-\frac{4}{9}\pi^2$ (d) $\frac{4}{9\sqrt{3}}\pi^2$

100. Let $y = y(x)$ be the solution of the differential equation $\frac{dy}{dx} + 2y = f(x)$, where $f(x) = \begin{cases} 1, & x \in [0,1] \\ 0, & otherwise \end{cases}$

If $y(0) = 0$, then $y\left(\frac{3}{2}\right)$ is **[Online April 15, 2018]**

(a) $\frac{e^2-1}{2e^3}$ (b) $\frac{e^2-1}{e^3}$

(c) $\frac{1}{2e}$ (d) $\frac{e^2+1}{2e^4}$

101. The curve satisfying the differential equation, $(x^2 - y^2)\, dx + 2xydy = 0$ and passing through the point (1, 1) is **[Online April 15, 2018]**

(a) a circle of radius two (b) a circle of radius one

(c) a hyprbola (d) an ellipse

CHAPTER-25 : Vector Algebra

TOPIC-1

102. If the position vectors of the vertices A, B and C of a ΔABC are respectively $4\hat{i}+7\hat{j}+8\hat{k}$, $2\hat{i}+3\hat{j}+4\hat{k}$ and $2\hat{i}+5\hat{j}+7\hat{k}$, then the position vector of the point, where the bisector of $\angle A$ meets BC is **[Online April 15, 2018]**

(a) $\frac{1}{2}(4\hat{i}+8\hat{j}+11\hat{k})$ (b) $\frac{1}{3}(6\hat{i}+13\hat{j}+18\hat{k})$

(c) $\frac{1}{4}(8\hat{i}+14\hat{j}+9\hat{k})$ (d) $\frac{1}{3}(6\hat{i}+11\hat{j}+15\hat{k})$

TOPIC-2

103. Let $\vec{u}$ be a vector coplanar with the vectors $\vec{a}=2\hat{i}+3\hat{j}-\hat{k}$ and $\vec{b}=\hat{j}+\hat{k}$. If $\vec{u}$ is perpendicular to $\vec{a}$ and $\vec{u}\cdot\vec{b}-24$, then $|\vec{u}|^2$ is equal to: **[2018]**

(a) 315 (b) 256
(c) 84 (d) 336

TOPIC-3

104. Let $\vec{a}=\hat{i}+\hat{j}+\hat{k}, \vec{c}=\hat{j}-\hat{k}$ and a vector $\vec{b}$ be such that $\vec{a}\times\vec{b}=\vec{c}$ and $\vec{a}\cdot\vec{b}=3$. Then $|\vec{b}|$ equals? **[Online April 16, 2018]**

(a) $\sqrt{\frac{11}{3}}$ (b) $\frac{\sqrt{11}}{3}$

(c) $\frac{11}{\sqrt{3}}$ (d) $\frac{11}{3}$

105. If $\vec{a}, \vec{b}$, and $\vec{c}$ are unit vectors such that $\vec{a}+2\vec{b}+2\vec{c}=\vec{0}$, then $|\vec{a}\times\vec{c}|$ is equal to **[Online April 15, 2018]**

(a) $\frac{1}{4}$ (b) $\frac{\sqrt{15}}{4}$

(c) $\frac{15}{16}$ (d) $\frac{\sqrt{15}}{16}$

CHAPTER-26 : Three Dimensional Geometry

TOPIC-1

106. An angle between the lines whose direction cosines are given by the equations, $l+3m+5n=0$ and $5lm-2mn+6nl=0$, is **[Online April 15, 2018]**

(a) $\cos^{-1}\left(\frac{1}{8}\right)$ (b) $\cos^{-1}\left(\frac{1}{6}\right)$

(c) $\cos^{-1}\left(\frac{1}{3}\right)$ (d) $\cos^{-1}\left(\frac{1}{4}\right)$

TOPIC-2

107. If the angle between the lines, $\frac{x}{2}=\frac{y}{2}=\frac{z}{1}$ and $\frac{5-x}{-2}=\frac{7y-14}{P}=\frac{z-3}{4}$ is $\cos^{-1}\left(\frac{2}{3}\right)$, then P is equal to **[Online April 16, 2018]**

(a) $-\frac{7}{4}$ (b) $\frac{2}{7}$

(c) $-\frac{4}{7}$ (d) $\frac{7}{2}$

TOPIC-3

108. The length of the projection of the line segment joining the points (5, –1, 4) and (4, –1, 3) on the plane, $x+y+z=7$ is: **[2018]**

(a) $\frac{2}{3}$ (b) $\frac{1}{3}$

(c) $\sqrt{\frac{2}{3}}$ (d) $\frac{2}{\sqrt{3}}$

109. If L_1 is the line of intersection of the planes $2x-2y+3z-2=0$, $x-y+z+1=0$ and L_2 is the line of intersection of the planes $x+2y-z-3=0$, $3x-y+2z-1=0$, then the distance of the origin from the plane, containing the lines L_1 and L_2, is: **[2018]**

(a) $\frac{1}{3\sqrt{2}}$ (b) $\frac{1}{2\sqrt{2}}$

(c) $\frac{1}{\sqrt{2}}$ (d) $\frac{1}{4\sqrt{2}}$

110. The sum of the intercepts on the coordinate axes of the plane passing through the point (– 2, – 2, 2) and containing the line joining the points (1, – 1, 2) and (1, 1, 1) is **[Online April 16, 2018]**

(a) 12 (b) – 8
(c) – 4 (d) 4

111. A variable plane passes through a fixed point (3, 2, 1) and meets x, y and z axes at A, B and C respectively. A plane is drawn parallel to yz – *plane* through A, a second plane is drawn parallel zx – *plane* through B and a third plane is drawn parallel to xy – *plane* through C. Then the locus of the point of intersection of these three planes, is **[Online April 15, 2018]**

(a) $x+y+z=6$ (b) $\frac{x}{3}+\frac{y}{2}+\frac{z}{1}=1$

(c) $\frac{3}{x}+\frac{2}{y}+\frac{1}{z}=1$ (d) $\frac{1}{x}+\frac{1}{y}+\frac{1}{z}=\frac{11}{6}$

112 An angle between the plane, $x + y + z = 5$ and the line of intersection of the planes, $3x + 4y + z - 1 = 0$ and $5x + 8y + 2z + 14 = 0$, is **[Online April 15, 2018]**

(a) $\cos^{-1}\left(\frac{3}{\sqrt{17}}\right)$ (b) $\cos^{-1}\left(\sqrt{\frac{3}{17}}\right)$

(c) $\sin^{-1}\left(\frac{3}{\sqrt{17}}\right)$ (d) $\sin^{-1}\left(\sqrt{\frac{3}{17}}\right)$

113. A plane bisects the line segment joining the points (1, 2, 3) and (– 3, 4, 5) at right angles. Then this plane also passes through the point. **[Online April 15, 2018]**

(a) $(-3, 2, 1)$ (b) $(3, 2, 1)$

(c) $(1, 2, -3)$ (d) $(-1, 2, 3)$

CHAPTER-27 : Probability

TOPIC-1

114. A bag contains 4 red and 6 black balls. A ball is drawn at random from the bag, its colour is observed and this ball along with two additional balls of the same colour are returned to the bag. If now a ball is drawn at random from the bag, then the probability that this drawn ball is red, is : **[2018]**

(a) $\frac{2}{5}$ (b) $\frac{1}{5}$

(c) $\frac{3}{4}$ (d) $\frac{3}{10}$

115. Let A, B and C be three events, which are pair-wise independence and $\overline{E}$ denotes the complement of an event E. If $P(A \cap B \cap C) = 0$ and $P(C) > 0$, then $P[(\overline{A} \cap \overline{B})|C]$ is equal to. **[Online April 16, 2018]**

(a) $P(A) + P(\overline{B})$ (b) $P(\overline{A}) - P(\overline{B})$

(c) $P(\overline{A}) - P(B)$ (d) $P(\overline{A}) + P(\overline{B})$

116. A player X has a biased coin whose probability of showing heads is p and a player Y has a fair coin. They start playing a game with their own coins and play alternately. The player who throws a head first is a winner. If X starts the game, and the probability of winning the game by both the players is equal, then the value of 'p' is **[Online April 15, 2018]**

(a) $\frac{1}{3}$ (b) $\frac{1}{5}$

(c) $\frac{1}{4}$ (d) $\frac{2}{5}$

CHAPTER-28 : Properties of Triangles

TOPIC-2

117. PQR is a triangular park with PQ = PR = 200 m. A T.V. tower stands at the mid-point of QR. If the angles of elevation of the top of the tower at P, Q and R are respectively 45°, 30° and 30°, then the height of the tower (in m) is : **[2018]**

(a) 50 (b) $100\sqrt{3}$

(c) $50\sqrt{2}$ (d) 100

118. A man on the top of a vertical tower observes a car moving at a uniform speed towards the tower on a horizontal road. If it takes 18 min, for the angle of depression of the car to change from 30° to 45°, then after this, the time taken (in min) by the car to reach the foot of the tower, is. **[Online April 16, 2018]**

(a) $9(1 + \sqrt{3})$ (b) $\frac{9}{2}(\sqrt{3} - 1)$

(c) $18(1 + \sqrt{3})$ (d) $18(\sqrt{3} - 1)$

119. An aeroplane flying at a constant speed, parallel to the horizontal ground, $\sqrt{3}km$ above it, is observed at an elevation of 60° from a point on the ground. If, after five seconds, its elevation from the same point, is 30°, then the speed (in km/hr) of the aeroplane is **[Online April 15, 2018]**

(a) 1500 (b) 750

(c) 720 (d) 1440

120. A tower T_1 of height 60 m is located exactly opposite to a tower T_2 of height 80 m on a straight road. From the top of T_1, if the angle of depression of the foot of T_2 is twice the angle of elevation of the top of T_2, then the width (in m) of the road between the feet of the towers T_1 and T_2 is **[Online April 15, 2018]**

(a) $20\sqrt{2}$ (b) $10\sqrt{2}$

(c) $10\sqrt{3}$ (d) $20\sqrt{3}$

Hints and Solutions

1. **(b)** **Case-I:** $x \in [0,9]$

$$2(3-\sqrt{x})+x-6\sqrt{x}+6=0$$

$$\Rightarrow x-8\sqrt{x}+12=0 \Rightarrow \sqrt{x}=4,2$$

$$\Rightarrow x=16,4$$

Since $x \in [0,9]$

$\therefore$ $x=4$

Case-II: $x \in [9,\infty]$

$$2(\sqrt{x}-3)+x-6\sqrt{x}+6=0$$

$$\Rightarrow x-4\sqrt{x}=0 \Rightarrow x=16,0$$

Since $x \in [9,\infty]$

$\therefore x=16$

Hence, $x=4$ & 16

2. **(a)** $\because$ $8\cos x\left(\cos^2\frac{\pi}{6}-\sin^2 x-\frac{1}{2}\right)=1$

$$\Rightarrow \quad 8\cos x\left(\frac{3}{4}-\frac{1}{2}-\sin^2 x\right)=1$$

$$\Rightarrow \quad 8\cos x\left(\frac{1}{4}-(1-\cos^2 x)\right)=1$$

$$\Rightarrow \quad 8\cos x\left(\frac{1}{4}-1+\cos^2 x\right)=1$$

$$\Rightarrow \quad 8\cos x\left(\cos^2 x-\frac{3}{4}\right)=1$$

$$\Rightarrow \quad 8\left(\frac{4\cos^3 x-3\cos x}{4}\right)=1$$

$$\Rightarrow \quad 2(4\cos^3 x-3\cos x)=1$$

$$\Rightarrow \quad 2\cos 3x=1 \Rightarrow \cos 3x=\frac{1}{2}$$

$$\therefore \quad 3x=2n\pi\pm\frac{\pi}{3}, n\in I$$

$$\Rightarrow \quad x=\frac{2n\pi}{3}\pm\frac{\pi}{9}$$

In $x\in[0,\pi]: x=\frac{\pi}{9},\frac{2\pi}{3}+\frac{\pi}{9},\frac{2\pi}{3}-\frac{\pi}{9}$, only

Sum of all the solutions of the equation

$$=\left(\frac{1}{9}+\frac{2}{3}+\frac{1}{9}+\frac{2}{3}-\frac{1}{9}\right)\pi=\frac{13}{9}\pi$$

3. **(d)** $\sin 3x=\cos 2x$

$$\Rightarrow 3\sin x-4\sin^3 x=1-2\sin^2 x$$

$$\Rightarrow 4\sin^3 x-2\sin^2 x-3\sin x+1=0$$

$$\Rightarrow \sin x=1, \frac{-2\pm 2\sqrt{5}}{8}$$

In the interval $\left(\frac{\pi}{2},\pi\right)$, $\sin x=\frac{-2+2\sqrt{5}}{8}$

So, there is only one solution.

4. **(a)** $\because |z|=1$ & $Re\, z\neq 1$

Suppose $z=x+iy \Rightarrow x^2+y^2=1$ .....(i)

Now, $w=\dfrac{1+(1-8\alpha)z}{1-z}$

$$\Rightarrow w=\frac{1+(1-8\alpha)(x+iy)}{1-(x+iy)}$$

$$\Rightarrow w=\frac{1+(1-8\alpha)(x+iy))((1-x)+iy)}{1-(x+iy))((1-x)+iy)}$$

$$\Rightarrow \quad w=\frac{[(1+x(1-8\alpha)(1-x)-(1-8\alpha)y^2]}{(1-x)^2+y^2}$$

$$+i\frac{[(1+x(1-8\alpha))y-(1-8\alpha)y(1-x)]}{(1-x)^2+y^2}$$

As, w is purely imaginary. So,

$$Re\, w=\frac{[(1+x(1-8\alpha))(1-x)-(1-8\alpha)y^2]}{(1-x)^2+y^2}=0$$

$$\Rightarrow (1-x)+x(1-8\alpha)(1-x)=(1-8\alpha)y^2$$

$$\Rightarrow (1-x)+x(1-8\alpha)-x^2(1-8\alpha)=(1-8x)y^2$$

$$\Rightarrow (1-x)+x(1-8\alpha)=1-8\alpha \text{ [From (i), } x^2+y^2=1]$$

$$\Rightarrow 1-8\alpha=1$$

$$\Rightarrow \alpha=0$$

$$\therefore \alpha\in\{0\}$$

5. **(d)** If a and -1 are the roots of the polynomial, then we get

$$f(x)=x^2+(1-a)x-a.$$

$\therefore$ $f(1)=2-2a$

and $f(2)=6-3a$

As, $f(1)+f(2)=0 \Rightarrow 2-2a+6-3a=0 \Rightarrow a=\frac{8}{5}$

Therefore, the other root is $\frac{8}{5}$

6. (d) Let $l = \left(\frac{1+i\sqrt{3}}{1-i\sqrt{3}}\right)$.

$\therefore l = \left(\frac{1+i\sqrt{3}}{1-i\sqrt{3}}\right) \times \left(\frac{1+i\sqrt{3}}{1+i\sqrt{3}}\right) = \left(\frac{-2+i2\sqrt{3}}{4}\right) = \left(\frac{1-i\sqrt{3}}{-2}\right)$

Also,

$l = \left(\frac{1+i\sqrt{3}}{1-i\sqrt{3}}\right) \times \left(\frac{1-i\sqrt{3}}{1-i\sqrt{3}}\right) = \left(\frac{4}{-2-i2\sqrt{3}}\right) = \left(\frac{-2}{1+i\sqrt{3}}\right)$

Now, $\left(\frac{1+i\sqrt{3}}{1-i\sqrt{3}}\right)^3 = \left(\frac{1+i\sqrt{3}}{1-i\sqrt{3}}\right) \times \left(\frac{1+i\sqrt{3}}{1-i\sqrt{3}}\right) \times \left(\frac{1+i\sqrt{3}}{1-i\sqrt{3}}\right)$

$= \left(\frac{1+i\sqrt{3}}{1-i\sqrt{3}}\right) \times \left(\frac{-2}{1+i\sqrt{3}}\right) \times \left(\frac{1-i\sqrt{3}}{-2}\right) = 1$

$\therefore$ least positive integer n is 3.

7. (b) $|z-(3-2i)| \le 4$ represents a circle whose centre is $(3,-2)$ and radius $= 4$.
$|z| = |z-0|$ represents the distance of point 'z' from origin $(0, 0)$

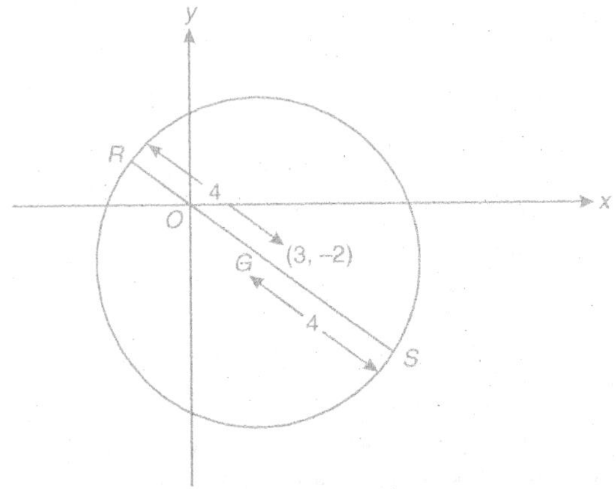

Suppose RS is the normal of the circle passing through origin 'O' and G is its center $(3,-2)$.
Here, OR is the least distance
and OS is the greatest distance
$OR = RG - OG$ and $OS = OG + GS$ ...(1)
As, $RG = GS = 4$

$OG = \sqrt{3^2+(-2)^2} = \sqrt{9+4} = \sqrt{13}$

From (1), $OR = 4-\sqrt{13}$ and $OS = 4+\sqrt{13}$

So, required difference $= \left(4+\sqrt{13}\right) - \left(4-\sqrt{13}\right)$

$= \sqrt{13}+\sqrt{13} = 2\sqrt{13}$

8. (b) α, β are roots of $x^2 - x + 1 = 0$

$\therefore \quad \alpha = -\omega$ and $\beta = -\omega^2$

where ω is cube root of unity

$\therefore \quad \alpha^{101} + \beta^{107} = (-\omega)^{101} + (-\omega)^{107}$
$= -[\omega^2 + \omega] = -[-1] = 1$

9. (b) $\frac{1}{x+p} + \frac{1}{x+q} = \frac{1}{r}$

$\frac{x+p+x+q}{(x+p)(x+q)} = \frac{1}{r}$

$(2x+p+q)r = x^2 + px + qx + pq$
$x^2 + (p+q-2r)x + pq - pr - qr = 0$
Let α and β be the roots.
$\therefore \alpha + \beta = -(p+q-2r)$ .... (i)
& $\alpha\beta = pq - pr - qr$ .... (ii)
$\because \alpha = -\beta$ (given)
$\therefore$ in eq. (1), we get
$\Rightarrow \quad -(p+q-2r) = 0$ ... (iii)
Now, $\alpha^2 + \beta^2 = (\alpha+\beta)^2 - 2\alpha\beta$
$= (-(p+q-2r))^2 - 2(pq - pr - qr)$ .... (from (i) and (ii))
$= p^2 + q^2 + 4r^2 + 2pq - 4pr - 4qr - 2pq + 2pr + 2qr$
$= p^2 + q^2 + 4r^2 - 2pr - 2qr$
$= p^2 + q^2 + 2r(2r - p - q)$ ... (from (iii))
$= p^2 + q^2 + 0$
$= p^2 + q^2$

10. (b) Here, $9x^2 + 27x + 20 = 0$

$\therefore x = \frac{-b \pm \sqrt{b^2 - 4ac}}{2a}$

$\Rightarrow x = \frac{-27 \pm \sqrt{27^2 - 4 \times 9 \times 20}}{2 \times 9}$

$\Rightarrow x = -\frac{4}{3}, -\frac{5}{3}$

Given, $\cos A = -\frac{3}{5}$

$\therefore \sec A = \frac{1}{\cos A} = -\frac{5}{3}$

Here, A is an obtuse angle.

$\therefore \tan A = -\sqrt{\sec^2 A - 1} = -\frac{4}{3}$.

Hence, roots of the equation are $\sec A$ and $\tan A$.

11. (b) Let, the roots of the equation, $x^2 + (2-\lambda)x + (10-\lambda) = 0$ are α and β.
Also roots of the given equation are

$\frac{\lambda - 2 \pm \sqrt{4 - 4\lambda + \lambda^2 - 40 + 4\lambda}}{2} = \frac{\lambda - 2 \pm \sqrt{\lambda^2 - 36}}{2}$

The magnitude of the difference of the roots is $\left|\sqrt{\lambda^2 - 36}\right|$

So, $\alpha^3+\beta^3=\frac{(\lambda-2)^3}{4}+\frac{3(\lambda-2)(\lambda^2-36)}{4}$

$=\frac{(\lambda-2)(4\lambda^2-4\lambda-104)}{4}=(\lambda-2)(\lambda^2-\lambda-26)=f(\lambda)$

As $f(\lambda)$ attains its minimum value at $\lambda=4$.

Therefore, the magintude of the difference of the roots is

$|i\sqrt{20}|=2\sqrt{5}$

12. (b) As tan A and tan B are the roots of $3x^2-10x-25=0$,

So, $\tan(A+B)=\frac{\tan A+\tan B}{1-\tan A\tan B}=\frac{\frac{10}{3}}{1+\frac{25}{3}}=\frac{10/3}{28/3}=\frac{5}{14}$

Now, $\cos 2(A+B)=-1+2\cos^2(A+B)$

$=\frac{1-\tan^2(A+B)}{1+\tan^2(A+B)}\Rightarrow\cos^2(A+B)=\frac{196}{221}$

$\therefore 3\sin^2(A+B)-10\sin(A+B)\cos(A+B)-25\cos^2(A+B)$
$=\cos^2(A+B)[3\tan^2(A+B)-10\tan(A+B)-25]$

$=\frac{75-700-4900}{196}\times\frac{196}{221}=-\frac{5525}{196}\times\frac{196}{221}=-25$

13. (a) The thousands place can only be filled with 2, 3 or 4, since the number is greater than 2000.
For the remaining 3 places, we have pick out digits such that the resultant number is divisible by 3.
It the sum of digits of the number is divisible by 3, then the number itself is divisible by 3.

Case 1: If we take 2 at thousands place.

The remaining digits can be filled as:

0, 1 and 3 as $2+1+0+3=6$ is divisible by 3.

0, 3 and 4 as $2+3+0+4=9$ is divisible by 3.

In both the above combinations the remaining three digits can be arranged in 3! ways.

$\therefore$ Total number of numbers in this case $=2\times 3!=12$.

Case 2: If we take 3 at thousands place. The remaining digits can be filled as:

0, 1 and 2 as $3+1+0+2=6$ is divisible by 3.

0, 2 and 4 as $3+2+0+4=9$ is divisible by 3.

In both the above combinations, the remaining three digits can be arranged in 3! ways. Total number of numbers in this case $=2\times 3!=12$.

Case 3: If we take 4 at thousands place.

The remaining digits can be filled as:

0, 2 and 3 as $4+2+0+3=9$ is divisible by 3.

In the above combination, the remaining three digits can be arranged in 3! ways.

$\therefore$ Total number of numbers in this case $=3!=6$.

$\therefore$ Total number of numbers between 2000 and 5000 divisible by 3 are $12+12+6=30$.

14. (d) Required n digit numbers is 3^n as each place can be filled by 2, 5, 7.
So smallest value of n such that $3^n>900$. Therefore $n=7$.

15. (d) $\therefore$ Required number of ways $={}^6C_4\times{}^3C_1\times 4!$
$=15\times 3\times 24=1080$

16. (d) If all four letters are different then the number of words ${}^5C_4\times 4!=120$
If two letters are R and other two different letters are chosen from B, A, C, K then the number of words
$={}^4C_2\times\frac{4!}{2!}=72$
If two letters are A and other two different letters are chosen from B, R, C, K then the number of words
$={}^4C_2\times\frac{4!}{2!}=72$
If word is formed using two R's and two A's then the number of words $=\frac{4!}{2!2!}=6$
Therefore, the number of four-letter words that can be formed $=120+72+72+6=270$

17. (c) Since we know that,
$(x+a)^5+(x-a)^5$
$=2[{}^5C_0x^5+{}^5C_2x^3\cdot a^2+{}^5C_4x\cdot a^4]$
$\therefore\quad\left(x+\sqrt{x^3-1}\right)^5+\left(x-\sqrt{x^3-1}\right)^5$
$=2[{}^5C_0x^5+{}^5C_2x^3(x^3-1)+{}^5C_4x(x^3-1)^2]$
$\Rightarrow\quad 2[x^5+10x^6-10x^3+5x^7-10x^4+5x]$
$\therefore$ Sum of coefficients of odd degree terms $=2$.

18. (a) Let $a=((1+2x+3x^2)^6+(1-4x^2)^6)$
$\therefore$ Coefficient of x^2 in the expansion of the product $(2-x^2)((1+2x+3x^2)^6+(1-4x^2)^6)$
$=2$ (Coefficient of x^2 in a) -1 (Constant of expansion)
In the expansion of $((1+2x+3x^2)^6+(1-4x^2)^6)$.
Constant $=1+1=2$
Coefficient of $x^2=$ [Coefficient of x^2 in $({}^6C_0(1+2x)^6(3x^2)^0)$] + [Cofficient of x^2 in $({}^6C_1(1+2x)^5(3x^2)^1)$]
$-[{}^6C_1(4x^2)]$
$=60+6\times 3-24=54$
$\therefore$ The coefficient of x^2 in $(2-x^2)((1+2x+3x^2)^6+(1-4x^2)^6)$
$=2\times 54-1(2)=108-2=106$

19. (d) $\left[\frac{1}{\sqrt{5x^3+1}-\sqrt{5x^3-1}}\right]^8+\left[\frac{1}{\sqrt{5x^3+1}+\sqrt{5x^3-1}}\right]^8$

After rationalise the polynomial we get

$$\left[\frac{1}{\sqrt{5x^3+1}-\sqrt{5x^3-1}}\times\frac{\sqrt{5x^3+1}+\sqrt{5x^3-1}}{\sqrt{5x^3+1}+\sqrt{5x^3-1}}\right]^8$$

$$+\left[\frac{1}{\sqrt{5x^3+1}+\sqrt{5x^3-1}}\times\frac{\sqrt{5x^3+1}-\sqrt{5x^3-1}}{\sqrt{5x^3+1}-\sqrt{5x^3-1}}\right]^8$$

$$=\left[\frac{\sqrt{5x^3+1}+\sqrt{5x^3-1}}{(5x^3+1)-(5x^3-1)}\right]^8+\left[\frac{\sqrt{5x^3+1}-\sqrt{5x^3-1}}{(5x^3+1)-(5x^3-1)}\right]^8$$

$$=\frac{1}{2^8}\left[\left(\sqrt{5x^3+1}+\sqrt{5x^3-1}\right)^8+\left(\sqrt{5x^3+1}-\sqrt{5x^3-1}\right)^8\right]$$

$$=\frac{1}{2^8}\left[\begin{array}{l}{}^8C_0\left(\sqrt{5x^3+1}\right)^8+{}^8C_2\left(\sqrt{5x^3+1}\right)^6\left(\sqrt{5x^3-1}\right)^2\\+{}^8C_4\left(\sqrt{5x^3+1}\right)^4\left(\sqrt{5x^3-1}\right)^4\\+{}^8C_6\left(\sqrt{5x^3+1}\right)^2\left(\sqrt{5x^3-1}\right)^6+{}^8C_8\left(\sqrt{5x^3-1}\right)^8\end{array}\right]$$

$$=\frac{1}{2^8}\left[\begin{array}{l}{}^8C_0(5x^3+1)^4+{}^8C_2(5x^3+1)^3(5x^3-1)+8_{C_4}\\(5x^3+1)^2(5x^3-1)^2\\+{}^8C_6(5x^3+1)(5x^3-1)^3+8_{C_8}(5x^3-1)^4\end{array}\right]$$

So, the degree of polynomial is 12,

Now, coefficient of $x^{12}=[{}^8C_05^4+{}^8C_25^4+{}^8C_45^4+{}^8C_65^4+{}^8C_85^4]$

$$=5^4\times\frac{2^8}{2}=5^4\times2^4\times\frac{2^4}{2}$$

$$=10^4\times2^3=8(10)^4$$

20. (a) $\because(1+x)^2=1+2x+x^2$,

$(1+x^2)^3=1+3x^2+3x^4+x^6$,

and $(1+x^3)^4=1+4x^3+6x^6+4x^9+x^{12}$

So, the possible combinations for x^{10} are:

$x\,.\,x^9, x\,.\,x^6\,.\,x^3, x^2\,.\,x^2\,.\,x^6, x^4\,.\,x^6$

Corresponding coefficients are 2×4, $2\times1\times4$, $1\times3\times6$, 3×6 or 8, 8, 18, 18.

$\therefore$ Sum of the coefficient is $8+8+18+18=52$

Therefore, the coefficient of x^{10} in the expansion of $(1+x)^2(1+x^2)^3(1+x^3)^4$ is 52.

21. (b) $\because\sum_{k=0}^{12}a_{4k+1}=416\Rightarrow\frac{13}{2}[2a_1+48d]=416$

$\Rightarrow a_1+24d=32$ ...(1)

Now, $a_9+a_{43}=66\Rightarrow2a_1+50d=66$ ...(2)

From eq. (1) & (2) we get; $d=1$ and $a_1=8$

Also, $\sum_{r=1}^{17}a_r^2=\sum_{r=1}^{17}[8+(r-1)1]^2=140\text{ m}$

$$\Rightarrow\sum_{r=1}^{17}(r+7)^2=140\text{ m}$$

$$\Rightarrow\sum_{r=1}^{17}(r^2+14r+49)=140\text{ m}$$

$$\Rightarrow\left(\frac{17\times18\times35}{6}\right)+14\left(\frac{17\times18}{2}\right)+(49\times17)=140$$

$$\Rightarrow m=34$$

22. (c) $\because\frac{1}{x_1},\frac{1}{x_2},\frac{1}{x_3},.....,\frac{1}{x_n}$ are in A.P

$x_1=4$ and $x_{21}=20$

Let 'd' be the common difference of this A.P

$\therefore$ its 21st term $=\frac{1}{x_{21}}=\frac{1}{x_1}+[(21-1)\times d]$

$$\Rightarrow d=\frac{1}{20}\times\left(\frac{1}{20}-\frac{1}{4}\right)\quad\Rightarrow d=-\frac{1}{100}$$

Also $x_n>50$ (given).

$$\therefore\frac{1}{x_n}=\frac{1}{x_1}+[(n-1)\times d]$$

$$\Rightarrow x_n=\frac{x_1}{1+(n-1)\times d\times x_1}$$

$$\therefore\frac{x_1}{1+(n-1)\times d\times x_1}>50$$

$$\Rightarrow\frac{4}{1+(n-1)\times\left(-\frac{1}{100}\right)\times4}>50$$

$$\Rightarrow1+(n-1)\times\left(-\frac{1}{100}\right)\times4<\frac{4}{50}$$

$$\Rightarrow-\frac{1}{100}(n-1)<-\frac{23}{100}$$

$$\Rightarrow n-1>23\quad\Rightarrow n>24$$

Therefore, $n=25$.

$$\Rightarrow\sum_{i=1}^{25}\frac{1}{x_i}=\frac{25}{2}\left[\left(2\times\frac{1}{4}\right)+(25-1)\times\left(-\frac{1}{100}\right)\right]=\frac{13}{4}$$

23. (a) Suppose d_1 is the common difference of the A.P. $x_1, x_2, ... x_n$ then

$$\because x_8 - x_3 = 5d_1 = 12 \Rightarrow d_1 = \frac{12}{5} = 2.4$$

$$\Rightarrow x_5 = x_3 + 2d_1 = 8 + 2 \times \frac{12}{5} = 12.8$$

Suppose d_2 is the common difference of the A.P $\frac{1}{h_1}, \frac{1}{h_2}, ... \frac{1}{h_n}$ then

$$5d_2 = \frac{1}{20} - \frac{1}{8} = \frac{-3}{40} \Rightarrow d_2 = \frac{-3}{200}$$

$$\because \frac{1}{h_{10}} = \frac{1}{h_7} + 3d_2 = \frac{1}{200} \Rightarrow h_{10} = 200$$

$$\Rightarrow x_5 . h_{10} = 12.8 \times 200 = 2560$$

24. (c) First term $= b$ and common ratio $= r$

For infinite series, Sum $= \frac{b}{1-r} = 5$

$\Rightarrow b = 5(1 - r)$

So, interval of $b = (0, 10)$ as, $-1 < r < 1$ for infinite G.P.

25. (b) $A_n = \left(\frac{3}{4}\right) - \left(\frac{3}{4}\right)^2 + \left(\frac{3}{4}\right)^3 - ... + (-1)^{n-1}\left(\frac{3}{4}\right)^n$

Which is a G.P. with $a = \frac{3}{4}, r = \frac{-3}{4}$ and number of terms $= n$

$$\therefore A_n = \frac{\frac{3}{4} \times \left(1 - \left(\frac{-3}{4}\right)^n\right)}{1 - \left(\frac{-3}{4}\right)} = \frac{\frac{3}{4} \times \left(1 - \left(\frac{-3}{4}\right)^n\right)}{\frac{7}{4}}$$

$$\Rightarrow A_n = \frac{3}{7}\left[1 - \left(\frac{-3}{4}\right)^n\right] \quad (1)$$

As, $B_n = 1 - A_n$

For least odd natural number p, such that $B_n > A_n$

$$\Rightarrow 1 - A_n > A_n \quad \Rightarrow 1 > 2 \times A_n \quad \Rightarrow A_n < \frac{1}{2}$$

From eqn. (1), we get

$$\frac{3}{7} \times \left[1 - \left(\frac{-3}{4}\right)^n\right] < \frac{1}{2} \quad \Rightarrow 1 - \left(\frac{-3}{4}\right)^n < \frac{7}{6}$$

$$\Rightarrow 1 - \frac{7}{6} < \left(\frac{-3}{4}\right)^n \quad \Rightarrow \frac{-1}{6} < \left(\frac{-3}{4}\right)^n$$

As n is odd, then $\left(\frac{-3}{4}\right)^n = -\frac{3^n}{4}$

So $\frac{-1}{6} < -\left(\frac{3}{4}\right)^n \quad \Rightarrow \frac{1}{6} > \left(\frac{3}{4}\right)^n$

$$\log\left(\frac{1}{6}\right) = n \log\left(\frac{3}{4}\right) \quad \Rightarrow 6.228 < n$$

Hence, n should be 7.

26. (d) $\because a, b, c$ are in A.P. then

$a + c = 2b$

also it is given that,

$$a + b + c = \frac{3}{4} \quad ...(1)$$

$$\Rightarrow 2b + b = \frac{3}{4} \quad \Rightarrow b = \frac{1}{4} ...(2)$$

Again it is given that, a^2, b^2, c^2 are in G.P. then

$$(b^2)^2 = a^2c^2 \Rightarrow ac = \pm\frac{1}{16} \quad ...(3)$$

From (1), (2) and (3), we get;

$$a \pm \frac{1}{16a} = \frac{1}{2} \Rightarrow 16a^2 - 8a \pm 1 = 0$$

Case I: $16a^2 - 8a + 1 = 0$

$\Rightarrow a = \frac{1}{4}$ (not possible as $a < b$)

Case II: $16a^2 - 8a - 1 = 0 \Rightarrow a = \frac{8 \pm \sqrt{128}}{32}$

$$\Rightarrow a = \frac{1}{4} \pm \frac{1}{2\sqrt{2}}$$

$$\therefore a = \frac{1}{4} - \frac{1}{2\sqrt{2}} \quad (\because a < b)$$

27. (a) Here, B – 2A =

$$\sum_{n=1}^{40} a_n - 2\sum_{n=1}^{20} a_n = \sum_{n=21}^{40} a_n - 2\sum_{n=1}^{20} a_n$$

$B - 2A = (21^2 + 2.22^2 + 23^2 + 2.24^2 + ... + 40^2) - (1^2 + 2.2^2 + 3^2 + 2.4^2 ..... + 20^2)$

$= 20[22 + 2.24 + 26 + 2.28 + ... + 60]$

$$= 20\left[\underbrace{(22 + 24 + 26....60)}_{20 \text{ terms}} + \underbrace{(24 + 28 + ... + 60)}_{10 \text{ terms}}\right]$$

$$20\left[\frac{20}{2}(22 + 60) + \frac{10}{2}(24 + 60)\right]$$

$= 10[20.82 + 10.84]$

$= 100[164 + 84] = 100.248$

28. (d) The general term of the given series $= \frac{2\times 2^r - 1}{2^r}$,

where $r \geq 0$

$\therefore$ req. sum $= 1 + \sum_{r=1}^{19} \frac{2\times 2^r - 1}{2^r}$

Now, $\sum_{r=1}^{19}\left(\frac{2\times 2^r - 1}{2^r}\right) = \sum_{r=1}^{19}\left(2 - \frac{1}{2^r}\right)$

$$= 2(19) - \frac{\frac{1}{2}\left(1-\left(\frac{1}{2}\right)^{19}\right)}{1-\frac{1}{2}} = 38 + \frac{\left(\frac{1}{2}\right)^{19} - 1}{1}$$

$$= 38 + \left(\frac{1}{2}\right)^{19} - 1 = 37 + \left(\frac{1}{2}\right)^{19}$$

$\therefore$ req. sum $= 1 + 37 + \left(\frac{1}{2}\right)^{19} = 38 + \left(\frac{1}{2}\right)^{19}$

29. (b) Since Orthocentre of the triangle is A(–3, 5) and centriod of the triangle is B(3, 3), then

$AB = \sqrt{40} = 2\sqrt{10}$

A B C

Centroid divides orthocentre and circumcentre of the triangle in ratio 2 : 1

$\therefore$ AB : BC = 2 : 1

Now, $AB = \frac{2}{3}AC$

$\Rightarrow \quad AC = \frac{3}{2}AB = \frac{3}{2}(2\sqrt{10}) \Rightarrow AC = 3\sqrt{10}$

$\therefore$ Radius of circle with AC as diametre

$$= \frac{AC}{2} = \frac{3}{2}\sqrt{10} = 3\sqrt{\frac{5}{2}}$$

30. (b) Equation of PQ is

$$\frac{x}{h} + \frac{y}{k} = 1 \qquad ...(1)$$

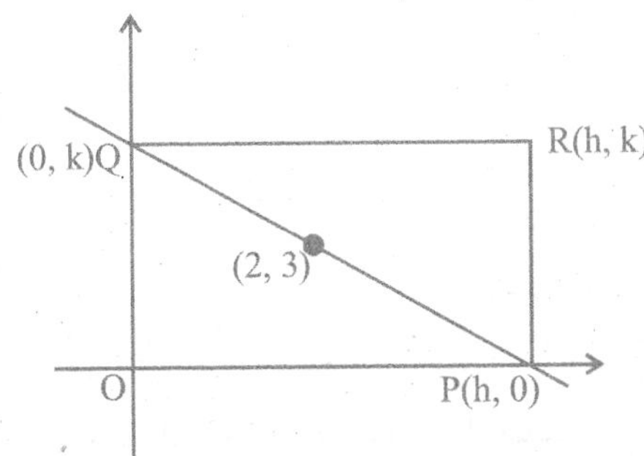

Since, (1) passes through the fixed point (2, 3) Then,

$$\frac{2}{h} + \frac{3}{k} = 1$$

Then, the locus of R is $\frac{2}{x} + \frac{3}{y} = 1$ or $3x + 2y = xy$.

31. (b) Median through C is $x = 4$

So the x coordianate of C is 4. let $C \equiv (4, y)$, then the midpoint of A (1, 2) and C (4, y) is D which lies on the median through B.

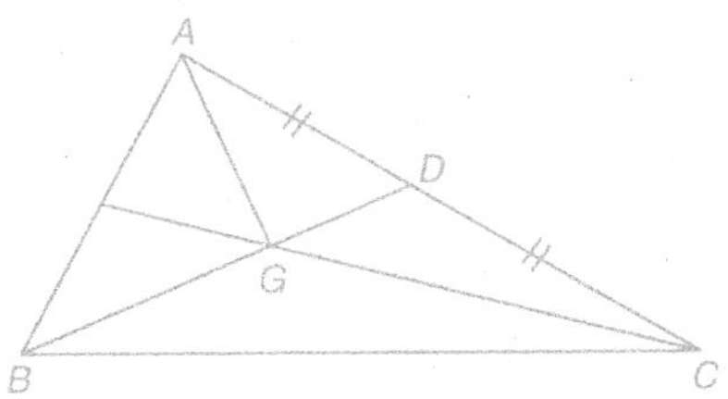

$\therefore \quad D \equiv \left(\frac{1+4}{2}, \frac{2+y}{2}\right)$

Now, $\frac{1+4+2+y}{2} = 5 \Rightarrow y = 3$.

So, $C \equiv (4, 3)$.

The centroid of the triangle is the intersection of the mesians. Here the medians $x = 4$ and $x + 4$ and $x + y = 5$ intersect at G (4, 1).

The area of triangle $\Delta ABC = 3 \times \Delta AGC$

$$= 3 \times \frac{1}{2}[1(1-3) + 4(3-2) + 4(2-1)] = 9.$$

32. (d) Equation of the line, which is perpendicular to the line, $3x + y = \lambda (\lambda \neq 0)$ and passing through origin, is given by

$$\frac{x-0}{3} = \frac{y-0}{1} = r$$

For foot of perpendicular

$$r = \frac{-((3\times 0) + (1\times 0) - \lambda)}{3^2 + 1^2} = \frac{\lambda}{10}$$

So, foot of perpendicular $P = \left(\frac{3\lambda}{10}, \frac{\lambda}{10}\right)$

Given the line meets X-axis at $A = \left(\frac{\lambda}{3}, 0\right)$ and meets Y-axis at $B = (0, \lambda)$

So, $BP = \sqrt{\left(\frac{3\lambda}{10}\right)^2 + \left(\frac{\lambda}{10} - \lambda\right)^2} \Rightarrow BP = \sqrt{\frac{9\lambda^2}{100} + \frac{81\lambda^2}{100}}$

$$\Rightarrow BP = \sqrt{\frac{90\lambda^2}{100}}$$

Now, $PA = \sqrt{\left(\frac{\lambda}{3} - \frac{3\lambda}{10}\right)^2 + \left(0 - \frac{\lambda}{10}\right)^2}$

$$\Rightarrow PA\sqrt{\frac{\lambda^2}{900} + \frac{\lambda^2}{100}} \Rightarrow PA = \sqrt{\frac{10\lambda^2}{900}}$$

Therefore $BP : PA = 3 : 1$

33. (d) Let the coordinate A be $(0, c)$
Equations of the given lines are
$x-y+2=0$ and
$7x-y+3=0$
We know that the diagonals of the rhombus will be parallel to the angle bisectors of the two given lines; $y=x+2$ and $y=7x+3$
$\therefore$ equation of angle bisectors is given as:

$$\frac{x-y+2}{\sqrt{2}}=\pm\frac{7x-y+3}{5\sqrt{2}}$$

$5x-5y+10=\pm(7x-y+3)$
$\therefore$ Parallel equations of the diagonals are $2x+4y-7=0$ and $12x-6y+13=0$

$\therefore$ slopes of diagonals are $\frac{-1}{2}$ and 2.

Now, slope of the diagonal from $A(0, c)$ and passing through $P(1, 2)$ is $(2-c)$
$\therefore 2-c=2 \Rightarrow c=0$ (not possible)

$\therefore 2-c=\frac{-1}{2} \Rightarrow c=\frac{5}{2}$

$\therefore$ ordinate of A is $\frac{5}{2}$.

34. (c) Equation of tangent at (1, 7) to $x^2=y-6$ is $2x-y+5=0$.

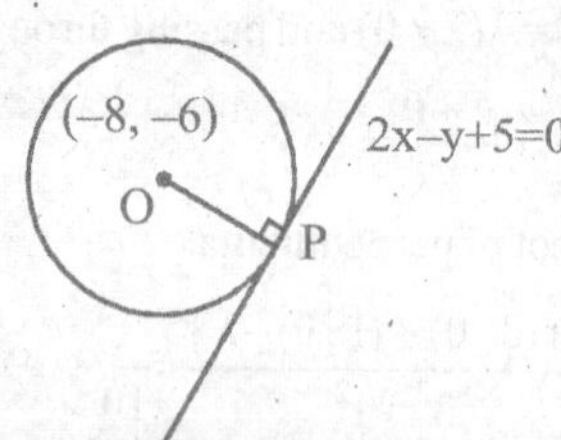

Now, perpendicular from centre O(–8, –6) to $2x-y+5=0$ should be equal to radius of the circle

$$\therefore \left|\frac{-16+6+5}{\sqrt{5}}\right|=\sqrt{64+36-C}$$

$\Rightarrow \sqrt{5}=\sqrt{100-c}$
$\Rightarrow c=95$

35. (d) Given circle is:
$x^2+y^2+2x-4y-4=0$
$\therefore$ its centre is $(-1, 2)$ and radius is 3 units.
Let $A=(x, y)$ be the centre of the circle C

$\therefore \frac{x-1}{2}=2 \Rightarrow x=5$ and $\frac{y+2}{2}=2 \Rightarrow y=2$

So the centre of C is (5, 2) and its radius is 3
$\therefore$ equation of centre C is:
$x^2+y^2-10x-4y+20=0$
$\therefore$ The length of the intercept it cuts on the x-axis

$=2\sqrt{g^2-c}=2\sqrt{25-20}=2\sqrt{5}$

36. (c) Equation of the line passing through the points (2, 3) and (4, 5) is

$$y-3=\left(\frac{5-3}{4-2}\right)x-2 \Rightarrow x-y+1=0 \text{ ..... (1)}$$

Equation of the perpendicular line passing through the midpoint (3, 4) is $x+y-7=0$ ..... (2)
Lines (1) and (2) intersect at the center of the circle. So, the center of the circle is (3, 4)
Therefore, the radius is

$$\sqrt{(x_2-x_1)^2+(y_2-y_1)^2}=\sqrt{(2-3)^2+(3-4)^2}=\sqrt{2} \text{ units.}$$

37. (c) As origin is the only common point to x-axis and y-axis, so, origin is the common vertex
Let the equation of two of parabolas be $y^2=4ax$ and $x^2=4by$
Now latus rectum of both parabolas = 3
$\therefore 4a=4b=3$

$\Rightarrow a=b=\frac{3}{4}$

$\therefore$ Two parabolas are $y^2=3x$ and $x^2=3y$
Suppose $y=mx+c$ is the common tangent.
$\therefore y^2=3x \Rightarrow (mx+c)^2=3x \Rightarrow m^2x^2+(2mc-3)x+c^2=0$
As, the tangent touches at one point only
So, $b^2-4ac=0$
$\Rightarrow (2mc-3)^2-4m^2c^2=0$
$\Rightarrow 4m^2c^2+9-12mc-4m^2c^2=0$

$\Rightarrow c=\frac{9}{12m}=\frac{3}{4m}$ .... (i)

$\therefore x^2=3y \Rightarrow x^2=3(mx+c) \Rightarrow x^2-3mx-3c=0$
Again, $b^2-4ac=0$
$\Rightarrow 9m^2-4(1)(-3c)=0$
$\Rightarrow 9m^2=-12c$ ..... (ii)
Form (i) and (ii)

$$m^2=\frac{-4c}{3}=\frac{-4}{3}\left(\frac{3}{4m}\right)$$

$\Rightarrow m^3=-1 \Rightarrow m=-1 \Rightarrow c=\frac{-3}{4}$

Hence, $y=mx+c=-x-\frac{3}{4}$

$\Rightarrow 4(x+y)+3=0$

38. (a) Here, equation of tangent on C_1 at (2, 1) is:
$2x+y-(x+2)-1=0$
Or $x+y=3$
If it cuts off the chord of the circle C_2 then the equation of the chord is:

$x+y=3$

$\therefore$ distance of the chord from (3, – 2) is :

$$d=\left|\frac{3-2-3}{\sqrt{2}}\right|=\sqrt{2}$$

Also, length of the chord is $l=4$

$$\therefore \text{ radius of } C_2=r=\sqrt{\left(\frac{l}{2}\right)^2+d^2}$$

$$=\sqrt{(2)^2+(\sqrt{2})^2}=\sqrt{6}$$

39. (a) Equation of tnagent at P(16, 16) is given as:
$x-2y+16=0$

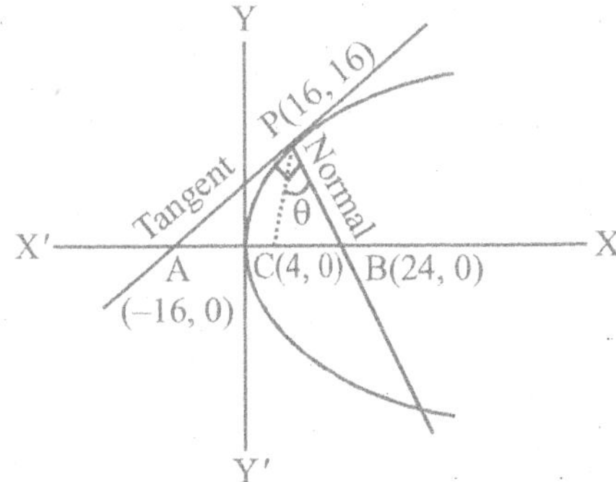

Slope of PC $(m_1)=\frac{4}{3}$

Slope of PB $(m_2)=-2$

Hence, $\tan\theta=\left|\frac{m_1-m_2}{1+m_1\cdot m_2}\right|=\left|\frac{\frac{4}{3}+2}{1-\frac{4}{3}\cdot 2}\right|$

$\Rightarrow$ $\tan\theta=2$

40. (a) Equation of the chord of contact PQ is given by:
$T=0$
or $T\equiv yy_1-4(x+x_1)$, where $(x_1,y_1)\equiv(-8,0)$
$\therefore$ Equation becomes: $x=8$
& Chord of contact is $x=8$
$\therefore$ Coordinates of point P and Q are (8, 8) and (8, – 8) and focus of the parabola is F (2, 0)

$\therefore$ Area of triangle $PQF=\frac{1}{2}\times(8-2)\times(8+8)=48$ sq. units

41. (a) $A=\{(a,b)\in R\times R:|a-5|<1,|b-5|<1\}$

Let $a-5,=x$, $b-5=y$

Set A contains all points inside $|x|<1,|y|<1$

$B=\{(a,b)\in R\times R:4(a-6)^2+9(B-5)^2\le 36\}$

Set B contains all points inside or on

$$\frac{(x-1)^2}{9}+\frac{y^2}{4}=1$$

42. (d) Let for ellipse coordinates of focus and vertex are $(ae, 0)$ and $(a, 0)$ respectively.

$\therefore$ Distance between focus and vertex $=a(1-e)=\frac{3}{2}$ (given)

$$\Rightarrow a-\frac{3}{2}=ae$$

$$\Rightarrow a^2+\frac{9}{4}-3a=a^2e^2 \quad ...(i)$$

Length of latus rectum $=\frac{2b^2}{a}=4$

$$\Rightarrow b^2=2a \quad ...(ii)$$

$$e^2=1-\frac{b^2}{a^2}$$

$$\Rightarrow e^2=1-\frac{2a}{a^2} \quad \text{(from (ii))}$$

$$\Rightarrow e^2=1-\frac{2}{a} \quad ...(iii)$$

Substituting the value of e^2 in eq. (i) we get;

$$\Rightarrow a^2+\frac{9}{4}-3a=a^2\left(1-\frac{2}{a}\right)$$

$$\Rightarrow a=\frac{9}{4}$$

$\therefore$ from eq. (iii) we get;

$$e^2=1-\frac{2}{a}=1-\frac{8}{9}=\frac{1}{9}$$

$$\Rightarrow e=\frac{1}{3}$$

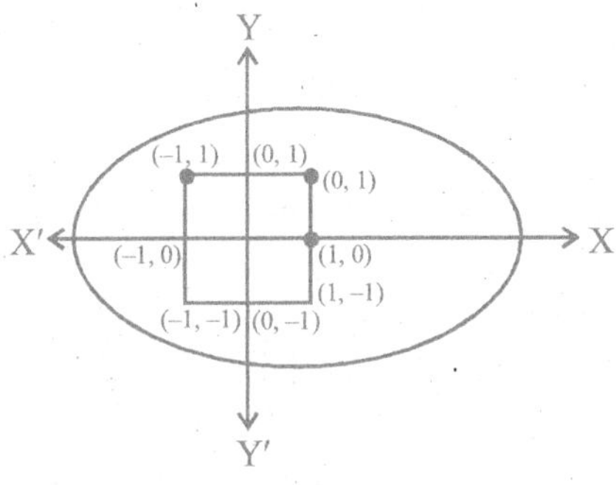

$\therefore$ $(\pm1,\pm1)$ lies inside the ellipse.

Hence, $A\subset B$.

43. (d) Here equation of hyperbola is $\frac{x^2}{9}-\frac{y^2}{36}=1$

Now, PQ is the chord of contant

$\therefore$ Equation of PQ is : $\frac{x(0)}{9}-\frac{y(3)}{36}=1$

$\Rightarrow$ $y=-12$

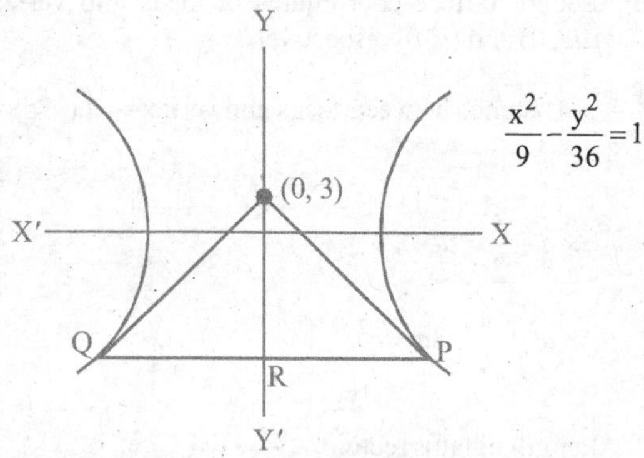

$\therefore$ Area of $\Delta PQT=\frac{1}{2}\times TR\times PQ$

$\because$ $P\equiv(3\sqrt{5},-12)$ $\therefore$ $TR=3+12=15$,

$\therefore$ Area of $\Delta PQT=\frac{1}{2}\times15\times6\sqrt{5}=45\sqrt{5}$ sq. units

44. (a) Here, lines are:

$\sqrt{2}x-y+4\sqrt{2}k=0$

$\Rightarrow \sqrt{2}x+4\sqrt{2}k=y$ ...(i)

and $\sqrt{2}kx+ky-4\sqrt{2}=0$ ...(ii)

Put the value of y from (i) in (ii) we get;

$\Rightarrow 2\sqrt{2}kx+4\sqrt{2}\left(k^2-1\right)=0$

$\Rightarrow x=\frac{2(1-k^2)}{k}, y=\frac{2\sqrt{2}(1+k^2)}{k}$

$\therefore \left(\frac{y}{4\sqrt{2}}\right)^2-\left(\frac{x}{4}\right)^2=1$

$\therefore$ length of transverse axis

$2a=2\times 4\sqrt{2}=8\sqrt{2}$

Hence, the locus is a hyperbola with length of its transverse axis equal to $8\sqrt{2}$

45. (b) Since, $\lim_{x\to0^+} x\left(\left[\frac{1}{x}\right]+\left[\frac{2}{x}\right]+...+\left[\frac{15}{x}\right]\right)$

$=\lim_{x\to0^+} x\left(\frac{1+2+3+...+15}{x}\right)-\left(\left\{\frac{1}{x}\right\}+\left\{\frac{2}{x}\right\}+...+\left\{\frac{15}{x}\right\}\right)$

$\because 0\le\left\{\frac{r}{x}\right\}<1 \Rightarrow 0\le x\left\{\frac{r}{x}\right\}<x$

$\therefore \lim_{x\to0^+} x\left(\frac{1+2+3+...+15}{x}\right)=\frac{15\times16}{2}=120$

46. (d) Let, $L=\lim_{x\to0}\frac{(x\tan2x-2x\tan x)}{(1-\cos2x)^2}=\lim_{x\to0}K$ (say)

$$\Rightarrow K=\frac{x\left[\frac{2\tan x}{1-(\tan x)^2}\right]-2x\tan x}{(1-(1-2\sin^2x))^2}$$

$$=\frac{2x\tan x-[2x\tan x-2x\tan^3x]}{4\sin^4x\times(1-\tan^2x)}$$

$$=\frac{2x\tan^3x}{4\sin^4x\times(1-\tan^2x)}$$

$$=\frac{2x\tan^3x}{4\sin^4x\times\left(\frac{\cos^2x-\sin^2x}{\cos^2x}\right)}$$

$$=\frac{2x\frac{\sin^3x}{\cos^3x}}{4\sin^4x\times\left(\frac{\cos^2x-\sin^2x}{\cos^2x}\right)}$$

$$\Rightarrow K=\frac{x}{2\sin x\times(\cos^2x-\sin^2x)\cos x}$$

$$\therefore L=\lim_{x\to0}\frac{x}{2\sin x}\times\lim_{x\to0}\frac{1}{\cos x(\cos^2x-\sin^2x)}$$

$$=\lim_{x\to0}\frac{x}{2\sin x}\times\lim_{x\to0}\frac{1}{\cos0(\cos^20-\sin^20)}$$

$$=\frac{1}{2}$$

47. (c) Let $L=\lim_{x\to0}\frac{(27+x)^{\frac{1}{3}}-3}{9-(27+x)^{\frac{2}{3}}}$

Here 'L' is in the indeterminate form i.e., $\frac{0}{0}$

$\therefore$ using the L'Hospital rule we get:

$$L=\lim_{x\to0}\frac{\frac{1}{3}(27+x)^{\frac{-2}{3}}}{-\frac{2}{3}(27+x)^{\frac{-1}{3}}}=\frac{\frac{1}{3}\times(27)^{\frac{-2}{3}}}{\frac{-2}{3}\times27^{\frac{-1}{3}}}=-\frac{1}{6}$$

48. (d) $\because f(x)$ has extremum values at $x=1$ and $x=2$

$\because f'(1)=0$ and $f'(2)=0$

As, $f(x)$ is a polynomial of degree 4.

Suppose $f(x)=Ax^4+Bx^3+Cx^2+Dx+E$

$\because \lim_{x\to0}\left(\frac{f(x)}{x^2}+1\right)=3$

$\Rightarrow \lim_{x\to0}\left(\frac{Ax^4+Bx^3+Cx^2+Dx+E}{x^2}+1\right)=3$

$$\Rightarrow \lim_{x\to 0}\left(Ax^2+Bx+C+\frac{D}{x}+\frac{E}{x^2}+1\right)=3$$

As limit has finite value, so $D=0$ and $E=0$

Now $A(0)^2+B(0)+C+0+0+1=3$

$\Rightarrow c+1=3 \Rightarrow c=2$

$f'(x)=4Ax^3+3Bx^2+2Cx+D$

$f'(1)=0 \Rightarrow 4A(1)+3B(1)+2C(1)+D=0$

$\Rightarrow 4A+3B=-4$ ...(1)

$f'(2)=0 \Rightarrow 4A(8)+3B(4)+2C(2)+D=0$

$\Rightarrow 8A+3B=-2$ ...(2)

From equations (1) and (2), we get

$A=\frac{1}{2}$ and $B=-2$

So, $f(x)=\frac{x^4}{2}-2x^3+2x^2$

Therefore, $f(-1)=\frac{(-1)^4}{2}-2(-1)^3+2(-1)^2$

$=\frac{1}{2}+2+2=\frac{9}{2}$

Hence $f(-1)=\frac{9}{2}$

49. (d) $\sim(p\vee q)\vee(\sim p\wedge q)$

$\Rightarrow(\sim p\wedge\sim q)\vee(\sim p\wedge q)$

$\Rightarrow\sim p\wedge(\sim q\vee q)$

$\Rightarrow\sim p\wedge t\equiv\sim p$

50. (d)

p	q	$\sim p$	$\sim q$	$\sim p\vee\sim q$	$p\to(\sim p\vee\sim q)$
T	T	F	F	F	F
T	F	F	T	T	T
F	T	T	F	T	T
F	F	T	T	T	T

From the truth table,

$p\to(\sim p\vee\sim q)$ is false only when p and q both are true.

51. (b) As the truth table for the $(p\wedge\sim q)\wedge(p\wedge r)\to\sim p\vee q$ is false, then only possible values of (p, q, r) is (T, F, T)

p	q	r	$\sim q$	$p\wedge\sim q$	$p\wedge r$	$\sim p$	$\sim p\vee q$	$(p\wedge\sim q)\wedge(p\wedge r)$	$(p\wedge\sim q)\wedge(p\wedge r)\to\sim p\vee q$
T	T	T	F	F	T	F	T	F	T
T	F	T	T	T	T	F	F	T	F
T	T	F	F	F	F	F	T	F	T
F	T	T	F	F	F	T	T	F	T
F	F	T	T	F	F	T	T	F	T
F	T	F	F	F	F	T	T	F	T
T	F	F	T	T	F	F	F	F	T
F	F	F	T	F	F	T	T	F	T

52. (a) Statement p:

$$\sin 120°=\cos 30°=\frac{\sqrt{3}}{2}\Rightarrow 2\sin 120°=\sqrt{3}$$

$$\text{So, }\sqrt{1+\sin 240°}-\sqrt{1-\sin 240°}=\sqrt{\frac{1-\sqrt{3}}{2}}-\sqrt{\frac{1+\sqrt{3}}{2}}$$

$$\neq\sqrt{3}$$

Statement q:

$$\text{So, }A+B+C+D=2\pi\Rightarrow\frac{A+C}{2}+\frac{B+D}{2}=\pi$$

$$\Rightarrow\cos\left(\frac{A+C}{2}\right)+\cos\left(\frac{B+D}{2}\right)$$

$$=\cos\left(\frac{A+C}{2}\right)-\cos\left(\frac{A+C}{2}\right)=0$$

Therefore, statement p is false and statement q is true.

53. (b) As mean is a linear operation, so if each observation is multiplied by λ and decreased by 25 then the mean becomes $75\ \lambda-25$.

According to the question,

$75\lambda-25=75\Rightarrow\lambda=\frac{4}{3}$.

54. (b) Given $\sum_{i=1}^{9}(x_i-5)=9\Rightarrow\sum_{i=1}^{9}x_i=54$ ...(i)

Also, $\sum_{i=1}^{9}(x_i-5)^2=45$

$\Rightarrow\ \sum_{i=1}^{9}x_i^2-10\sum_{i=1}^{9}x_i+9(25)=45$ ...(ii)

From (i) and (ii) we get,

$$\sum_{i=1}^{9} x_i^2 = 360$$

Since, variance $= \frac{\sum x_i^2}{9} - \left(\frac{\sum x_i}{9}\right)^2$

$$= \frac{360}{9} - \left(\frac{54}{9}\right)^2 = 40 - 36 = 4$$

$\therefore$ Standard deviation $= \sqrt{\text{Variance}} = 2$

55. **(c)** Here mean $= \bar{x} = 9$

$\Rightarrow \bar{x} = \frac{\Sigma x_i}{n} = 9$

$\Rightarrow \Sigma x_i = 9 \times 5 = 45$

Now, standard deviation = 0

$\therefore$ all the five terms are same i.e.; 9.

Now for changed observation

$\bar{x}_{new} = \frac{36 + x_5}{5} = 10$

$\Rightarrow x_5 = 14$

$\therefore \sigma_{new} = \sqrt{\frac{\Sigma(x_i - \bar{x}_{new})^2}{n}}$

$= \sqrt{\frac{4(9-10)^2 + (14-10)^2}{5}} = 2$

56. **(d)** $\bar{x} = \frac{7+8+9+7+8+7+\lambda+8}{8} = 8$

$\Rightarrow \frac{54+\lambda}{8} = 8 \Rightarrow \lambda = 10$

Now variance $= \sigma^2$

$$= \frac{(7-8)^2+(8-8)^2+(9-8)^2+(7-8)^2+(8-8)^2 + (7-8)^2+(10-8)^2+(8-8)^2}{8}$$

$\Rightarrow \sigma^2 = \frac{1+0+1+1+0+1+4+0}{8} = \frac{8}{8} = 1$

Hence, the variance is 1.

57. **(d)** Let the number of children in each family be x.

Thus the total number of children in both the families are $2x$

Now, it is given that 3 tickets are distributed amongst the children of these two families.

Thus, the probability that all the three tickets go to the children in family B

$= \frac{{}^{x}C_3}{{}^{2x}C_3} = \frac{1}{12}$

$\Rightarrow \frac{x(x-1)(x-2)}{2x(2x-1)(2x-2)} = \frac{1}{12}$

$\Rightarrow \frac{(x-2)}{(2x-1)} = \frac{1}{6}$

$\Rightarrow x = 5$

Thus, the number of children in each family is 5.

58. **(a)** Probability of drawing a white ball and then a red ball from bag B is given by $\frac{{}^{4}C_1 \times {}^{2}C_1}{{}^{9}C_2} = \frac{2}{9}$

Probability of drawing a white ball and then a red ball from bag A is given by $\frac{{}^{2}C_1 \times {}^{3}C_1}{{}^{7}C_2} = \frac{2}{7}$

Hence, the probability of drawing a white ball and then a red ball from bag $B = \frac{\frac{2}{9}}{\frac{2}{7}+\frac{2}{9}} = \frac{2 \times 7}{18+14} = \frac{7}{16}$

59. **(c)** Here,

$R_1 = \{(x, y) \in N \times N : 2x + y = 10\}$ and

$R_2 = \{(x, y) \in N \times N : x + 2y = 10\}$

For R_1; $2x + y = 10$ and $x, y \in N$

So, possible values for x and y are:

$x = 1, y = 8$ i.e. $(1, 8)$;

$x = 2, y = 6$ i.e. $(2, 6)$;

$x = 3, y = 4$ i.e. $(3, 4)$ and

$x = 4, y = 2$ i.e. $(4, 2)$.

$R_1 = \{(1, 8), (2, 6), (3, 4), (4, 2)\}$

Therefore, Range of R_1 is $\{2, 4, 6, 8\}$

R_1 is not symmetric

Also, R_1 is not transitive because $(3, 4), (4, 2) \in R_1$ but $(3, 2) \notin R_1$

Thus, options A, B and D are incorrect.

For R_2; $x + 2y = 10$ and $x, y \in N$

So, possible values for x and y are:

$x = 8, y = 1$ i.e. $(8, 1)$;

$x = 6, y = 2$ i.e. $(6, 2)$;

$x = 4, y = 3$ i.e. $(4, 3)$ and

$x = 2, y = 4$ i.e. $(2, 4)$

$R_2 = \{(8, 1), (6, 2), (4, 3), (2, 4)\}$

Therefore, Range of R_2 is $\{1, 2, 3, 4\}$

R_2 is not symmetric and transitive.

60. **(a)** Both R_1 and R_2 are symmetric as

For any $(x, y) \in R_1$, we have

$(y, x) \in R_1$ and similarly for R_2

Now, for R_2, $(b, a) \in R_2$, $(a, c) \in R_2$ but $(b, c) \notin R_2$.

Similarly, for R_1, $(b, c) \in R_1$, $(c, a) \in R_1$ but $(b, a) \notin R_1$.

Therefore, neither R_1 nor R_2 is transitive.

61. **(d)** Suppose $y = f(x)$

$\Rightarrow y = \frac{x-1}{x-2}$

$\Rightarrow yx - 2y = x - 1$

$\Rightarrow (y-1)x = 2y - 1$

$\Rightarrow x = f^{-1}(y) = \dfrac{2y-1}{y-1}$

As the function is invertible on the given domain and its inverse can be obtained as above.

62. (c) Here $A = \begin{bmatrix} 1 & 0 & 0 \\ 1 & 1 & 0 \\ 1 & 1 & 1 \end{bmatrix}$

$\therefore \quad A^2 = A.A = \begin{bmatrix} 1 & 0 & 0 \\ 1 & 1 & 0 \\ 1 & 1 & 1 \end{bmatrix} \times \begin{bmatrix} 1 & 0 & 0 \\ 1 & 1 & 0 \\ 1 & 1 & 1 \end{bmatrix}$

$= \begin{bmatrix} 1 & 0 & 0 \\ 2 & 1 & 0 \\ 3 & 2 & 1 \end{bmatrix}$

also $A^3 = A^2.A = \begin{bmatrix} 1 & 0 & 0 \\ 2 & 1 & 0 \\ 3 & 2 & 1 \end{bmatrix} \times \begin{bmatrix} 1 & 0 & 0 \\ 1 & 1 & 0 \\ 1 & 1 & 1 \end{bmatrix}$

$= \begin{bmatrix} 1 & 0 & 0 \\ 3 & 1 & 0 \\ 6 & 3 & 1 \end{bmatrix}$

and, $A^4 = A^3.A = \begin{bmatrix} 1 & 0 & 0 \\ 3 & 1 & 0 \\ 6 & 3 & 1 \end{bmatrix} \times \begin{bmatrix} 1 & 0 & 0 \\ 1 & 1 & 0 \\ 1 & 1 & 1 \end{bmatrix}$

$= \begin{bmatrix} 1 & 0 & 0 \\ 4 & 1 & 0 \\ 10 & 4 & 1 \end{bmatrix}$

On observing the pattern, we come to a conclusion that,

$$A = \begin{bmatrix} 1 & 0 & 0 \\ n & 1 & 0 \\ \dfrac{n(n+1)}{2} & n & 1 \end{bmatrix}$$

$\therefore \quad A^{20} = \begin{bmatrix} 1 & 0 & 0 \\ 20 & 1 & 0 \\ 210 & 20 & 1 \end{bmatrix}$

Therefore, sum of first column of $A^{20} = [1 + 20 + 210]$ $= 231$

63. (b) Here, $\begin{vmatrix} x-4 & 2x & 2x \\ 2x & x-4 & 2x \\ 2x & 2x & x-4 \end{vmatrix} = (A+Bx)(x-A)^2$

Put $x = 0 \Rightarrow \begin{vmatrix} -4 & 0 & 0 \\ 0 & -4 & 0 \\ 0 & 0 & -4 \end{vmatrix} = A^3 \Rightarrow A^3 = (-4)^3$

$\Rightarrow A = -4$

$\Rightarrow \begin{vmatrix} x-4 & 2x & 2x \\ 2x & x-4 & 2x \\ 2x & 2x & x-4 \end{vmatrix} = (Bx-4)(x+4)^2$

Now take x common from both the sides

$\therefore \begin{vmatrix} 1-\dfrac{4}{x} & 2x & 2x \\ 2x & 1-\dfrac{4}{x} & 2x \\ 2x & 2x & 1-\dfrac{4}{x} \end{vmatrix} = (B-\dfrac{4}{x})(1+\dfrac{4}{x})^2$

Now take $x \to \infty$, then $\dfrac{1}{x} \to 0$

$\Rightarrow \begin{vmatrix} 1 & 2 & 2 \\ 2 & 1 & 2 \\ 2 & 2 & 1 \end{vmatrix} = B \Rightarrow B = 5$

64. (d) Since $A.\begin{bmatrix} 1 & 2 \\ 0 & 3 \end{bmatrix}$ is a scalar matrix and $|3A| = 108$

suppose the scalar matrix is $\begin{bmatrix} k & 0 \\ 0 & k \end{bmatrix}$

$\therefore A.\begin{bmatrix} 1 & 2 \\ 0 & 3 \end{bmatrix} = \begin{bmatrix} k & 0 \\ 0 & k \end{bmatrix}$

$\Rightarrow A = \begin{bmatrix} k & 0 \\ 0 & k \end{bmatrix} \begin{bmatrix} 1 & 2 \\ 0 & 3 \end{bmatrix}^{-1}$

$[\therefore AB = C \Rightarrow ABB^{-1} = CB^{-1} \Rightarrow A = CB^{-1}]$

$\Rightarrow A = \dfrac{1}{3}\begin{bmatrix} k & 0 \\ 0 & k \end{bmatrix} \begin{bmatrix} 3 & -2 \\ 0 & 1 \end{bmatrix}$

$\Rightarrow A = \begin{bmatrix} k & 0 \\ 0 & k \end{bmatrix} \begin{bmatrix} 1 & -\dfrac{2}{3} \\ 0 & \dfrac{1}{3} \end{bmatrix}$

$$\Rightarrow A=\begin{bmatrix} k & -\frac{2}{3}k \\ 0 & \frac{k}{3} \end{bmatrix} \quad ...(1)$$

$\because |3A| = 108$

$$\Rightarrow 108 = \begin{vmatrix} 3k & -2k \\ 0 & k \end{vmatrix} \quad \Rightarrow 3k^2 = 108 \Rightarrow k^2 = 36$$

$\Rightarrow k = \pm 6$

For $k = 6$

$$A=\begin{bmatrix} 6 & -4 \\ 0 & 2 \end{bmatrix} \quad ... \text{From (1)}$$

$$\Rightarrow A^2=\begin{bmatrix} 36 & -32 \\ 0 & 4 \end{bmatrix}$$

For $k = -6$

$$\Rightarrow A=\begin{bmatrix} -6 & 4 \\ 0 & -2 \end{bmatrix} \quad .... \text{From (1)}$$

$$\Rightarrow A^2=\begin{bmatrix} 36 & -32 \\ 0 & 4 \end{bmatrix}$$

65. **(a)** We have

$(A-3I)(A-5I)=O$

$\Rightarrow A^2-8A+15I=O$

Multiplying both sides by A^{-1}, we get;

$A^{-1}A.A-8A^{-1}A+15A^{-1}I=A^{-1}O$

$\Rightarrow A-8I+15A^{-1}=O$

$A+15A^{-1}=8I$

$$\frac{A}{2}+\frac{15A^{-1}}{2}=4I$$

$$\therefore \alpha+\beta=\frac{1}{2}+\frac{15}{2}=\frac{16}{2}=8$$

66. **(a)** For non zero solution of the system of linear equations;

$$\begin{vmatrix} 1 & k & 3 \\ 3 & k & -2 \\ 2 & 4 & -3 \end{vmatrix}=0$$

$\Rightarrow k=11$

Now equations become

$x+11y+3z=0 \quad ...(1)$

$3x+11y-2z=0 \quad ...(2)$

$2x+4y-3z=0 \quad ...(3)$

Adding equations (1) & (3) we get

$3x+15y=0$

$\Rightarrow x=-5y$

Now put $x=-5y$ in equation (1), we get

$-5y+11y+3z=0$

$\Rightarrow z=-2y$

$$\therefore \frac{xz}{y^2}=\frac{(-5y)(-2y)}{y^2}=10$$

67. **(c)** Here, the equations are;

$(k+2)x+10y=k$

& $kx+(k+3)y=k-1$.

These equations can be written in the form of $Ax=B$ as

$$\begin{bmatrix} k+2 & 10 \\ k & k+3 \end{bmatrix}\begin{bmatrix} x \\ y \end{bmatrix}=\begin{bmatrix} k \\ k-1 \end{bmatrix}$$

For the system to have no solution

$|A|=0$

$$\Rightarrow \begin{bmatrix} k+2 & 10 \\ k & k+3 \end{bmatrix}=0 \Rightarrow (k+2)(k+3)-k\times 10=0$$

$\Rightarrow k^2-5k+6=(k-2)(k-3)=0$

$\therefore k=2, 3$

For $k=2$, equations become:

$4x+10y=2$

& $2x+5y=1$

& hence infinite number of solutions.

For $k=3$, equations becomes;

$5x+10y=3$

$3x+6y=2$

& hence no solution.

$\therefore$ req. number of values of k is 1

68. **(b)** The system of linear equations is:

$x+y+z=2$

$2x+y-z=3$

$3x+2y+kz=4$

As, system has unique solution.

$$\text{So, } \begin{vmatrix} 1 & 1 & 1 \\ 2 & 1 & -1 \\ 3 & 2 & k \end{vmatrix}\neq 0$$

$\Rightarrow k+2-(2k+3)+1\neq 0$

$\Rightarrow k\neq 0$

Hence, $k\in R-\{0\}\equiv S$

69. **(d)** As the system of equations has no solution then Δ should be zero and at least one of Δ_1, Δ_2 and Δ_3 should not be zero. **[Online April 15, 2018]**

$$\therefore \Delta=\begin{vmatrix} 1 & a & 1 \\ 1 & 2 & 2 \\ 1 & 5 & 3 \end{vmatrix}=0$$

$\Rightarrow -a-1=0 \Rightarrow a=-1$

$$\Delta_2=\begin{vmatrix} 1 & 3 & 1 \\ 1 & 6 & 2 \\ 1 & b & 3 \end{vmatrix}\neq 0$$

$\Rightarrow b\neq 9$

70. (a) If the function is continuous at $x = 0$, then $\lim_{x\to 0} f(x)$ will exist and $f(0) = \lim_{x\to 0} f(x)$

Now, $\lim_{x\to 0} f(x) = \lim_{x\to 0}\left(\frac{1}{x} - \frac{k-1}{e^{2x}-1}\right)$

$$= \lim_{x\to 0}\left(\frac{e^{2x}-1-kx+x}{(x)(e^{2x}-1)}\right)$$

$$= \lim_{x\to 0}\left[\frac{\left(1+2x+\frac{(2x)^2}{2!}+\frac{(2x)^3}{3!}+...\right)-1-kx+x}{(x)\left(\left(1+2x+\frac{(2x)^2}{2!}+\frac{(2x)^3}{3!}+...\right)-1\right)}\right]$$

$$= \lim_{x\to 0}\left[\frac{(3-k)x+\frac{4x^2}{2!}+\frac{8x^3}{3!}+...}{\left(2x^2+\frac{4x^3}{2!}+\frac{8x^3}{3!}+...\right)}\right]$$

For the limit to exist, power of x in the numerator should be greater than or equal to the power of x in the denominator. Therefore, coefficient of x in numerator is equal to zero

$\Rightarrow 3 - k = 0$

$\Rightarrow k = 3$

So the limit reduces to

$$\lim_{x\to 0}\frac{(x^2)\left(\frac{4}{2!}+\frac{8x}{3!}+...\right)}{(x^2)\left(2+\frac{4x}{2!}+\frac{8x^2}{3!}+...\right)}$$

$$= \lim_{x\to 0}\frac{\frac{4}{2!}+\frac{8x}{3!}+...}{2+\frac{4x}{2!}+\frac{8x^2}{3!}+...} = 1$$

Hence, $f(0) = 1$

71. (c) Since $f(x)$ is continuous at $x = 2$.

$\therefore \lim_{x\to 2} f(x) = f(2)$

$\Rightarrow \lim_{x\to 2}(x-1)^{\frac{1}{2-x}} = k$ $\quad (1^{\infty}$ form)

$\therefore e^{l} = k$

where $l = \lim_{x\to 2}(x-1-1)\times\frac{1}{2-x} = \lim_{x\to 2}\frac{x-2}{2-x}$

$$= \lim_{x\to 2}\left(\frac{x-2}{x-2}\right)$$

$\Rightarrow k = e^{-1}$

72. (d) $f(x) = |x-\pi|(e^{|x|}-1)\sin|x|$

Check differentiability of f(x) at $x = \pi$ and $x = 0$

at $x = \pi$:

$$\text{R.H.D.} = \lim_{h\to 0}\frac{|\pi+h-\pi|(e^{|\pi+h|}-1)\sin|\pi+h|-0}{h}$$

$$\text{L.H.D} = \lim_{h\to 0}\frac{|\pi-h-\pi|(e^{|\pi-h|}-1)\sin|\pi-h|-0}{-h} = 0$$

$\because$ RHD = LHD

Therefore, function is differentiable at $x = \pi$

at $x = 0$:

$$\text{R.H.D.} = \lim_{h\to 0}\frac{|h-\pi|(e^{|h|}-1)\sin|h|-0}{h} = 0$$

$$\text{L.H.D.} = \lim_{h\to 0}\frac{|-h-\pi|(e^{|-h|}-1)\sin|-h|-0}{-h} = 0$$

$\therefore$ RHD = LHD

Therefore, function is differentiable.

at $x = 0$.

Since, the function f(x) is differentiable at all the points including π and 0.

i.e., f(x) is every where differentiable.

Therefore, there is no element in the set S.

$\Rightarrow S = \phi$ (an empty set)

73. (a) $S = \{(\lambda, \mu) \in R\times R : f(t) = (|\lambda|e^{|t|} - \mu)\sin(2|t|), t \in R$

$f(t) = (|\lambda|e^{|t|} - \mu)\sin(2|t|)$

$$= \begin{cases}(|\lambda|e^{t}-\mu)\sin 2t, & t>0\\ (|\lambda|e^{-t}-\mu)(-\sin 2t), & t<0\end{cases}$$

$$f'(t) = \begin{cases}(|\lambda|e^{t})\sin 2t + (|\lambda|e^{t}-\mu)(2\cos 2t), & t>0\\ |\lambda|e^{-t}\sin 2t + (|\lambda|e^{-t}-\mu)(-2\cos 2t), & t<0\end{cases}$$

As, $f(t)$ is differentiable

$\therefore$ LHD = RHD at $t = 0$

$\Rightarrow |\lambda|.\sin 2(0) + (|\lambda|e^{0}-\mu)2\cos(0)$

$= |\lambda|e^{-0}.\sin 2(0) - 2\cos(0)(|\lambda|e^{-0}-\mu)$

$\Rightarrow 0 + (|\lambda|-\mu)2 = 0 - 2(|\lambda|-\mu)$

$\Rightarrow 4(|\lambda|-\mu) = 0$

$\Rightarrow |\lambda| = \mu$

So, $S \equiv (\lambda, \mu) = \{\lambda \in R \,\&\, \mu \in [0, \infty)\}$

Therefore set S is subset of $R \times [0, \infty)$

74. (b) Here, $\frac{dx}{dt} = \frac{1}{2\sqrt{2^{\text{cosec}^{-1}t}}}2^{\text{cosec}^{-1}t}\log 2.\frac{-1}{x\sqrt{x^2-1}}$

$$\frac{dy}{dt} = \frac{1}{2\sqrt{2^{\sec^{-1}t}}}2^{\sec^{-1}t}\log 2.\frac{1}{x\sqrt{x^2-1}}$$

$$\therefore \quad \frac{dy}{dx}=\frac{\frac{dy}{dt}}{\frac{dx}{dt}}=\frac{-\sqrt{2^{\operatorname{cosec}^{-1}t}}}{\sqrt{2^{\sec^{-1}t}}}\frac{2^{\sec^{-1}t}}{2^{\operatorname{cosec}^{-1}t}}$$

$$\frac{dy}{dx}=\frac{\frac{dy}{dt}}{\frac{dx}{dt}}=-\sqrt{\frac{2^{\sec^{-1}t}}{2^{\operatorname{cosec}^{-1}t}}}=\frac{-y}{x}$$

75. **(a)** $f(x)=\begin{vmatrix}\cos x & x & 1\\ 2\sin x & x^2 & 2x\\ \tan x & x & 1\end{vmatrix}$

$= \cos x\,(x^2-2x^2)-x\,(2\sin x-2x\tan x)$
$\qquad +1(2x\sin x-x^2\tan x)$
$=-x^2\cos x-2x\sin x+2x^2\tan x+2x\sin x-x^2\tan x$
$=x^2\tan x-x^2\cos x \quad =x^2(\tan x-\cos x)$
$\Rightarrow f'(x)=2x(\tan x-\cos x)+x^2(\sec^2 x+\sin x)$

$\therefore \quad \lim_{x\to 0}\frac{f'(x)}{x}=$

$\lim_{x\to 0}\frac{2x(\tan x-\cos x)+x^2(\sec^2 x+\sin x)}{x}$

$=\lim_{x\to 0}(\tan x-\cos x)+x(\sec^2 x+\sin x)$
$=2(0-1)+0=-2$

So, $\lim_{x\to 0}\frac{f'(x)}{x}=-2$

76. **(a)** Since $f(x)=\sin\left(\frac{2\times 3^x}{1+9^x}\right)$

Suppose $3^x=\tan t$

$\Rightarrow f(x)=\sin^{-1}\left(\frac{2\tan t}{1+\tan^2 t}\right)=\sin^{-1}(\sin 2t)=2t$

$=2\tan^{-1}(3x)$

So, $f'(x)=\frac{2}{1+(3^x)^2}\times 3^x.\log_e 3$

$\therefore \quad f'\left(-\frac{1}{2}\right)=\frac{2}{1+\left(3^{-\frac{1}{2}}\right)^2}\times 3^{-\frac{1}{2}}.\log_e 3$

$=\frac{1}{2}\times\sqrt{3}\times\log_e 3 \;=\; \sqrt{3}\times\log_e\sqrt{3}$

77. **(a)** Given, $x^2+y^2+\sin y=4$

After differentiating the above equation w. r. t. x we get

$2x+2y\frac{dy}{dx}+\cos y\frac{dy}{dx}=0 \qquad ...(1)$

$\Rightarrow 2x+(2y+\cos y)\frac{dy}{dx}=0$

$\Rightarrow \frac{dy}{dx}=\frac{-2x}{2y+\cos y}$

At $(-2,0)$, $\left(\frac{dy}{dx}\right)_{(-2,0)}=\frac{-2\times -2}{2\times 0+\cos 0}$

$\Rightarrow \left(\frac{dy}{dx}\right)_{(-2,0)}=\frac{4}{0+1}$

$\Rightarrow \left(\frac{dy}{dx}\right)_{(-2,0)}=4 \qquad ...(2)$

Again differentiating equation (1) w. r. t to x, we get

$2+2\left(\frac{dy}{dx}\right)^2+2y\frac{d^2y}{dx^2}-\sin y\left(\frac{dy}{dx}\right)^2+\cos y\frac{d^2y}{dx^2}=0$

$\Rightarrow 2+(2-\sin y)\left(\frac{dy}{dx}\right)^2+(2y+\cos y)\frac{d^2y}{dx^2}=0$

$\Rightarrow (2y+\cos y)\frac{d^2y}{dx^2}=-2-(2-\sin y)\left(\frac{dy}{dx}\right)^2$

$\Rightarrow \frac{d^2y}{dx^2}=\frac{-2-(2-\sin y)\left(\frac{dy}{dx}\right)^2}{2y+\cos y}$

So, at $(-2,0)$,

$\frac{d^2y}{dx^2}=\frac{-2-(2-0)\times 4^2}{2\times 0+1}$

$\Rightarrow \frac{d^2y}{dx^2}=\frac{-2-2\times 16}{1}$

$\Rightarrow \frac{d^2y}{dx^2}=-34$

78. **(c)** Let curve intersect each other at point $P(x_1, y_1)$

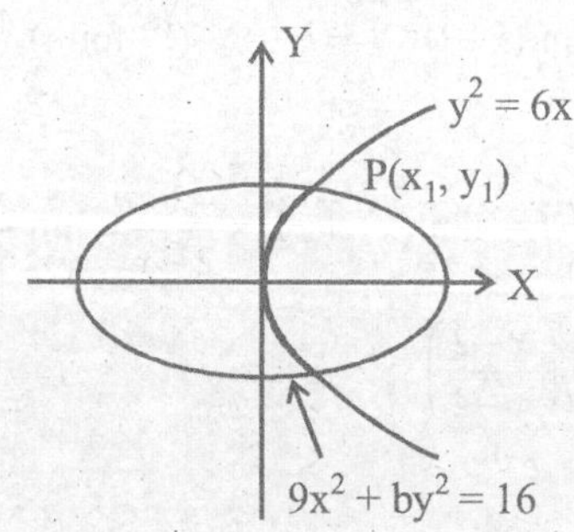

Since, point of intersection is on both the curves, then

$y_1^2 = 6x_1$ ...(i)

and $9x_1^2 + by_1^2 = 16$ ...(ii)

Now, find the slope of tangent to both the curves at the point of intersection $P(x_1, y_1)$

For slope of curves:

curve (i):

$$\left(\frac{dy}{dx}\right)_{(x_1,y_1)} = m_1 = \frac{3}{y_1}$$

curve (ii):

and $\left(\frac{dy}{dx}\right)_{(x_1,y_1)} = m_2 = -\frac{9x_1}{by_1}$

Since, both the curves intersect each other at right angle then,

$$m_1m_2 = -1 \Rightarrow \frac{27x_1}{by_1^2} = 1 \Rightarrow b = 27\frac{x_1}{y_1^2}$$

$\therefore$ from equation (i), $b = 27 \times \frac{1}{6} = \frac{9}{2}$

79. **(c)** Let $P(2t, t^2)$ be any point on the parabola.

Centre of the given circle $C = (-g, -f) = (-3, 0)$

For PC to be minimum, it must be the normal to the parabola at P.

Slope of line $PC = \frac{y_2 - y_1}{x_2 - x_1} = \frac{t^2 - 0}{2t + 3}$

Also, slope of tangent to parabola at $P = \frac{dy}{dx} = \frac{x}{2} = t$

$\therefore$ Slope of normal $= \frac{-1}{t}$

$\therefore \frac{t^2 - 0}{2t + 3} = \frac{-1}{t}$

$\Rightarrow t^3 + 2t + 3 = 0$

$\Rightarrow (t+1)(t^2 - t + 3) = 0$

$\therefore$ Real roots of above equation is

$t = -1$

Coordinate of $P = (2t, t^2) = (-2, 1)$

Slope of tangent to parabola at $P = t = -1$

Therefore, equation of tangent is:

$(y - 1) = (-1)(x + 2)$

$\Rightarrow x + y + 1 = 0$

80. **(d)** Equation of hyperbola is :

$4y^2 = x^2 + 1 \Rightarrow -x^2 + 4y^2 = 1$

$$\Rightarrow -\frac{x^2}{1^2} + \frac{y^2}{\left(\frac{1}{2}\right)^2} = 1$$

$\therefore a = 1, b = \frac{1}{2}$

Now, tangent to the curve at point (x_1, y_1) is given by

$$4 \times 2y_1\frac{dy}{dx} = 2x_1$$

$$\Rightarrow \frac{dy}{dx} = \frac{2x_1}{8y_1} = \frac{x_1}{4y_1}$$

Equation of tangent at (x_1, y_1) is

$y = mx + c$

$$\Rightarrow y = \frac{x_1}{4y_1} \cdot x + c$$

As tangent passes through (x_1, y_1)

$$\therefore y_1 = \frac{x_1 x_1}{4y_1} + c$$

$$\Rightarrow C = \frac{4y_1^2 - x_1^2}{4y_1} = \frac{1}{4y_1}$$

Therefore, $y = \frac{x_1}{4y_1}x + \frac{1}{4y_1} \Rightarrow 4y_1y = x_1x + 1$

which intersects x axis at $A\left(\frac{-1}{x_1}, 0\right)$ and y axis at $B\left(0, \frac{1}{4y_1}\right)$

Let midpoint of AB is (h, k)

$$\therefore h = \frac{-1}{2x_1}$$

$$\Rightarrow x_1 = \frac{-1}{2h} \;\&\; y_1 = \frac{1}{8k}$$

Thus, $4\left(\frac{1}{8k}\right)^2 = \left(\frac{-1}{2h}\right)^2 + 1 \Rightarrow \frac{1}{16k^2} = \frac{1}{4h^2} + 1$

$$\Rightarrow 1 = \frac{16k^2}{4h^2} + 16k^2 \Rightarrow h^2 = 4k^2 + 16h^2k.$$

So, required equation is

$x^2 - 4y^2 - 16x^2y^2 = 0$

81. **(b)** Since, $x^2 + 3y^2 = 9$

$$\Rightarrow 2x + 6y\frac{dy}{dx} = 0$$

$$\Rightarrow \frac{dy}{dx} = \frac{-x}{3y}$$

Slope of normal is $-\frac{dx}{dy} = \frac{3y}{x}$

$$\Rightarrow \left(-\frac{dx}{dy}\right)_{(3\cos\theta,\sqrt{3}\sin\theta)} = \frac{3\sqrt{3}\sin\theta}{3\cos\theta} = \sqrt{3}\tan\theta = m_1$$

$$\& \left(-\frac{dx}{dy}\right)_{(-3\sin\theta,\sqrt{3}\cos\theta)}$$

$$= \frac{3\sqrt{3}\cos\theta}{-3\sin\theta} = -\sqrt{3}\cot\theta = m_2$$

As, β is the anagle between the normals to the given ellipse then

$$\tan\beta = \left|\frac{m_1 - m_2}{1 + m_1 m_2}\right|$$

$$= \left|\frac{\sqrt{3}\tan\theta + \sqrt{3}\cot\theta}{1 - 3\tan\theta\cot\theta}\right| = \left|\frac{\sqrt{3}\tan\theta + \sqrt{3}\cot\theta}{1-3}\right|$$

$$\text{So, } \tan\beta = \frac{\sqrt{3}}{2}|\tan\theta + \cot\theta|$$

$$\Rightarrow \frac{1}{\cot\beta} = \frac{\sqrt{3}}{2}\left|\frac{\sin\theta}{\cos\theta} + \frac{\cos\theta}{\sin\theta}\right|$$

$$\Rightarrow \frac{1}{\cot\beta} = \frac{\sqrt{3}}{2}\left|\frac{1}{\sin\theta\cos\theta}\right|$$

$$\Rightarrow \frac{1}{\cot\beta} = \frac{\sqrt{3}}{\sin 2\theta} \Rightarrow \frac{2\cot\beta}{\sin 2\theta} = \frac{2}{\sqrt{3}}$$

82. **(c)** Given, $4x^2 - 9y^2 = 36$

After differentiating w.r.t. x, we get

$$4.2.x - 9.2.y.\frac{dy}{dx} = 0$$

$$\Rightarrow \text{Slope of tangent} = \frac{dy}{dx} = \frac{4x}{9y}$$

$$\text{So, slope of normal} = \frac{-9y}{4x}$$

Now, equation of normal at point (x_0, y_0) is given by

$$y - y_0 = \frac{-9y_0}{4x_0}(x - x_0)$$

As normal intersects X axis at A, Then

$$A \equiv \left(\frac{13x_0}{9}, 0\right) \text{ and } B \equiv \left(0, \frac{13y_0}{4}\right)$$

As $OABP$ is a parallelogram

$$\therefore \text{ midpoint of } OB \equiv \left(0, \frac{13y_0}{8}\right) \equiv \text{Midpoint of } AP$$

$$\text{So, } P(x, y) \equiv \left(\frac{-13x_0}{9}, \frac{13y_0}{4}\right) \quad \text{...(i)}$$

$\because (x_0, y_0)$ lies on hyperbola, therefore

$$4(x_0)^2 - 9(y_0)^2 = 36 \quad \text{...(ii)}$$

From equation (i): $x_0 = \frac{-9x}{13}$ and $y_0 = \frac{4y}{13}$

From equation (ii), we get

$9x^2 - 4y^2 = 169$

Hence, locus of point P is : $9x^2 - 4y^2 = 169$

83. **(c)** Here, $h(x) = \dfrac{x^2 + \frac{1}{x^2}}{x - \frac{1}{x}} = \left(x - \frac{1}{x}\right) + \dfrac{2}{x - \frac{1}{x}}$

When $x - \frac{1}{x} < 0$

$$\therefore \quad x - \frac{1}{x} + \frac{2}{x - \frac{1}{x}} \le -2\sqrt{2}$$

Hence, $-2\sqrt{2}$ will be local maximum value of h(x).

When $x - \frac{1}{x} > 0$

$$\therefore \quad x - \frac{1}{x} + \frac{2}{x - \frac{1}{x}} \ge 2\sqrt{2}$$

Hence, $2\sqrt{2}$ will be local minimum value of h(x).

84. **(a)** Here, $f(x) = 2x^3 - 9x^2 + 12x + 5$

$\Rightarrow \quad f'(x) = 6x^2 - 18x + 12 = 0$

For maxima or minima put $f'(x) = 0$

$\Rightarrow x^2 - 3x + 2 = 0$

$\Rightarrow x = 1$ or $x = 2$

Now, $f''(x) = 12x - 18$

$\Rightarrow \quad f''(1) = 12(1) - 18 = -6 < 0$

Hence, $f(x)$ has maxima at $x = 1$

$\therefore$ maximum value $= M = f(1) = 2 - 9 + 12 + 5 = 10$.

And, $f''(2) = 12(2) - 18 = 6 > 0$.

Hence, $f(x)$ has minima at $x = 2$.

$\therefore$ minimum value $= m = f(2) = 2(8) - 9(4) + 12(2) + 5 = 9$

$\therefore M - m = 10 - 9 = 1$

85. **(a)** Sphere of radius $r = 3$ *cm*

Let b, h be base radius and height of cone respectively.

$$\text{So, volume of cone} = \frac{1}{2}\pi b^2 h$$

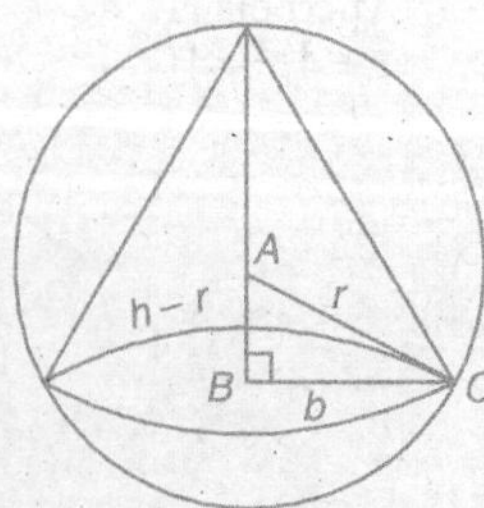

In right angled ΔABC by Pythagoras theorem

$(h-r)^2 + b^2 = r^2$

$\Rightarrow b^2 = r^2 - (h-r)^2 = r^2 - (h^2 - 2hr + r^2) = 2hr - h^2$

$\therefore$ Volume $(v) = \frac{1}{3}\pi h\left[2hr - h^2\right] = \frac{1}{3}\left[2h^2r - h^3\right]$

$\frac{dv}{dh} = \frac{1}{3}\left[4hr - 3h^2\right] = 0 \Rightarrow h(4r - 3h) = 0$

$\frac{d^2v}{dh^2} = \frac{1}{3}[4r - 6h]$

At $h = \frac{4r}{3}, \frac{d^2v}{dh^2} = \frac{1}{3}\left[4r - \frac{4r}{3}\times 6\right] = \frac{1}{3}[4r - 8r] < 0$

$\Rightarrow$ maximum volume ocurs at $h = \frac{4r}{3} = \frac{4}{3}\times 3 = 4\ cm$

As from (1),

$(h-r)^2 + b^2 = r^2$

$\Rightarrow b^2 = 2hr - h^2 = 2\cdot\frac{4r}{3}r - \frac{16r^2}{9} = \frac{8r^2}{3} - \frac{16r^2}{9}$

$= \frac{(24-16)r^2}{9} = \frac{8r^2}{9}$

$\Rightarrow b = \frac{2\sqrt{2}}{3}r = 2\sqrt{2}\ cm$

Therefore curved surface area $= \pi bl$

$= \pi b\sqrt{h^2 + r^2} = \pi 2\sqrt{2}\sqrt{4^2 + 8} = 8\sqrt{3}\pi\ cm^2$

86. **(a)** Let I

$= \int \frac{\sin^2 x\cos^2 x}{(\sin^5 x + \cos^3 x\sin^2 x + \sin^3 x\cos^2 x + \cos^5 x)^2}dx$

$= \int \frac{\sin^2 x\cos^2 x}{[(\sin^2 x + \cos^2 x)(\sin^3 x + \cos^3 x)]^2}dx$

$= \int \frac{\sin^2 x\cos^2 x}{(\sin^3 x + \cos^3 x)^2}dx = \int \frac{\tan^2 x\cdot\sec^2 x}{(1+\tan^3 x)^2}dx$

Now, put $(1 + \tan^3 x) = t$

$\Rightarrow$ $3\tan^2 x\sec^2 x\, dx = dt$

$\therefore$ $I = \frac{1}{3}\int\frac{dt}{t^2} = -\frac{1}{3t} + C = \frac{-1}{3(1+\tan^3 x)} + C$

87. **(a)** Let $I = \int \frac{\tan x}{1 + \tan x + \tan^2 x}dx$

$\Rightarrow I = \int \frac{\tan x + 1 + \tan^2 x}{\tan x + 1 + \tan^2 x}dx - \int \frac{(1+\tan^2 x)}{1 + \tan x + \tan^2 x}$

$\Rightarrow I = x - \int \frac{\sec^2 x dx}{1 + \tan x + \tan^2 x}$

Put $\tan x = t \Rightarrow \sec^2 x\, .\, dx = dt$

$\therefore I = x - \int \frac{dt}{t^2 + t + \frac{1}{4} + 1 - \frac{1}{4}}$

$= x - \int \frac{dt}{\left(t + \frac{1}{2}\right)^2 + \left(\frac{\sqrt{3}}{2}\right)^2}$

$\Rightarrow I = x - \frac{2}{\sqrt{3}}\tan^{-1}\left(\frac{t + \frac{1}{2}}{\frac{\sqrt{3}}{2}}\right) + C$

$\Rightarrow I = x - \frac{2}{\sqrt{3}}\tan^{-1}\left(\frac{2\tan x + 1}{\sqrt{3}}\right) + C$

$\therefore$ $A = 3$ and $K = 2$

88. **(b)** Suppose, $\frac{x-4}{x+2} = y \Rightarrow x - 4 = y(x+2)$

$\Rightarrow x(1-y) = 2y + 4 \Rightarrow x = \frac{2y+4}{1-y}$

So, $f(y) = 2\left(\frac{2y+4}{1-y}\right) + 1$

Now, $f(x) = 2\left(\frac{2x+4}{1-x}\right) + 1 = \frac{3x+9}{1-x}$

$= \frac{3(x+3)}{1-x} = \frac{3(x-1+4)}{1-x} = -3 + \frac{12}{1-x}$

$\therefore \int f(x)\,dx = -12\log_e|1-x| - 3x + c$

89. **(a)** $\because 7 - 6x - x^2 = 16 - (x+3)^2$

and $\frac{d}{dx}(7 - 6x - x^2) = -2x - 6$

So, $\int \frac{2x+5}{\sqrt{7-6x-x^2}}dx = \int \frac{2x+6}{\sqrt{7-6x-x^2}}dx$

$-\int \frac{1}{\sqrt{16-(x+3)^2}}dx$

$= -2\sqrt{7-6x-x^2} - \sin^{-1}\left(\frac{x+3}{4}\right) + C$

Therefore, $A = -2$, & $B = -1$.

90. (c) Let, $I = \int_{-\pi/2}^{\pi/2} \frac{\sin^2 x}{1+2^x} dx$ ...(i)

Using, $\int_a^b f(x)dx = \int_a^b f(a+b-x)dx$, we get :

$I = \int_{-\pi/2}^{\pi/2} \frac{\sin^2 x}{1+2^{-x}} dx$ ...(ii)

Adding (i) and (ii), we get;

$2I = \int_{-\pi/2}^{\pi/2} \sin^2 x\, dx \Rightarrow 2I = 2\cdot \int_0^{x/2} \sin^2 x\, dx$

$\Rightarrow \quad 2I = 2\times\frac{\pi}{4} \Rightarrow I = \frac{\pi}{4}$

91. (a) $f(x) = \int_0^x t(\sin x - \sin t)\cdot dt$

$= \sin x \int_0^x t\cdot dt - \int_0^x t \sin t \cdot dt$

$= \frac{x^2}{2} \sin x + [t \cos t]_0^x + \sin x$

$\Rightarrow f(x) = \frac{x^2}{2} \sin x + x \cos x + \sin x$

$f'(x) = \frac{x^2}{2} \cos x + 2 \cos x$

$f''(x) = x \cos x - \frac{x^2}{2} \sin x - 2 \sin x$

$f'''(x) = \cos x - 2x \sin x - \frac{x^2}{2} \cos x - 2 \cos x$

$\therefore f'''(x) + f'(x) = \cos x - 2x \sin x$

92. (a) Let $I = \int_{\frac{\pi}{4}}^{\frac{3\pi}{4}} \frac{x}{1+\sin x} dx$

also let $K = \frac{x}{1+\sin x}$

Multiplying numerator and denominator by $(1 - \sin x)$, we get;

$K = \frac{x(1-\sin x)}{1-(\sin x)^2} = \frac{x(1-\sin x)}{(\cos x)^2}$

$= x(1 - \sin x)\sec^2 x$

$= x \sec^2 x - x \sin x \sec^2 x = x \sec^2 x - x \tan x \sec x$

Now, $I = \int_{\frac{\pi}{4}}^{\frac{3\pi}{4}} x \sec^2 x dx - \int_{\frac{\pi}{4}}^{\frac{3\pi}{4}} x \sec x \tan x dx$

$= \left[x \tan x - \int \frac{dx}{dx} \tan x dx\right]_{\frac{\pi}{4}}^{\frac{3\pi}{4}} - \left[x \sec x - \int \frac{dx}{dx} \sec x dx\right]_{\frac{\pi}{4}}^{\frac{3\pi}{4}}$

$= [x \tan x - \ln|\sec x|]_{\frac{\pi}{4}}^{\frac{3\pi}{4}}$

$-[x \sec x - \ln|\sec x + \tan x|]_{\frac{\pi}{4}}^{\frac{3\pi}{4}} + c$

$\Rightarrow I = \left\{\left[\frac{3\pi}{4} \tan \frac{3\pi}{4} - \ln\left|\frac{3\pi}{4}\right|\right.\right.$

$\left.\left. - \left[\frac{3\pi}{4} \sec \frac{3\pi}{4} - \ln\left|\sec \frac{3\pi}{4} + \tan \frac{3\pi}{4}\right|\right]\right]\right\}$

$-\left\{\left[\frac{\pi}{4} \tan \frac{\pi}{4} - \ln\left|\frac{\pi}{4}\right|\right.\right.$

$\left.\left. - \left[\frac{\pi}{4} \sec \frac{\pi}{4} - \ln\left|\sec \frac{\pi}{4} + \tan \frac{\pi}{4}\right|\right]\right]\right\}$

$= \frac{\pi}{2}(\sqrt{2} + 1)$

93. (d) Given:

$I_1 = \int_0^1 e^{-x} \cos^2 x\, dx;$

$I_2 = \int_0^1 e^{-x^2} \cos^2 x\, dx$ and

$I_3 = \int_0^1 e^{-x^3} dx$

For $x \in (0, 1)$

$\Rightarrow x > x^2$ or $-x < -x^2$

and $x^2 > x^3$ or $-x^2 < -x^3$

$\therefore e^{-x^2} < e^{-x^3}$ and $e^{-x} < e^{-x^2}$

$\Rightarrow e^{-x} < e^{-x^2} < e^{-x^3}$

$\Rightarrow e^{-x^3} > e^{-x^2} > e^{-x}$

$\Rightarrow I_3 > I_2 > I_1$

94. (c) Let

$I = \int_{-\frac{\pi}{2}}^{\frac{\pi}{2}} \sin^4 x\left(1 + \log\left(\frac{2+\sin x}{2-\sin x}\right)\right) dx$ ..... (1)

$\Rightarrow I = \int_{-\frac{\pi}{2}}^{\frac{\pi}{2}} \sin^4(-x))\left(1 + \log\left(\frac{2+\sin(-x)}{2-\sin(-x)}\right)\right)\cdot dx$

$= \left[\because \int_a^b f(x).dx = \int_a^b f(a+b-x).dx\right]$

$= \int_{-\frac{\pi}{2}}^{\frac{\pi}{2}} (\sin^4 x)\left(1 + \log\left(\frac{2-\sin x}{2+\sin x}\right)\right).dx$

$$= \int_{-\frac{\pi}{2}}^{\frac{\pi}{2}} \sin^4 x \left(1 - \log\left(\frac{2+\sin x}{2-\sin x}\right)\right).dx \text{.....(2)}$$

After adding equation (1) and (2) we get,

$$2I = 2\int_{-\frac{\pi}{2}}^{\frac{\pi}{2}} \sin^4 x\,.dx$$

$$2I = 4\int_{0}^{\frac{\pi}{2}} \sin^4 x\,.dx$$

$$I = 2\int_{0}^{\frac{\pi}{2}} \sin^4 x\,.dx = \frac{2\times\frac{3}{2}\times\frac{1}{2}\times\pi}{2\times2} = \frac{3\pi}{8}$$

[By Gamma function]

95. **(d)** Here, $18x^2 - 9\pi x + \pi^2 = 0$

$\Rightarrow (3x - \pi)(6x - \pi) = 0$

$\Rightarrow \alpha = \frac{\pi}{6}, \beta = \frac{\pi}{3}$

Also, $gof(x) = \cos x$

$\therefore$ Req. area $= \int_{\pi/6}^{\pi/3} \cos x dx = \frac{\sqrt{3}-1}{2}$

96. **(b)** The intersection point of $y = x^2$ and $y = \frac{1}{x}$ is (1, 1)

Area bounded by the curves is the region ABCDA is given as:

$$\text{Area} = \int_0^1 x^2\,dx + \int_1^t \frac{1}{x}\,dx$$

$$= \left[\frac{x^3}{3}\right]_0^1 + [\ln(x)]_1^t = \frac{1}{3} + \ln(t)$$

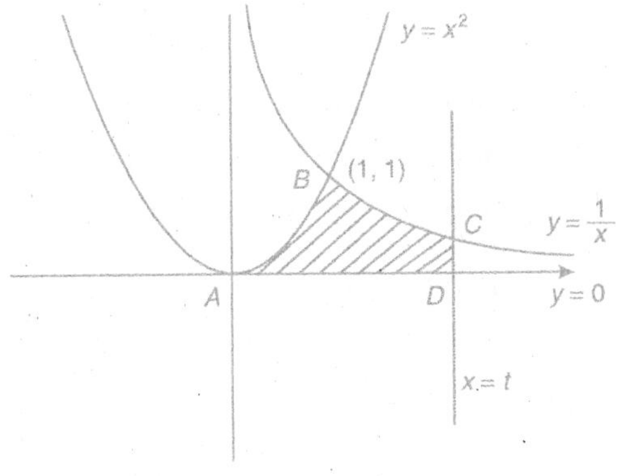

$\because$ area = 1.

$\Rightarrow \frac{1}{3} + \ln(t) = 1 \quad \Rightarrow \ln(t) = \frac{2}{3} \quad \Rightarrow t = e^{\frac{2}{3}}$

97. **(b)** The intersection point of $y = x - 2$ and $y = \sqrt{x}$ is (4, 2). The required area

$$= \int_0^4 \sqrt{x}dx - \frac{1}{2}\times2\times2 = \frac{16}{3} - 2 = \frac{10}{3}$$

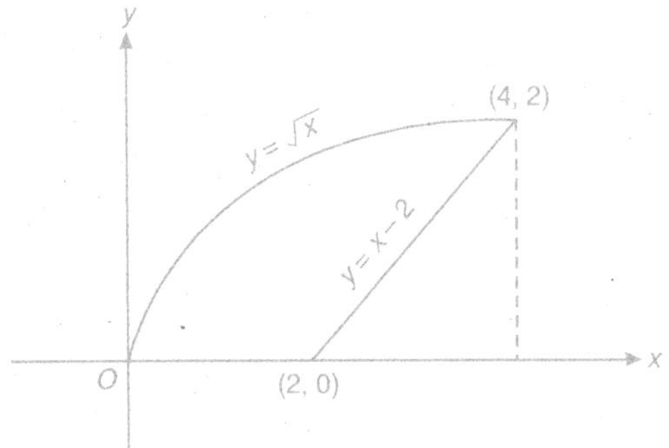

98. **(c)** $\frac{x^2}{a^2} + \frac{y^2}{b^2} = 1$

Since, it passes through (0, 3)

$\therefore \frac{0}{a^2} + \frac{9}{b^2} = 1$

$\Rightarrow b^2 = 9$

$\therefore$ eq. of ellipse becomes:

$$\frac{x^2}{a^2} + \frac{y^2}{9} = 1$$

differential w.r.t. x, we get;

$$\frac{2x}{a^2} + \frac{2y}{9}\frac{dy}{dx} = 0$$

$$\Rightarrow \frac{y}{x}\left(\frac{dy}{dx}\right) = \frac{-9}{a^2}$$

Again differentiating w.r.t. x, we get;

$$\frac{y}{x}\frac{d^2y}{dx^2} + \frac{x\frac{dy}{dx} - y}{x^2}\frac{dy}{dx} = 0$$

$\Rightarrow xyy'' + x(y')^2 - yy' = 0$

99. **(b)** Consider the given differential equation the $\sin x dy + y\cos x dx = 4x dx$

$\Rightarrow d(y.\sin x) = 4x dx$

Integrate both sides

$\Rightarrow y.\sin x = 2x^2 + C$ ...(1)

$\Rightarrow y(x) = \frac{2x^2}{\sin x} + c$ ...(2)

$\because$ eq. (2) passes through $\left(\frac{\pi}{2}, 0\right)$

$$\Rightarrow 0 = \frac{\pi^2}{2} + C$$

$$\Rightarrow C = -\frac{\pi^2}{2}$$

Now, put the value of C in (1)

Then, $y \sin x = 2x^2 - \frac{\pi^2}{2}$ is the solution

$$\therefore y\left(\frac{\pi}{6}\right) = \left(2.\frac{\pi^2}{36} - \frac{\pi^2}{2}\right)2 = -\frac{8\pi^2}{9}$$

100. (a) When $x \in [0, 1]$, then $\frac{dy}{dx} + 2y = 1 \Rightarrow y = \frac{1}{2} + C_1 e^{-2x}$

$$\because y(0) = 0 \Rightarrow y(x) = \frac{1}{2} - \frac{1}{2}e^{-2x}$$

Here, $y(1) = \frac{1}{2} - \frac{1}{2}e^{-2} = \frac{e^2 - 1}{2e^2}$

When $x \notin [0, 1]$, then $\frac{dy}{dx} + 2y = 0 \Rightarrow y = c_2 e^{-2x}$

$$\because y(1) = \frac{e^2 - 1}{2} \Rightarrow \frac{e^2 - 1}{2} = c^2 e^{-2} \Rightarrow C_2 = \frac{e^2 - 1}{2}$$

$$\therefore y(x)\left(\frac{e^2 - 1}{2}\right)e^{-2x} \Rightarrow y\left(\frac{3}{2}\right) = \frac{e^2 - 1}{2e^3}$$

101. (b) $(x^2 - y^2)\,dx + 2xydy = 0$

$$\Rightarrow \frac{dy}{dx} = \frac{y^2 - x^2}{2xy}$$

Let $y = vx$

$$\frac{dy}{dx} = v + x\frac{dv}{dx}$$

$$\Rightarrow v + x\frac{dv}{dx} = \frac{v^2x^2 - x^2}{2vx^2} \Rightarrow v + x\frac{dv}{dx} = \frac{v^2 - 1}{2v}$$

$$\Rightarrow x\frac{dv}{dx} = \frac{-v^2 - 1}{2v}$$

$$\Rightarrow \frac{2vdv}{v^2 + 1} = -\frac{dx}{x}$$

After integrating, we get

$ln\,|v^2 + 1| = -ln\,|x| + lnc$

$$\frac{y^2}{x^2} + 1 = \frac{c}{x}$$

As curve passes through the point (1, 1), so $1 + 1 = c$

$\Rightarrow c = 2$

$x^2 + y^2 - 2x = 0$, which is a circle of radius one.

102. (b) Suppose angular bisector of A meets BC at D (x, y, z)

Using angular bisector theorem,

$$\frac{AB}{AC} = \frac{BD}{DC}$$

$$\frac{BD}{DC} = \frac{\sqrt{(4-2)^2 + (7-3)^2 + (8-4)^2}}{\sqrt{(4-2)^2 + (7-5)^2 + (8-7)^2}}$$

$$= \frac{\sqrt{2^2 + 4^2 + 4^2}}{\sqrt{2^2 + 2^2 + 1^2}} = \frac{6}{3} = 2$$

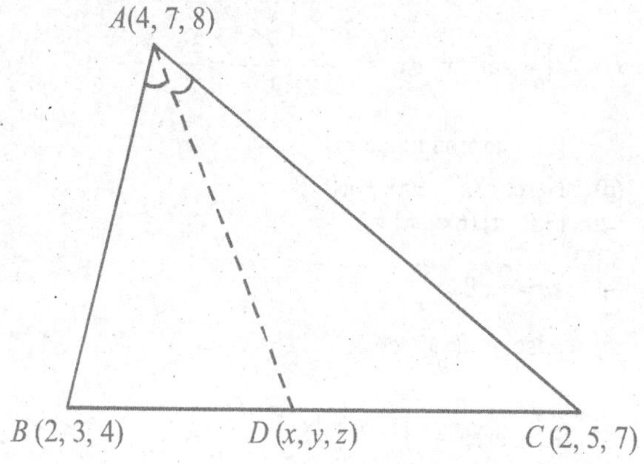

$$\text{So, } D(x, y, z) \equiv \left(\frac{(2)(2) + (1)(2)}{2+1}, \frac{(2)(5) + (1)(3)}{2+1}, \frac{(2)(7) + (1)(4)}{2+1}\right)$$

$$D(x, y, z) \equiv \left(\frac{6}{3}, \frac{13}{3}, \frac{18}{3}\right)$$

Therefore, position vector of point $P = \frac{1}{3}(6i + 13j + 18k)$

103. (d) $\because \vec{u}, \vec{a}$ & $\vec{b}$ are coplanar

$$\therefore \vec{u} = \lambda(\vec{a} \times \vec{b}) \times \vec{a} = \lambda\{\vec{a}^2.\vec{b} - (\vec{a}.\vec{b})\vec{a}\}$$

$$= \lambda\{-4\hat{i} + 8\hat{j} + 16\hat{k}\} = \lambda'\{-\hat{i} + 2\hat{j} + 4\hat{k}\}.$$

Also, $\vec{u}.\vec{b} = 24 \Rightarrow \lambda' = 4$

$$\therefore \quad \vec{u} = -4\hat{i} + 8\hat{j} + 16\hat{k}$$

$$\Rightarrow \quad |\vec{u}|^2 = 336$$

104. (a) $\because \vec{a} = \hat{i} + \hat{j} + \hat{k} \Rightarrow |\vec{a}| = \sqrt{3}$

& $\vec{c} = \hat{j} - \hat{k} \Rightarrow |\vec{c}|\sqrt{2}$

Now, $\vec{a} \times \vec{b} = \vec{c}$ (Given)

$$\Rightarrow |\vec{a}||\vec{b}| \sin\theta = |\vec{c}|$$

$\Rightarrow |\vec{a}||\vec{b}|\sin\theta = \sqrt{2}$ ...[i]

Also $\vec{a}\cdot\vec{b} = 3$

$\Rightarrow |\vec{a}||\vec{b}|\cos\theta = 3$ ....[ii]

Dividing [i] by [ii], we get

$\tan\theta = \frac{\sqrt{2}}{3} \quad \therefore \sin\theta = \frac{\sqrt{2}}{\sqrt{11}}$

Substituting value of $\sin\theta$ in [i] we get

$\sqrt{3}|\vec{b}|\frac{\sqrt{2}}{\sqrt{11}} = \sqrt{2}$

$|\vec{b}| = \frac{\sqrt{11}}{\sqrt{3}}$

105. (b) $\because \vec{a} + 2\vec{b} + 2\vec{c} = \vec{0}$ [Given]

$\Rightarrow \vec{a} + 2\vec{c} = -2\vec{b} \Rightarrow (\vec{a}+2\vec{c})\cdot(\vec{a}+2\vec{c}) = (-2\vec{b})(-2\vec{b})$

$\Rightarrow \vec{a}\cdot\vec{a} + 4\vec{c}\cdot\vec{c} + 4\vec{a}\cdot\vec{c} = 4\vec{b}\cdot\vec{b} \Rightarrow 1 + 4 + 4\vec{a}\cdot\vec{c} = 4$

$\Rightarrow \vec{a}\cdot\vec{c} = \frac{-1}{4}$

$\because |\vec{a}\cdot\vec{c}|^2 + |\vec{a}\times\vec{c}|^2 = 1$ ($\vec{a}$ is unit vector)

$\Rightarrow \frac{1}{16} + |\vec{a}\times\vec{c}|^2 = 1$

$\Rightarrow |\vec{a}\times\vec{c}|^2 = \frac{15}{16} \Rightarrow |\vec{a}\times\vec{c}| = \frac{\sqrt{15}}{4}$

106. (b) Given

$l + 3m + 5n = 0$ (1)

and $5lm - 2mn + 6nl = 0$ (2)

From eq. (1) we have

$l = -3m - 5n$

Put the value of l in eq. (2), we get;

$5(-3m - 5n)m - 2mn + 6n(-3m - 5n) = 0$

$\Rightarrow 15m^2 + 45mn + 30n^2 = 0$

$\Rightarrow m^2 + 3mn + 2n^2 = 0$

$\Rightarrow m^2 + 2mn + mn + 2n^2 = 0$

$\Rightarrow (m+n)(m+2n) = 0$

$\therefore m = -n$ or $m = -2n$

For $m = -n, l = -2n$

And for $m = -2n, l = n$

$\therefore (l, m, n) = (-2n, -n, n)$ Or $(l, m, n) = (n, -2n, n)$

$\Rightarrow (l, m, n) = (-2, -1, 1)$ Or $(l, m, n) = (1, -2, 1)$

Therefore, angle between the lines is given as:

$$\cos(\theta) = \frac{(-2)(1) + (-1).(-2) + (1)(1)}{\sqrt{6}.\sqrt{6}}$$

$$\Rightarrow \cos(\theta) = \frac{1}{6} \Rightarrow \theta = \cos^{-1}\left(\frac{1}{6}\right)$$

107. (d) Let θ be the angle between the two lines

Here direction cosines of $\frac{x}{2} = \frac{y}{2} = \frac{z}{1}$ are 2, 2, 1

Also second line can be written as:

$$\frac{x-5}{2} = \frac{y-2}{\frac{P}{7}} = \frac{z-3}{4}$$

$\therefore$ its direction cosines are $2, \frac{P}{7}, 4$

Also, $\cos\theta = \frac{2}{3}$ (Given)

$$\because \cos\theta = \left|\frac{a_1a_2 + b_1b_2 + c_1c_2}{\sqrt{a_1^2 + b_1^2 + c_1^2}\sqrt{a_2^2 + b_2^2 + c_2^2}}\right|$$

$$\Rightarrow \frac{2}{3} = \left|\frac{(2\times 2) + \left(2\times\frac{P}{7}\right) + (1\times 4)}{\sqrt{2^2 + 2^2 + 1^2}\sqrt{2^2 + \frac{P^2}{49} + 4^2}}\right|$$

$$= \frac{4 + \frac{2P}{7} + 4}{3\times\sqrt{2^2 + \frac{P^2}{49} + 4^2}}$$

$$\Rightarrow \left(4 + \frac{P}{7}\right)^2 = 20 + \frac{P^2}{49} \Rightarrow 16 + \frac{8P}{7} + \frac{P^2}{49} = 20 + \frac{P^2}{49}$$

$$\Rightarrow \frac{8P}{7} = 4 \Rightarrow P = \frac{7}{2}$$

108. (c)

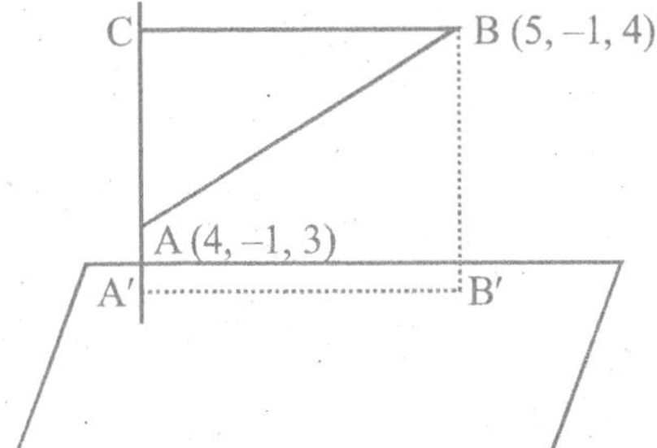

$$AC = \overrightarrow{AB}.\hat{AC} = (\hat{i} + \hat{k}).\frac{(\hat{i} + \hat{j} + \hat{k})}{\sqrt{3}} = \frac{2}{\sqrt{3}}$$

Now, $A'B' = BC = \sqrt{AB^2 - AC^2} = \sqrt{2 - \frac{4}{3}} = \sqrt{\frac{2}{3}}$

$\therefore$ Length of projection $= \sqrt{\frac{2}{3}}$

109. (a) Equation of plane passing through the line of intersection of first two planes is:

$$(2x-2y+3z-2)+\lambda(x-y+z+1)=0$$

or $x(\lambda+2)-y(2+\lambda)+z(\lambda+3)+(\lambda-2)=0$ ...(i)

is having infinite number of solution with $x+2y-z-3=0$ and $3x-y+2z-1=0$, then

$$\begin{vmatrix} (\lambda+2) & -(\lambda+2) & (\lambda+3) \\ 1 & 2 & -1 \\ 3 & -1 & 2 \end{vmatrix}=0$$

$\Rightarrow \lambda=5$

Now put $\lambda=5$ in (i), we get

$7x-7y+8z+3=0$

Now perpendicular distance from (0, 0, 0) to the place containing L_1 and $L_2=\frac{3}{\sqrt{162}}=\frac{1}{3\sqrt{2}}$

110. (c) Equation of plane passing through three given points is:

$$\begin{vmatrix} x-x_1 & y-y_1 & z-z_1 \\ x_2-x_1 & y_2-y_1 & z_2-z_1 \\ x_3-x_1 & y_3-y_1 & z_3-z_1 \end{vmatrix}=0$$

$$\Rightarrow \begin{vmatrix} x+2 & y+2 & z-2 \\ 1+2 & -1+2 & 2-2 \\ 1+2 & 1+2 & 1-2 \end{vmatrix}=0$$

$$\Rightarrow \begin{vmatrix} x+2 & y+2 & z-2 \\ 3 & 1 & 0 \\ 3 & 3 & -1 \end{vmatrix}=0$$

$\Rightarrow -x+3y+6z-8=0$

$\Rightarrow \frac{x}{8}-\frac{3y}{8}-\frac{6z}{8}+\frac{8}{8}=0$

$\Rightarrow \frac{x}{8}-\frac{y}{\frac{8}{3}}-\frac{z}{\frac{8}{6}}=-1$

$\Rightarrow \frac{x}{-8}+\frac{y}{\frac{8}{3}}+\frac{z}{\frac{8}{6}}=1$

$\therefore$ Sum of intercepts $=-8+\frac{8}{3}+\frac{8}{6}=-4$

111. (c) If a, b, c are the intercepts of the variable plane on the x, y, z axes respectively, then the equation of the plane is

$\frac{x}{a}+\frac{y}{b}+\frac{z}{c}=1$

And the point of intersection of the planes parallel to the xy, yz and zx planes is (a, b, c).

As the point (3, 2, 1) lies on the variable plane, so

$\frac{3}{a}+\frac{2}{b}+\frac{1}{c}=1$

Therefore, the required locus is $\frac{3}{x}+\frac{2}{y}+\frac{1}{z}=1$

112. (d) Normal to $3x+4y+z=1$ is $3\hat{i}+4\hat{j}+\hat{k}$.

Normal to $5x+8y+2z=-14$ is $5\hat{i}+8\hat{j}+2\hat{k}$

The line of intersection of the planes is perpendicular to both normals, so, direction ratios of the intersection line are directly proportional to the cross product of the normal vectors.

Therefore the direction ratios of the line is $-\hat{j}+4\hat{k}$

Hence the angle between the plane $x+y+z+5=0$ and the intersection line is $\sin^{-1}\left(\frac{-1+4}{\sqrt{17}\sqrt{3}}\right)=\sin^{-1}\left(\sqrt{\frac{3}{17}}\right)$

113. (a) Since the plane bisects the line joining the points (1, 2, 3) and (–3, 4, 5) then the plane passes through the midpoint of the line which is :

$$\left(\frac{1-3}{2},\frac{2+4}{2},\frac{5+3}{2}\right)\equiv\left(\frac{-2}{2},\frac{6}{2},\frac{8}{2}\right)\equiv(-1,3,4).$$

As plane cuts the line segment at right angle, so the direction cosines of the normal of the plane are $(-3-1, 4-2, 5-3)=(-4, 2, 2)$

So the equation of the plane is : $-4x+2y+2z=\lambda$

As plane passes through (– 1, 3, 4) so

$-4(-1)+2(3)+2(4)=\lambda \Rightarrow \lambda=18$

Therefore, equation of plane is : $-4x+2y+2z=18$

Now, only (– 3, 2, 1) satisfies the given plane as $-4(-3)+2(2)+2(1)=18$

114. (a) Let R_t be the even of drawing red ball in t^{th} draw and B_t be the event of drawing black ball in t^{th} draw.

Now, in the given bag there are 4 red and 6 black balls.

$\therefore \quad P(R_1)=\frac{4}{10}$ and $P(B_1)=\frac{6}{10}$

And, $P\left(\frac{R_2}{R_1}\right)=\frac{6}{12}$ and $P\left(\frac{R_2}{B_1}\right)=\frac{4}{12}$

Now, required probability

$=P(R_1)\times P\left(\frac{R_2}{R_1}\right)+P(B_1)\times P\left(\frac{R_2}{B_1}\right)$

$=\left(\frac{4}{10}\times\frac{6}{12}\right)+\left(\frac{6}{10}\times\frac{4}{12}\right)=\frac{2}{5}$

115. (c) Here, $P(\bar{A} \cap \bar{B} | C) = \dfrac{P(\bar{A} \cap \bar{B} \cap C)}{P(C)}$.

$$= \frac{P(C) - P(A \cap C - P(B \cap C) + P(A \cap B \cap C))}{P(C)}$$

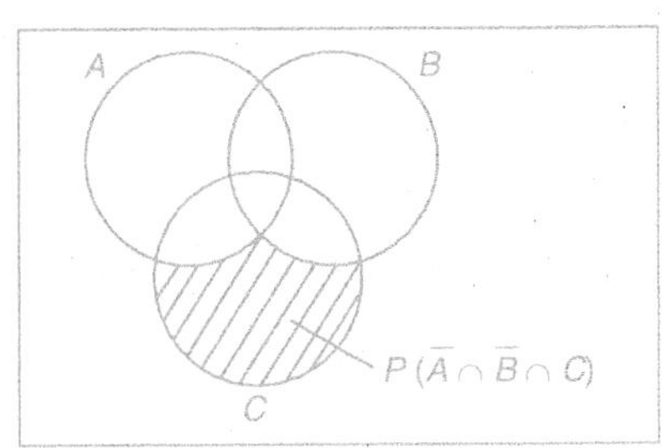

$$= 1 - \left[\frac{P(A).P(C) + P(B).P(C)}{P(C)}\right]$$

$= 1 - P(A) - P(B) = P(\bar{A}) - P(B)(\because P(A \cap B \cap C) = 0)$

116. (a) If the outcome is one of the following: *H, TTH, TTTTH*, ..., then *X* wins.
As subsequent tosses are independent, so the probability that *X* wins is

$$p + \frac{p}{4} + \frac{p}{16} + ... = \frac{4p}{3}.$$

Similarly *Y* wins if the outcome is one of the following: *TH, TTTH, TTTTTH*, ...
Therefore, the probability that *Y* wins is

$$\frac{1-p}{2} + \frac{1-p}{8} + \frac{1-p}{32} = \frac{2(1-p)}{3}$$

Since, the probability of winning the game by both the players is equal then, we have

$$\frac{4p}{3} = \frac{2(1-p)}{3} \Rightarrow p = \frac{1}{3}$$

117. (d)

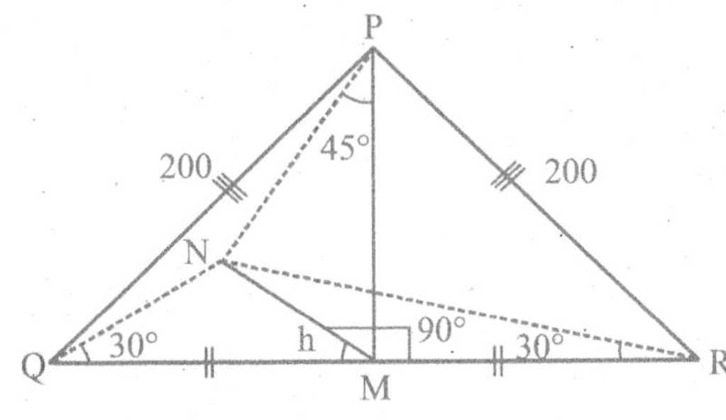

Let height of tower MN = h
In ΔQMN we have

$$\tan 30° = \frac{MN}{QM}$$

$\therefore$ $QM = \sqrt{3}h = MR$ ...(1)

Now in ΔMNP
MN = PM ...(2)
In ΔPMQ we have :

$$MP = \sqrt{(200)^2 - (\sqrt{3}h)^2}$$

$\therefore$ From (2), we get :

$$\sqrt{(200)^2 - (\sqrt{3}h)^2} = h \Rightarrow h = 100m$$

118. (a) Here; $\angle DOA = 45°$; $\angle DOB = 60°$
Now, let height of tower = *h*.

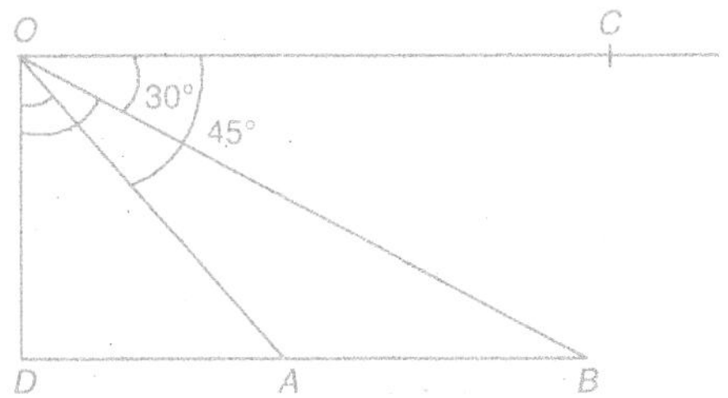

In ΔDOA, $\tan(\angle DOA) = \dfrac{DA}{OD}$

$$\Rightarrow \tan 45° = \frac{DA}{h} \Rightarrow h = DA$$

Now, in Δ DOB

$$\tan(\angle DOB) = \frac{BD}{OD}$$

$$\Rightarrow \tan 60° = \frac{BD}{h} \Rightarrow BD = \sqrt{3}\,h.$$

$\therefore$ speed for the distance BA $= \dfrac{BD - AD}{18} = \dfrac{(\sqrt{3}-1)h}{18}$

$\therefore$ required time taken

$$= \frac{AD}{\text{speed}} = \frac{h \times 18}{(\sqrt{3}-1)h} = \frac{18}{\sqrt{3}-1} = 9(\sqrt{3}+1)$$

119. (d) For Δ OA, A, $OA_1 = \dfrac{\sqrt{3}}{\tan 60°} = 1$ km.

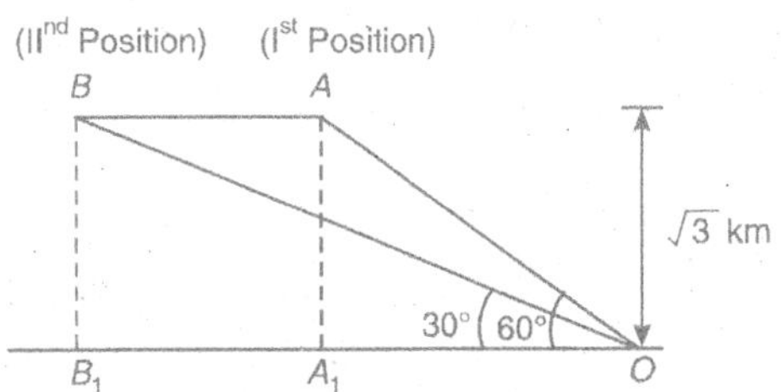

For Δ OB_1, B, $OB_1 = \dfrac{\sqrt{3}}{\tan 30°} = 3$ *km*.

As, a distance of 3 – 1 = 2 km is covered in 5 seconds. Therefore the speed of the plane is

$$\frac{2 \times 3600}{5} = 1440 \text{ km/hr}$$

120. (d) Let the distance between T_1 and T_2 be x

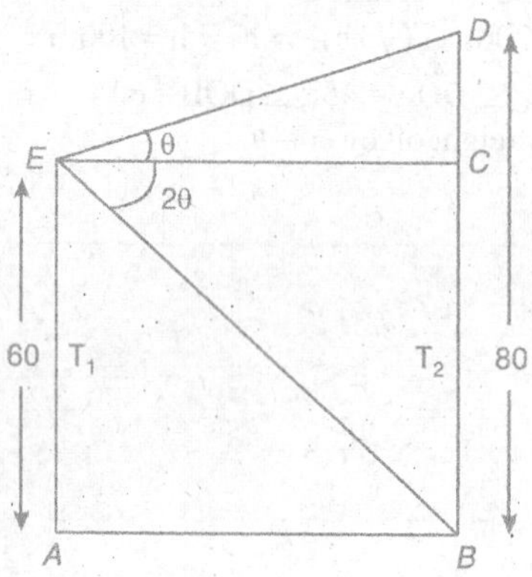

From the figure

$EA = 60$ m (T_1) and $DB = 80$ m (T_2)

$\angle DEC = \theta$ and $\angle BEC = 2\theta$

Now in ΔDEC,

$$\tan\theta = \frac{DC}{AB} = \frac{20}{x}$$

and in ΔBEC,

$$\tan 2\theta = \frac{BC}{CE} = \frac{60}{x}$$

We know that

$$\tan 2\theta = \frac{2\tan\theta}{1-(\tan\theta)^2}$$

$$\Rightarrow \frac{60}{x} = \frac{2\left(\frac{20}{x}\right)}{1-\left(\frac{20}{x}\right)^2}$$

$$\Rightarrow x^2 = 1200 \Rightarrow x = 20\sqrt{3}$$

Sets

TOPIC-1 : Sets, Types of Sets, Disjoint Sets, Complementary Sets, Subsets, Power Set, Cardinal Number of Sets, Operations on Sets

1. If $f(x) + 2f\left(\frac{1}{x}\right) = 3x, x \neq 0$ and

   $S = \{x \in R : f(x) = f(-x)\}$; then S: **[2016]**
   (a) contains exactly two elements.
   (b) contains more than two elements.
   (c) is an empty set.
   (d) contains exactly one element.

2. Let $P = \{\theta : \sin\theta - \cos\theta = \sqrt{2}\cos\theta\}$ and $Q = \{\theta : \sin\theta + \cos\theta = \sqrt{2}\sin\theta\}$ be two sets. Then : **[Online April 10, 2016]**
   (a) $P \subset Q$ and $Q - P \neq \phi$
   (b) $Q \not\subset P$
   (c) $P = Q$
   (d) $P \not\subset Q$

3. A relation on the set $A = \{x : |x| < 3, x \in Z\}$, where Z is the set of integers is defined by $R = \{(x, y) : y = |x|, x \neq -1\}$. Then the number of elements in the power set of R is: **[Online April 12, 2014]**
   (a) 32 (b) 16
   (c) 8 (d) 64

4. Let $X = \{1,2,3,4,5\}$. The number of different ordered pairs (Y,Z) that can formed such that $Y \subseteq X$, $Z \subseteq X$ and $Y \cap Z$ is empty is : **[2012]**
   (a) 5^2 (b) 3^5
   (c) 2^5 (d) 5^3

5. If *A*, *B* and *C* are three sets such that $A \cap B = A \cap C$ and $A \cup B = A \cup C$, then **[2009]**
   (a) $A = C$ (b) $B = C$
   (c) $A \cap B = \phi$ (d) $A = B$

TOPIC- 2 : Venn Diagrams, Algebraic Operations on Sets, De Morgan's Law, Number of Elements in Different Sets

6. In a certain town, 25% of the families own a phone and 15% own a car; 65% families own neither a phone nor a car and 2,000 families own both a car and a phone. Consider the following three statements : **[Online April 10, 2015]**
   (A) 5% families own both a car and a phone
   (B) 35% families own either a car or a phone
   (C) 40,000 families live in the town

   Then,
   (a) Only (A) and (C) are correct.
   (b) Only (B) and (C) are correct.
   (c) All (A), (B) and (C) are correct.
   (d) Only (A) and (B) are correct.

Hints & Solutions

1. **(a)** $f(x)+2f\left(\frac{1}{x}\right)=3x$ ....(1)

$f\left(\frac{1}{x}\right)+2f(x)=\frac{3}{x}$ ....(2)

Adding (1) and (2) $\Rightarrow f(x)+f\left(\frac{1}{x}\right)=x+\frac{1}{x}$

Substracting (1) from (2) $\Rightarrow f(x)-f\left(\frac{1}{x}\right)=\frac{3}{x}-3x$

On adding the above equations

$\Rightarrow f(x)=\frac{2}{x}-x$

$f(x)=f(-x)\Rightarrow\frac{2}{x}-x=\frac{-2}{x}+x\Rightarrow x=\frac{2}{x}$

$x^2=2$ or $x=\sqrt{2},-\sqrt{2}$.

2. **(c)** $\sin\theta-\cos\theta=\sqrt{2}\cos\theta$

$\Rightarrow\ \sin\theta=\cos\theta+\sqrt{2}\cos\theta$

$=(\sqrt{2}+1)\cos\theta=\left(\frac{2-1}{\sqrt{2}-1}\right)\cos\theta$

$\Rightarrow\ (\sqrt{2}-1)\sin\theta=\cos\theta$

$\Rightarrow\ \sin\theta+\cos\theta=\sqrt{2}\sin\theta$

$\therefore\ P=Q$

3. **(b)** $A=\{x:|x|<3,\ x\in Z\}$

$A=\{-2,-1,0,1,2\}$

$R=\{(x,y):y=|x|,\ x\neq-1\}$

$R=\{(-2,2),(0,0),(1,1),(2,2)\}$

R has four elements

Number of elements in the power set of R

$=2^4=16$

4. **(b)** Let $X=\{1,2,3,4,5\}$

Total no. of elements = 5

Each element has 3 options. Either set Y or set Z or none. ($\because Y\cap Z=\phi$)

So, number of ordered pairs = 3^5

5. **(b)** Let $x\in A$ and $x\in B\Leftrightarrow x\in A\cup B$

$\Leftrightarrow x\in A\cup C\quad(\because A\cup B=A\cup C)$

$\Leftrightarrow x\in C$

$\therefore\ B=C.$

Let $x\in A$ and $x\in B\Leftrightarrow x\in A\cap B$

$\Leftrightarrow x\in A\cap C\quad(\because A\cap B=A\cap C)$

$\Leftrightarrow x\in C$

$\therefore B=C$

6. **(c)** $n(P)=25\%$

$n(C)=15\%$

$n(P'\cup C')=65\%$

$\Rightarrow n(P\cup C)'=65\%$

$n(P\cup C)=35\%$

$n(P\cap C)=n(P)+n(C)-n(P\cup C)$

$25+15-35=5\%$

$x\times5\%=2000$

$x=40{,}000$

Chapter 2 Relations and Functions

TOPIC-1 : Relations, Domain, Codomain and Range of a Relation, Functions, Domain, Codomain and Range of a Function

1. The range of the function

$f(x)=\frac{x}{1+|x|}$, $x \in R$, is **[Online May 7, 2012]**

(a) R (b) $(-1, 1)$

(c) $R-\{0\}$ (d) $[-1, 1]$

2. The domain of the function $f(x)=\frac{1}{\sqrt{|x|-x}}$ is **[2011]**

(a) $(0, \infty)$ (b) $(-\infty, 0)$

(c) $(-\infty, \infty)-\{0\}$ (d) $(-\infty, \infty)$

3. Domain of definition of the function

$f(x)=\frac{3}{4-x^2}+\log_{10}(x^3-x)$, is **[2003]**

(a) $(-1,0)\cup(1,2)\cup(2,\infty)$ (b) $(a,2)$

(c) $(-1,0)\cup(a,2)$ (d) $(1,2)\cup(2,\infty)$.

TOPIC-2 : Even and Odd Functions, Explicit and Implicit Functions, Greatest Integer Function, Periodic Functions, Value of a Function, Equal Functions, Algebraic Operations on Functions.

4. Let $f(n)=\left[\frac{1}{3}+\frac{3n}{100}\right]n$, where [n] denotes the greatest integer less than or equal to n. Then $\sum_{n=1}^{56} f(n)$ is equal to:

[Online April 19, 2014]

(a) 56 (b) 689

(c) 1287 (d) 1399

5. Let f be an odd function defined on the set of real numbers such that for $x \geq 0$,

$f(x) = 3 \sin x + 4 \cos x$.

Then f(x) at $x = -\frac{11\pi}{6}$ is equal to:

[Online April 11, 2014]

(a) $\frac{3}{2}+2\sqrt{3}$ (b) $-\frac{3}{2}+2\sqrt{3}$

(c) $\frac{3}{2}-2\sqrt{3}$ (d) $-\frac{3}{2}-2\sqrt{3}$

6. A real valued function $f(x)$ satisfies the functional equation

$f(x-y)=f(x)f(y)-f(a-x)f(a+y)$

where a is a given constant and $f(0) = 1$, $f(2a-x)$ is equal to **[2005]**

(a) $-f(x)$ (b) $f(x)$

(c) $f(a)+f(a-x)$ (d) $f(-x)$

7. The graph of the function $y=f(x)$ is symmetrical about the line $x=2$, then **[2004]**

(a) $f(x)=-f(-x)$ (b) $f(2+x)=f(2-x)$

(c) $f(x)=f(-x)$ (d) $f(x+2)=f(x-2)$

8. If $f: R \to R$ satisfies $f(x+y)=f(x)+f(y)$, for all x, $y \in R$ and $f(1)=7$, then $\sum_{r=1}^{n} f(r)$ is **[2003]**

(a) $\frac{7n(n+1)}{2}$ (b) $\frac{7n}{2}$

(c) $\frac{7(n+1)}{2}$ (d) $7n+(n+1)$.

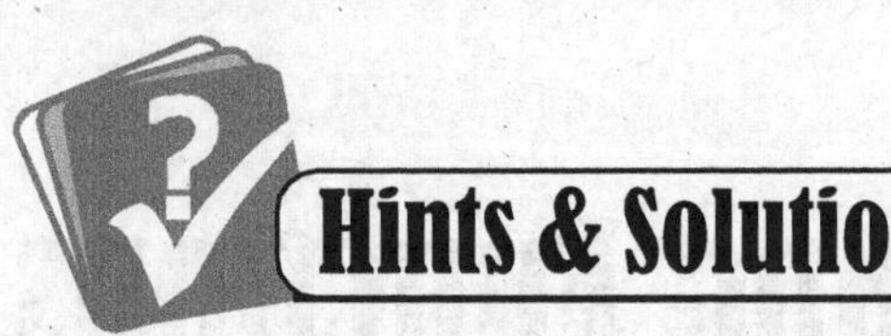

1. (b) $f(x)=\frac{x}{1+|x|}, x \in R$

If $x>0, |x|=x \Rightarrow f(x)=\frac{x}{1+x}$

which is not defined for $x=-1$

If $x<0, |x|=-x \Rightarrow f(x)=\frac{x}{1-x}$

which is not defined for $x=1$

Thus $f(x)$ defined for all values of R except 1 and – 1

Hence, range = (– 1, 1).

2. (b) $f(x)=\frac{1}{\sqrt{|x|-x}}$, define if $|x|-x>0$

$\Rightarrow |x|>x, \Rightarrow x<0$

Hence domain of $f(x)$ is $(-\infty, 0)$

3. (a) $f(x)=\frac{3}{4-x^2}+\log_{10}(x^3-x)$

$4-x^2 \neq 0;\ x^3-x>0;$

$x \neq \pm\sqrt{4}$ and $-1<x<0$ or $1<x<\infty$

– + – +
–1 0 1

$\therefore D=(-1, 0)\cup(1, \infty)-\{\sqrt{4}\}$

$D=(-1, 0)\cup(1, 2)\cup(2, \infty)$.

4. (d) Let $f(n)=\left[\frac{1}{3}+\frac{3n}{100}\right]n$

where $[n]$ is greatest integer function,

$=\left[0.33+\frac{3n}{100}\right]n$

For n = 1, 2, ..., 22, we get $f(n)$ = 0

and for n = 23, 24, ..., 55, we get $f(n)$ = 1

For n = 56, $f(n)$ = 2

So, $\sum_{n=1}^{56} f(n)=1(23)+1(24)+...+1(55)+2(56)$

$=(23+24+...+55)+112$

$=\frac{33}{2}[46+32]+112$

$=\frac{33}{2}(78)+112=1399.$

5. (c) Given f be an odd function

$f(x) = 3\sin x + 4\cos x$

Now,

$f\left(\frac{-11\pi}{6}\right) = 3\sin\left(\frac{-11\pi}{6}\right)+4\cos\left(\frac{-11\pi}{6}\right)$

$f\left(\frac{-11\pi}{6}\right) = 3\sin\left(-2\pi+\frac{\pi}{6}\right)+4\cos\left(-2\pi+\frac{\pi}{6}\right)$

$f\left(\frac{-11\pi}{6}\right) = 3\sin\left\{-\left(2\pi-\frac{\pi}{6}\right)\right\}+4\cos\left\{-\left(2\pi-\frac{\pi}{6}\right)\right\}$

$\left\{\text{For odd functions } \begin{array}{l}\sin(-\theta)=-\sin\theta \\ \text{and} \cos(-\theta)=-\cos\theta\end{array}\right\}$

$\therefore f\left(\frac{-11\pi}{6}\right) = -3\sin\left(2\pi-\frac{\pi}{6}\right)-4\cos\left(2\pi-\frac{\pi}{6}\right)$

$\Rightarrow f\left(\frac{-11\pi}{6}\right) = +3\sin\left(\frac{\pi}{6}\right)-4\cos\frac{\pi}{6}$

$\Rightarrow f\left(\frac{-11\pi}{6}\right) = 3\times\frac{1}{2}-4\times\frac{\sqrt{3}}{2}$

or $f\left(\frac{-11\pi}{6}\right)=\frac{3}{2}-2\sqrt{3}$

6. **(a)** $f(2a-x)=f(a-(x-a))$

$=f(a)f(x-a)-f(0)f(x)=f(a)f(x-a)-f(x)$

$=-f(x)$

$[\because x=0, y=0,\ f(0)=f^2(0)-f^2(a)$

$\Rightarrow f^2(a)=0 \Rightarrow f(a)=0$

$\Rightarrow f(2a-x)=-f(x)$

7. **(b)** Let us consider a graph symm. with respect to line $x=2$ as shown in the figure.

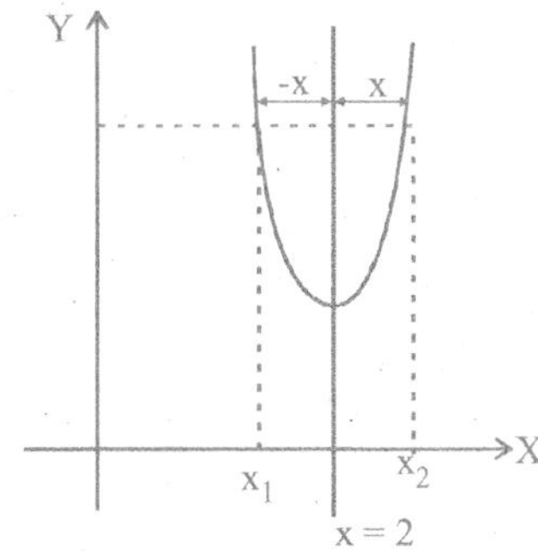

From the figure

$f(x_1)=f(x_2)$, where $x_1=2-x$ and $x_2=2+x$

$\therefore f(2-x)=f(2+x)$

8. **(a)** $f(x+y)=f(x)+f(y)$.

Function should be $f(x)=mx$

$f(1)=7;\ \therefore m=7,\ f(x)=7x$

$\sum_{r=1}^{n} f(r)=7\sum_{1}^{n} r=\frac{7n(n+1)}{2}$

Chapter 3

Trigonometric Functions

TOPIC-1 : Circular System, Trigonometric Ratios, Domain and Range of Trigonometric Functions, Trigonometric Ratios of Allied Angles

1. Let $f_k(x)=\frac{1}{k}\left(\sin^k x+\cos^k x\right)$ where $x\in R$ and $k\geq 1$.

Then $f_4(x)-f_6(x)$ equals **[2014]**

(a) $\frac{1}{4}$ (b) $\frac{1}{12}$

(c) $\frac{1}{6}$ (d) $\frac{1}{3}$

2. If $2\cos q+\sin q=1\left(\theta\neq\frac{\pi}{2}\right)$,

then $7\cos\theta+6\sin\theta$ is equal to: **[Online April 11, 2014]**

(a) $\frac{1}{2}$ (b) 2

(c) $\frac{11}{2}$ (d) $\frac{46}{5}$

3. The expression $\frac{\tan A}{1-\cot A}+\frac{\cot A}{1-\tan A}$

can be written as : **[2013]**

(a) $\sin A\cos A+1$ (b) $\sec A\,\mathrm{cosec}A+1$

(c) $\tan A+\cot A$ (d) $\sec A+\mathrm{cosec}A$

4. The value of $\cos 255°+\sin 195°$ is **[Online May 26, 2012]**

(a) $\frac{\sqrt{3}-1}{2\sqrt{2}}$ (b) $\frac{\sqrt{3}-1}{\sqrt{2}}$

(c) $-\left(\frac{\sqrt{3}-1}{\sqrt{2}}\right)$ (d) $\frac{\sqrt{3}+1}{\sqrt{2}}$

5. Let $f(x)=\sin x$, $g(x)=x$.

Statement 1: $f(x)\leq g(x)$ for x in $(0,\infty)$

Statement 2: $f(x)\leq 1$ for x in $(0,\infty)$ but $g(x)\to\infty$ as $x\to\infty$. **[Online May 7, 2012]**

(a) Statement 1 is true, Statement 2 is false.

(b) Statement 1 is true, Statement 2 is true, Statement 2 is a correct explanation for Statement 1.

(c) Statement 1 is true, Statement 2 is true, Statement 2 is not a correct explanation for Statement 1.

(d) Statement 1 is false, Statement 2 is true.

6. A triangular park is enclosed on two sides by a fence and on the third side by a straight river bank. The two sides having fence are of same length x. The maximum area enclosed by the park is **[2006]**

(a) $\frac{3}{2}x^2$ (b) $\sqrt{\frac{x^3}{8}}$

(c) $\frac{1}{2}x^2$ (d) πx^2

TOPIC-2 : Trigonometric Identities, Conditional Trigonometric Identities, Greatest and Least Value of Trigonometric Expressions

7. If $5(\tan^2 x-\cos^2 x)=2\cos 2x+9$, then the value of $\cos 4x$ is : **[2017]**

(a) $-\frac{7}{9}$ (b) $-\frac{3}{5}$

(c) $\frac{1}{3}$ (d) $\frac{2}{9}$

8. If m and M are the minimum and the maximum values of

$4+\frac{1}{2}\sin^2 2x-2\cos^4 x, x\in R$, then $M-m$ is equal to : **[Online April 9, 2016]**

(a) $\frac{9}{4}$ (b) $\frac{15}{4}$

(c) $\frac{7}{4}$ (d) $\frac{1}{4}$

9. If $\cos\alpha+\cos\beta=\frac{3}{2}$ and $\sin\alpha+\sin\beta\ \frac{1}{2}$ and θ is the the arithmetic mean of α and β, then $\sin 2\theta+\cos 2\theta$ is equal to : **[Online April 11, 2015]**

(a) $\frac{3}{5}$ (b) $\frac{7}{5}$

(c) $\frac{4}{5}$ (d) $\frac{8}{5}$

10. If $\operatorname{cosec}\theta = \frac{p+q}{p-q}$ $(p \neq q \neq 0)$, then $\left|\cot\left(\frac{\pi}{4}+\frac{\theta}{2}\right)\right|$ is equal to: **[Online April 9, 2014]**

(a) $\sqrt{\frac{p}{q}}$ (b) $\sqrt{\frac{q}{p}}$

(c) $\sqrt{pq}$ (d) pq

11. If $A = \sin^2 x + \cos^4 x$, then for all real x : **[2011]**

(a) $\frac{13}{16} \leq A \leq 1$ (b) $1 \leq A \leq 2$

(c) $\frac{3}{4} \leq A \leq \frac{13}{16}$ (d) $\frac{3}{4} \leq A \leq 1$

12. Let $\cos(\alpha+\beta) = \frac{4}{5}$ and $\sin(\alpha-\beta) = \frac{5}{13}$, where $0 \leq \alpha, \beta \leq \frac{\pi}{4}$. Then $\tan 2\alpha$ = **[2010]**

(a) $\frac{56}{33}$ (b) $\frac{19}{12}$

(c) $\frac{20}{7}$ (d) $\frac{25}{16}$

13. Let **A** and **B** denote the statements

A : $\cos\alpha + \cos\beta + \cos\gamma = 0$

B : $\sin\alpha + \sin\beta + \sin\gamma = 0$

If $\cos(\beta-\gamma) + \cos(\gamma-\alpha) + \cos(\alpha-\beta) = -\frac{3}{2}$, then : **[2009]**

(a) **A** is false and **B** is true
(b) both **A** and **B** are true
(c) both **A** and **B** are false
(d) **A** is true and **B** is false

14. If p and q are positive real numbers such that $p^2 + q^2 = 1$, then the maximum value of $(p+q)$ is **[2007]**

(a) $\frac{1}{2}$ (b) $\frac{1}{\sqrt{2}}$

(c) $\sqrt{2}$ (d) 2.

15. If $0 < x < \pi$ and $\cos x + \sin x = \frac{1}{2}$, then $\tan x$ is **[2006]**

(a) $\frac{(1-\sqrt{7})}{4}$ (b) $\frac{(4-\sqrt{7})}{3}$

(c) $-\frac{(4+\sqrt{7})}{3}$ (d) $\frac{(1+\sqrt{7})}{4}$

16. If $u = \sqrt{a^2\cos^2\theta + b^2\sin^2\theta} + \sqrt{a^2\sin^2\theta + b^2\cos^2\theta}$ then the difference between the maximum and minimum values of u^2 is given by **[2004]**

(a) $(a-b)^2$ (b) $2\sqrt{a^2+b^2}$

(c) $(a+b)^2$ (d) $2(a^2+b^2)$

17. Let α, β be such that $\pi < \alpha - \beta < 3\pi$.

If $\sin\alpha + \sin\beta = -\frac{21}{65}$ and $\cos\alpha + \cos\beta = -\frac{27}{65}$, then the value of $\cos\frac{\alpha-\beta}{2}$ **[2004]**

(a) $\frac{-6}{65}$ (b) $\frac{3}{\sqrt{130}}$

(c) $\frac{6}{65}$ (d) $-\frac{3}{\sqrt{130}}$

18. The function $f(x) = \log\left(x+\sqrt{x^2+1}\right)$, is **[2003]**

(a) neither an even nor an odd function
(b) an even function
(c) an odd function
(d) a periodic function.

19. The period of $\sin^2\theta$ is **[2002]**

(a) π^2 (b) π
(c) 2π (d) $\pi/2$

20. Which one is not periodic? **[2002]**

(a) $|\sin 3x| + \sin^2 x$ (b) $\cos\sqrt{x} + \cos^2 x$
(c) $\cos 4x + \tan^2 x$ (d) $\cos 2x + \sin x$

TOPIC-3 : Solutions of Trigonometric Equations

21. If $0 \leq x < 2\pi$, then the number of real values of x, which satisfy the equation
$\cos x + \cos 2x + \cos 3x + \cos 4x = 0$ is: **[2016]**

(a) 7 (b) 9
(c) 3 (d) 5

22. The number of $x \in [0, 2\pi]$ for which

$$\left|\sqrt{2\sin^4 x + 18\cos^2 x} - \sqrt{2\cos^4 x + 18\sin^2 x}\right| = 1 \text{ is}$$

[Online April 9, 2016]

(a) 2 (b) 6
(c) 4 (d) 8

23. The number of values of α in $[0, 2\pi]$ for which $2\sin^3\alpha - 7\sin^2\alpha + 7\sin\alpha = 2$, is:

[Online April 9, 2014]

(a) 6 (b) 4
(c) 3 (d) 1

24. Let $A = \{\theta : \sin(\theta) = \tan(\theta)\}$ and $B = \{\theta : \cos(\theta) = 1\}$ be two sets. Then : **[Online April 25, 2013]**

(a) $A = B$
(b) $A \not\subset B$
(c) $B \not\subset A$
(d) $A \subset B$ and $B - A \neq \phi$

25. The number of solutions of the equation $\sin 2x - 2\cos x + 4\sin x = 4$ in the interval $[0, 5\pi]$ is :

[Online April 23, 2013]

(a) 3 (b) 5
(c) 4 (d) 6

26. **Statement-1:** The number of common solutions of the trigonometric equations $2\sin^2\theta - \cos 2\theta = 0$ and $2\cos^2\theta - 3\sin\theta = 0$ in the interval $[0, 2\pi]$ is two.

Statement-2: The number of solutions of the equation, $2\cos^2\theta - 3\sin\theta = 0$ in the interval $[0, \pi]$ is two.

[Online April 22, 2013]

(a) Statement-1 is true; Statement-2 is true; Statement-2 is a correct explanation for statement-1.
(b) Statement-1 is true; Statement-2 is true; Statement-2 is **not** a correct explanation for statement-1.
(c) Statement-1 is false; Statement-2 is true.
(d) Statement-1 is true; Statement-2 is false.

27. The equation $e^{\sin x} - e^{-\sin x} - 4 = 0$ has : **[2012]**

(a) infinite number of real roots
(b) no real roots
(c) exactly one real root
(d) exactly four real roots

28. The possible values of $\theta \in (0, \pi)$ such that $\sin(\theta) + \sin(4\theta) + \sin(7\theta) = 0$ are **[2011RS]**

(a) $\frac{\pi}{4}, \frac{5\pi}{12}, \frac{\pi}{2}, \frac{2\pi}{3}, \frac{3\pi}{4}, \frac{8\pi}{9}$

(b) $\frac{2\pi}{9}, \frac{\pi}{4}, \frac{\pi}{2}, \frac{2\pi}{3}, \frac{3\pi}{4}, \frac{35\pi}{36}$

(c) $\frac{2\pi}{9}, \frac{\pi}{4}, \frac{\pi}{2}, \frac{2\pi}{3}, \frac{3\pi}{4}, \frac{8\pi}{9}$

(d) $\frac{2\pi}{9}, \frac{\pi}{4}, \frac{4\pi}{9}, \frac{\pi}{2}, \frac{3\pi}{4}, \frac{8\pi}{9}$

29. The number of values of x in the interval $[0, 3\pi]$ satisfying the equation $2\sin^2 x + 5\sin x - 3 = 0$ is **[2006]**

(a) 4 (b) 6
(c) 1 (d) 2

30. The number of solution of $\tan x + \sec x = 2\cos x$ in $[0, 2\pi)$ is **[2002]**

(a) 2 (b) 3
(c) 0 (d) 1

Hints & Solutions

1. **(b)** Let $f_k(x)=\frac{1}{k}(\sin^k x+\cos^k x)$

Consider

$f_4(x)-f_6(x)=\frac{1}{4}(\sin^4 x+\cos^4 x)$

$-\frac{1}{6}(\sin^6 x+\cos^6 x)$

$=\frac{1}{4}[1-2\sin^2 x\cos^2 x]-\frac{1}{6}[1-3\sin^2 x\cos^2 x]$

$=\frac{1}{4}-\frac{1}{6}=\frac{1}{12}$

2. **(d)** Given $2\cos\theta+\sin\theta=1$

Squaring both sides, we get

$(2\cos\theta+\sin\theta)^2=1^2$

$\Rightarrow 4\cos^2\theta+\sin^2\theta+4\sin\theta\cos\theta=1$

$\Rightarrow 3\cos^2\theta+(\cos^2\theta+\sin^2\theta)+4\sin\theta\cos\theta=1$

$\Rightarrow 3\cos^2\theta+\cancel{1}+4\sin\theta\cos\theta=\cancel{1}$

$\Rightarrow 3\cos^2\theta+4\sin\theta\cos\theta=0$

$\Rightarrow \cos\theta(3\cos\theta+4\sin\theta)=0$

$\Rightarrow 3\cos\theta+4\sin\theta=0\Rightarrow 3\cos\theta=-4\sin\theta$

$\Rightarrow \frac{-3}{4}=\tan\theta=\sqrt{\sec^2\theta-1}=\frac{-3}{4}$

$\left(\because \tan\theta=\sqrt{\sec^2\theta-1}\right)$

$\Rightarrow \sec^2\theta-1=\left(\frac{-3}{4}\right)^2=\frac{9}{16}$

$\Rightarrow \sec^2\theta=\frac{9}{16}+1=\frac{25}{16}\Rightarrow \sec\theta=\frac{5}{4}$

or $\boxed{\cos\theta=\frac{4}{5}}$ ...(1)

Now, $\sin^2\theta+\cos^2\theta=1\Rightarrow \sin^2\theta+\left(\frac{4}{5}\right)^2=1$

$\sin^2\theta+\frac{4}{5}=1\Rightarrow \sin^2\theta=1-\frac{16}{25}=\frac{9}{25}$

$\sin\theta=\pm\frac{3}{5}$ ...(2)

Taking $\left(\sin\theta=+\frac{3}{5}\right)$ because $\left(\sin\theta=-\frac{3}{5}\right)$ cannot satisfy the given equation.

Therefore; $7\cos\theta+6\sin\theta$

$=7\times\frac{4}{5}+6\times\frac{3}{5}=\frac{28}{5}+\frac{18}{5}=\frac{46}{5}$

3. **(b)** Given expression can be written as

$\frac{\sin A}{\cos A}\times\frac{\sin A}{\sin A-\cos A}+\frac{\cos A}{\sin A}\times\frac{\cos A}{\cos A-\sin A}$

$\left(\because \tan A=\frac{\sin A}{\cos A} \text{ and } \cot A=\frac{\cos A}{\sin A}\right)$

$=\frac{1}{\sin A-\cos A}\left\{\frac{\sin^3 A-\cos^3 A}{\cos A\sin A}\right\}$

$=\frac{\sin^2 A+\sin A\cos A+\cos^2 A}{\sin A\cos A}$

$=1+\sec A\operatorname{cosec} A$

4. **(c)** Consider $\cos 255^\circ+\sin 195^\circ$

$=\cos(270^\circ-15^\circ)+\sin(180^\circ+15^\circ)$

$=-\sin 15^\circ-\sin 15^\circ$

$=-2\sin 15^\circ=-2\left(\frac{\sqrt{3}-1}{2\sqrt{2}}\right)=-\left(\frac{\sqrt{3}-1}{\sqrt{2}}\right)$

5. **(c)** Let $f(x)=\sin x$ and $g(x)=x$

Statement-1: $f(x)\le g(x)\,\forall x\in(0,\infty)$

i.e., $\sin x\le x\,\forall x\in(0,\infty)$

which is true

Statement-2: $f(x)\le 1\;\forall\; x\in(0,\infty)$

i.e., $\sin x\le 1\;\forall\; x\in(0,\infty)$

It is true and

$g(x)=x\to\infty$ as $x\to\infty$ also true.

6. **(c)** Area $=\frac{1}{2}x^2\sin\theta$

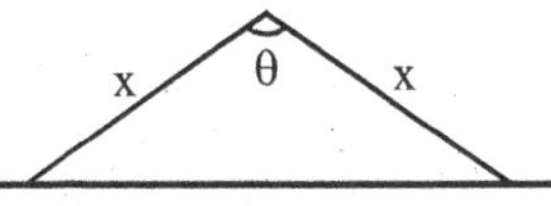

Maximum value of $\sin\theta$ is 1 at $\theta=\frac{\pi}{2}$

$A_{max}=\frac{1}{2}x^2$

7. **(a)** We have

$5\tan^2 x - 5\cos^2 x = 2(2\cos^2 x - 1) + 9$

$\Rightarrow 5\tan^2 x - 5\cos^2 x = 4\cos^2 x - 2 + 9$

$\Rightarrow 5\tan^2 x = 9\cos^2 x + 7$

$\Rightarrow 5(\sec^2 x - 1) = 9\cos^2 x + 7$

Let $\cos^2 x = t$

$\Rightarrow \frac{5}{t} - 9t - 12 = 0$

$\Rightarrow 9t^2 + 12t - 5 = 0$

$\Rightarrow 9t^2 + 15t - 3t - 5 = 0$

$\Rightarrow (3t-1)(3t+5) = 0$

$\Rightarrow t = \frac{1}{3}$ as $t \neq -\frac{5}{3}$.

$\cos 2x = 2\cos^2 x - 1 = 2\left(\frac{1}{3}\right) - 1 = -\frac{1}{3}$

$\cos 4x = 2\cos^2 2x - 1 = 2\left(-\frac{1}{3}\right)^2 - 1 = -\frac{7}{9}$

8. **(b)** $4 + \frac{1}{2}\sin^2 2x - 2\cos^4 x$

$4 + 2(1 - \cos^2 x)\cos^2 x - 2\cos^4 x$

$-4\left\{\cos^4 x - \frac{\cos^2 x}{2} - 1 + \frac{1}{16} - \frac{1}{16}\right\}$

$-4\left\{\left(\cos^2 x - \frac{1}{4}\right)^2 - \frac{17}{16}\right\}$

$0 \le \cos^2 x \le 1$

$-\frac{1}{4} \le \cos^2 x - \frac{1}{4} \le \frac{3}{4}$

$0 \le \left(\cos^2 x - \frac{1}{4}\right)^2 \le \frac{9}{16}$

$-\frac{17}{16} \le \left(\cos^2 x - \frac{1}{4}\right)^2 - \frac{17}{16} \le \frac{9}{16} - \frac{17}{16}$

$\frac{17}{4} \ge -4\left\{\left(\cos^2 x - \frac{1}{4}\right)^2 - \frac{17}{16}\right\} \ge \frac{1}{2}$

$M = \frac{17}{4}$

$m = \frac{1}{2}$

$M - m = \frac{17}{4} - \frac{2}{4} = \frac{15}{4}$

9. **(b)** Let $\cos\alpha + \cos\beta = \frac{3}{2}$

$\Rightarrow 2\cos\frac{\alpha+\beta}{2}\cos\frac{\alpha-\beta}{2} = \frac{3}{2}$ ...(i)

and $\sin\alpha + \sin\beta = \frac{1}{2}$

$\Rightarrow 2\sin\frac{\alpha+\beta}{2}\cos\frac{\alpha-\beta}{2} = \frac{1}{2}$ ...(ii)

On dividing (ii) by (i), we get

$\tan\left(\frac{\alpha+\beta}{2}\right) = \frac{1}{3}$

Given : $\theta = \frac{\alpha+\beta}{2} \Rightarrow 2\theta = \alpha + \beta$

Consider $\sin 2\theta + \cos 2\theta = \sin(\alpha+\beta) + \cos(\alpha+\beta)$

$= \frac{\frac{2}{3}}{1+\frac{1}{9}} + \frac{1-\frac{1}{9}}{1+\frac{1}{9}} = \frac{6}{10} + \frac{8}{10} = \frac{7}{5}$

10. **(b)** $\text{cosec}\theta = \frac{p+q}{p-q}$, $\sin\theta = \frac{p-q}{p+q}$

$\cos\theta = \pm\sqrt{1-\sin^2\theta} = \sqrt{1 - \left(\frac{p-q}{p+q}\right)^2} = \frac{2\sqrt{pq}}{(p+q)}$

$\left|\cot\left(\frac{\pi}{4} + \frac{\theta}{2}\right)\right| = \left|\frac{\cot\frac{\pi}{4}\cot\frac{\theta}{2} - 1}{\cot\frac{\pi}{4} + \cot\frac{\theta}{2}}\right| = \left|\frac{\cot\frac{\theta}{2} - 1}{\cot\frac{\theta}{2} + 1}\right|$

$= \left|\frac{\cos\frac{\theta}{2} - \sin\frac{\theta}{2}}{\cos\frac{\theta}{2} + \sin\frac{\theta}{2}}\right|$

On rationalizing denominator, we get

$\left|\left(\frac{\cos\frac{\theta}{2} - \sin\frac{\theta}{2}}{\cos\frac{\theta}{2} + \sin\frac{\theta}{2}}\right)\left(\frac{\cos\frac{\theta}{2} + \sin\frac{\theta}{2}}{\cos\frac{\theta}{2} + \sin\frac{\theta}{2}}\right)\right|$

$= \left|\frac{\cos\theta}{\sin^2\frac{\theta}{2} + \cos^2\frac{\theta}{2} + 2\sin\frac{\theta}{2}\cos\frac{\theta}{2}}\right|$

$= \left|\frac{\cos\theta}{1+\sin\theta}\right| = \left|\frac{2\sqrt{pq}/(p+q)}{1 + \frac{(p-q)}{p+q}}\right| = \frac{\sqrt{pq}}{p} = \sqrt{\frac{q}{p}}$

11. **(d)** $A = \sin^2 x + \cos^4 x$

$= \sin^2 x + \cos^2 x(1 - \sin^2 x)$

$= \sin^2 x + \cos^2 x - \frac{1}{4}(2\sin x.\cos x)^2$

$= 1 - \frac{1}{4}\sin^2(2x)$

Now $0 \le \sin^2(2x) \le 1$

$\Rightarrow 0 \ge -\frac{1}{4}\sin^2(2x) \ge -\frac{1}{4}$

$\Rightarrow 1 \ge 1-\frac{1}{4}\sin^2(2x) \ge 1-\frac{1}{4}$

$\Rightarrow 1 \ge A \ge \frac{3}{4}$

12. (a) $\cos(\alpha+\beta) = \frac{4}{5} \Rightarrow \tan(\alpha+\beta) = \frac{3}{4}$

$\sin(\alpha-\beta) = \frac{5}{13} \Rightarrow \tan(\alpha-\beta) = \frac{5}{12}$

$\tan 2\alpha = \tan[(\alpha+\beta)+(\alpha-\beta)]$

$$= \frac{\frac{3}{4}+\frac{5}{12}}{1-\frac{3}{4}\cdot\frac{5}{12}} = \frac{56}{33}$$

13. (b) We have
$\cos(\beta-\gamma)+\cos(\gamma-\alpha)+\cos(\alpha-\beta)$

$$= -\frac{3}{2}$$

$\Rightarrow 2[\cos(\beta-\gamma)+\cos(\gamma-\alpha) + \cos(\alpha-\beta)]+3=0$

$\Rightarrow 2[\cos(\beta-\gamma)+\cos(\gamma-\alpha)+\cos(\alpha-\beta)] + \sin^2\alpha+\cos^2\alpha+\sin^2\beta+\cos^2\beta + \sin^2\gamma+\cos^2\alpha=0$

$\Rightarrow [\sin^2\alpha+\sin^2\beta+\sin^2\gamma+2\sin\alpha\sin\beta+2\sin\beta\sin\gamma+ 2\sin\gamma\sin\alpha]+[\cos^2\alpha+\cos^2\beta+\cos^2\gamma+2\cos\alpha\cos\beta + 2\cos\beta\cos\gamma+2\cos\gamma\cos\alpha]=0$

$\Rightarrow [\sin\alpha+\sin\beta+\sin\gamma]^2+(\cos\alpha+\cos\beta+\cos\gamma)^2=0$

$\Rightarrow \sin\alpha+\sin\beta+\sin\gamma=0$ and $\cos\alpha+\cos\beta+\cos\gamma=0$

$\therefore$ A and B both are true.

14. (c) Given that $p^2+q^2=1$

$\therefore\ p=\cos\theta$ and $q=\sin\theta$

Then $p+q=\cos\theta+\sin\theta$

We know that

$-\sqrt{a^2+b^2} \le a\cos\theta+b\sin\theta \le \sqrt{a^2+b^2}$

$\therefore -\sqrt{2} \le \cos\theta+\sin\theta \le \sqrt{2}$

Hence max. value of $p+q$ is $\sqrt{2}$

15. (c) $\cos x+\sin x = \frac{1}{2} \Rightarrow 1+\sin 2x = \frac{1}{4}$

$\Rightarrow \sin 2x = -\frac{3}{4}$, so x is obtuse and

$\frac{2\tan x}{1+\tan^2 x} = -\frac{3}{4}$

$\Rightarrow 3\tan^2 x+8\tan x+3=0$

$\therefore\ \tan x = \frac{-8\pm\sqrt{64-36}}{6} = -\frac{-4\pm\sqrt{7}}{3}$

as $\tan x<0$ $\quad\therefore\ \tan x = \frac{-4-\sqrt{7}}{3}$

16. (a) $u^2 = a^2+b^2+2\sqrt{(a^4+b^4)\cos^2\theta\sin^2\theta + a^2b^2(\cos^4\theta+\sin^4\theta)}$ ...(1)

Now $(a^4+b^4)\cos^2\theta\sin^2\theta$

$+a^2b^2(\cos^4\theta+\sin^4\theta)$

$=(a^4+b^4)\cos^2\theta\sin^2\theta$

$+a^2b^2(1-2\cos^2\theta\sin^2\theta)$

$=(a^4+b^4-2a^2b^2)\cos^2\theta\sin^2\theta+a^2b^2$

$=(a^2-b^2)^2.\frac{\sin^2 2\theta}{4}+a^2b^2$ ...(2)

$\because 0 \le \sin^2 2\theta \le 1$

$\Rightarrow 0 \le (a^2-b^2)^2\frac{\sin^2 2\theta}{4} \le \frac{(a^2-b^2)^2}{4}$

$\Rightarrow a^2b^2 \le (a^2-b^2)^2\frac{\sin^2 2\theta}{4}+a^2b^2$

$\le (a^2-b^2)^2.\frac{1}{4}+a^2b^2$ ....(3)

$\therefore$ from (1), (2) and (3)
Minimum value of

$u^2 = a^2+b^2+2\sqrt{a^2b^2} = (a+b)^2$

Maximum value of u^2

$= a^2+b^2+2\sqrt{\left(a^2-b^2\right)^2.\frac{1}{4}+a^2b^2}$

$= a^2+b^2+\frac{2}{2}\sqrt{(a^2+b^2)^2} = 2(a^2+b^2)$

$\therefore$ Max value - Min value

$= 2(a^2+b^2)-(a+b^2)=(a-b)^2$

17. (d) $\pi<\alpha-\beta<3\pi$

$\Rightarrow \frac{\pi}{2}<\frac{\alpha-\beta}{2}<\frac{3\pi}{2} \Rightarrow \cos\frac{\alpha-\beta}{2}<0$

$\sin\alpha+\sin\beta=-\frac{21}{65}$

$\Rightarrow 2\sin\frac{\alpha+\beta}{2}\cos\frac{\alpha-\beta}{2}=-\frac{21}{65}$ ....(1)

$\cos\alpha+\cos\beta=-\frac{27}{65}$

$\Rightarrow 2\cos\frac{\alpha+\beta}{2}\cos\frac{\alpha-\beta}{2}=-\frac{27}{65}$ ....(2)

Square and add (1) and (2)

$4\cos^2\frac{\alpha-\beta}{2}=\frac{(21)^2+(27)^2}{(65)^2}=\frac{1170}{65\times65}$

$\therefore \cos^2\frac{\alpha-\beta}{2}=\frac{9}{130}\Rightarrow\cos\frac{\alpha-\beta}{2}=-\frac{3}{\sqrt{130}}$

18. (c) $f(x)=\log(x+\sqrt{x^2+1})$

$f(-x)=\log\left\{-x+\sqrt{x^2+1}\right\}=\log\left\{\frac{-x^2+x^2+1}{x+\sqrt{x^2+1}}\right\}$

$=-\log(x+\sqrt{x^2+1})=-f(x)$

$\Rightarrow f(x)$ is an odd function.

19. (b) $\sin^2\theta=\frac{1-\cos 2\theta}{2}$; Period $=\frac{2\pi}{2}=\pi$

20. (b) $\because \cos\sqrt{x}$ is non periodic

$\therefore \cos\sqrt{x}+\cos^2 x$ can not be periodic.

21. (a) $\cos x+\cos 2x+\cos 3x+\cos 4x=0$

$\Rightarrow 2\cos 2x\cos x+2\cos 3x\cos x=0$

$\Rightarrow 2\cos x\left(2\cos\frac{5x}{2}\cos\frac{x}{2}\right)=0$

$\cos x=0,\ \cos\frac{5x}{2}=0,\ \cos\frac{x}{2}=0$

$x=\pi,\frac{\pi}{2},\frac{3\pi}{2},\frac{\pi}{5},\frac{3\pi}{5},\frac{7\pi}{5},\frac{9\pi}{5}$

22. (d) $\left|\sqrt{2\sin^4 x+18\cos^2 x}-\sqrt{2\cos^4 x+18\sin^2 x}\right|=1$

$\sqrt{2\sin^4 x+18\cos^2 x}-\sqrt{2\cos^4 x+18\sin^2 x}=\pm1$

$\sqrt{2\sin^4 x+18\cos^2 x}=\pm1+\sqrt{2\cos^4 x+18\sin^2 x}$

by squaring both the sides we will get 8 solutions

23. (c) $2\sin^3\alpha-7\sin^2\alpha+7\sin\alpha-2=0$

$\Rightarrow 2\sin^2\alpha(\sin\alpha-1)-5\sin\alpha(\sin\alpha-1)+2(\sin\alpha-1)=0$

$\Rightarrow(\sin\alpha-1)(2\sin^2\alpha-5\sin\alpha+2)=0$

$\Rightarrow \sin\alpha-1=0$ or $2\sin^2\alpha-5\sin\alpha+2=0$

$\sin\alpha=1$ or $\sin\alpha=\frac{5\pm\sqrt{25-16}}{4}=\frac{5\pm3}{4}$

$\alpha=\frac{\pi}{2}$ or $\sin\alpha=\frac{1}{2},2$

Now, $\sin\alpha\neq2$

for, $\sin\alpha=\frac{1}{2}$

$\alpha=\frac{\pi}{3},\frac{2\pi}{3}$

There are three values of α between $[0,2\pi]$

24. (b) Let $A=\{\theta:\sin\theta=\tan\theta\}$

and $B=\{\theta:\cos\theta=1\}$

Now, $A=\left\{\theta:\sin\theta=\frac{\sin\theta}{\cos\theta}\right\}$

$=\{\theta:\sin\theta(\cos\theta-1)=0\}$

$=\{\theta=0,\pi,2\pi,3\pi,.....\}$

For $B:\cos\theta=1\Rightarrow\theta=\pi,2\pi,4\pi,......$

This shows that A is not contained in B. i.e. $A\not\subset B$. but $B\subset A$.

25. (a) $\sin 2x-2\cos x+4\sin x=4$

$\Rightarrow 2\sin x.\cos x-2\cos x+4\sin x-4=0$

$\Rightarrow(\sin x-1)(\cos x-2)=0$

$\because \cos x-2\neq0,\ \therefore\ \sin x=1$

$\therefore\ x=\frac{\pi}{2},\frac{5\pi}{2},\frac{9\pi}{2}$

26. (b) $2\sin^2\theta-\cos 2\theta=0$

$\Rightarrow 2\sin^2\theta-(1-2\sin^2\theta)=0$

$\Rightarrow 2\sin^2\theta-1+2\sin^2\theta=0$

$\Rightarrow 4\sin^2\theta=1\Rightarrow\sin\theta=\pm\frac{1}{2}$

$\therefore\ \theta=\frac{\pi}{4},\frac{3\pi}{4},\frac{5\pi}{4},\frac{7\pi}{4},\theta\in[0,2\pi]$

$\therefore\ \theta=\frac{\pi}{6},\frac{5\pi}{6},\frac{7\pi}{6},\frac{11\pi}{6}$

Now $2\cos^2\theta-3\sin\theta=0$

$\Rightarrow\ 2(1-\sin^2\theta)-3\sin\theta=0$

$\Rightarrow\ -2\sin^2\theta-3\sin\theta+2=0$

$\Rightarrow\ -2\sin^2\theta-4\sin\theta+\sin\theta+2=0$

$\Rightarrow\ 2\sin^2\theta-\sin\theta+4\sin\theta-2=0$

$\Rightarrow\ \sin\theta(2\sin\theta-1)+2(2\sin\theta-1)=0$

$\Rightarrow\ \sin\theta=\frac{1}{2},-2$

But $\sin\theta=-2$, is not possible

$\therefore\ \sin\theta=\frac{1}{2},-2\ \Rightarrow\ \theta=\frac{\pi}{6},\frac{5\pi}{6}$

Hence, there are two common solution, there each of the statement-1 and 2 are true but statement-2 is not a correct explanation for statement-1.

27. **(b)** Given equation is $e^{\sin x} - e^{-\sin x} - 4 = 0$

Put $e^{\sin x} = t$ in the given equation, we get

$t^2 - 4t - 1 = 0$

$$\Rightarrow \quad t = \frac{4 \pm \sqrt{16+4}}{2} = \frac{4 \pm \sqrt{20}}{2}$$

$$= \frac{4 \pm 2\sqrt{5}}{2} = 2 \pm \sqrt{5}$$

$$\Rightarrow \quad e^{\sin x} = 2 \pm \sqrt{5} \left(\because\ t = e^{\sin x}\right)$$

$$\Rightarrow \quad e^{\sin x} = 2 - \sqrt{5} \text{ and } e^{\sin x} = 2 + \sqrt{5}$$

$$\Rightarrow \quad e^{\sin x} = 2 - \sqrt{5} < 0$$

and $\sin x = \ln\left(2 + \sqrt{5}\right) > 1$

So, rejected.

Hence given equation has no solution.

$\therefore$ The equation has no real roots.

28. **(d)** $\sin 4\theta + 2\sin 4\theta \cos 3\theta = 0$

$\sin 4\theta\left(1 + 2\cos 3\theta\right) = 0$

$\sin 4\theta = 0$ or $\cos 3\theta = -\dfrac{1}{2}$

$4\theta = n\pi;\ n \in I$

or $3\theta = 2n\pi \pm \dfrac{2\pi}{3}, n \in I$

$\theta = \dfrac{\pi}{4}, \dfrac{\pi}{2}, \dfrac{3\pi}{4}$ or $\theta = \dfrac{2\pi}{9}, \dfrac{8\pi}{9}, \dfrac{4\pi}{9}$

$[\because\ \theta, \in (0, \pi)]$

29. **(a)**

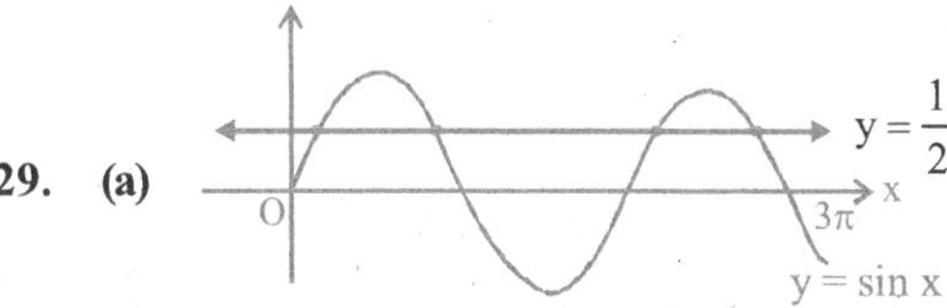

$2\sin^2 x + 5\sin x - 3 = 0$

$\Rightarrow \ (\sin x + 3)(2\sin x - 1) = 0$

$\Rightarrow \ \sin x = \dfrac{1}{2}$ and $\sin x \neq -3$

$\therefore$ In $[0, 3\pi]$, x has 4 values.

30. **(b)** The given equation is $\tan x + \sec x = 2\cos x$;

$\Rightarrow \sin x + 1 = 2\cos^2 x$

$\Rightarrow \sin x + 1 = 2(1 - \sin^2 x)$;

$\Rightarrow 2\sin^2 x + \sin x - 1 = 0$;

$\Rightarrow (2\sin x - 1)(\sin x + 1) = 0$

$\Rightarrow \sin x = \dfrac{1}{2}, -1.$;

$\Rightarrow x = 30°, 150°, 270°.$

Principle of Mathematical Induction

TOPIC-1 : Problems Based on Sum of Series, Problems Based on Inequality and Divisibility

1. Let $S(K)=1+3+5...+(2K-1)=3+K^2$. Then which of the following is true **[2004]**
   (a) Principle of mathematical induction can be used to prove the formula
   (b) $S(K) \Rightarrow S(K+1)$
   (c) $S(K) \nRightarrow S(K+1)$
   (d) $S(1)$ is correct

2. If $a_n=\sqrt{7+\sqrt{7+\sqrt{7+......}}}$ having n radical signs then by methods of mathematical induction which is true **[2002]**
   (a) $a_n > 7 \ \forall \ n \geq 1$ (b) $a_n < 7 \ \forall \ n \geq 1$
   (c) $a_n < 4 \ \forall \ n \geq 1$ (d) $a_n < 3 \ \forall \ n \geq 1$

Hints & Solutions

1. **(b)** $S(K) = 1+3+5+...+(2K-1) = 3+K^2$

$S(1): 1 = 3+1,$ which is not true

$\because$ $S(1)$ is not true.

$\therefore$ P.M.I cannot be applied

Let $S(K)$ is true, i.e.

$1+3+5....+(2K-1) = 3+K^2$

$\Rightarrow 1+3+5....+(2K-1)+2K+1$

$= 3+K^2+2K+1 = 3+(K+1)^2$

$\therefore S(K) \Rightarrow S(K+1)$

2. **(b)** $a_1 = \sqrt{7} < 7$. Let $a_m < 7$

Then $a_{m+1} = \sqrt{7+a_m} \Rightarrow a^2_{m+1} = 7+a_m < 7+7 < 14.$

$\Rightarrow a_{m+1} < \sqrt{14} < 7;$ So by the principle of mathematical induction $a_n < 7 \ \forall \ n.$

$\therefore$ r = 0,8,16,24,........256 , total 33 values.

Complex Numbers and Quadratic Equations

TOPIC-1 : Integral Powers of Iota, Algebraic Operations of Complex Numbers, Conjugate, Modulus and Argument or Amplitude of a Complex Number

1. A value of θ for which $\frac{2+3i\sin\theta}{1-2i\sin\theta}$ is purely imaginary, is: **[2016]**
(a) $\sin^{-1}\left(\frac{\sqrt{3}}{4}\right)$ (b) $\sin^{-1}\left(\frac{1}{\sqrt{3}}\right)$
(c) $\frac{\pi}{3}$ (d) $\frac{\pi}{6}$

2. If z is a non-real complex number, then the minimum value of $\frac{Imz^5}{(Imz)^5}$ is : **[Online April 11, 2015]**
(a) –1 (b) –4
(c) –2 (d) –5

3. If z is a complex number such that $|z| \geq 2$, then the minimum value of $\left|z+\frac{1}{2}\right|$: **[2014]**
(a) is strictly greater than $\frac{5}{2}$
(b) is strictly greater than $\frac{3}{2}$ but less than $\frac{5}{2}$
(c) is equal to $\frac{5}{2}$
(d) lie in the interval (1, 2)

4. For all complex numbers z of the form $1+i\alpha$, $\alpha \in R$, if $z^2 = x+iy$, then **[Online April 19, 2014]**
(a) $y^2-4x+2=0$
(b) $y^2+4x-4=0$
(c) $y^2-4x-4=0$
(d) $y^2+4x+2=0$

5. Let $z \neq -i$ be any complex number such that $\frac{z-i}{z+i}$ is a purely imaginary number. Then $z+\frac{1}{z}$ is: **[Online April 12, 2014]**
(a) 0
(b) any non-zero real number other than 1.
(c) any non-zero real number.
(d) a purely imaginary number.

6. If z_1, z_2 and z_3, z_4 are 2 pairs of complex conjugate numbers, then $\arg\left(\frac{z_1}{z_4}\right)+\arg\left(\frac{z_2}{z_3}\right)$ equals: **[Online April 11, 2014]**
(a) 0 (b) $\frac{\pi}{2}$
(c) $\frac{3\pi}{2}$ (d) π

7. Let w (Im w ≠ 0) be a complex number. Then the set of all complex number z satisfying the equation $w-\overline{w}z = k(1-z)$, for some real number k, is **[Online April 9, 2014]**
(a) $\{z : |z| = 1\}$ (b) $\{z : z = \overline{z}\}$
(c) $\{z : z \neq 1\}$ (d) $\{z : |z| = 1, z \neq 1\}$

8. If z is a complex number of unit modulus and argument θ, then $\arg\left(\frac{1+z}{1+\overline{z}}\right)$ equals: **[2013]**
(a) $-\theta$ (b) $\frac{\pi}{2}-\theta$
(c) θ (d) $\pi-\theta$

9. Let z satisfy $|z| = 1$ and $z = 1-\overline{z}$.
Statement 1 : z is a real number.
Statement 2 : Principal argument of z is $\frac{\pi}{3}$ **[Online April 25, 2013]**
(a) Statement 1 is true Statement 2 is true; Statement 2 is a correct explanation for Statement 1.
(b) Statement 1 is false; Statement 2 is true
(c) Statement 1 is true, Statement 2 is false.
(d) Statement 1 is true; Statement 2 is true; Statement 2 is not a correct explanation for Statement 1.

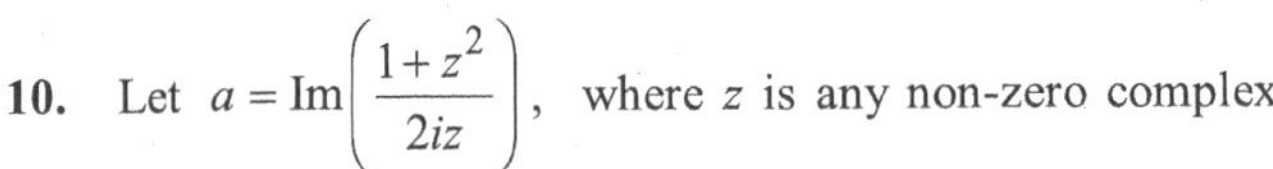

10. Let $a = \text{Im}\left(\frac{1+z^2}{2iz}\right)$, where z is any non-zero complex number. **[Online April 23, 2013]**

The set A = $\{a : |z| = 1 \text{ and } z \neq \pm 1\}$ is equal to:

(a) $(-1, 1)$ (b) $[-1, 1]$
(c) $[0, 1)$ (d) $(-1, 0]$

11. If $Z_1 \neq 0$ and Z_2 be two complex numbers such that $\frac{Z_2}{Z_1}$ is a purely imaginary number, then $\left|\frac{2Z_1 + 3Z_2}{2Z_1 - 3Z_2}\right|$ is equal to : **[Online April 9, 2013]**

(a) 2 (b) 5
(c) 3 (d) 1

12. $|z_1 + z_2|^2 + |z_1 - z_2|^2$ is equal to **[Online May 26, 2012]**

(a) $2(|z_1| + |z_2|)$ (b) $2(|z_1|^2 + |z_2|^2)$
(c) $|z_1||z_2|$ (d) $|z_1|^2 + |z_2|^2$

13. Let Z and W be complex numbers such that $|Z| = |W|$, and arg Z denotes the principal argument of Z. **[Online May 19, 2012]**

Statement 1: If arg Z + arg $W = \pi$, then $Z = -\overline{W}$.

Statement 2: $|Z| = |W|$, implies arg Z – arg $\overline{W} = \pi$.

(a) Statement 1 is true, Statement 2 is false.
(b) Statement 1 is true, Statement 2 is true, Statement 2 is a correct explanation for Statement 1.
(c) Statement 1 is true, Statement 2 is true, Statement 2 is not a correct explanation for Statement 1.
(d) Statement 1 is false, Statement 2 is true.

14. Let Z_1 and Z_2 be any two complex number.

Statement 1: $|Z_1 - Z_2| \geq |Z_1| - |Z_2|$

Statement 2: $|Z_1 + Z_2| \leq |Z_1| + |Z_2|$ **[Online May 7, 2012]**

(a) Statement 1 is true, Statement 2 is true, Statement 2 is a correct explanation of Statement 1.
(b) Statement 1 is true, Statement 2 is true, Statement 2 is not a correct explanation of Statement 1.
(c) Statement 1 is true, Statement 2 is false.
(d) Statement 1 is false, Statement 2 is true.

15. The number of complex numbers z such that $|z-1| = |z+1| = |z-i|$ equals **[2010]**

(a) 1 (b) 2
(c) ∞ (d) 0

16. The conjugate of a complex number is $\frac{1}{i-1}$ then that complex number is **[2008]**

(a) $\frac{-1}{i-1}$ (b) $\frac{1}{i+1}$
(c) $\frac{-1}{i+1}$ (d) $\frac{1}{i-1}$

17. If $z = x - i\,y$ and $z^{\frac{1}{3}} = p + iq$, then $\left(\frac{x}{p} + \frac{y}{q}\right) \Big/ (p^2 + q^2)$ is equal to **[2004]**

(a) -2 (b) -1
(c) 2 (d) 1

18. Let z and w be complex numbers such that $\overline{z} + i\,\overline{w} = 0$ and arg $zw = \pi$. Then arg z equals **[2004]**

(a) $\frac{5\pi}{4}$ (b) $\frac{\pi}{2}$
(c) $\frac{3\pi}{4}$ (d) $\frac{\pi}{4}$

19. If $\left(\frac{1+i}{1-i}\right)^x = 1$ then **[2003]**

(a) $x = 2n+1$, where n is any positive integer
(b) $x = 4n$, where n is any positive integer
(c) $x = 2n$, where n is any positive integer
(d) $x = 4n+1$, where n is any positive integer.

20. If z and ω are two non-zero complex numbers such that $|z\omega| = 1$ and $Arg(z) - Arg(\omega) = \frac{\pi}{2}$, then $\bar{z}\omega$ is equal to

(a) -1 (b) 1 **[2003]**
(c) $-i$ (d) i

21. If $|z-4| < |z-2|$, its solution is given by **[2002]**

(a) Re(z) > 0 (b) Re(z) < 0
(c) Re(z) > 3 (d) Re(z) > 2

22. z and w are two non zero complex numbers such that $|z| = |w|$ and Arg z + Arg w = π then z equals **[2002]**

(a) $\overline{\omega}$ (b) $-\overline{\omega}$
(c) ω (d) $-\omega$

TOPIC-2 : Rotational Theorem, Square Root of a Complex Number, Cube Roots of Unity, Geometry of Complex Numbers, De-moiver's Theorem, Powers of Complex Numbers

23. The point represented by 2 + i in the Argand plane moves 1 unit eastwards, then 2 units northwards and finally from there $2\sqrt{2}$ units in the south–westwards direction. Then its new position in the Argand plane is at the point represented by : **[Online April 9, 2016]**

(a) 1 + i (b) 2 + 2i
(c) –2 – 2i (d) –1 – i

24. A complex number z is said to be unimodular if $|z| = 1$. Suppose z_1 and z_2 are complex numbers such that $\frac{z_1 - 2z_2}{2 - z_1\bar{z}_2}$ is unimodular and z_2 is not unimodular. Then the point z_1 lies on a: **[2015]**
(a) circle of radius 2.
(b) circle of radius $\sqrt{2}$.
(c) straight line parallel to x-axis
(d) straight line parallel to y-axis.

25. If $z \neq 1$ and $\frac{z^2}{z-1}$ is real, then the point represented by the complex number z lies : **[2012]**
(a) either on the real axis or on a circle passing through the origin.
(b) on a circle with centre at the origin
(c) either on the real axis or on a circle not passing through the origin.
(d) on the imaginary axis.

26. If $\omega(\neq 1)$ is a cube root of unity, and $(1+\omega)^7 = A + B\omega$. Then (A, B) equals **[2011]**
(a) (1, 1) (b) (1, 0)
(c) (–1, 1) (d) (0, 1)

27. If $|z + 4| \leq 3$, then the maximum value of $|z+1|$ is **[2007]**
(a) 6 (b) 0
(c) 4 (d) 10

28. If $\omega = \frac{z}{z - \frac{1}{3}i}$ and $|\omega| = 1$, then z lies on **[2005]**
(a) an ellipse (b) a circle
(c) a straight line (d) a parabola

29. If z_1 and z_2 are two non- zero complex numbers such that $|z_1 + z_2| = |z_1| + |z_2|$, then $\arg z_1 - \arg z_2$ is equal to **[2005]**
(a) $\frac{\pi}{2}$ (b) $-\pi$
(c) 0 (d) $\frac{-\pi}{2}$

30. If the cube roots of unity are **1**, ω, ω^2 then the roots of the equation $(x-1)^3 + 8 = 0$, are **[2005]**
(a) $-1, -1+2\omega, -1-2\omega^2$
(b) $-1, -1, -1$
(c) $-1, 1-2\omega, 1-2\omega^2$
(d) $-1, 1+2\omega, 1+2\omega^2$

31. If $|z^2 - 1| = |z|^2 + 1$, then z lies on **[2004]**
(a) an ellipse (b) the imaginary axis
(c) a circle (d) the real axis

32. The locus of the centre of a circle which touches the circle $|z - z_1| = a$ and $|z - z_2| = b$ externally(z, z_1 & z_2 are complex numbers) will be **[2002]**
(a) an ellipse (b) a hyperbola
(c) a circle (d) none of these

TOPIC-3 : Solutions of Quadratic Equations, Sum and Product of Roots, Nature of Roots, Relation Between Roots and Co-efficients, Formation of an Equation with Given Roots.

33. If, for a positive integer n, the quadratic equation,
$x(x+1) + (x+1)(x+2) + \ldots + (x+\overline{n-1})(x+n) = 10n$
has two consecutive integral solutions, then n is equal to : **[2017]**
(a) 11 (b) 12
(c) 9 (d) 10

34. The sum of all the real values of x satisfying the equation $2^{(x-1)(x^2+5x-50)} = 1$ is : **[Online April 9, 2017]**
(a) 16 (b) 14
(c) –4 (d) –5

35. Let p(x) be a quadratic polynomial such that p(0)=1. If p(x) leaves remainder 4 when divided by x–1 and it leaves remainder 6 when divided by x+1; then : **[Online April 8, 2017]**
(a) p(2) = 11 (b) p(2) = 19
(c) p(–2) = 19 (d) p(–2) = 11

36. The sum of all real values of x satisfying the equation $(x^2 - 5x + 5)^{x^2+4x-60} = 1$ is : **[2016]**
(a) 6 (b) 5
(c) 3 (d) –4

37. If x is a solution of the equation, $\sqrt{2x+1} - \sqrt{2x-1} = 1, \left(x \geq \frac{1}{2}\right)$, then $\sqrt{4x^2 - 1}$ is equal to : **[Online April 10, 2016]**
(a) $\frac{3}{4}$ (b) $\frac{1}{2}$
(c) $2\sqrt{2}$ (d) 2

38. Let α and β be the roots of equation $x^2 - 6x - 2 = 0$. If $a_n = \alpha^n - \beta^n$, for $n \geq 1$, then the value of $\frac{a_{10} - 2a_8}{2a_9}$ is equal to : **[2015]**
(a) 3 (b) –3
(c) 6 (d) –6

39. If the two roots of the equation, $(a-1)(x^4+x^2+1)+(a+1)(x^2+x+1)^2=0$ are real and distinct, then the set of all values of 'a' is : **[Online April 11, 2015]**

(a) $\left(0,\frac{1}{2}\right)$ (b) $\left(-\frac{1}{2},0\right)\cup\left(0,\frac{1}{2}\right)$

(c) $\left(-\frac{1}{2},0\right)$ (d) $(-\infty,-2)\cup(2,\infty)$

40. If $2+3i$ is one of the roots of the equation $2x^3-9x^2+kx-13=0, k\in R$, then the real root of this equation : **[Online April 10, 2015]**

(a) exists and is equal to $-\frac{1}{2}$.

(b) exists and is equal to $\frac{1}{2}$.

(c) exists and is equal to 1.

(d) does not exist.

41. If $a\in R$ and the equation

$-3(x-[x])^2+2(x-[x])+a^2=0$

(where $[x]$ denotes the greatest integer $\le x$) has no integral solution, then all possible values of a lie in the interval: **[2014]**

(a) $(-2,-1)$ (b) $(-\infty,-2)\cup(2,\infty)$

(c) $(-1,0)\cup(0,1)$ (d) $(1,2)$

42. The equation $\sqrt{3x^2+x+5}=x-3$, where x is real, has; **[Online April 19, 2014]**

(a) no solution
(b) exactly one solution
(c) exactly two solution
(d) exactly four solution

43. The sum of the roots of the equation, $x^2+|2x-3|-4=0$, is: **[Online April 12, 2014]**

(a) 2 (b) -2

(c) $\sqrt{2}$ (d) $-\sqrt{2}$

44. If α and β are roots of the equation,

$x^2-4\sqrt{2}kx+2e^{4\ln k}-1=0$ for some k, and $\alpha^2+\beta^2=66$, then $\alpha^3+\beta^3$ is equal to: **[Online April 11, 2014]**

(a) $248\sqrt{2}$ (b) $280\sqrt{2}$

(c) $-32\sqrt{2}$ (d) $-280\sqrt{2}$

45. If $\frac{1}{\sqrt{\alpha}}$ and $\frac{1}{\sqrt{\beta}}$ are the roots of the equation, $ax^2+bx+1=0$ ($a\ne 0$, a, b, $\in$ R), then the equation, $x\left(x+b^3\right)+\left(a^3-3abx\right)=0$ as roots : **[Online April 9, 2014]**

(a) $\alpha^{3/2}$ and $\beta^{3/2}$ (b) $\alpha\beta^{1/2}$ and $\alpha^{1/2}\beta$

(c) $\sqrt{\alpha\beta}$ and $\alpha\beta$ (d) $\alpha^{-\frac{3}{2}}$ and $\beta^{-\frac{3}{2}}$

46. If p and q are non-zero real numbers and $\alpha^3+\beta^3=-p, \alpha\beta=q$, then a quadratic equation whose roots are $\frac{\alpha^2}{\beta},\frac{\beta^2}{\alpha}$ is : **[Online April 25, 2013]**

(a) $px^2-qx+p^2=0$ (b) $qx^2+px+q^2=0$
(c) $px^2+qx+p^2=0$ (d) $qx^2-px+q^2=0$

47. If α and β are roots of the equation $x^2+px+\frac{3p}{4}=0$, such that $|\alpha-\beta|=\sqrt{10}$, then p belongs to the set : **[Online April 22, 2013]**

(a) $\{2,-5\}$ (b) $\{-3,2\}$
(c) $\{-2,5\}$ (d) $\{3,-5\}$

48. If a complex number z statisfies the equation $z+\sqrt{2}|z+1|+i=0$, then $|z|$ is equal to : **[Online April 22, 2013]**

(a) 2 (b) $\sqrt{3}$

(c) $\sqrt{5}$ (d) 1

49. Let $p, q, r\in R$ and $r>p>0$. If the quadratic equation $px^2+qx+r=0$ has two complex roots α and β, then $|\alpha|+|\beta|$ is **[Online May 19, 2012]**

(a) equal to1
(b) less than 2 but not equal to 1
(c) greater than 2
(d) equal to 2

50. If the sum of the square of the roots of the equation $x^2-(\sin\alpha-2)x-(1+\sin\alpha)=0$ is least, then α is equal to **[Online May 12, 2012]**

(a) $\frac{\pi}{6}$ (b) $\frac{\pi}{4}$

(c) $\frac{\pi}{3}$ (d) $\frac{\pi}{2}$

51. The value of k for which the equation $(k-2)x^2+8x+k+4=0$ has both roots real, distinct and negative is **[Online May 7, 2012]**

(a) 6 (b) 3
(c) 4 (d) 1

52. Let for $a \neq a_1 \neq 0$,

$f(x) = ax^2 + bx + c$, $g(x) = a_1x^2 + b_1x + c_1$

and $p(x) = f(x) - g(x)$.

If $p(x) = 0$ only for $x = -1$ and $p(-2) = 2$, then the value of $p(2)$ is : **[2011 RS]**

(a) 3 (b) 9
(c) 6 (d) 18

53. Sachin and Rahul attempted to solve a quadratic equation. Sachin made a mistake in writing down the constant term and ended up in roots (4,3). Rahul made a mistake in writing down coefficient of x to get roots (3,2). The correct roots of equation are : **[2011 RS]**

(a) 6, 1 (b) 4, 3
(c) $-6, -1$ (d) $-4, -3$

54. Let α, β be real and z be a complex number. If $z^2 + \alpha z + \beta = 0$ has two distinct roots on the line Re $z = 1$, then it is necessary that : **[2011]**

(a) $\beta \in (-1, 0)$ (b) $|\beta| = 1$
(c) $\beta \in (1, \infty)$ (d) $\beta \in (0, 1)$

55. If α and β are the roots of the equation $x^2 - x + 1 = 0$, then $\alpha^{2009} + \beta^{2009} =$ **[2010]**

(a) -1 (b) 1
(c) 2 (d) -2

56. If the roots of the equation $bx^2 + cx + a = 0$ be imaginary, then for all real values of x, the expression $3b^2x^2 + 6bcx + 2c^2$ is : **[2009]**

(a) less than $4ab$ (b) greater than $-4ab$
(c) less than $-4ab$ (d) greater than $4ab$

57. If the difference between the roots of the equation $x^2 + ax + 1 = 0$ is less than $\sqrt{5}$, then the set of possible values of a is **[2007]**

(a) $(3, \infty)$ (b) $(-\infty, -3)$
(c) $(-3, 3)$ (d) $(-3, \infty)$

58. All the values of m for which both roots of the equation $x^2 - 2mx + m^2 - 1 = 0$ are greater than -2 but less than 4, lie in the interval **[2006]**

(a) $-2 < m < 0$ (b) $m > 3$
(c) $-1 < m < 3$ (d) $1 < m < 4$

59. If the roots of the quadratic equation $x^2 + px + q = 0$ are $\tan 30°$ and $\tan 15°$, respectively, then the value of $2 + q - p$ is **[2006]**

(a) 2 (b) 3
(c) 0 (d) 1

60. If $z^2 + z + 1 = 0$, where z is complex number, then the value of $\left(z+\frac{1}{z}\right)^2 + \left(z^2+\frac{1}{z^2}\right)^2 + \left(z^3+\frac{1}{z^3}\right)^2 + \ldots\ldots + \left(z^6+\frac{1}{z^6}\right)^2$ is

(a) 18 (b) 54 **[2006]**
(c) 6 (d) 12

61. In a triangle PQR, $\angle R = \frac{\pi}{2}$. If $\tan\left(\frac{P}{2}\right)$ and $-\tan\left(\frac{Q}{2}\right)$ are the roots of $ax^2 + bx + c = 0$, $a \neq 0$ then **[2005]**

(a) $a = b + c$ (b) $c = a + b$
(c) $b = c$ (d) $b = a + c$

62. If the roots of the equation $x^2 - bx + c = 0$ be two consecutive integers, then $b^2 - 4c$ equals **[2005]**

(a) -2 (b) 3
(c) 2 (d) 1

63. If one root of the equation $x^2 + px + 12 = 0$ is 4, while the equation $x^2 + px + q = 0$ has equal roots, then the value of 'q' is **[2004]**

(a) 4 (b) 12
(c) 3 (d) $\frac{49}{4}$

64. If $(1-p)$ is a root of quadratic equation $x^2 + px + (1-p) = 0$ then its root are **[2004]**

(a) $-1, 2$ (b) $-1, 1$
(c) $0, -1$ (d) $0, 1$

65. The number of real solutions of the equation $x^2 - 3|x| + 2 = 0$ is **[2003]**

(a) 3 (b) 2
(c) 4 (d) 1

66. The value of 'a' for which one root of the quadratic equation $(a^2 - 5a + 3)x^2 + (3a - 1)x + 2 = 0$ is twice as large as the other is **[2003]**

(a) $-\frac{1}{3}$ (b) $\frac{2}{3}$
(c) $-\frac{2}{3}$ (d) $\frac{1}{3}$

67. Let Z_1 and Z_2 be two roots of the equation $Z^2 + aZ + b = 0$, Z being complex. Further, assume that the origin, Z_1 and Z_2 form an equilateral triangle. Then **[2003]**

(a) $a^2 = 4b$ (b) $a^2 = b$
(c) $a^2 = 2b$ (d) $a^2 = 3b$

68. If p and q are the roots of the equation $x^2 + px + q = 0$, then **[2002]**

(a) $p = 1, q = -2$ (b) $p = 0, q = 1$
(c) $p = -2, q = 0$ (d) $p = -2, q = 1$

69. Product of real roots of the equation $t^2 x^2 + |x| + 9 = 0$ **[2002]**

(a) is always positive (b) is always negative
(c) does not exist (d) none of these

70. Difference between the corresponding roots of $x^2+ax+b=0$ and $x^2+bx+a=0$ is same and $a \neq b$, then **[2002]**

(a) $a + b + 4 = 0$ (b) $a + b - 4 = 0$
(c) $a - b - 4 = 0$ (d) $a - b + 4 = 0$

71. If $\alpha \neq \beta$ but $\alpha^2 = 5\alpha - 3$ and $\beta^2 = 5\beta - 3$ then the equation having α/β and β/α as its roots is **[2002]**

(a) $3x^2 - 19x + 3 = 0$ (b) $3x^2 + 19x - 3 = 0$
(c) $3x^2 - 19x - 3 = 0$ (d) $x^2 - 5x + 3 = 0$.

TOPIC-4 : Condition for Common Roots, Maximum and Minimum value of Quadratic Equation, Quadratic Expression in two Variables, Solution of Quadratic Inequalities.

72. If the equations $x^2 + bx - 1 = 0$ and $x^2 + x + b = 0$ have a common root different from -1, then $|b|$ is equal to : **[Online April 9, 2016]**

(a) 2 (b) 3
(c) $\sqrt{3}$ (d) $\sqrt{2}$

73. If non-zero real numbers b and c are such that min f(x) > max g(x), where $f(x) = x^2 + 2bx + 2c^2$ and $g(x) = -x^2 - 2cx + b^2$ $(x \in R)$;

then $\left|\frac{c}{b}\right|$ lies in the interval: **[Online April 19, 2014]**

(a) $\left(0, \frac{1}{2}\right)$ (b) $\left[\frac{1}{2}, \frac{1}{\sqrt{2}}\right)$

(c) $\left[\frac{1}{\sqrt{2}}, \sqrt{2}\right]$ (d) $\left(\sqrt{2}, \infty\right)$

74. If equations $ax^2 + bx + c = 0$ $(a, b, c \in R, a \neq 0)$ and $2x^2 + 3x + 4 = 0$ have a common root, then a : b : c equals: **[Online April 9, 2014]**

(a) 1 : 2 : 3 (b) 2 : 3 : 4
(c) 4 : 3 : 2 (d) 3 : 2 : 1

75. If the equations $x^2 + 2x + 3 = 0$ and $ax^2 + bx + c = 0$, $a,b,c \in R$, have a common root, then $a : b : c$ is **[2013]**

(a) 1 : 2 : 3 (b) 3 : 2 : 1
(c) 1 : 3 : 2 (d) 3 : 1 : 2

76. The least integral value α of x such that $\frac{x-5}{x^2 + 5x - 14} > 0$, satisfies : **[Online April 23, 2013]**

(a) $\alpha^2 + 3\alpha - 4 = 0$ (b) $\alpha^2 - 5\alpha + 4 = 0$
(c) $\alpha^2 - 7\alpha + 6 = 0$ (d) $\alpha^2 + 5\alpha - 6 = 0$

77. The values of 'a' for which one root of the equation $x^2 - (a+1)x + a^2 + a - 8 = 0$ exceeds 2 and the other is lesser than 2, are given by : **[Online April 9, 2013]**

(a) $3 < a < 10$ (b) $a \geq 10$
(c) $-2 < a < 3$ (d) $a \leq -2$

78. If $\left|z - \frac{4}{z}\right| = 2$, then the maximum value of $|z|$ is equal to : **[2009]**

(a) $\sqrt{5} + 1$ (b) 2
(c) $2 + \sqrt{2}$ (d) $\sqrt{3} + 1$

79. The quadratic equations $x^2 - 6x + a = 0$ and $x^2 - cx + 6 = 0$ have one root in common. The other roots of the first and second equations are integers in the ratio 4 : 3. Then the common root is **[2009]**

(a) 1 (b) 4
(c) 3 (d) 2

80. If x is real, the maximum value of $\frac{3x^2 + 9x + 17}{3x^2 + 9x + 7}$ is **[2006]**

(a) $\frac{1}{4}$ (b) 41
(c) 1 (d) $\frac{17}{7}$

81. If both the roots of the quadratic equation $x^2 - 2kx + k^2 + k - 5 = 0$ are less than 5, then k lies in the interval **[2005]**

(a) $(5, 6]$ (b) $(6, \infty)$
(c) $(-\infty, 4)$ (d) $[4, 5]$

82. The value of a for which the sum of the squares of the roots of the equation $x^2 - (a-2)x - a - 1 = 0$ assume the least value is **[2005]**

(a) 1 (b) 0
(c) 3 (d) 2

Hints & Solutions

1. (b) Rationalizing the given expression

$$\frac{(2+3i\sin\theta)(1+2i\sin\theta)}{1+4\sin^2\theta}$$

For the given expression to be purely imaginary, real part of the above expression should be equal to zero.

$$\Rightarrow \frac{2-6\sin^2\theta}{1+4\sin^2\theta}=0 \quad \Rightarrow \sin^2\theta=\frac{1}{3}$$

$$\Rightarrow \sin\theta=\pm\frac{1}{\sqrt{3}}$$

2. (b) Let $z=re^{i\theta}$

Consider $\frac{\text{Im}z^5}{(\text{Im}z)^5}=\frac{r^5(\sin 5\theta)}{r^5(\sin\theta)^5}$

$(\because e^{i\theta}=\cos\theta+i\sin\theta)$

$$=\frac{\sin 5\theta}{\sin^5\theta}=\frac{16\sin^5\theta-20\sin^3\theta+5\sin\theta}{\sin^5\theta}$$

$$=\frac{16\sin^5\theta}{\sin^5\theta}-\frac{20\sin^3\theta}{\sin^5\theta}+\frac{5\sin\theta}{\sin^5\theta}$$

$= 5\,\text{cosec}^4\theta - 20\,\text{cosec}^2\theta + 16$

minimum value of $\frac{\text{Im}\,z^5}{(\text{Im}z)^5}$ is -4.

3. (d) We know minimum value of $|Z_1+Z_2|$ is $||Z_1|-|Z_2||$

Thus minimum value of $\left|Z+\frac{1}{2}\right|$ is $\left||Z|-\frac{1}{2}\right|$

$$\le\left|Z+\frac{1}{2}\right|\le|Z|+\frac{1}{2}$$

Since, $|Z|\ge 2$ therefore

$$2-\frac{1}{2}<\left|Z+\frac{1}{2}\right|<2+\frac{1}{2}$$

$$\Rightarrow \frac{3}{2}<\left|Z+\frac{1}{2}\right|<\frac{5}{2}$$

4. (b) Let $z = 1+i\alpha,\ \alpha\in R$

$z^2 = (1+i\alpha)(1+i\alpha)$

$x+iy = (1+2i\alpha-\alpha^2)$

On comparing real and imaginary parts, we get

$x = 1-\alpha^2,\ y = 2\alpha$

Now, consider option (b), which is

$y^2+4x-4=0$

LHS : $y^2+4x-4 = (2\alpha)^2+4(1-\alpha^2)-4$

$= 4\alpha^2+4-4\alpha^2-4$

$= 0 = $ R.H.S.

Hence, $y^2+4x-4=0$

5. (c) Let $z = x+iy$

$\frac{z-i}{z+i}$ is purely imaginary means its real part is zero.

$$\frac{x+iy-i}{x+iy+i}=\frac{x+i(y-1)}{x+i(y+1)}\times\frac{x-i(y+1)}{x-i(y+1)}$$

$$=\frac{x^2-2ix(y+1)+xi(y-1)+y^2-1}{x^2+(y+1)^2}$$

$$=\frac{x^2+y^2-1}{x^2+(y+1)^2}-\frac{2xi}{x^2+(y+1)^2}$$

for pure imaginary, we have

$$\frac{x^2+y^2-1}{x^2+(y+1)^2}=0$$

$\Rightarrow x^2+y^2=1$

$\Rightarrow (x+iy)(x-iy)=1$

$\Rightarrow x+iy=\frac{1}{x-iy}=z$

and $\frac{1}{z}=x-iy$

$$z+\frac{1}{z}=(x+iy)+(x-iy)=2x$$

$\left(z+\frac{1}{z}\right)$ is any non-zero real number

6. (a) Consider $\arg\left(\frac{z_1}{z_4}\right)+\arg\left(\frac{z_2}{z_3}\right)$

$= \arg(z_1)-\arg(z_4)+\arg(z_2)-\arg(z_3)$

$= (\arg(z_1)+\arg(z_2))-(\arg(z_3)+\arg(z_4))$

given $\begin{pmatrix} z_2=\bar{z}_1\ \& \\ z_4=\bar{z}_3 \end{pmatrix}$

$= (\arg(z_1)+\arg(\bar{z}_1))-(\arg(z_3)+\arg(\bar{z}_3))$

$\begin{Bmatrix}\text{also } (\arg(\bar{z}_1)=-\arg(z_1)) \\ \arg(\bar{z}_3)=-\arg(z_3)\end{Bmatrix}$

$= (\arg(z_1)-\arg(z_1))-(\arg(z_3)-\arg(z_3))$

$= 0-0=0$

7. (d) Consider the equation

$$w - \bar{w}z = k(1-z), k \in R$$

Clearly $z \neq 1$ and $\frac{w - \bar{w}z}{1-z}$ is purely real

$$\therefore \overline{\frac{w - \bar{w}z}{1-z}} = \frac{w - \bar{w}z}{1-z}$$

$$\Rightarrow \frac{\bar{w} - w\bar{z}}{1-\bar{z}} = \frac{w - \bar{w}z}{1-z}$$

$$\Rightarrow \bar{w} - \bar{w}z - w\bar{z} + wz\bar{z} = w - w\bar{z} - \bar{w}z + \bar{w}z\bar{z}$$

$$\Rightarrow \bar{w} + w|z|^2 = w + \bar{w}|z|^2$$

$$\Rightarrow (w - \bar{w})(|z|^2) = w - \bar{w}$$

$\Rightarrow |z|^2 = 1$ $(\because \text{Im } w \neq 0)$

$\Rightarrow |z| = 1$ and $z \neq 1$

$\therefore$ The required set is $\{z : |z| = 1, z \neq 1\}$

8. (c) Given $|z| = 1$, $\arg z = \theta$

As we know, $\bar{z} = \frac{1}{z}$

$$\therefore \arg\left(\frac{1+z}{1+\bar{z}}\right) = \arg\left(\frac{1+z}{1+\frac{1}{z}}\right) = \arg(z) = \theta.$$

9. (b) Let $z = x + iy$, $\bar{z} = x - iy$

Now, $z = 1 - \bar{z}$

$\Rightarrow x + iy = 1 - (x - iy)$

$\Rightarrow 2x = 1 \Rightarrow x = \frac{1}{2}$

Now, $|z| = 1 \Rightarrow x^2 + y^2 = 1 \Rightarrow y^2 = 1 - x^2$

$\Rightarrow y = \pm\frac{\sqrt{3}}{2}$

Now, $\tan\theta = \frac{y}{x}$ (θ is the argument)

$= \frac{\sqrt{3}}{2} \div \frac{1}{2}$ (+ve since only principal argument)

$= \sqrt{3}$

$\Rightarrow \theta = \tan^{-1}\sqrt{3} = \frac{\pi}{3}$

Hence, z is not a real number

So, statement-1 is false and 2 is true.

10. (a) Let $z = x + iy \Rightarrow z^2 = x^2 - y^2 + 2ixy$

$$\text{Now, } \frac{1+z^2}{2iz} = \frac{1+x^2-y^2+2ixy}{2i(x+iy)} = \frac{(x^2-y^2+1)+2ixy}{2ix-2y}$$

$$= \frac{(x^2-y^2+1)+2ixy}{-2y+2ix} \times \frac{-2y-2ix}{-2y-2ix}$$

$$= \frac{y(x^2+y^2-1)+x(x^2+y^2+1)i}{2(x^2+y^2)}$$

$$a = \frac{x(x^2+y^2+1)}{2(x^2+y^2)}$$

Since, $|z| = 1 \Rightarrow \sqrt{x^2+y^2} = 1$

$\Rightarrow x^2 + y^2 = 1$

$$\therefore a = \frac{x(1+1)}{2\times 1} = x$$

Also $z \neq 1 \Rightarrow x + iy \neq 1$

$\therefore A = (-1, 1)$

11. (d) Let $z_1 = 1 + i$ and $z_2 = 1 - i$

$$\frac{z_2}{z_1} = \frac{1-i}{1+i} = \frac{(1-i)(1-i)}{(1+i)(1-i)} = -i$$

$$\frac{2z_1+3z_2}{2z_1-3z_2} = \frac{2+3\left(\frac{z_2}{z_1}\right)}{2-3\left(\frac{z_2}{z_1}\right)} = \frac{2-3i}{2+3i}$$

$$\left|\frac{2z_1+3z_2}{2z_1-3z_2}\right| = \left|\frac{2-3i}{2+3i}\right| = \frac{|2-3i|}{|2+3i|} \quad \left[\because \left|\frac{z_1}{z_2}\right| = \frac{|z_1|}{|z_2|}\right]$$

$$= \frac{\sqrt{4+9}}{\sqrt{4+9}} = 1$$

12. (b) $|z_1+z_2|^2 + |z_1-z_2|^2$

$$= |z_1|^2 + |z_2|^2 + 2|z_1||z_2| + |z_1|^2 + |z_2|^2 - 2|z_1||z_2|$$

$$= 2|z_1|^2 + 2|z_2|^2 = 2\left[|z_1|^2 + |z_2|^2\right]$$

13. (a) Let $|Z| = |W| = r$

$\Rightarrow Z = re^{i\theta}$, $W = re^{i\phi}$

where $\theta + \phi = \pi$

$\therefore \bar{W} = re^{-i\phi}$

Now, $Z = re^{i(\pi-\phi)} = re^{i\pi} \times e^{-i\phi} = -re^{-i\phi}$

$= -\bar{W}$

Thus, statement-1 is true but statement-2 is false.

14. (b) Statement - 1 and 2 both are true.

It is fundamental property.

But Statement - 2 is not correct explanation for Statement - 1.

15. (a) Let $z = x + iy$

$$|z-1| = |z+1| \Rightarrow (x-1)^2 + y^2 = (x+1)^2 + y^2$$

$\Rightarrow \text{Re } z = 0 \quad \Rightarrow x = 0$

$$|z-1| = |z-i| \Rightarrow (x-1)^2 + y^2 = x^2 + (y-1)^2$$

$\Rightarrow x = y$

$$|z+1| = |z-i| \Rightarrow (x+1)^2 + y^2 = x^2 + (y-1)^2$$

Only (0, 0) will satisfy all conditions.

$\Rightarrow$ Number of complex number $z = 1$

16. (c) $\left(\frac{1}{i-1}\right)=\frac{1}{-i-1}=\frac{-1}{i+1}$

17. (a) $z^{\frac{1}{3}}=p+iq \Rightarrow z=p^3+(iq)^3+3p(iq)(p+iq)$

$\Rightarrow x-iy=p^3-3pq^2+i(3p^2q-q^3)$

$\therefore x=p^3-3pq^2 \Rightarrow \frac{x}{p}=p^2-3q^2$

$y=q^3-3p^2q \Rightarrow \frac{y}{q}=q^2-3p^2$

$\therefore \frac{x}{p}+\frac{y}{q}=-2p^2-2q^2 \therefore \left(\frac{x}{p}+\frac{y}{q}\right)\Big/(p^2+q^2)=-2$

18. (c) $\arg zw=\pi \Rightarrow \arg z+\arg w=\pi$...(1)

$\bar{z}+i\bar{w}=0 \Rightarrow \bar{z}=-i\bar{w}$

$\therefore z=iw \Rightarrow \arg z=\frac{\pi}{2}+\arg w$

$\Rightarrow \arg z=\frac{\pi}{2}+\pi-\arg z$ (from (1))

$\therefore \arg z=\frac{3\pi}{4}$

19. (b) $\left(\frac{1+i}{1-i}\right)^x=1 \Rightarrow \left[\frac{(1+i)^2}{1-i^2}\right]^x=1$

$\left(\frac{1+i^2+2i}{1+1}\right)^x=1 \Rightarrow (i)^x=1;\ \therefore x=4n;\ n\in I^+$

20. (a) $|\bar{z}\omega|=|\bar{z}||\omega|=|z||\omega|=|z\omega|=1$

$\text{Arg}(\bar{z}\omega)=\arg(\bar{z})+\arg(\omega)$

$=-\arg(z)+\arg\omega=-\frac{\pi}{2}$ $\qquad \therefore \bar{z}\omega=-1$

ALTERNATE SOLUTION

Let $z=r_1e^{i\theta}$ and $w=r_2e^{i\phi}$, $\therefore\ \bar{z}=r_1e^{-i\theta}$

Now $|z\omega|=1 \Rightarrow \left|r_1r_2e^{i(\theta+\phi)}\right|=1 \Rightarrow r_1r_2=1$

Also $\arg(z)-\arg(\omega)=\frac{\pi}{2} \Rightarrow \theta-\phi=\frac{\pi}{2}$

Now $\bar{z}\omega=r_1e^{-i\theta}.r_2e^{i\phi}$

$=r_1r_2e^{-i(\theta-\phi)}=e^{-\frac{i\pi}{2}}=-1$

21. (c) Given $|z-4|<|z-2|$ Let $z=x+iy$

$\Rightarrow |(x-4)+iy)|<|(x-2)+iy|$

$\Rightarrow (x-4)^2+y^2<(x-2)^2+y^2$

$\Rightarrow x^2-8x+16<x^2-4x+4 \Rightarrow 12<4x$

$\Rightarrow x>3 \Rightarrow \text{Re}(z)>3$

22. (b) Let $|z|=|\omega|=r$

$\therefore z=re^{i\theta},\ \omega=re^{i\phi}$ where $\theta+\phi=\pi$.

$\therefore z=re^{i(\pi-\phi)}=re^{i\pi}.e^{-i\phi}=-re^{-i\phi}=-\bar{\omega}$.

$[\because \bar{\omega}=re^{-i\phi}]$

23. (a)

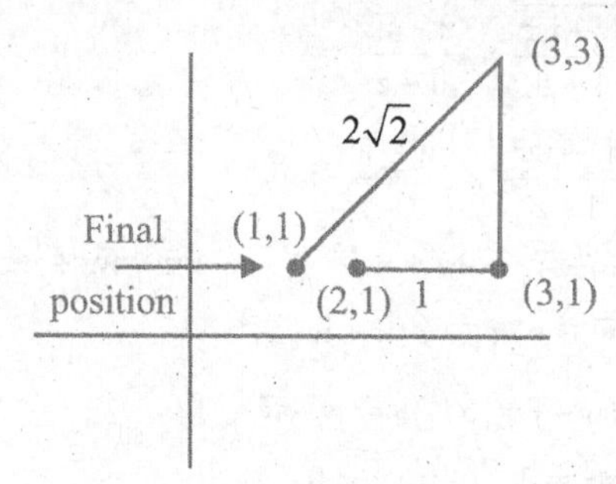

So new position is at the point $1+i$

24. (a) $\left|\frac{z_1-2z_2}{2-z_1\bar{z}_2}\right|=1$

$\Rightarrow |z_1-2z_2|^2=|2-z_1\bar{z}_2|^2$

$\Rightarrow (z_1-2z_2)\overline{(z_1-2z_2)}=(2-z_1\bar{z}_2)\overline{(2-z_1\bar{z}_2)}$

$\Rightarrow (z_1-2z_2)(\bar{z}_1-2\bar{z}_2)=(2-z_1\bar{z}_2)(2-\bar{z}_1z_2)$

$\Rightarrow (z_1\bar{z}_1)-2z_1\bar{z}_2-2\bar{z}_1z_2+4z_2\bar{z}_2$

$=4-2\bar{z}_1z_2-2z_1\bar{z}_2+z_1\bar{z}_1z_2\bar{z}_2$

$\Rightarrow |z_1|^2+4|z_2|^2=4+|z_1|^2|z_2|^2$

$\Rightarrow |z_1|^2+4|z_2|^2-4-|z_1|^2|z_2|^2=0$

$\left(|z_1|^2-4\right)\left(1-|z_2|^2\right)=0$

$\because |z_2|\neq 1$

$\therefore |z_1|^2=4$

$\Rightarrow |z_1|=2$

$\Rightarrow$ Point z_1 lies on circle of radius 2.

25. (a) Since we know $z=\bar{z}$ if z is real.

Therefore, $\frac{z^2}{z-1}=\frac{\bar{z}^2}{\bar{z}-1}$

$\Rightarrow z\bar{z}z-z^2=z.\bar{z}.\bar{z}-\bar{z}^2$

$\Rightarrow |z|^2.z-z^2=|z|^2.\bar{z}-\bar{z}^2$

$\Rightarrow |z|^2(z-\bar{z})-(z-\bar{z})(z+\bar{z})=0$

$\Rightarrow (z-\bar{z})\left(|z|^2-(z+\bar{z})\right)=0$

Either $z-\bar{z}=0$ or $|z|^2-(z+\bar{z})=0$

Either $z=\bar{z} \Rightarrow$ real axis

or $|z|^2=z+\bar{z} \Rightarrow z\bar{z}-z-\bar{z}=0$

represents a circle passing through origin.

26. **(a)** $(1+\omega)^7=A+B\omega$

$(-\omega^2)^7=A+B\omega$

$-\omega^2=A+B\omega$

$1+\omega=A+B\omega$

$\Rightarrow A=1, B=1.$

27. **(a)** z lies on or inside the circle with centre (–4, 0) and radius 3 units.

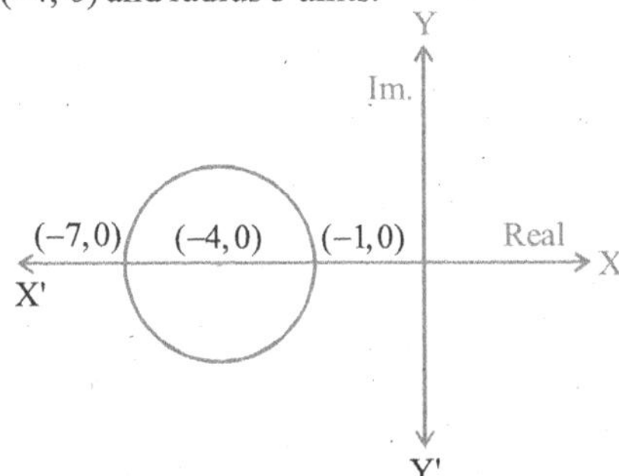

From the Argand diagram maximum value of $|z+1|$ is 6

ALTERNATE SOLUTION $|z+1|=|z+4-3|$

$\le |z+4|+|-3| \le |3|+|-3|$

$\Rightarrow |z+1| \le 6 \Rightarrow |z+1|_{max}=6$

28. **(c)** As given $w=\dfrac{z}{z-\frac{1}{3}i}$

$\Rightarrow |w|=\dfrac{|z|}{|z-\frac{1}{3}i|}=1$

$\Rightarrow |z|=\left|z-\frac{1}{3}i\right|$

$\Rightarrow$ distance of z from origin and point $\left(0, \frac{1}{3}\right)$ is same

hence z lies on bisector of the line joining points (0, 0) and (0, 1/3).

Hence z lies on a straight line.

29. **(c)** $|z_1+z_2|=|z_1|+|z_2| \Rightarrow z_1$ and z_2 are collinear and are to the same side of origin; hence arg z_1 – arg $z_2=0$.

30. **(c)** $(x-1)^3+8=0 \Rightarrow (x-1)=(-2)(1)^{1/3}$

$\Rightarrow x-1=-2$ or -2ω or $-2\omega^2$

or $x=-1$ or $1-2\omega$ or $1-2\omega^2$.

31. **(b)** $|z^2-1|=|z|^2+1 \Rightarrow |z^2-1|^2=(z\bar{z}+1)^2$

$\Rightarrow (z^2-1)(\bar{z}^2-1)=(z\bar{z}+1)^2$

$\Rightarrow z^2\bar{z}^2-z^2-\bar{z}^2+1=z^2\bar{z}^2+2z\bar{z}+1$

$\Rightarrow z^2+2z\bar{z}+\bar{z}^2=0 \Rightarrow (z+\bar{z})^2=0 \Rightarrow z=-\bar{z}$

$\Rightarrow z$ is purely imaginary

ALTERNATE SOLUTION 1

Let $z=r(\cos\theta+i\sin\theta)$

Then $|z^2-1|=|r^2(\cos 2\theta+i\sin 2\theta)-1|$

$=\sqrt{r^4-2r^2\cos 2\theta+1}$ and $|z^2-1|^2=(|z|^2+1)^2$

$\Rightarrow r^4-2r^2\cos 2\theta+1=r^4+2r^2+1$

$\Rightarrow 2\cos^2\theta=0 \Rightarrow \cos\theta=\pm\frac{\pi}{2}$

$\therefore z$ lies on imaginary axis.

ALTERNATE SOLUTION 2

We know that, if $|z_1+z_2|=|z_1|+|z_2|$

then origin, z_1 and z_2 are collinear

$\Rightarrow \arg(z_1)=\arg(z_2)$

As per question $\left|z^2+(-1)\right|=\left|z^2\right|+|-1|$

$\Rightarrow \arg\left(z^2\right)=\arg(-1)$

$\Rightarrow 2\arg(z)=\pi \Rightarrow \arg(z)=\frac{\pi}{2}$

$\Rightarrow z$ lies on imaginary axis.

32. **(b)** Let the circle be $|z-z_0|=r$. Then according to given conditions $|z_0-z_1|=r+a$ and $|z_0-z_2|=r+b$. Eliminating r, we get $|z_0-z_1|-|z_0-z_2|=a-b$.

$\therefore$ Locus of centre z_0 is $|z-z_1|-|z-z_2|=a-b$, which represents a hyperbola.

33. **(a)** We have

$\sum_{r=1}^{n}(x+r-1)(x+r)=10n$

$\sum_{r=1}^{n}(x^2+xr+(r-1)x+r^2-r=10n$

$\Rightarrow \sum_{r=1}^{n}(x^2+(2r-1)x+r(r-1)=10n$

$\Rightarrow nx^2+\{1+3+5+....+(2n-1)\}x+\{1.2+2.3+....+(n-1)n\}=10n$

$\Rightarrow nx^2+n^2x+\dfrac{(n-1)n(n+1)}{3}=10n$

$\Rightarrow x^2+nx+\dfrac{n^2-31}{3}=0$

Let α and α + 1 be its two solutions

(∵ it has two consequtive integral solutions)

$\Rightarrow \quad \alpha+(\alpha+1)=-n$

$\Rightarrow \quad \alpha=\dfrac{-n-1}{2}$ ...(a)

Also $\alpha(\alpha+1)=\dfrac{n^2-31}{3}$ ...(b)

Putting value of (a) in (b), we get

$-\left(\dfrac{n+1}{2}\right)\left(\dfrac{1-n}{2}\right)=\dfrac{n^2-31}{3}$

$\Rightarrow n^2=121$

$\Rightarrow n=11$

34. (c) $(x-1)(x^2+5x-50)=0$

$\Rightarrow (x-1)(x+10)(x-5)=0$

$\Rightarrow \quad x=1,5,-10$

Sum $=-4$

35. (c) Let $p(x)=ax^2+bx+c$

$\because \; p(0)=1 \Rightarrow c=1$

Also, $p(1)=4$ & $p(-1)=6$

$\Rightarrow \; a+b+1=4$ & $a-b+1=6$

$\Rightarrow \; a+b=3$ & $a-b=5$

$\Rightarrow \; a=4$ & $b=-1$

$p(x)=4x^2-x+1$

$p(b)=16-2+1=15$

$p(-2)=16+2+1=19$

36. (c) $(x^2-5x+5)^{x^2+4x-60}=1$

Case I

$x^2-5x+5=1$ and $x^2+4x-60$ can be any real number

$\Rightarrow x=1,4$

Case II

$x^2-5x+5=-1$ and $x^2+4x-60$ has to be an even number

$\Rightarrow x=2,3$

where 3 is rejected because for $x=3$, $x^2+4x-60$ is odd.

Case III

x^2-5x+5 can be any real number and $x^2+4x-60=0$

$\Rightarrow x=-10,6$

$\Rightarrow$ Sum of all values of $x=-10+6+2+1+4=3$

37. (a) $\sqrt{2x+1}-\sqrt{2x-1}=1$ .....(a)

$\Rightarrow \; 2x+1+2x-1-2\sqrt{4x^2-1}=1$

$\Rightarrow \; 4x-1=2\sqrt{4x^2-1}$

$\Rightarrow \; 16x^2-8x+1=16x^2-4$

$\Rightarrow \; 8x=5$

$\Rightarrow \; x=\dfrac{5}{8}$ which satisfies equation (a)

So, $\sqrt{4x^2-1}=\dfrac{3}{4}$

38. (a) $\alpha,\beta=\dfrac{6\pm\sqrt{36+8}}{2}=3\pm\sqrt{11}$

$\alpha=3+\sqrt{11},\ \beta=3-\sqrt{11}$

$\therefore\ a_n=\left(3+\sqrt{11}\right)^n-\left(3-\sqrt{11}\right)^n$

$\dfrac{a_{10}-2a_8}{2a_9}$

$=\dfrac{\left(3+\sqrt{11}\right)^{10}-\left(3-\sqrt{11}\right)^{10}-2\left(3+\sqrt{11}\right)^8+2\left(3-\sqrt{11}\right)^8}{2\left[\left(3+\sqrt{11}\right)^9-\left(3-\sqrt{11}\right)^9\right]}$

$=\dfrac{\left(3+\sqrt{11}\right)^8\left[\left(3+\sqrt{11}\right)^2-2\right]+\left(3-\sqrt{11}\right)^8\left[2-\left(3-\sqrt{11}\right)^2\right]}{2\left[\left(3+\sqrt{11}\right)^9-\left(3-\sqrt{11}\right)^9\right]}$

$=\dfrac{\left(3+\sqrt{11}\right)^8\left(9+11+6\sqrt{11}-2\right)+\left(3-\sqrt{11}\right)^8\left(2-9-11+6\sqrt{11}\right)}{2\left[\left(3+\sqrt{11}\right)^9-\left(3-\sqrt{11}\right)^9\right]}$

$=\dfrac{6\left(3+\sqrt{11}\right)^9-6\left(3-\sqrt{11}\right)^9}{2\left[\left(3+\sqrt{11}\right)^9-\left(3-\sqrt{11}\right)^9\right]}=\dfrac{6}{2}=3$

39. (b) $(a-1)(x^4+x^2+1)+(a+1)(x^2+x+1)^2=0$

$\Rightarrow (a-1)(x^2+x+1)(x^2-x+1)+(a+1)(x^2+x+1)^2=0$

$\Rightarrow (x^2+x+1)[(a-1)(x^2-x+1)+(a+1)(x^2+x+1)]=0$

$\Rightarrow (x^2+x+1)(ax^2+x+a)=0$

For roots to be distinct and real, $a\neq 0$ and $1-4a^2>0$

$\Rightarrow a\neq 0$ and $a^2<\dfrac{1}{4}$

$\Rightarrow a\in\left(-\dfrac{1}{2},0\right)\cup\left(0,\dfrac{1}{2}\right)$

40. (b) $\alpha=2+3i;\ \beta=2-3i,\ \gamma=?$

$\alpha\beta\gamma=\dfrac{13}{2}$ $\left[\text{since product of roots}=\dfrac{d}{a}\right]$

$\Rightarrow (4+9)\gamma=\dfrac{13}{2}\Rightarrow \gamma=\dfrac{1}{2}$

41. (c) Consider $-3(x-[x])^2+2[x-[x])+a^2=0$

$\Rightarrow \; 3\{x\}^2-2\{x\}-a^2=0 \quad (\because x-[x]=\{x\})$

$\Rightarrow \; 3\left(\{x\}^2-\dfrac{2}{3}\{x\}\right)=a^2, a\neq 0$

$\Rightarrow \; a^2=3\{x\}\left(\{x\}-\dfrac{2}{3}\right)$

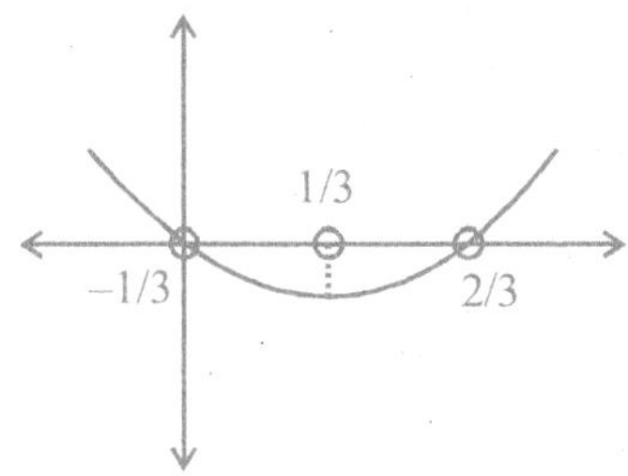

Now, $\{x\} \in (0,1)$ and $\frac{-2}{3} \le a^2 < 1$ (by graph)

Since, x is not an integer

$\therefore \quad a \in (-1,1) - \{0\}$

$\Rightarrow a \in (-1,0) \cup (0,1)$

42. (a) Consider $\sqrt{3x^2+x+5} = x-3$

Squaring both the sides, we get

$3x^2 + x + 5 = (x-3)^2$

$\Rightarrow 3x^2+x+5 = x^2+9-6x$

$\Rightarrow 2x^2+7x-4 = 0$

$\Rightarrow 2x^2+8x-x-4 = 0$

$\Rightarrow 2x(x+4)-1(x+4) = 0$

$\Rightarrow x = \frac{1}{2}$ or $x = -4$

For $x = \frac{1}{2}$ and $x = -4$

L.H.S. $\neq$ R.H.S. of equation, $\sqrt{3x^2+x+5} = x-3$

Also, for every $x \in R$, LHS $\neq$ RHS of the given equation.

$\therefore$ Given equation has no solution.

43. (c) $x^2 + |2x-3| - 4 = 0$

$$|2x-3| = \begin{cases} (2x-3) & \text{if } x > \frac{3}{2} \\ -(2x-3) & \text{if } x < \frac{3}{2} \end{cases}$$

for $x > \frac{3}{2}$, $x^2+2x-3-4 = 0$

$x^2 + 2x - 7 = 0$

$$x = \frac{-2\pm\sqrt{4+28}}{2} = \frac{-2\pm 4\sqrt{2}}{2} = -1\pm 2\sqrt{2}$$

Here $x = 2\sqrt{2}-1 \quad \left\{2\sqrt{2}-1 < \frac{3}{2}\right\}$

for $x < \frac{3}{2}$

$x^2 - 2x + 3 - 4 = 0$

$\Rightarrow \quad x^2 - 2x - 1 = 0$

$$\Rightarrow \quad x = \frac{2\pm\sqrt{4+4}}{2} = \frac{2\pm 2\sqrt{2}}{2} = 1\pm\sqrt{2}$$

Here $x = 1-\sqrt{2} \quad \left\{(1-\sqrt{2}) < \frac{3}{2}\right\}$

Sum of roots : $(2\sqrt{2}-1)+(1-\sqrt{2}) = \sqrt{2}$

44. (d) $x^2 - 4\sqrt{2}kx + 2e^{4\ln k} - 1 = 0$

or, $x^2 - 4\sqrt{2}kx + 2k^4 - 1 = 0$

$\alpha+\beta = 4\sqrt{2}k$ and $\alpha.\beta = 2k^4 - 1$

Squaring both sides, we get

$(\alpha+\beta)^2 = (4\sqrt{2}k)^2 \Rightarrow \alpha^2+\beta^2+2\alpha\beta = 32k^2$

$66 + 2\alpha\beta = 32k^2$

$66 + 2(2k^4-1) = 32k^2$

$66 + 4k^4 - 2 = 32k^2 \Rightarrow 4k^4 - 32k^2 + 64 = 0$

or, $k^4 - 8k^2 + 16 = 0 \Rightarrow (k^2)^2 - 8k^2 + 16 = 0$

$\Rightarrow (k^2-4)(k^2-4) = 0 \Rightarrow k^2 = 4, k^2 = 4$

$\Rightarrow k = \pm 2$

Now, $\alpha^3+\beta^3 = (\alpha+\beta)(\alpha^2+\beta^2-\alpha\beta)$

$\therefore \alpha^3+\beta^3 = (4\sqrt{2}k)\,[66-(2k^4-1)]$

Putting $k = -2$, ($k = +2$ cannot be taken because it does not satisfy the above equation)

$\therefore \alpha^3+\beta^3 = (4\sqrt{2}(-2))[66-2(-2)^4-1]$

$\alpha^3+\beta^3 = (-8\sqrt{2})\,(66-32+1) = (-8\sqrt{2})\,(35)$

$\therefore \alpha^3+\beta^3 = -280\sqrt{2}$

45. (a) Let $\frac{1}{\sqrt{\alpha}}$ and $\frac{1}{\sqrt{\beta}}$ be the roots of $ax^2+bx+1=0$

$$\frac{1}{\sqrt{\alpha}}+\frac{1}{\sqrt{\beta}} = \left(\frac{\sqrt{\alpha}+\sqrt{\beta}}{\sqrt{\alpha\beta}}\right) = -\frac{b}{a}$$

$$\frac{1}{\sqrt{\alpha}\sqrt{\beta}} = \frac{1}{a} \Rightarrow a = \sqrt{\alpha\beta}$$

$$b = -\left(\sqrt{\alpha}+\sqrt{\beta}\right)$$

$$x(x+b^3)+(a^3-3abx) = 0$$

$$\Rightarrow \quad x^2+(b^3-3ab)x+a^3 = 0$$

Putting values of a and b, we get

$$x^2+\left[\left(-\sqrt{\alpha}+\sqrt{\beta}\right)^3+3\left(\sqrt{\alpha\beta}\right)\left(\sqrt{\alpha}+\sqrt{\beta}\right)\right]+(\alpha\beta)^{3/2} = 0$$

$$\Rightarrow x^2-\left[\alpha^{3/2}+\beta^{3/2}+3\sqrt{\alpha\beta}\left(\sqrt{\alpha}+\sqrt{\beta}\right)-3\sqrt{\alpha\beta}(\sqrt{\alpha}+\sqrt{\beta})\right]x+(\alpha\beta)^{3/2} = 0$$

$$\Rightarrow \quad x^2-(\alpha^{3/2}+\beta^{3/2})x+\alpha^{3/2}\beta^{3/2} = 0$$

Roots of this equation are $\alpha^{3/2}, \beta^{3/2}$

46. **(b)** Given $\alpha^3+\beta^3=-p$ and $\alpha\beta=q$

Let $\frac{\alpha^2}{\beta}$ and $\frac{\beta^2}{\alpha}$ be the root of required quadratic equation.

So, $\frac{\alpha^2}{\beta}+\frac{\beta^2}{\alpha}=\frac{\alpha^3+\beta^3}{\alpha\beta}=\frac{-p}{q}$

and $\frac{\alpha^2}{\beta}\times\frac{\beta^2}{\alpha}=\alpha\beta=q$

Hence, required quadratic equation is

$x^2-\left(\frac{-p}{q}\right)x+q=0$

$\Rightarrow x^2+\frac{p}{q}x+q=0 \Rightarrow qx^2+px+q^2=0$

47. **(c)** Given quadratic eqn. is

$x^2+px+\frac{3p}{4}=0$

So, $\alpha+\beta=-p, \alpha\beta=\frac{3p}{4}$

Now, given $|\alpha-\beta|=\sqrt{10}$

$\Rightarrow \alpha-\beta=\pm\sqrt{10}$

$\Rightarrow (\alpha-\beta)^2=10 \Rightarrow \alpha^2+\beta^2-2\alpha\beta=10$

$\Rightarrow (\alpha+\beta)^2-4\alpha\beta=10$

$\Rightarrow p^2-4\times\frac{3p}{4}=10 \Rightarrow p^2-3p-10=0$

$\Rightarrow p=-2, 5 \Rightarrow p\in\{-2, 5\}$

48. **(c)** Given equation is

$z+\sqrt{2}|z+1|+i=0$

put $z=x+iy$ in the given equation.

$(x+iy)+\sqrt{2}\,|x+iy+1|+i=0$

$\Rightarrow x+iy+\sqrt{2}\left[\sqrt{(x+1)^2+y^2}\right]+i=0$

Now, equating real and imaginary part, we get

$x+\sqrt{2}\sqrt{(x+1)^2+y^2}=0$ and

$y+1=0 \Rightarrow y=-1$

$\Rightarrow x+\sqrt{2}\sqrt{(x+1)^2+(-1)^2}=0 \quad (\because y=-1)$

$\Rightarrow \sqrt{2}\sqrt{(x+1)^2+1}=-x$

$\Rightarrow 2[(x+1)^2+1]=x^2$

$\Rightarrow x^2+4x+4=0$

$\Rightarrow x=-2$

Thus, $z=-2+i(-1) \Rightarrow |z|=\sqrt{5}$

49. **(c)** Given quadratic equation is

$px^2+qx+r=0$ ...(1)

$D=q^2-4pr$

Since α and β are two complex root

$\therefore \beta=\bar{\alpha} \Rightarrow |\beta|=|\bar{\alpha}| \Rightarrow |\beta|=|\alpha| (\because |\bar{\alpha}|=|\alpha|)$

Consider

$|\alpha|+|\beta|=|\alpha|+|\alpha|$ $(\because |\beta|=|\alpha|)$

$=2\,|\alpha|>2.1=2$ $(\because |\alpha|>1)$

Hence, $|\alpha|+|\beta|$ is greater than 2.

50. **(d)** Given equation is

$x^2-(\sin\alpha-2)x-(1+\sin\alpha)=0$

Let x_1 and x_2 be two roots of quadratic equation.

$\therefore x_1+x_2=\sin\alpha-2$ and $x_1x_2=-(1+\sin\alpha)$

$(x_1+x_2)^2=(\sin\alpha-2)^2=\sin^2\alpha+4-4\sin\alpha$

$\Rightarrow x_1^2+x_2^2=\sin^2\alpha+4-4\sin\alpha-2x_1x_2$

$=\sin^2\alpha+4-4\sin\alpha+2(1+\sin\alpha)$

$=\sin^2\alpha-2\sin\alpha+6$ ...(A)

Now, By putting

$\alpha=\frac{\pi}{6}, \alpha=\frac{\pi}{4}, \alpha=\frac{\pi}{3}$ and $\alpha=\frac{\pi}{2}$ in (A) one by one

We get least value of $x_1^2+x_2^2$ at $\frac{\pi}{2}$

Hence, $\alpha=\frac{\pi}{2}$

51. **(b)** $(k-2)x^2+8x+k+4=0$

If real roots then,

$8^2-4(k-2)(k+4)>0$

$\Rightarrow k^2+2k-8<16$

$\Rightarrow k^2+6k-4k-24<0$

$\Rightarrow (k+6)(k-4)<0$

$\Rightarrow -6<k<4$

If both roots are negative

then $\alpha\beta$ is +ve

$\Rightarrow \frac{k+4}{k-2}>0 \Rightarrow k>-4$

Also, $\frac{k-2}{k+4}>0 \Rightarrow k>2$

Roots are real so, $-6<k<4$

So, 6 and 4 are not correct.

Since, $k>2$, so 1 is also not correct value of k.

$\therefore k=3$

52. **(d)** $p(x)=0$

$\Rightarrow f(x)=g(x)$

$\Rightarrow ax^2+bx+c=a_1x^2+b_1x+c_1$

$\Rightarrow (a-a_1)x^2+(b-b_1)x+(c-c_1)=0.$

It has only one solution, $x=-1$

$\Rightarrow b-b_1=a-a_1+c-c_1$ ...(1)

vertex $=(-1,0)$

$\Rightarrow \quad \dfrac{b-b_1}{2(a-a_1)}=-1$

$\Rightarrow \quad b-b_1=2(a-a_1)$ ...(2)

Now $p(-2)=2$

$\Rightarrow \quad f(-2)-g(-2)=2$

$\Rightarrow \quad 4a-2b+c-4a_1+2b_1-c_1=2$

$\Rightarrow \quad 4(a-a_1)-2(b-b_1)+(c-c_1)=2$ ...(3)

From equations, (1), (2) and (3)

$$a-a_1=c-c_1=\frac{1}{2}(b-b_1)=2$$

Now, $p(2)=f(2)-g(2)$

$$=4(a-a_1)+2(b-b_1)+(c-c_1)$$

$$=8+8+2=18$$

53. (a) Let the correct equation be

$ax^2+bx+c=0$

Now Sachin's equation

$ax^2+bx+c'=0$

Roots found by Sachin's are 4 and 3

Rahul's equation, $ax^2+b'x+c=0$

Roots found by Rahul's are 3 and 2

$-\dfrac{b}{a}=7$ ....(i)

$\dfrac{c}{a}=6$ ...(ii)

From (i) and (ii), roots of the correct equation $x^2-7x+6=0$ are 6 and 1.

54. (c) Since both the roots lie in the line $Re\ z=1$ i.e., $x=1$, hence real part of both the roots are 1.

Let both roots be $1+i\alpha$ and $1-i\alpha$

Product of the roots, $1+\alpha^2=\beta$

$\because \alpha^2+1\geq 1$

$\therefore \beta\geq 1 \Rightarrow \because \beta\in(1,\infty)$

55. (b) $x^2-x+1=0 \Rightarrow x=\dfrac{1\pm\sqrt{1-4}}{2}$

$$x=\frac{1\pm\sqrt{3}i}{2}$$

$$\alpha=\frac{1}{2}+i\frac{\sqrt{3}}{2}=-\omega^2$$

$$\beta=\frac{1}{2}-\frac{i\sqrt{3}}{2}=-\omega$$

$$\alpha=\cos\frac{\pi}{3}+i\sin\frac{\pi}{3},\quad \beta=\cos\frac{\pi}{3}-i\sin\frac{\pi}{3}$$

$$\alpha^{2009}+\beta^{2009}=(-\omega^2)^{2009}+(-\omega)^{2009}$$

$$=-\omega^2-\omega=1$$

56. (b) Given that roots of the equation $bx^2+cx+a=0$ are imaginary

$\therefore \quad c^2-4ab<0$ ....(i)

Let $y=3b^2x^2+6\,bc\,x+2c^2$

$\Rightarrow \quad 3b^2x^2+6\,bc\,x+2c^2-y=0$

As x is real, $D\geq 0$

$\Rightarrow \quad 36\,b^2c^2-12\,b^2(2c^2-y)\geq 0$

$\Rightarrow \quad 12\,b^2(3\,c^2-2\,c^2+y)\geq 0$

$\Rightarrow \quad c^2+y\geq 0 \quad\Rightarrow\quad y\geq -c^2$

But from eqn. (i), $c^2<4ab$ or $-c^2>-4ab$

$\therefore$ we get $y\geq -c^2>-4ab$

$\Rightarrow \quad y>-4\,ab$

57. (c) Let α and β are roots of the equation $x^2+ax+1=0$

$\alpha+\beta=-a$ and $\alpha\beta=1$

given $|\alpha-\beta|<\sqrt{5}$

$\Rightarrow \sqrt{(\alpha+\beta)^2-4\alpha\beta}<\sqrt{5}$

$\left(\because (\alpha-\beta)^2=(\alpha+\beta)^2-4\alpha\beta\right)$

$\Rightarrow \sqrt{a^2-4}<\sqrt{5} \Rightarrow a^2-4<5$

$\Rightarrow a^2-9<0 \Rightarrow a^2<9 \Rightarrow -3<a<3$

$\Rightarrow a\in(-3,3)$

58. (c) Equation $x^2-2mx+m^2-1=0$

$(x-m)^2-1=0$ or $(x-m+1)(x-m-1)=0$

$x=m-1, m+1$

$m-1>-2$ and $m+1<4$

$\Rightarrow m>-1$ and $m<3$ or, $-1<m<3$

59. (b) $x^2+px+q=0$

Sum of roots $=\tan 30°+\tan 15°=-p$

Product of roots $=\tan 30°.\tan 15°=q$

$$\tan 45°=\frac{\tan 30°+\tan 15°}{1-\tan 30°.\tan 15°}=\frac{-p}{1-q}=1$$

$\Rightarrow -p=1-q \Rightarrow q-p=1$

$\therefore 2+q-p=3$

60. (d) $z^2+z+1=0 \Rightarrow z=\omega$ or ω^2

So, $z+\dfrac{1}{z}=\omega+\omega^2=-1$

$z^2+\dfrac{1}{z^2}=\omega^2+\omega=-1,\quad z^3+\dfrac{1}{z^3}=\omega^3+\omega^3=2$

$z^4+\dfrac{1}{z^4}=-1,\quad z^5+\dfrac{1}{z^5}=-1$

and $z^6+\dfrac{1}{z^6}=2$

$\therefore$ The given sum $=1+1+4+1+1+4$
$=12$

61. **(b)** $\tan\left(\frac{P}{2}\right), \tan\left(\frac{Q}{2}\right)$ are the roots of $ax^2+bx+c=0$

$$\tan\left(\frac{P}{2}\right)+\tan\left(\frac{Q}{2}\right)=-\frac{b}{a}$$

$$\tan\left(\frac{P}{2}\right)\cdot\tan\left(\frac{Q}{2}\right)=\frac{c}{a}$$

$$\frac{\tan\left(\frac{P}{2}\right)+\tan\left(\frac{Q}{2}\right)}{1-\tan\left(\frac{P}{2}\right)\tan\left(\frac{Q}{2}\right)}=\tan\left(\frac{P}{2}+\frac{Q}{2}\right)=1$$

$$\Rightarrow \frac{-\frac{b}{a}}{1-\frac{c}{a}}=1 \Rightarrow -\frac{b}{a}=\frac{a}{a}-\frac{c}{a}$$

$\Rightarrow -b=a-c$ or $c=a+b$.

62. **(d)** Let α, $\alpha+1$ be roots
Then $\alpha+\alpha+1=b=$ sum of roots
$\alpha(\alpha+1)=c=$ product of roots
$\therefore\ b^2-4c=(2\alpha+1)^2-4\alpha(\alpha+1)=1$.

63. **(d)** 4 is a root of $x^2+px+12=0$

$\Rightarrow 16+4p+12=0 \Rightarrow p=-7$

Now, the equation $x^2+px+q=0$
has equal roots.

$$\therefore p^2-4q=0 \Rightarrow q=\frac{p^2}{4}=\frac{49}{4}$$

64. **(c)** Let the second root be α.
Then $\alpha+(1-p)=-p \Rightarrow \alpha=-1$
Also $\alpha.(1-p)=1-p$
$\Rightarrow (\alpha-1)(1-p)=0 \Rightarrow p=1 [\because \alpha=-1]$
$\therefore$ Roots are $\alpha=-1$ and $p-1=0$

65. **(c)** $x^2-3|x|+2=0 \Rightarrow |x|^2-3|x|+2=0$
$(|x|-2)(|x|-1)=0$
$|x|=1,2$ or $x=\pm1,\pm2$
$\therefore$ No.of solution $=4$

66. **(b)** Let the roots of given equation be α and 2α then

$$\alpha+2\alpha=3\alpha=\frac{1-3a}{a^2-5a+3}$$

and $\alpha.2\alpha=2\alpha^2=\dfrac{2}{a^2-5a+3}$

$$\Rightarrow \alpha=\frac{1-3a}{3(a^2-5a+3)}$$

$$\therefore\ 2\left[\frac{1}{9}\frac{(1-3a)^2}{(a^2-5a+3)^2}\right]=\frac{2}{a^2-5a+3}$$

$$\frac{(1-3a)^2}{(a^2-5a+3)}=9 \text{ or } 9a^2-6a+1$$

$$=9a^2-45a+27$$

or $39a=26$ or $a=\dfrac{2}{3}$

67. **(d)** $Z^2+aZ+b=0$; $Z_1+Z_2=-a$ & $Z_1Z_2=b$
$0, Z_1, Z_2$ form an equilateral Δ
$\therefore\ 0^2+Z_1^2+Z_2^2=0.Z_1+Z_1.Z_2+Z_2.0$
(for an equilateral triangle,
$Z_1^2+Z_2^2+Z_3^2=Z_1Z_2+Z_2Z_3+Z_3Z_1$)
$\Rightarrow Z_1^2+Z_2^2=Z_1Z_2 \Rightarrow (Z_1+Z_2)^2=3Z_1Z_2$
$\therefore\ a^2=3b$

68. **(a)** $p+q=-p$ and $pq=q \Rightarrow q(p-1)=0$
$\Rightarrow q=0$ or $p=1$.
If $q=0$, then $p=0$. i.e. $p=q$
$\therefore p=1$ and $q=-2$.

69. **(a)** Product of real roots $=\dfrac{9}{t^2}>0,\ \forall\, t\in R$
$\therefore$ Product of real roots is always positive.

70. **(a)** Let α, β and γ, δ be the roots of the equations $x^2+ax+b=0$ and
$x^2+bx+a=0$ respectively.
$\therefore \alpha+\beta=-a, \alpha\beta=b$ and $\gamma+\delta=-b, \gamma\delta=a$.
Given $|\alpha-\beta|=|\gamma-\delta| \Rightarrow (\alpha-\beta)^2=(\gamma-\delta)^2$
$\Rightarrow (\alpha+\beta)^2-4\alpha\beta=(\gamma+\delta)^2-4\gamma\delta$
$\Rightarrow a^2-4b=b^2-4a$
$\Rightarrow (a^2-b^2)+4(a-b)=0$
$\Rightarrow a+b+4=0\ (\because a\neq b)$

71. **(a)** We have $\alpha^2=5\alpha-3$ and $\beta^2=5\beta-3$;
$\Rightarrow \alpha$ & β are roots of equation, $x^2=5x-3$
or $x^2-5x+3=0$
$\therefore \alpha+\beta=5$ and $\alpha\beta=3$

Thus, the equation having $\dfrac{\alpha}{\beta}$ & $\dfrac{\beta}{\alpha}$ as its roots is

$$x^2-x\left(\frac{\alpha}{\beta}+\frac{\beta}{\alpha}\right)+\frac{\alpha\beta}{\alpha\beta}=0$$

$$\Rightarrow x^2-x\left(\frac{\alpha^2+\beta^2}{\alpha\beta}\right)+1=0$$

or $3x^2-19x+3=0$

72. **(c)** $x^2+bx-1=0$ common root

$x^2+x+b=0$

$- \quad - \quad -$

$x=\frac{b+1}{b-1}$

Put $x=\frac{b+1}{b-1}$ in equation ...(b)

$\left(\frac{b+1}{b-1}\right)^2+\left(\frac{b+1}{b-1}\right)+b=0$

$(b+1)^2+(b+1)(b-1)+b(b-1)^2=0$

$b^2+1+2b+b^2-1+b(b^2-2b+1)=0$

$2b^2+2b+b^3-2b^2+b=0$

$b^3+3b=0$

$b(b^2+3)=0$

$b^2=-3$

$b=\pm\sqrt{3}i$

$|b|=\sqrt{3}$

73. **(d)** We have

$f(x) = x^2+2bx+2c^2$

and $g(x) = -x^2-2cx+b^2,(x\in R)$

$\Rightarrow f(x) = (x+b)^2+2c^2-b^2$

and $g(x) = -(x+c)^2+b^2+c^2$

Now, $f_{min} = 2c^2 - b^2$ and $g_{max} = b^2 + c^2$

Given : min $f(x) >$ max $g(x)$

$\Rightarrow 2c^2-b^2>b^2+c^2$

$\Rightarrow c^2>2b^2$

$\Rightarrow |c| > |b|\sqrt{2}$

$\Rightarrow \frac{|c|}{|b|}>\sqrt{2} \Rightarrow \left|\frac{c}{b}\right|>\sqrt{2}$

$\Rightarrow \left|\frac{c}{b}\right|\in(\sqrt{2},\infty)$.

74. **(b)** Let α, β be the common roots of both the equations.

For first equation $ax^2+bx+c=0$, we have

$\alpha+\beta = \frac{-b}{a}$ ...(1)

$\alpha.\beta = \frac{c}{a}$ ...(2)

For second equation $2x^2+3x+4=0$, we have

$\alpha+\beta = \frac{-3}{2}$ ...(3)

$\alpha.\beta = \frac{2}{1}$ ...(4)

Now, from (1) & (3) & from (2) & (4)

$\frac{-b}{a}=\frac{-3}{2}$ $\qquad \frac{c}{a}=\frac{2}{1}$

$\frac{b}{a}=\frac{3/2}{1}$

Therefore on comparing we get $a = 1$, $b = \frac{3}{2}$ & $c = 2$

putting these values in first equation, we get

$x^2+\frac{3}{2}x+2=0$ or $2x^2+3x+4=0$

from this, we get $a = 2$, $b = 3$; $c = 4$

or $a : b : c = 2 : 3 : 4$

75. **(a)** Given equations are

$x^2+2x+3=0$ ...(i)

$ax^2+bx+c=0$ ...(ii)

Roots of equation (i) are imaginary roots.

According to the question (ii) will also have both roots same as (i). Thus

$\frac{a}{1}=\frac{b}{2}=\frac{c}{3}=\lambda$ (say)

$\Rightarrow a=\lambda, b=2\lambda, c=3\lambda$

Hence, required ratio is 1 : 2 : 3

76. **(a)** $\frac{x-5}{x^2+5x-14}>0 \Rightarrow x^2+5x-14<x-5$

$\Rightarrow x^2+4x-9<0$

$\Rightarrow \alpha=-5,-4,-3,-2,-1,0,1$

$\alpha=-5$ does not satisfy any of the options

$\alpha=-4$ satisfy the option (a) $\alpha^2+3\alpha-4=0$

77. **(c)** $x^2-(a+1)x+a^2+a-8=0$

Since roots are different, therefore D > 0

$\Rightarrow (a+1)^2-4(a^2+a-8)>0$

$\Rightarrow (a-3)(3a+1)<0$

There are two cases arises.

Case I. $a-3>0$ and $3a+1<0$

$\Rightarrow a>3$ and $a<-\frac{11}{3}$

Hence, no solution in this case

Case II : $a-3<0$ and $3a+11>0$

$\Rightarrow a<3$ and $a>-\frac{11}{3}$

$\therefore -\frac{11}{3}<a<3 \Rightarrow -2<a<3$

78. **(a)** Given that $\left|z-\frac{4}{z}\right|=2$

Now $|z| = \left|z-\frac{4}{z}+\frac{4}{z}\right| \le \left|z-\frac{4}{z}\right|+\frac{4}{|z|}$

$\Rightarrow |z| \le 2+\frac{4}{|z|}$

$\Rightarrow |z|^2-2|z|-4\le 0$

$\Rightarrow \left(|z|-\frac{2+\sqrt{20}}{2}\right)\left(|z|-\frac{2-\sqrt{20}}{2}\right)\le 0$

$\Rightarrow \left(|z|-(1+\sqrt{5})\right)\left(|z|-(1-\sqrt{5})\right)\le 0$

$\Rightarrow \left(-\sqrt{5}+1\right)\le |z| \le \left(\sqrt{5}+1\right)$

$\Rightarrow |z|_{max}=\sqrt{5}+1$ Hence T is an equivalence relation.

79. **(d)** Let the roots of equation $x^2-6x+a=0$ be α and 4β and that of the equation $x^2-cx+6=0$ be α and 3β. Then

$\alpha+4\beta=6;\quad 4\alpha\beta=a$

and $\alpha+3\beta=c;\quad 3\alpha\beta=6$

$\Rightarrow a=8$

$\therefore$ The equation becomes $x^2-6x+8=0$

$\Rightarrow (x-2)(x-4)=0$

$\Rightarrow$ roots are 2 and 4

$\Rightarrow \alpha=2, \beta=1$ $\therefore$ Common root is 2.

80. **(b)** $y=\frac{3x^2+9x+17}{3x^2+9x+7}$

$3x^2(y-1)+9x(y-1)+7y-17=0$

$D\ge 0$ $\because$ x is real

$81(y-1)^2-4\times 3(y-1)(7y-17)\ge 0$

$\Rightarrow (y-1)(y-41)\le 0 \Rightarrow 1\le y\le 41$

$\therefore$ Max value of y is 41

ALTERNATE SOLUTION

Given $f(x)=\frac{3x^2+9x+17}{3x^2+9x+7}$

$\Rightarrow f(x)=1+\frac{10}{3x^2+9x+7}$

Clearly $f(x)$ is maximum when $g(x)=3x^2+9x+7$ is min.

Here $g(x)=3\left(x^2+3x+\frac{9}{4}\right)+7-\frac{27}{4}$

$=3\left(x+\frac{3}{2}\right)^2+\frac{1}{4}$

which is minimum when $x=\frac{-3}{2}$

$\therefore f_{max}=1+\frac{10}{3\times\frac{9}{4}-9\times\frac{3}{2}+7}=1+\frac{10\times 4}{27-54+28}=41$

81. **(c)** both roots are less than 5

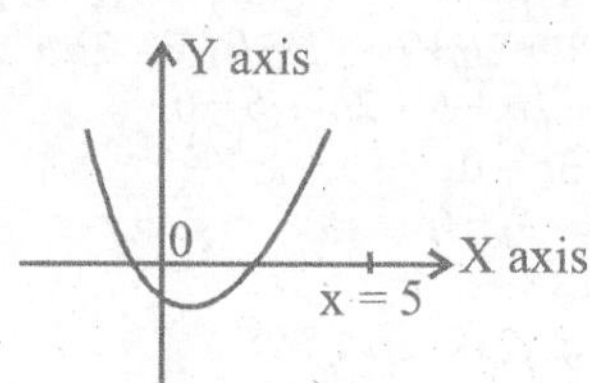

then (i) Discriminant ≥ 0

(ii) $p(5)>0$

(iii) $\frac{\text{Sum of roots}}{2}<5$

Hence (i) $4k^2-4(k^2+k-5)\ge 0$

$4k^2-4k^2-4k+20\ge 0$

$4k\le 20\Rightarrow k\le 5$

(ii) $\Rightarrow f(5)>0;\ 25-10k+k^2+k-5>0$

or $k^2-9k+20>0$

or $k(k-4)-5(k-4)>0$

or $(k-5)(k-4)>0$

$\Rightarrow k\in(-\infty,4)\cup(-\infty,5)$

(iii) $\Rightarrow \frac{\text{Sum of roots}}{2}=-\frac{b}{2a}=\frac{2k}{2}<5$

The intersection of (i), (ii) & (iii) gives $k\in(-\infty,4)$.

82. **(a)** $x^2-(a-2)x-a-1=0$

$\Rightarrow \alpha+\beta=a-2;\ \alpha\beta=-(a+1)$

$\alpha^2+\beta^2=(\alpha+\beta)^2-2\alpha\beta=a^2-2a+6=(a-1)^2+5$

For min. value of $\alpha^2+\beta^2$ where α is an integer

$\Rightarrow a=1.$

Chapter 6

Linear Inequalities

TOPIC : Solution of Linear Inequality and System of Linear Inequalities, Representation of Solution of Linear Inequality in One Variable on a Number Line, Representation of Solution of a Linear Inequality and System of Linear Inequalities in a Cartesian Plane, Equations and Inequations Involving Absolute Value Functions, Greatest Integer Functions, Logarithmic Functions

1. If $f(x)=\left(\frac{3}{5}\right)^x+\left(\frac{4}{5}\right)^x-1$, $x\in R$, then the equation $f(x)=0$ has : **[Online April 9, 2014]**
   (a) no solution
   (b) one solution
   (c) two solutions
   (d) more than two solutions
2. If *a*, *b*, *c* are distinct +ve real numbers and $a^2+b^2+c^2=1$ then $ab+bc+ca$ is **[2002]**
   (a) less than 1 (b) equal to 1
   (c) greater than 1 (d) any real no.

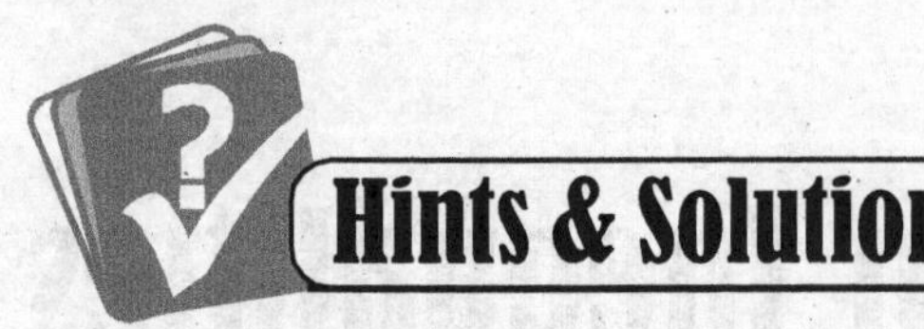

Hints & Solutions

1. (b) $f(x)=\left(\frac{3}{5}\right)^x+\left(\frac{4}{5}\right)^x-1$

Put $f(x)=0$

$\Rightarrow\ 0=\left(\frac{3}{5}\right)^x+\left(\frac{4}{5}\right)^x-1$

$\Rightarrow\ \left(\frac{3}{5}\right)^x+\left(\frac{4}{5}\right)^x=1$

$\Rightarrow\ 3^x+4^x=5^x$ ...(1)

For $x=1$

$3^1+4^1>5^1$

For $x=3$

$3^3+4^3=91<5^3$

Only for $x=2$, equation (1) Satisfy

So, only one solution ($x=2$)

2. (a) $\because (a-b)^2+(b-c)^2+(c-a)^2>0$

$\Rightarrow 2(a^2+b^2+c^2-ab-bc-ca)>0$

$\Rightarrow 2>2(ab+bc+ca) \Rightarrow ab+bc+ca<1$

Permutations and Combinations

TOPIC-1 : Fundamental Principle of Counting, Factorials, Permutations, Counting Formula for Permutations, Permutations in Which Things may be Repeated, Permutations in Which all Things are Different, Number of Permutations Under Certain Restricted Conditions, Circular Permutations

1. The number of ways in which 5 boys and 3 girls can be seated on a round table if a particular boy B_1 and a particular girl G_1 never sit adjacent to each other, is : **[Online April 9, 2017]**
   (a) $5 \times 6!$ (b) $6 \times 6!$
   (c) $7!$ (d) $5 \times 7!$

2. If all the words, with or without meaning, are written using the letters of the word QUEEN and are arranged as in English dictionary, then the position of the word QUEEN is : **[Online April 8, 2017]**
   (a) 44th (b) 45th
   (c) 46th (d) 47th

3. If all the words (with or without meaning) having five letters, formed using the letters of the word SMALL and arranged as in a dictionary; then the position of the word SMALL is : **[2016]**
   (a) 52nd (b) 58th
   (c) 46th (d) 59th

4. The sum $\sum_{r=1}^{10}(r^2+1)\times(r!)$ is equal to : **[Online April 10, 2016]**
   (a) $11 \times (11!)$ (b) $10 \times (11!)$
   (c) $(11!)$ (d) $101 \times (10!)$

5. If the four letter words (need not be meaningful) are to be formed using the letters from the word "MEDITERRANEAN" such that the first letter is R and the fourth letter is E, then the total number of all such words is : **[Online April 9, 2016]**
   (a) 110 (b) 59
   (c) $\frac{11!}{(2!)^3}$ (d) 56

6. The number of points, having both co-ordinates as integers, that lie in the interior of the triangle with vertices (0, 0), (0, 41) and (41, 0) is : **[2015]**
   (a) 820 (b) 780
   (c) 901 (d) 861

7. The number of integers greater than 6,000 that can be formed, using the digits 3, 5, 6, 7 and 8, without repetition, is : **[2015]**
   (a) 120 (b) 72
   (c) 216 (d) 192

8. The number of ways of selecting 15 teams from 15 men and 15 women, such that each team consists of a man and a woman, is: **[Online April 10, 2015]**
   (a) 1120 (b) 1880
   (c) 1960 (d) 1240

9. Two women and some men participated in a chess tournament in which every participant played two games with each of the other participants. If the number of games that the men played between themselves exceeds the number of games that the men played with the women by 66, then the number of men who participated in the tournament lies in the interval: **[Online April 19, 2014]**
   (a) [8, 9] (b) [10, 12)
   (c) (11, 13] (d) (14, 17)

10. 8-digit numbers are formed using the digits 1, 1, 2, 2, 2, 3, 4, 4. The number of such numbers in which the odd digits do no occupy odd places, is: **[Online April 12, 2014]**
    (a) 160 (b) 120
    (c) 60 (d) 48

11. An eight digit number divisible by 9 is to be formed using digits from 0 to 9 without repeating the digits. The number of ways in which this can be done is: **[Online April 11, 2014]**
    (a) 72(7!) (b) 18(7!)
    (c) 40(7!) (d) 36(7!)

12. The sum of the digits in the unit's place of all the 4-digit numbers formed by using the numbers 3, 4, 5 and 6, without repetition, is: **[Online April 9, 2014]**
    (a) 432 (b) 108
    (c) 36 (d) 18

13. 5 - digit numbers are to be formed using 2, 3, 5, 7, 9 without repeating the digits. If p be the number of such numbers that exceed 20000 and q be the number of those that lie between 30000 and 90000, then $p : q$ is : **[Online April 25, 2013]**
    (a) 6 : 5 (b) 3 : 2
    (c) 4 : 3 (d) 5 : 3

14. Assuming the balls to be identical except for difference in colours, the number of ways in which one or more balls can be selected from 10 white, 9 green and 7 black balls is : **[2012]**

(a) 880 (b) 629
(c) 630 (d) 879

15. If seven women and seven men are to be seated around a circular table such that there is a man on either side of every woman, then the number of seating arrangements is **[Online May 26, 2012]**

(a) 6! 7! (b) $(6!)^2$
(c) $(7!)^2$ (d) 7!

16. If the letters of the word SACHIN are arranged in all possible ways and these words are written out as in dictionary, then the word SACHIN appears at serial number **[2005]**

(a) 601 (b) 600
(c) 603 (d) 602

17. How many ways are there to arrange the letters in the word GARDEN with vowels in alphabetical order **[2004]**

(a) 480 (b) 240
(c) 360 (d) 120

18. The range of the function $f(x) = {}^{7-x}P_{x-3}$ is **[2004]**

(a) $\{1,2,3,4,5\}$ (b) $\{1,2,3,4,5,6\}$
(c) $\{1,2,3,4,\}$ (d) $\{1,2,3,\}$

19. The number of ways in which 6 men and 5 women can dine at a round table if no two women are to sit together is given by **[2003]**

(a) $6! \times 5!$ (b) 6×5
(c) 30 (d) 5×4

20. The sum of integers from 1 to 100 that are divisible by 2 or 5 is **[2002]**

(a) 3000 (b) 3050
(c) 3600 (d) 3250

21. Number greater than 1000 but less than 4000 is formed using the digits 0, 1, 2, 3, 4 (repetition allowed). Their number is **[2002]**

(a) 125 (b) 105
(c) 375 (d) 625

22. Total number of four digit odd numbers that can be formed using 0, 1, 2, 3, 5, 7 (using repetition allowed) are **[2002]**

(a) 216 (b) 375
(c) 400 (d) 720

TOPIC-2 : Combinations, Counting Formula for Combinations, Division and Distribution of Objects, Dearrangement Theorem, Sum of Numbers, Important Result About Point

23. A man X has 7 friends, 4 of them are ladies and 3 are men. His wife Y also has 7 friends, 3 of them are ladies and 4 are men. Assume X and Y have no common friends. Then the total number of ways in which X and Y together can throw a party inviting 3 ladies and 3 men, so that 3 friends of each of X and Y are in this party, is : **[2017]**

(a) 484 (b) 485
(c) 468 (d) 469

24. If $\dfrac{{}^{n+2}C_6}{{}^{n-2}P_2} = 11$, then n satisfies the equation : **[Online April 10, 2016]**

(a) $n^2+n-110=0$ (b) $n^2+2n-80=0$
(c) $n^2+3n-108=0$ (d) $n^2+5n-84=0$

25. The value of $\sum_{r=1}^{15} r^2\left(\dfrac{{}^{15}C_r}{{}^{15}C_{r-1}}\right)$ is equal to : **[Online April 9, 2016]**

(a) 1240 (b) 560
(c) 1085 (d) 680

26. Let A and B be two sets containing four and two elements respectively. Then the number of subsets of the set A × B, each having at least three elements is : **[2015]**

(a) 275 (b) 510
(c) 219 (d) 256

27. If in a regular polygon the number of diagonals is 54, then the number of sides of this polygon is **[Online April 11, 2015]**

(a) 12 (b) 6
(c) 10 (d) 9

28. Let A and B two sets containing 2 elements and 4 elements respectively. The number of subsets of A × B having 3 or more elements is **[2013]**

(a) 256 (b) 220
(c) 219 (d) 211

29. Let T_n be the number of all possible triangles formed by joining vertices of an n-sided regular polygon. If $T_{n+1} - T_n = 10$, then the value of n is : **[2013]**

(a) 7 (b) 5
(c) 10 (d) 8

30. On the sides AB, BC, CA of a ΔABC, 3, 4, 5 distinct points (excluding vertices A, B, C) are respectively chosen. The number of triangles that can be constructed using these chosen points as vertices are : **[Online April 23, 2013]**

(a) 210 (b) 205
(c) 215 (d) 220

31. The number of ways in which an examiner can assign 30 marks to 8 questions, giving not less than 2 marks to any question, is : **[Online April 22, 2013]**

(a) ${}^{30}C_7$ (b) ${}^{21}C_8$
(c) ${}^{21}C_7$ (d) ${}^{30}C_8$

32. A committee of 4 persons is to be formed from 2 ladies, 2 old men and 4 young men such that it includes at least 1 lady, at least 1 old man and at most 2 young men. Then the total number of ways in which this committee can be formed is : **[Online April 9, 2013]**

(a) 40 (b) 41
(c) 16 (d) 32

33. The number of arrangements that can be formed from the letters a, b, c, d, e, f taken 3 at a time without repetition and each arrangement containing at least one vowel, is **[Online May 19, 2012]**

(a) 96 (b) 128
(c) 24 (d) 72

34. If $n = {}^mC_2$, then the value of ${}^nC_2$ is given by **[Online May 19, 2012]**

(a) $3({}^{m+1}C_4)$ (b) ${}^{m-1}C_4$
(c) ${}^{m+1}C_4$ (d) $2({}^{m+2}C_4)$

35. **Statement 1:** If A and B be two sets having p and q elements respectively, where $q > p$. Then the total number of functions from set A to set B is q^p. **[Online May 12, 2012]**
Statement 2: The total number of selections of p different objects out of q objects is ${}^qC_p$.
(a) Statement 1 is true, Statement 2 is false.
(b) Statement 1 is true, Statement 2 is true, Statement 2 is not a correct explanation of Statement 1.
(c) Statement 1 is false, Statement 2 is true
(d) Statement 1 is true, Statement 2 is true, Statement 2 is a correct explanation of Statement 1.

36. If the number of 5-element subsets of the set $A = \{a_1, a_2, ..., a_{20}\}$ of 20 distinct elements is k times the number of 5-element subsets containing a_4, then k is **[Online May 7, 2012]**

(a) 5 (b) $\frac{20}{7}$
(c) 4 (d) $\frac{10}{3}$

37. There are 10 points in a plane, out of these 6 are collinear. If N is the number of triangles formed by joining these points. Then : **[2011RS]**
(a) $N \le 100$ (b) $100 < N \le 140$
(c) $140 < N \le 190$ (d) $N > 190$

38. **Statement-1:** The number of ways of distributing 10 identical balls in 4 distinct boxes such that no box is empty is ${}^9C_3$.
Statement-2: The number of ways of choosing any 3 places from 9 different places is ${}^9C_3$. **[2011]**
(a) Statement-1 is true, Statement-2 is true; Statement-2 is not a correct explanation for Statement-1.
(b) Statement-1 is true, Statement-2 is false.
(c) Statement-1 is false, Statement-2 is true.
(d) Statement-1 is true, Statement-2 is true; Statement-2 is a correct explanation for Statement-1.

39. There are two urns. Urn A has 3 distinct red balls and urn B has 9 distinct blue balls. From each urn two balls are taken out at random and then transferred to the other. The number of ways in which this can be done is **[2010]**
(a) 36 (b) 66
(c) 108 (d) 3

40. From 6 different novels and 3 different dictionaries, 4 novels and 1 dictionary are to be selected and arranged in a row on a shelf so that the dictionary is always in the middle. Then the number of such arrangement is: **[2009]**
(a) at least 500 but less than 750
(b) at least 750 but less than 1000
(c) at least 1000
(d) less than 500

41. How many different words can be formed by jumbling the letters in the word MISSISSIPPI in which no two S are adjacent? **[2008]**
(a) $8.{}^6C_4.{}^7C_4$ (b) $6.7.{}^8C_4$
(c) $6.8.{}^7C_4$. (d) $7.{}^6C_4.{}^8C_4$

42. The set $S = \{1, 2, 3, ..., 12\}$ is to be partitioned into three sets A, B, C of equal size.
Thus $A \cup B \cup C = S$, $A \cap B = B \cap C = A \cap C = \phi$. The number of ways to partition S is **[2007]**

(a) $\frac{12!}{(4!)^3}$ (b) $\frac{12!}{(4!)^4}$

(c) $\frac{12!}{3!(4!)^3}$ (d) $\frac{12!}{3!(4!)^4}$

43. At an election, a voter may vote for any number of candidates, not greater than the number to be elected. There are 10 candidates and 4 are of be selected, if a voter votes for at least one candidate, then the number of ways in which he can vote is **[2006]**
(a) 5040 (b) 6210
(c) 385 (d) 1110

44. The value of ${}^{50}C_4 + \sum_{r=1}^{6} {}^{56-r}C_3$ is **[2005]**

(a) ${}^{55}C_4$ (b) ${}^{55}C_3$
(c) ${}^{56}C_3$ (d) ${}^{56}C_4$

45. The number of ways of distributing 8 identical balls in 3 distinct boxes so that none of the boxes is empty is

(a) ${}^8C_3$ (b) 21 **[2004]**
(c) 3^8 (d) 5

46. A student is to answer 10 out of 13 questions in an examination such that he must choose at least 4 from the first five questions. The number of choices available to him is **[2003]**
(a) 346 (b) 140
(c) 196 (d) 280

47. If ${}^nC_r$ denotes the number of combination of n things taken r at a time, then the expression ${}^nC_{r+1} + {}^nC_{r-1} + 2 \times {}^nC_r$ equals **[2003]**

(a) ${}^{n+1}C_{r+1}$ (b) ${}^{n+2}C_r$
(c) ${}^{n+2}C_{r+1}$ (d) ${}^{n+1}C_r$

48. Five digit number divisible by 3 is formed using 0, 1, 2, 3, 4, 6 and 7 without repetition. Total number of such numbers are **[2002]**
(a) 312 (b) 3125
(c) 120 (d) 216

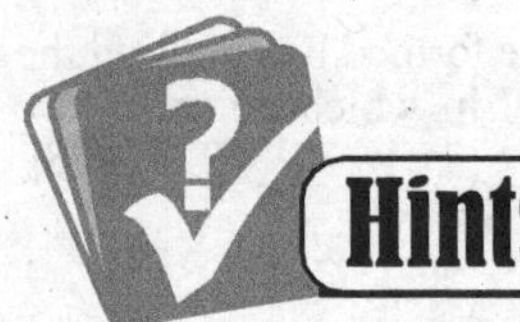

Hints & Solutions

1. (a) 4 boys and 2 girls in circle

$\Rightarrow 5! \times \dfrac{6!}{4!2!} \times 2!$

$\Rightarrow 5 \times 6!$

2. (c) E, E, N, Q, U

(i) E................ $= 4! = 24$

(ii) N................ $= \dfrac{4!}{2} = 12$

(iii) QE.............. $= 3! = 6$

(iv) QN.............. $= \dfrac{3!}{2!} = 3$

(v) QUEEN $= 1$

$\therefore$ Required rank

$= (24) + (12) + (6) + (c) + (a) = 46$th

3. (b) ALLMS

No. of words starting with

A : $\underline{A}$ _ _ _ _ $\dfrac{4!}{2!} = 12$

L : $\underline{L}$ _ _ _ _ $4! = 24$

M : $\underline{M}$ _ _ _ _ $\dfrac{4!}{2!} = 12$

S : $\underline{S}\,\underline{A}$ _ _ _ _ $\dfrac{3!}{2!} = 3$

: $\underline{S}\,\underline{L}$ _ _ _ $3! = 6$

SMALL $\rightarrow 58^{\text{th}}$ word

4. (b) $\sum_{R-1}^{10} (r^2+1)\underline{|r}$

$T_1 = (r^2 + 1 + r - r)\underline{|r} = (r^2 + r)\underline{|r} - (r - r)\underline{|r}$

$T_1 = r\underline{|r+r} - (r-1)\underline{|r}$

$T_1 = 1\underline{|2} - 0$

$T_2 = 2\underline{|3} - 1\underline{|2}$

$T_3 = 3\underline{|4} - 2\underline{|3}$

$T_{10} = 10\underline{|11} - 9\underline{|10}$

$\sum_{R-1}^{10} (r^2+1)\underline{|r} = 10\underline{|11}$

5. (b) M, EEE, D. I, T, RR, AA, NN

R – – E

Two empty places can be filled with identical letters [EE, AA, NN] $\Rightarrow$ 3 ways

Two empty places, can be filled with distinct letters [M, E, D, I, T, R, A, N] $\Rightarrow {}^8P_2$

$\therefore$ Number of words $3 + {}^8P_2 = 59$

6. (b) Total number of integral points inside the square OABC $= 40 \times 40 = 1600$

No. of integral points on AC

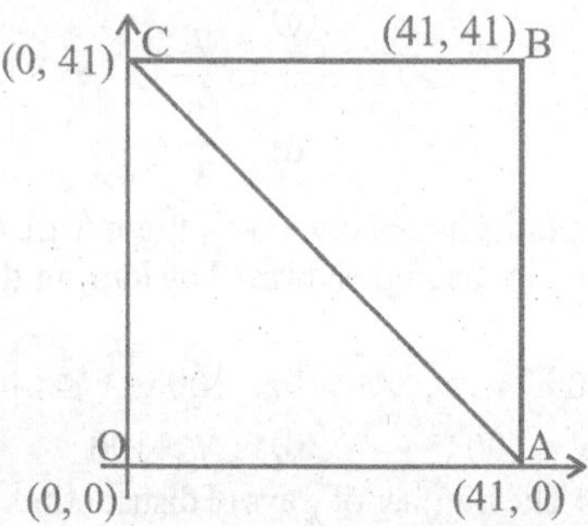

= No. of integral points on OB

$= 40$ [namely (1, 1), (2, 2) ... (40, 40)]

$\therefore$ No. of integral points inside the ΔOAC

$= \dfrac{1600 - 40}{2} = 780$

7. (d) Four digits number can be arranged in $3 \times 4!$ ways.

Five digits number can be arranged in 5! ways.

Number of integers $= 3 \times 4! + 5! = 192$.

8. (d) Number of ways of selecting a man and a woman for a team from 15 men and 15 women

$= 15 \times 15 = (15)^2$

Number of ways of selecting a man and a woman for next team out of the remaining 14 men and 14 women.

$= 14 \times 14 = (14)^2$

Similarly for other teams

Hence required number of ways

$= (15)^2 + (14)^2 + ... + (1)^2 = \dfrac{15 \times 16 \times 31}{6} = 1240$

9. (b) Let no. of men $= n$

No. of women $= 2$

Total participants $= n + 2$

No. of games that M_1 plays with all other men

$= 2(n-1)$

These games are played by all men

$M_2, M_3, \ldots\ldots, M_n$.

So, total no. of games among men $= n.2(n-1)$.

However, we must divide it by '2', since each game is counted twice (for both players).

So, total no. of games among all men

$= n(n-1)$ .... (1)

Now, no. of games M_1 plays with W_1 and $W_2 = 4$ (2 games with each)

Total no. of games that $M_1, M_2, \ldots.., M_n$ play with W_1 and $W_2 = 4n$ .... (2)

Given : $n(n-1) - 4n = 66$

$\Rightarrow \quad n = 11, -6$

As the number of men can't be negative.

So, $n = 11$

10. (b) In 8 digits numbers, 4 places are odd places.

Also, in the given 8 digits, there are three odd digits 1, 1 and 3.

No. of ways three odd digits arranged at four even places $= \frac{4P_3}{2!} = \frac{4!}{2!}$

No. of ways the remaining five digits 2, 2, 2, 4 and 4 arranged at remaining five places $= \frac{5!}{3!2!}$

Hence, required number of 8 digits number

$= \frac{4!}{2!} \times \frac{5!}{3!2!} = 120$

11. (d) We know that any number is divisible by 9 if sum of the digits of the number is divisible by 9.

Now sum of the digits from 0 to 9

$= 0 + 1 + 2 + 3 + 4 + 5 + 6 + 7 + 8 + 9 = 45$

Hence to form 8 digits numbers which are divisible by 9, a pair of digits either 0 and 9, 1 and 8, 2 and 7, 3 and 6 or 4 and 5 are not used.

Digits which are not used to form 8 digits number divisible by 9	Number of 8 digits numbers which are divisible by 9
0 and 9	$8 \times 7!$
1 and 8	$7 \times 7!$
2 and 7	$7 \times 7!$
3 and 6	$7 \times 7!$
4 and 5	$7 \times 7!$

Hence total number of 8 digits numbers which are divisible by 9

$= 8 \times (7!) + 7 \times (7!) + 7 \times (7!) + 7 \times (7!) + 7 \times (7!)$

$= 36 \times (7!)$

12. (b) With 3 at unit place,

total possible four digit number (without repetition) will be $3! = 6$

With 4 at unit place,

total possible four digit numbers will be $3! = 6$

With 5 at unit place,

total possible four digit numbers will be $3! = 6$

With 6 at unit place,

total possible four digit numbers will be $3! = 6$

Sum of unit digits of all possible numbers

$= 6 \times 3 + 6 \times 4 + 6 \times 5 + 6 \times 6$

$= 6\,[3 + 4 + 5 + 6]$

$= 6\,[18]$

$= 108$

13. (d) p :

0	0	0	0	0	place
5	4	3	2	1	ways

Total no. of ways $= 5! = 120$

Since all numbers are $> 20{,}000$

$\therefore$ all numbers 2, 3, 5, 7, 9 can come at first place.

q :

0	0	0	0	0	place
3	4	3	2	1	ways

Total no. of ways $= 3 \times 4! = 72$

($\because$ 2 and 9 can not be put at first place)

So, $p : q = 120 : 72 = 5 : 3$

14. (d) Number of white balls = 10

Number of green balls = 9

and Number of black balls = 7

$\therefore$ Required probability

$= (10+1)(9+1)(7+1) - 1$

$= 11.10.8 - 1 = 879$

[$\because$ The total number of ways of selecting one or more items from p identical items of one kind, q identical items of second kind; r identical items of third kind is $(p+1)(q+1)(r+1) - 1$]

15. (a) 7 women can be arranged around a circular table in 6! ways.

Among these 7 men can sit in 7! ways.

Hence, number of seating arrangement

$= 7! \times 6!$

16. (a) Alphabetical order is

A, C, H, I, N, S

No. of words starting with A – 5!

No. of words starting with C – 5!

No. of words starting with H – 5!

No. of words starting with I – 5!

No. of words starting with N – 5!

SACHIN – 1

$\therefore$ sachin appears at serial no 601

17. (c) Total number of arrangements of letters in the word GARDEN = 6 ! = 720 there are two vowels A and E, in half of the arrangements A preceeds E and other half A follows E.

So, vowels in alphabetical order in $\frac{1}{2} \times 720 = 360$

18. (d) ${}^{7-x}P_{x-3}$ is defined if

$7 - x \geq 0, x - 3 \geq 0$ and $7 - x \geq x - 3$

$\Rightarrow 3 \leq x \leq 5$ and $x \in \mathbf{I}$

$\therefore x = 3, 4, 5$

$\therefore f(3) = {}^{7-3}P_{3-3} = {}^{4}P_0 = 1$

$\therefore f(4) = {}^{7-4}P_{4-3} = {}^{3}P_1 = 3$

$\therefore f(5) = {}^{7-5}P_{5-3} = {}^{2}P_2 = 2$

Hence range = {1, 2, 3}

19. (a) No. of ways in which 6 men can be arranged at a round table = (6 - 1)! = 5!

Now women can be arranged in ${}^{6}P_5$

= 6! Ways.

Total Number of ways = 6! × 5!

20. (b) Required sum

$= (2 + 4 + 6 + ... + 100)$
$\quad + (5 + 10 + 15 + ... + 100)$
$\quad - (10 + 20 + ... + 100)$
$= 2550 + 1050 - 530 = 3050.$

21. (c) Required number of numbers = 3 × 5 × 5 × 5 = 375

22. (d) Required number of numbers

= 5 × 6 × 6 × 4 = 36 × 20 = 720.

23. (b) X → 4 ladies, 3 men; Y → 3 ladies, 4 men

Possible cases for X are
(a) 3 ladies, 0 man
(b) 2 ladies, 1 man
(c) 1 lady, 2 men
(d) 0 ladies, 3 men
Possible cases for Y are
(a) 0 ladies, 3 men
(b) 1 lady, 2 men
(c) 2 ladies, 1 man
(d) 3 ladies, 0 man

No. of ways $= {}^{4}C_3 . {}^{4}C_3 + ({}^{4}C_2 . {}^{3}C_1)^2 + ({}^{4}C_1 . {}^{3}C_2)^2 + ({}^{3}C_3)^2$

$= 16 + 324 + 144 + 1 = 485$

24. (c) $\frac{{}^{n+2}C_6}{{}^{n-2}P_2} = 11$

$\Rightarrow \frac{\frac{(n+2)(n+1)n(n-1)(n-2)(n-3)}{6.5.4.3.2.1}}{\frac{(n-2)(n-3)}{2.1}} = 11$

$\Rightarrow (n+2)(n+1)n(n-1) = 11 . 10 . 9 . 4$

$\Rightarrow n = 9$

$n^2 + 3n - 108 = (9)^2 + 3(9) - 108$
$= 81 + 27 - 108$
$= 108 - 108 = 0$

25. (d) $\sum_{r=1}^{15} r^2 \left(\frac{{}^{15}C_r}{{}^{15}C_{r-1}} \right)$

$\frac{{}^{15}C_r}{{}^{15}C_{r-1}} = \frac{\frac{\lfloor 15}{\lfloor 15-r \lfloor r}}{\frac{\lfloor 15}{\lfloor r-1 \lfloor 16-r}} = \frac{\frac{1}{\lfloor 15-r \lfloor r-1}}{\frac{1}{\lfloor r-1 \lfloor 15-r .(16-r)}}$

$= \frac{16-r}{r}$

$= \sum_{r=1}^{15} r^2 \left(\frac{16-r}{r} \right) = \sum_{r=1}^{15} r(16-r)$

$= 16 \sum_{r=1}^{15} r - \sum_{r=1}^{15} r^2$

$= \frac{16 \times 15 \times 16}{2} - \frac{15 \times 31 \times 16}{6}$

$= 8 \times 15 \times 16 - 5 \times 8 \times 31 = 1920 - 1240 = 680$

26. (c) n(A) = 4, n (B) = 2 ⇒ n(A × B) = 8

The number of subsets of A × B having atleast 3 = elements $= {}^{8}C_3 + {}^{8}C_4 + ... + {}^{8}C_8$

$= 2^8 - {}^{8}C_0 - {}^{8}C_1 - {}^{8}C_2$

$= 256 - 1 - 8 - 28 = 219$

27. (a) Number of diagonal = 54

$\Rightarrow \frac{n(n-3)}{2} = 54$

$\Rightarrow n^2 - 3n - 108 = 0 \Rightarrow n^2 - 12n + 9n - 108 = 0$

$\Rightarrow n(n - 12) + 9(n - 12) = 0$

$\Rightarrow n = 12, -9 \Rightarrow n = 12 \ (\because n \neq -9)$

28. (c) Given

$n(A) = 2, n(B) = 4, n(A \times B) = 8$

Required number of subsets =

${}^{8}C_3 + {}^{8}C_4 + ... + {}^{8}C_8 = 2^8 - {}^{8}C_0 - {}^{8}C_1 - {}^{8}C_2$

$= 256 - 1 - 8 - 28 = 219$

29. **(b)** We know,

$T_n = {}^nC_3,\ T_{n+1} = {}^{n+1}C_3$

ATQ, $T_{n+1} - T_n = {}^{n+1}C_3 - {}^nC_3 = 10$

$\Rightarrow {}^nC_2 = 10$

$\Rightarrow n = 5.$

30. **(b)** Required number of triangles

$= {}^{12}C_3 - ({}^3C_3 + {}^4C_3 + {}^5C_3) = 205$

31. **(c)** 30 marks to be alloted to 8 questions. Each question has to be given ≥ 2 marks

Let questions be a, b, c, d, e, f, g, h

and $a + b + c + d + e + f + g + h = 30$

Let $a = a_1 + 2$ so, $a_1 \geq 0$

$b = a_2 + 2$ so, $a_2 \geq 0, \ldots\ldots, a_8 \geq 0$

So, $\left.\begin{matrix} a_1 + a_2 + \ldots\ldots + a_8 \\ +2+2+\ldots\ldots+2 \end{matrix}\right\} = 30$

$\Rightarrow a_1 + a_2 + \ldots\ldots + a_8 = 30 - 16 = 14$

So, this is a problem of distributing 14 articles in 8 groups.

Number of ways $= {}^{14+8-1}C_{8-1} = {}^{21}C_7$

32. **(b)**

L	O	Y
2	2	4
≥1	≥1	2≤

⇒

L	O	Y
1	1	2
1	2	1
2	1	1
2	2	0

Required number of ways

$= {}^2C_1 \times {}^2C_1 \times {}^2C_2 + {}^2C_1 \times {}^2C_2 \times {}^4C_1 + {}^2C_2 \times {}^2C_1 \times {}^4C_1 + {}^2C_2 \times {}^2C_2 \times {}^4C_0$

$= 2 \times 2 \times \frac{4 \times 3}{2} + 2 \times 1 \times 4 + 1 \times 2 \times 4 + 1 \times 1 \times 1$

$= 24 + 8 + 8 + 1 = 41$

33. **(a)** There are 2 vowels and 4 consonants in the letters a, b, c, d, e, f.

If we select one vowel, then number of arrangements

$= {}^2C_1 \times {}^4C_2 \times 3! = 2 \times \frac{4 \times 3}{2} \times 3 \times 2 = 72$

If we select two vowels, then number of arrangements

$= {}^2C_2 \times {}^4C_1 \times 3! = 1 \times 4 \times 6 = 24$

Hence, total number of arrangements

$= 72 + 24 = 96$

34. **(a)** $n = {}^mC_2 = \frac{m(m-1)}{2}$

Since m and $(m - 1)$ are two consecutive natural numbers, therefore their product is an even natural number. So $\frac{m(m-1)}{2}$ is also a natural number.

Now $\frac{m(m-1)}{2} = \frac{m^2 - m}{2}$

$\therefore \frac{m(m-1)}{2}C_2 = \frac{\left(\frac{m^2-m}{2}\right)\left(\frac{m^2-m}{2} - 1\right)}{2}$

$= \frac{m(m-1)(m^2 - m - 2)}{8}$

$= \frac{m(m-1)[m^2 - 2m + m - 2]}{8}$

$= \frac{m(m-1)[m(m-2) + 1(m-2)]}{8}$

$= \frac{m(m-1)(m-2)(m+1)}{8}$

$= \frac{3 \times (m+1)m(m-1)(m-2)}{4 \times 3 \times 2 \times 1} = 3\left({}^{m+1}C_4\right)$

35. **(d)** **Statement - 1 :** $n(A) = p, n(B) = q, q > p$

Total number of functions from $A \to B = q^p$

It is a true statement.

Statement - 2 : The total number of selections of p different objects out of q objects is ${}^qC_p$.

It is also a true statement and it is a correct explanation for statement - 1 also.

36. **(c)** Set $A = \{a_1, a_2, \ldots.., a_{20}\}$ has 20 distinct elements.

We have to select 5-element subset.

$\therefore$ Number of 5-element subsets $= {}^{20}C_5$

According to question

$${}^{20}C_5 = \left({}^{19}C_4\right).k$$

$$\Rightarrow \frac{20!}{5!\ 15!} = k.\left(\frac{19!}{4!\ 15!}\right)$$

$$\Rightarrow \frac{20}{5} = k \Rightarrow k = 4$$

37. **(a)** Number of required triangles $= {}^{10}C_3 - {}^6C_3$

$= \frac{10 \times 9 \times 8}{6} - \frac{6 \times 5 \times 4}{6} = 120 - 20 = 100$

38. **(a)** The number of ways of distributing 10 identical balls in 4 distinct boxes such that no box empty is same as the number of ways of selecting $(r - 1)$ places out of $(n - 1)$ different places, that is ${}^{n-1}C_{r-1}$.

Hence require number of ways

$= {}^{10-1}C_{4-1} = {}^9C_3$

39. (c) Total number of ways = ${}^3C_2 \times {}^9C_2$

$= 3 \times \frac{9 \times 8}{2} = 3 \times 36 = 108$

40. (c) 4 novels, out of 6 novels and 1 dictionary out of 3 can be selected in ${}^6C_4 \times {}^3C_1$ ways

Then 4 novels with one dictionary in the middle can be arranged in 4! ways.

$\therefore$ Total ways of arrangement

$= {}^6C_4 \times {}^3C_1 \times 4! = 1080$

41. (d) First let us arrange M, I, I, I, I, P, P

Which can be done in $\frac{7!}{4!2!}$ ways

√M√I√I√I√I√P√P√

Now 4 S can be kept at any of the ticked places in ${}^8C_4$ ways so that no two *S* are adjacent.

Total required ways

$= \frac{7!}{4!2!}\,{}^8C_4 = \frac{7!}{4!2!}\,{}^8C_4 = 7 \times {}^6C_4 \times {}^8C_4$

42. (a) Set S = {1, 2, 3, ... 12}

$A \cup B \cup C = S,\ A \cap B = B \cap C = A \cap C = \phi$

$\therefore$ The number of ways to partition

$= {}^{12}C_4 \times {}^8C_4 \times {}^4C_4$

$= \frac{12!}{4!8!} \times \frac{8!}{4!4!} \times \frac{4!}{4!0!} = \frac{12!}{(4!)^3}$

43. (c) ${}^{10}C_1 + {}^{10}C_2 + {}^{10}C_3 + {}^{10}C_4$

$= 10 + 45 + 120 + 210 = 385$

44. (d) ${}^{50}C_4 + \sum_{r=1}^{6} {}^{56-r}C_3$

$= {}^{50}C_4 + \left[{}^{55}C_3 + {}^{54}C_3 + {}^{53}C_3 + {}^{52}C_3 + {}^{51}C_3 + {}^{50}C_3 \right]$

We know $\left[{}^nC_r + {}^nC_{r-1} = {}^{n+1}C_r \right]$

$= ({}^{50}C_4 + {}^{50}C_3)$

$+ {}^{51}C_3 + {}^{52}C_3 + {}^{53}C_3 + {}^{54}C_3 + {}^{55}C_3$

$= ({}^{51}C_4 + {}^{51}C_3) + {}^{52}C_3 + {}^{53}C_3 + {}^{54}C_3 + {}^{55}C_3$

Proceeding in the same way, we get

$= {}^{55}C_4 + {}^{55}C_3 = {}^{56}C_4.$

45. (b) We know that the number of ways of distributing n identical items among *r* persons, when each one of them receives at least one item is ${}^{n-1}C_{r-1}$

$\therefore$ The required number of ways

$= {}^{8-1}C_{3-1} = {}^7C_2 = \frac{7!}{2!5!} = \frac{7 \times 6}{2 \times 1} = 21$

46. (c) As for given question two cases are possible.

(i) Selecting 4 out of first five question and 6 out of remaining 8 question

$= {}^5C_4 \times {}^8C_6 = 140$ choices.

(ii) Selecting 5 out of first five question and 5 out of remaining 8 questions $= {}^5C_5 \times {}^8C_5 = 56$ choices.

Therefore, total number of choices
$= 140 + 56 = 196.$

47. (c) ${}^nC_{r+1} + {}^nC_{r-1} + 2\,{}^nC_r$

$= {}^nC_{r-1} + {}^nC_r + {}^nC_r + {}^nC_{r+1}$

$= {}^{n+1}C_r + {}^{n+1}C_{r+1} = {}^{n+2}C_{r+1}$

48. (d) We know that a number is divisible by 3 only when the sum of the digits is divisible by 3. The given digits are 0, 1, 2, 3, 4, 5.

Here the possible number of combinations of 5 digits out of 6 are ${}^5C_4 = 5$, which are as follows–

$1 + 2 + 3 + 4 + 5 = 15 = 3 \times 5$

$0 + 2 + 3 + 4 + 5 = 14$ (not divisible by 3)

$0 + 1 + 3 + 4 + 5 = 13$ (not divisible by 3)

$0 + 1 + 2 + 4 + 5 = 12 = 3 \times 4$

$0 + 1 + 2 + 3 + 5 = 11$ (not divisible by 3)

$0 + 1 + 2 + 3 + 4 = 10$ (not divisible by 3)

Thus the number should contain the digits 1, 2, 3, 4, 5 or the digits 0, 1, 2, 4, 5.

Taking 1, 2, 3, 4, 5, the 5 digit numbers are = 5! = 120

Taking 0, 1, 2, 4, 5, the 5 digit numbers are = 5! – 4! = 96

$\therefore$ Total number of numbers = 120 + 96 = 216

Chapter 8 Binomial Theorem

TOPIC-1 : Binomial Theorem for a Positive Integral Index 'x', Expansion of Binomial, General Term, Coefficient of any Power of 'x'

1. The coefficient of x^{-5} in the binomial expansion of $\left(\frac{x+1}{x^{\frac{2}{3}}-x^{\frac{1}{3}}+1}-\frac{x-1}{x-x^{\frac{1}{2}}}\right)^{10}$ where $x \neq 0, 1$, is : **[Online April 9, 2017]**
   (a) 1 (b) 4
   (c) −4 (d) −1

2. If $(27)^{999}$ is divided by 7, then the remainder is : **[Online April 8, 2017]**
   (a) 1 (b) 2
   (c) 3 (d) 6

3. If the coefficients of x^{-2} and x^{-4} in the expansion of $\left(x^{\frac{1}{3}}+\frac{1}{2x^{\frac{1}{3}}}\right)^{18}$, $(x > 0)$, are m and n respectively, then $\frac{m}{n}$ is equal to : **[Online April 10, 2016]**
   (a) 27 (b) 182
   (c) $\frac{5}{4}$ (d) $\frac{4}{5}$

4. If the coefficients of the three successive terms in the binomial expansion of $(1 + x)^n$ are in the ratio 1 : 7 : 42, then the first of these terms in the expansion is: **[Online April 10, 2015]**
   (a) 8th (b) 6th
   (c) 7th (d) 9th

5. If the coefficents of x^3 and x^4 in the expansion of $(1+ax+bx^2)(1-2x)^{18}$ in powers of x are both zero, then (a, b) is equal to: **[2014]**
   (a) $\left(14,\frac{272}{3}\right)$ (b) $\left(16,\frac{272}{3}\right)$
   (c) $\left(16,\frac{251}{3}\right)$ (d) $\left(14,\frac{251}{3}\right)$

6. If $X=\{4^n-3n-1 : n \in N\}$ and $Y=\{9(n-1): n \in N\}$, where N is the set of natural numbers, then $X \cup Y$ is equal to: **[2014]**
   (a) X (b) Y
   (c) N (d) $Y-X$

7. If $1+x^4+x^5=\sum_{i=0}^{5} a_i(1+x)^i$, for all x in R, then a_2 is: **[Online April 12, 2014]**
   (a) −4 (b) 6
   (c) −8 (d) 10

8. If $\left(2+\frac{x}{3}\right)^{55}$ is expanded in the ascending powers of x and the coefficients of powers of x in two consecutive terms of the expansion are equal, then these terms are: **[Online April 12, 2014]**
   (a) 7th and 8th (b) 8th and 9th
   (c) 28th and 29th (d) 27th and 28th

9. The number of terms in the expansion of $(1+x)^{101}(1+x^2-x)^{100}$ in powers of x is: **[Online April 9, 2014]**
   (a) 302 (b) 301
   (c) 202 (d) 101

10. If for positive integers $r > 1$, $n > 2$, the coefficients of the $(3r)^{th}$ and $(r+2)^{th}$ powers of x in the expansion of $(1+x)^{2n}$ are equal, then n is equal to : **[Online April 25, 2013]**
    (a) $2r+1$ (b) $2r-1$
    (c) $3r$ (d) $r+1$

11. The sum of the rational terms in the binomial expansion of $\left(2^{\frac{1}{2}}+3^{\frac{1}{5}}\right)^{10}$ is: **[Online April 23, 2013]**
    (a) 25 (b) 32
    (c) 9 (d) 41

12. If the 7th term in the binomial expansion of $\left(\frac{3}{\sqrt[3]{84}}+\sqrt{3}\ln x\right)^9, x>0$, is equal to 729, then x can be : **[Online April 22, 2013]**
(a) e^2 (b) e
(c) $\frac{e}{2}$ (d) $2e$

13. If n is a positive integer, then $\left(\sqrt{3}+1\right)^{2n}-\left(\sqrt{3}-1\right)^{2n}$ is : **[2012]**
(a) an irrational number
(b) an odd positive integer
(c) an even positive integer
(d) a rational number other than positive integers

14. The number of terms in the expansion of $\left(y^{1/5}+x^{1/10}\right)^{55}$, in which powers of x and y are free from radical signs are **[Online May 12, 2012]**
(a) six (b) twelve
(c) seven (d) five

15. If $f(y)=1-(y-1)+(y-1)^2-(y-1)^3+\ldots-(y-1)^{17}$, then the coefficient of y^2 in it is **[Online May 7, 2012]**
(a) $^{17}C_2$ (b) $^{17}C_3$
(c) $^{18}C_2$ (d) $^{18}C_3$

16. **Statement - 1 :** For each natural number n, $(n+1)^7-1$ is divisible by 7.
Statement - 2 : For each natural number n, n^7-n is divisible by 7. **[2011 RS]**
(a) Statement-1 is true, Statement-2 is true; Statement-2 is a correct explanation for Statement-1.
(b) Statement-1 is true, Statement-2 is true; Statement-2 is NOT a correct explanation for Statement-1
(c) Statement-1 is true, Statement-2 is false
(d) Statement-1 is false, Statement-2 is true

17. The coefficient of x^7 in the expansion of $(1-x-x^2+x^3)^6$ is **[2011]**
(a) –132 (b) –144
(c) 132 (d) 144

18. The remainder left out when $8^{2n}-(62)^{2n+1}$ is divided by 9 is: **[2009]**
(a) 2 (b) 7
(c) 8 (d) 0

19. **Statement -1 :** $\sum_{r=0}^{n}(r+1)\ {}^nC_r=(n+2)2^{n-1}$.
Statement-2: $\sum_{r=0}^{n}(r+1)\ {}^nC_rx^r=(1+x)^n+nx(1+x)^{n-1}$. **[2008]**
(a) Statement -1 is false, Statement-2 is true
(b) Statement -1 is true, Statement-2 is true; Statement -2 is a correct explanation for Statement-1
(c) Statement -1 is true, Statement-2 is true; Statement -2 is not a correct explanation for Statement-1
(d) Statement -1 is true, Statement-2 is false

20. In the binomial expansion of $(a-b)^n, n\geq 5$, the sum of 5th and 6th terms is zero, then a/b equals **[2007]**
(a) $\frac{n-5}{6}$ (b) $\frac{n-4}{5}$
(c) $\frac{5}{n-4}$ (d) $\frac{6}{n-5}$.

21. For natural numbers m, n if $(1-y)^m(1+y)^n=1+a_1y+a_2y^2+\ldots\ldots$ and $a_1=a_2=10$, then (m,n) is **[2006]**
(a) $(20,45)$ (b) $(35,20)$
(c) $(45,35)$ (d) $(35,45)$

22. If the coefficient of x^7 in $\left[ax^2+\left(\frac{1}{bx}\right)\right]^{11}$ equals the coefficient of x^{-7} in $\left[ax-\left(\frac{1}{bx^2}\right)\right]^{11}$, then a and b satisfy the relation **[2005]**
(a) $a-b=1$ (b) $a+b=1$
(c) $\frac{a}{b}=1$ (d) $ab=1$

23. The coefficient of x^n in expansion of $(1+x)(1-x)^n$ is **[2004]**
(a) $(-1)^{n-1}n$ (b) $(-1)^n(1-n)$
(c) $(-1)^{n-1}(n-1)^2$ (d) $(n-1)$

24. The number of integral terms in the expansion of $(\sqrt{3}+\sqrt[8]{5})^{256}$ is **[2003]**
(a) 35 (b) 32
(c) 33 (d) 34

25. r and n are positive integers $r>1$, $n>2$ and coefficient of $(r+2)^{th}$ term and $3r^{th}$ term in the expansion of $(1+x)^{2n}$ are equal, then n equals **[2002]**
(a) $3r$ (b) $3r+1$
(c) $2r$ (d) $2r+1$

26. The coefficients of x^p and x^q in the expansion of $(1+x)^{p+q}$ are **[2002]**
(a) equal
(b) equal with opposite signs
(c) reciprocals of each other
(d) none of these

TOPIC-2 : Middle Term, Greatest Term, Independent Term, Particular Term from end in Binomial Expansion, Greatest Binomial Coefficients

27. The term independent of x in the binomial expansion of $\left(1-\frac{1}{x}+3x^5\right)\left(2x^2-\frac{1}{x}\right)^8$ is : **(Online April 11, 2015)**
(a) 496 (b) –496
(c) 400 (d) –400

28. The term independent of x in expansion of $\left(\frac{x+1}{x^{2/3}-x^{1/3}+1}-\frac{x-1}{x-x^{1/2}}\right)^{10}$ is **[2013]**
(a) 4 (b) 120
(c) 210 (d) 310

29. The ratio of the coefficient of x^{15} to the term independent of x in the expansion of $\left(x^2+\frac{2}{x}\right)^{15}$ is : **[Online April 9, 2013]**
(a) 7 : 16 (b) 7 : 64
(c) 1 : 4 (d) 1 : 32

30. The middle term in the expansion of $\left(1-\frac{1}{x}\right)^n(1-x)^n$ in powers of x is **[Online May 26, 2012]**
(a) $-{}^{2n}C_{n-1}$ (b) $-{}^{2n}C_n$
(c) ${}^{2n}C_{n-1}$ (d) ${}^{2n}C_n$

31. The coefficient of the middle term in the binomial expansion in powers of x of $(1+\alpha x)^4$ and of $(1-\alpha x)^6$ is the same if α equals **[2004]**
(a) $\frac{3}{5}$ (b) $\frac{10}{3}$
(c) $\frac{-3}{10}$ (d) $\frac{-5}{3}$

TOPIC-3 : Properties of Binomial Coefficients, Number of Terms in the Expansion of (x+y+z)ⁿ, Binomial theorem for any Index, Multinomial theorem, Infinite Series

32. The value of
$({}^{21}C_1-{}^{10}C_1)+({}^{21}C_2-{}^{10}C_2)+({}^{21}C_3-{}^{10}C_3)+({}^{21}C_4-{}^{10}C_4)+....+({}^{21}C_{10}-{}^{10}C_{10})$ is : **[2017]**
(a) $2^{20}-2^{10}$ (b) $2^{21}-2^{11}$
(c) $2^{21}-2^{10}$ (d) $2^{20}-2^9$

33. If the number of terms in the expansion of $\left(1-\frac{2}{x}+\frac{4}{x^2}\right)^n$, $x \neq 0$, is 28, then the sum of the coefficients of all the terms in this expansion, is : **[2016]**
(a) 243 (b) 729
(c) 64 (d) 2187

34. The sum of coefficients of integral power of x in the binomial expansion $\left(1-2\sqrt{x}\right)^{50}$ is : **[2015]**
(a) $\frac{1}{2}\left(3^{50}-1\right)$ (b) $\frac{1}{2}\left(2^{50}+1\right)$
(c) $\frac{1}{2}\left(3^{50}+1\right)$ (d) $\frac{1}{2}\left(3^{50}\right)$

35. The coefficient of x^{1012} in the expansion of $(1+x^n+x^{253})^{10}$, (where $n \leq 22$ is any positive integer), is **[Online April 19, 2014]**
(a) 1 (b) ${}^{10}C_4$
(c) 4n (d) ${}^{253}C_4$

36. Let $S_1=\sum_{j=1}^{10} j(j-1)\,{}^{10}C_j$, $S_2=\sum_{j=1}^{10} j\,{}^{10}C_j$ and $S_3=\sum_{j=1}^{10} j^2\,{}^{10}C_j$. **[2010]**

Statement -1 : $S_3 = 55 \times 2^9$.

Statement - 2: $S_1 = 90 \times 2^8$ and $S_2 = 10 \times 2^8$.

(a) Statement -1 is true, Statement -2 is true ; Statement -2 is **not** a correct explanation for Statement -1.
(b) Statement -1 is true, Statement -2 is false.
(c) Statement -1 is false, Statement -2 is true .
(d) Statement - 1 is true, Statement 2 is true ; Statement -2 is a correct explanation for Statement -1.

37. In a shop there are five types of ice-creams available. A child buys six ice-creams.

Statement-1 : The number of different ways the child can buy the six ice-creams is $^{10}C_5$.

Statement -2 : The number of different ways the child can buy the six ice-creams is equal to the number of different ways of arranging 6 A's and 4 B's in a row. **[2008]**

(a) Statement -1 is false, Statement-2 is true

(b) Statement -1 is true, Statement-2 is true; Statement -2 is a correct explanation for Statement-1

(c) Statement -1 is true, Statement-2 is true; Statement -2 is not a correct explanation for Statement-1

(d) Statement -1 is true, Statement-2 is false

38. The sum of the series **[2007]**

$^{20}C_0 - {}^{20}C_1 + {}^{20}C_2 - {}^{20}C_3 + ... - ..... + {}^{20}C_{10}$ is

(a) 0 (b) $^{20}C_{10}$

(c) $-^{20}C_{10}$ (d) $\frac{1}{2}\,{}^{20}C_{10}$

39. If x is so small that x^3 and higher powers of x may be neglected, then $\dfrac{(1+x)^{\frac{3}{2}} - \left(1+\frac{1}{2}x\right)^3}{(1-x)^{\frac{1}{2}}}$ may be approximated as **[2005]**

(a) $1-\frac{3}{8}x^2$ (b) $3x+\frac{3}{8}x^2$

(c) $-\frac{3}{8}x^2$ (d) $\frac{x}{2}-\frac{3}{8}x^2$

40. If x is positive, the first negative term in the expansion of $(1+x)^{27/5}$ is **[2003]**

(a) 6th term (b) 7th term

(c) 5th term (d) 8th term

41. The positive integer just greater than $(1+0.0001)^{10000}$ is

(a) 4 (b) 5 **[2002]**

(c) 2 (d) 3

42. If the sum of the coefficients in the expansion of $(a+b)^n$ is 4096, then the greatest coefficient in the expansion is

(a) 1594 (b) 792 **[2002]**

(c) 924 (d) 2924

Hints & Solutions

1. (a) $\left[\frac{(x^{1/3}+1)(x^{2/3}-x^{1/3}+1)}{(x^{2/3}-x^{1/3}+1)}-\frac{(\sqrt{x}-1)(\sqrt{x}+1)}{\sqrt{x}(\sqrt{x}-1)}\right]^{10}$

$= \left(x^{1/3}+1-1-1/x^{1/2}\right)^{10}$

$= \left(x^{1/3}-1/x^{1/2}\right)^{10}$

$T_{r+1} = {}^{10}C_r\, x^{\frac{20-5r}{6}}$
for r = 10

$T_{11} = {}^{10}C_{10}\, x^{-5}$

Coefficient of $x^{-5} = {}^{10}C_{10}(1)(-1)^{10} = 1$

2. (d)

$\frac{(28-1)^{999}}{7} = \frac{28\lambda-1}{7}$

$\Rightarrow \frac{28\lambda-7+7-1}{7} = \frac{7(4\lambda-1)+6}{7}$

$\therefore$ Remainder = 6

3. (b) $T_{r+1} = {}^{18}C_r\left(x^{\frac{1}{3}}\right)^{18-r}\left(\frac{1}{2x^{\frac{1}{3}}}\right)^r = {}^{18}C_r x^{6-\frac{2r}{3}}\frac{1}{2^r}$

$\left\{\begin{array}{l} 6-\frac{2r}{3} = -2 \Rightarrow r = 12 \\ \& \; 6-\frac{2r}{3} = -4 \Rightarrow r = 15 \end{array}\right\}$

$\Rightarrow \frac{\text{coefficient of } x^{-2}}{\text{coefficient of } x^{-4}} = \frac{{}^{18}C_{12}\frac{1}{2^{12}}}{{}^{18}C_{15}\frac{1}{2^{15}}} = 182$

4. (c) $\frac{{}^nC_r}{1} = \frac{{}^nC_{r+1}}{7} = \frac{{}^nC_{r+2}}{42}$

By solving we get r = 6
so, it is 7th term.

5. (b) Consider $(1+ax+bx^2)(1-2x)^{18}$
$= (1+ax+bx^2)[{}^{18}C_0 - {}^{18}C_1(2x) + {}^{18}C_2(2x)^2 - {}^{18}C_3(2x)^3 + {}^{18}C_4(2x)^4 - ....]$
Coeff. of $x^3 = {}^{18}C_3(-2)^3 + a.(-2)^2.{}^{18}C_2 + b(-2).{}^{18}C_1 = 0$
Coeff. of $x^3 = -{}^{18}C_3.8 + a \times 4.\,{}^{18}C_2 - 2b \times 18 = 0$

$= -\frac{18\times17\times16}{6}.8 + \frac{4a+18\times17}{2} - 36b = 0$

$= -51\times16\times8 + a\times36\times17 - 36b = 0$
$= -34\times16 + 51a - 3b = 0$
$= 51a - 3b = 34\times16 = 544$
$= 51a - 3b = 544$ ....(i)
Only option number (b) satisfies the equation number (i)

6. (b) $4^n - 3n - 1 = (1+3)^n - 3n - 1$
$= [{}^nC_0 + {}^nC_1.3 + {}^nC_2.3^2 + ...+ {}^nC_n3^n] - 3n - 1$
$= 9\,[{}^nC_2 + {}^nC_3.3 + ... + {}^nC_n.3^{n-2}]$
$\therefore 4^n - 3n - 1$ is a multiple of 9 for all n.
$\therefore X = \{x : x \text{ is a multiple of } 9\}$
Also, $Y = \{9(n-1) : n \in \mathbf{N}\}$
$= \{\text{All multiples of } 9\}$
Clearly $X \subset Y$. $\therefore X \cup Y = Y$

7. (a) $1+x^4+x^5 = \sum_{i=0}^{5} a_i(1+x)^i$

$= a_0 + a_1(1+x)^1 + a_2(1+x)^2 + a_3(1+x)^3 + a_4(1+x)^4 + a_5(1+x)^5$

$\Rightarrow 1+x^4+x^5$
$= a_0 + a_1(1+x) + a_2(1+2x+x^2) + a_3(1+3x+3x^2+x^3) + a_4(1+4x+6x^2+4x^3+x^4) + a_5(1+5x+10x^2+10x^3+5x^4+x^5)$

$\Rightarrow 1+x^4+x^5$
$= a_0 + a_1 + a_1x + a_2 + 2a_2x + a_2x^2 + a_3 + 3a_3x + 3a_3x^2 + a_3x^3 + a_4 + 4a_4x + 6a_4x^2 + 4a_4x^3 + a_4x^4 + a_5 + 5a_5x + 10a_5x^2 + 10a_5x^3 + 5a_5x^4 + a_5x^5$

$\Rightarrow 1+x^4+x^5$
$= (a_0+a_1+a_2+a_3+a_4+a_5) + x(a_1+2a_2+3a_3+4a_4+5a_5) + x^2(a_2+3a_3+6a_4+10a_5) + x^3(a_3+4a_4+10a_5) + x^4(a_4+5a_5) + x^5(a_5)$

On comparing the like coefficients, we get

$\boxed{a_5 = 1}$ ...(1) ; $\boxed{a_4 + 5a_5 = 1}$ ...(2);

$\boxed{a_3 + 4a_4 + 10a_5 = 0}$ ...(3)

and $\boxed{a_2 + 3a_3 + 6a_4 + 10a_5 = 0}$ ...(4)

from (1) & (2), we get

$\boxed{a_4 = -4}$ ...(5) from (1), (3) & (5), we get

$\boxed{a_3 = +6}$ ...(6)

Now, from (1), (5) and (6), we get

$a_2 = -4$

8. (a) Let r^{th} and $(r+1)^{th}$ term has equal coefficient

$$\left(2+\frac{x}{3}\right)^{55} = 2^{55}\left(1+\frac{x}{6}\right)^{55}$$

$$r^{th} \text{ term} = 2^{55}\, {}^{55}C_r\left(\frac{x}{6}\right)^r$$

Coefficient of x^r is $2^{55}\, {}^{55}C_r \frac{1}{6^r}$

$$(r+1)^{th} \text{ term} = 2^{55}\, {}^{55}C_{r+1}\left(\frac{x}{6}\right)^{r+1}$$

Coefficient of x^{r+1} is $2^{55}\, {}^{55}C_{r+1} \cdot \frac{1}{6^{r+1}}$

Both coefficients are equal

$$2^{55}\, {}^{55}C_r \frac{1}{6^r} = 2^{55}\, {}^{55}C_{r+1} \frac{1}{6^{r+1}}$$

$$\frac{1}{\underline{|r}\,\underline{|55-r}} = \frac{1}{\underline{|r+1}\,\underline{|54-r}} \cdot \frac{1}{6}$$

$6(r+1) = 55 - r$

$6r + 6 = 55 - r$

$7r = 49$

$r = 7$

$(r+1) = 8$

Coefficient of 7th and 8th terms are equal.

9. (c) Given expansion is

$(1+x)^{101}(1-x+x^2)^{100}$

$= (1+x)(1+x)^{100}(1-x+x^2)^{100}$

$= (1+x)[(1+x)(1-x+x^2)]^{100}$

$= (1+x)[(1-x^3)^{100}]$

Expansion $(1-x^3)^{100}$ will have $100 + 1 = 101$ terms

So, $(1+x)(1-x^3)^{100}$ will have $2 \times 101 = 202$ terms

10. (a) Expansion of $(1+x)^{2n}$ is $1 + {}^{2n}C_1x + {}^{2n}C_2x^2 + ... + {}^{2n}C_r x^r + {}^{2n}C_{r+1}x^{r+1} + ... + {}^{2n}C_{2n}x^{2n}$

As given ${}^{2n}C_{r+2} = {}^{2n}C_{3r}$

$$\Rightarrow \frac{(2n)!}{(r+2)!(2n-r-2)!} = \frac{(2n)!}{(3r)!(2n-3r)!}$$

$$\Rightarrow (3r)!\,(2n-3r)! = (r+2)!\,(2n-r-2)! \quad ...(1)$$

Now, put value of n from the given choices.

Choice (a) put $n = 2r+1$ in (1)

LHS : $(3r)!\,(4r+2-3r)! = (3r)!\,(r+2)!$

RHS : $(r+2)!\,(3r)!$

$\Rightarrow$ LHS = RHS

11. (d) $(2^{1/2} + 3^{1/5})^{10} = {}^{10}C_0(2^{1/2})^{10} + {}^{10}C_1(2^{1/2})^9(3^{1/5}) + ... + {}^{10}C_{10}(3^{1/5})^{10}$

There are only two rational terms – first term and last term.

Now sum of two rational terms

$= (2)^5 + (3)^2 = 32 + 9 = 41$

12. (b) Let $r + 1 = 7 \Rightarrow r = 6$

Given expansion is

$$\left(\frac{3}{\sqrt[3]{84}} + \sqrt{3}\ln x\right)^9, x > 0$$

We have

$T_{r+1} = {}^nC_r (x)^{n-r} a^r$ for $(x+a)^n$.

$\therefore$ According to the question

$$729 = {}^9C_6\left(\frac{3}{\sqrt[3]{84}}\right)^3 .(\sqrt{3}\ln x)^6$$

$$\Rightarrow 3^6 = 84 \times \frac{3^3}{84} \times 3^3 \times (6 \ln x)$$

$\Rightarrow (\ln x)^6 = 1 \Rightarrow (\ln x)^6 = (\ln e)^6$

$\Rightarrow x = e$

13. (a) Consider $\left(\sqrt{3}+1\right)^{2n} - \left(\sqrt{3}-1\right)^{2n}$

$$= 2\left[{}^{2n}C_1\left(\sqrt{3}\right)^{2n-1} + {}^{2n}C_3\left(\sqrt{3}\right)^{2n-3} + {}^{2n}C_5\left(\sqrt{3}\right)^{2n-5} + ...\right]$$

(Using binomial expansion of $(a+b)^n$ and $(a-b)^n$)

= which is an irrational number.

14. (a) Given expansion is $\left(y^{1/5} + x^{1/10}\right)^{55}$

The general term is

$$T_{r+1} = {}^{55}C_r\left(y^{1/5}\right)^{55-r} \cdot \left(x^{\frac{1}{10}}\right)^r$$

T_{r+1} would free from radical sign if powers of y and x

are integers.

i.e. $\frac{55-r}{5}$ and $\frac{r}{10}$ are integer.

$\Rightarrow r$ is multiple of 10.

Hence, $r = 0, 10, 20, 30, 40, 50$

It is an A.P.

Thus, $50 = 0 + (k-1)\,10$

$50 = 10k - 10 \Rightarrow k = 6$

Thus, the six terms of the given expansion in which x and y are free from radical signs.

15. (d) Given function is

$f(y) = 1 - (y-1) + (y-1)^2 - (y-1)^3 + ... - (y-1)^{17}$

In the expansion of $(y-1)^n$

$T_{r+1} = {}^nC_r y^{n-r}(-1)^r$

coeff of y^2 in $(y-1)^2 = {}^2C_0$

coeff of y^2 in $(y-1)^3 = -{}^3C_1$

coeff of y^2 in $(y-1)^4 = {}^4C_2$

So, coeff of termwise is

${}^2C_0 + {}^3C_1 + {}^4C_2 + {}^5C_3 + ... + {}^{17}C_{15}$

$= 1 + {}^3C_1 + {}^4C_2 + {}^5C_3 + ... + {}^{17}C_{15}$

$= ({}^3C_0 + {}^3C_1) + {}^4C_2 + {}^5C_3 + ... + {}^{17}C_{15}$

$= {}^4C_1 + {}^4C_2 + {}^5C_3 + ... + {}^{17}C_{15}$

$= {}^5C_2 + {}^5C_3 + ... + {}^{17}C_{15}$

$= {}^{18}C_{15} = {}^{18}C_3$

16. (a) **Statement 2 :**

$P(n): n^7 - n$ is divisible by 7

Put $n = 1$, $1 - 1 = 0$ is divisible by 7, which is true

Let $n = k$, $P(k): k^7 - k$ is divisible by 7, true

Put $n = k + 1$

$\therefore \quad P(k+1): (k+1)^7 - (k+1)$ is div. by 7

$P(k+1): k^7 + {}^7C_1k^6 + {}^7C_2k^2 + ...+ {}^7C_6k + 1 - k - 1$, is div. by 7.

$P(k+1): (k^7 - k) + ({}^7C_1k^6 + {}^7C_2k^5 + ...+ {}^7C_6k)$ is div. by 7.

Since 7 is coprime with 1, 2, 3, 4, 5, 6.

So ${}^7C_1, {}^7C_2, ...{}^7C_6$ are all divisible by 7

$\therefore \quad P(k+1)$ is divisible by 7

Hence $P(n): n^7 - n$ is divisible by 7

Statement 1 : $n^7 - n$ is divisible by 7

$\Rightarrow \quad (n+1)^7 - (n+1)$ is divisible by 7

$\Rightarrow \quad (n+1)^7 - n^7 - 1 + (n^7 - n)$ is divisible by 7

$\Rightarrow \quad (n+1)^7 - n^7 - 1$ is divisible by 7

Hence both Statements 1 and 2 are correct and Statement 2 is the correct explanation of Statement -1.

17. (b) $(1 - x - x^2 + x^3)^6 = [(1-x) - x^2(1-x)]^6$

$= (1-x)^6(1-x^2)^6$

$= (1 - 6x + 15x^2 - 20x^3 + 15x^4 - 6x^5 + x^6)$

$\times (1 - 6x^2 + 15x^4 - 20x^6 + 15x^8 - 6x^{10} + x^{12})$

Coefficient of $x^7 = (-6)(-20) + (-20)(15) + (-6)(-6) = -144$

18. (a) $(8)^{2n} - (62)^{2n+1}$

$= (64)^n - (62)^{2n+1}$

$= (63+1)^n - (63-1)^{2n+1}$

$= \left[{}^nC_0(63)^n + {}^nC_1(63)^{n-1} + {}^nC_2(63)^{n-2} + ...+ {}^nC_{n-1}(63) + {}^nC_n\right]$

$= \left[{}^{2n+1}C_0(63)^{2n+1} - {}^{2n+1}C_1(63)^{2n} + {}^{2n+1}C_2(63)^{2n-1} - ....+ (-1)^{2n+1}\,{}^{2n+1}C_{2+1}\right]$

$= 63 \times$

$\left[{}^nC_0(63)^{n-1} + {}^nC_1(63)^{n-2} + {}^nC_2(63)^{n-3} + ...\right] + 1 - 63 \times$

$\left[{}^{2n+1}C_0(63)^{2n} - {}^{2n+1}C_1(63)^{2n-1} + ...\right] + 1$

$= 63 \times$ some integral value $+ 2$

$= 8^{2n} - (62)^{2n+1}$ when divided by 9 leaves 2 as the remainder.

19. (b) We have

$$\sum_{r=0}^{n}(r+1)\,{}^nC_r x^r = \sum_{r=0}^{n} r.\,{}^nC_r x^r + \sum_{r=0}^{n}{}^nC_r x^r$$

$$= \sum_{r=1}^{n} r\cdot\frac{n}{r}\,{}^{n-1}C_{r-1}x^r + (1+x)^n$$

$$= nx\sum_{r=1}^{n}{}^{n-1}C_{r-1}x^{r-1} + (1+x)^n$$

$= nx(1+x)^{n-1} + (1+x)^n = \text{RHS}$

$\therefore$ Statement 2 is correct.

Putting $x = 1$, we get

$$\sum_{r=0}^{n}(r+1)\,{}^nC_r = n\cdot 2^{n-1} + 2^n = (n+2)\cdot 2^{n-1}.$$

$\therefore$ Statement 1 is also true and statement 2 is a correct explanation for statement 1.

20. (b) $T_{r+1}=(-1)^r.{}^nC_r(a)^{n-r}.(b)^r$ is an expansion of $(a-b)^n$

$\therefore$ 5th term $=t_5=t_{4+1}$

$=(-1)^4.{}^nC_4(a)^{n-4}.(b)^4={}^nC_4.a^{n-4}.b^4$

6th term $=t_6=t_{5+1}=(-1)^5\,{}^nC_5(a)^{n-5}(b)^5$

Given $t_5+t_6=0$

$\therefore\ {}^nC_4.a^{n-4}.b^4+(-{}^nC_5.a^{n-5}.b^5)=0$

$$\Rightarrow \frac{n!}{4!(n-4)!}.\frac{a^n}{a^4}.b^4-\frac{n!}{5!(n-5)!}.\frac{a^nb^5}{a^5}=0$$

$$\Rightarrow \frac{n!.a^nb^4}{4!(n-5)!.a^4}\left[\frac{1}{(n-4)}-\frac{b}{5.a}\right]=0$$

or, $\frac{1}{n-4}-\frac{b}{5a}=0\Rightarrow\frac{a}{b}=\frac{n-4}{5}$

21. (d) $(1-y)^m(1+y)^n$

$=[1-{}^mC_1y+{}^mC_2y^2-......]$

$[1+{}^nC_1y+{}^nC_2y^2+.....]$

$$=1+(n-m)+\left\{\frac{m(m-1)}{2}+\frac{n(n-1)}{2}-mn\right\}y^2+.....$$

$\therefore\ a_1=n-m=10$

and $a_2=\frac{m^2+n^2-m-n-2mn}{2}=10$

So, $n-m=10$ and $(m-n)^2-(m+n)=20$

$\Rightarrow m+n=80$

$\therefore\ m=35, n=45$

22. (d) T_{r+1} in the expansion

$$\left[ax^2+\frac{1}{bx}\right]^{11}={}^{11}C_r(ax^2)^{11-r}\left(\frac{1}{bx}\right)^r$$

$={}^{11}C_r(a)^{11-r}(b)^{-r}(x)^{22-2r-r}$

For the Coefficient of x^7, we have

$22-3r=7\Rightarrow r=5$

$\therefore$ Coefficient of x^7

$={}^{11}C_5(a)^6\,(b)^{-5}$ ...(1)

Again T_{r+1} in the expansion

$$\left[ax-\frac{1}{bx^2}\right]^{11}={}^{11}C_r(ax^2)^{11-r}\left(-\frac{1}{bx^2}\right)^r$$

$={}^{11}C_r(a)^{11-r}(-1)^r\times(b)^{-r}(x)^{-2r}(x)^{11-r}$

For the Coefficient of x^{-7}, we have

Now $11-3r=-7\Rightarrow 3r=18\Rightarrow r=6$

$\therefore$ Coefficient of x^{-7}

$={}^{11}C_6\,a^5\times1\times(b)^{-6}$

$\therefore$ Coefficient of x^7 = Coefficient of x^{-7}

$\Rightarrow {}^{11}C_5(a)^6(b)^{-5}={}^{11}C_6\,a^5\times(b)^{-6}$

$\Rightarrow ab=1.$

23. (b) Coeff. of x^n in $(1+x)(1-x)^n$

= coeff of x^n in

$(1+x)(1-{}^nC_1x+{}^nC_2x^2-....+(-1)^{n}\,{}^nC_nx^n)$

$=(-1)^n\,{}^nC_n+(-1)^{n-1}\,{}^nC_{n-1}=(-1)^n+(-1)^{n-1}.n$

$=(-1)^n(1-n)$

ALTERNATE SOLUTION

Coeff of x^n in $(1+x)(1-x)^n$

= Coeff of x^n in

$(1-x)^n$ + Coeff of x^{n-1} in $(1-x)^n$

$=(-1)^n\,{}^nC_n+(-1)^{n-1}\,{}^nC_{n-1}$

$=(-1)^n1+(-1)^{n-1}n$

$=(-1)^n[1-n]$

24. (c) $T_{r+1}={}^{256}C_r(\sqrt{3})^{256-r}(\sqrt[8]{5})^r$

$={}^{256}C_r(3)^{\frac{256-r}{2}}(5)^{r/8}$

Terms will be integral if $\frac{256-r}{2}$ & $\frac{r}{8}$ both are +ve integer, which is so if r is an integral multiple of 8. As $0\le r\le 256$

25. (c) $t_{r+2}={}^{2n}C_{r+1}\,x^{r+1};t_{3r}={}^{2n}C_{3r-1}\,x^{3r-1}$

Given ${}^{2n}C_{r+1}={}^{2n}C_{3r-1}$;

$\Rightarrow {}^{2n}C_{2n-(r+1)}={}^{2n}C_{3r-1}$

$\Rightarrow 2n-r-1=3r-1\Rightarrow 2n=4r\Rightarrow n=2r$

26. (a) We have $t_{p+1}={}^{p+q}C_p\,x^p$ and $t_{q+1}={}^{p+q}C_q\,x^q$

${}^{p+q}C_p={}^{p+q}C_q$. [Remember ${}^nC_r={}^nC_{n-r}$]

27. (c) General term of $\left(2x^2-\frac{1}{x}\right)^8$ is

${}^8C_r(2x^2)^{8-r}\left(\frac{-1}{x}\right)^r$

$\therefore$ Given expression is equal to

$\left(1-\frac{1}{x}+3x^5\right){}^8C_r(2x^2)^{8-r}\left(-\frac{1}{x}\right)^r$

$$= {}^8C_r(2x^2)^{8-r}\left(-\frac{1}{x}\right)^r - \frac{1}{x}\,{}^8C_r(2x^2)^{8-r}\left(-\frac{1}{x}\right)^r$$

$$+3x^5.\,{}^8C_r(2x^2)^{8-r}\left(-\frac{1}{x}\right)^r$$

$$= {}^8C_r 2^{8-r}(-1)^r x^{16-3r} - {}^8C_r 2^{8-r}(-1)^r x^{15-3r}$$

$$+3.\,{}^8C_r 2^{(8-r)}\left(-\frac{1}{x}\right)^r (-1)^r x^{21-3r}$$

For the term independent of x, we should have

$16-3r=0,\ 15-3r=0,\ 21-3r=0$

From the simplification we get r = 5 and r = 7

$\therefore -{}^8C_5(2^3)(-1)^5 - 3.\,{}^8C_7.2$

$$+\left[\frac{8!}{5!3!}\times 8\right]-3\times\left[\frac{8!}{7!1!}\times 2\right]$$

$=(56\times 8)-48$

$=448-6\times 8=448-48=400$

28. **(c)** Given expression can be written as

$$\left((x^{1/3}+1)-\left(\frac{\sqrt{x}+1}{\sqrt{x}}\right)\right)^{10}$$

$$=\left(x^{1/3}+1-1-\frac{1}{\sqrt{x}}\right)^{10}$$

$=(x^{1/3}-x^{-1/2})^{10}$

General term $=T_{r+1}$

$={}^{10}C_r\,(x^{1/3})^{10-r}(-x^{-1/2})^r$

$$={}^{10}C_r\,x^{\frac{10-r}{3}}\cdot(-1)^r\cdot x^{-\frac{r}{2}}$$

$$={}^{10}C_r(-1)^r\cdot x^{\frac{10-r}{3}-\frac{r}{2}}$$

Term will be independent of x when $\frac{10-r}{3}-\frac{r}{2}=0$

$\Rightarrow r=4$

So, required term $=T_5={}^{10}C_4=210$

29. **(d)** $T_{r+1}={}^{15}C_r(x^2)^{15-r}.(2x^{-1})^r$

$={}^{15}C_r\times(2)^r\times x^{30-3r}$

For independent term, $30-3r=0 \Rightarrow r=10$

Hence the term independent of x,

$T_{11}={}^{15}C_{10}\times(2)^{10}$

For term involve x^{15}, $30-3r=15 \Rightarrow r=5$

Hence coefficient of $x^{15}={}^{15}C_5\times(2)^5$

$$\text{Required ratio}=\frac{{}^{15}C_5\times(2)^5}{{}^{15}C_{10}\times(2)^{10}}=\frac{\frac{15!}{10!5!}}{\frac{15!}{5!10!}\times(2)^5}$$

$=1:32$

30. **(d)** Given expansion can be written as

$$\left(\frac{x-1}{x}\right)^n.(1-x)^n=(-1)^n x^{-n}(1-x)^{2n}$$

Total number of terms will be $2n+1$ which is odd ($\because 2n$ is always even)

$$\therefore \text{Middle term}=\frac{2n+1+1}{2}=(n+1)\text{ th}$$

Now, $T_{r+1}={}^nC_r(1)^r x^{n-r}$

$$\text{So, }\frac{{}^{2n}C_n\cdot x^{2n-n}}{x^n.(-1)^n}={}^{2n}C_n.(-1)^n$$

Middle term is an odd term. So, $n+1$ will be odd. So, n will be even.

$\therefore$ Required answer is ${}^{2n}C_n$.

31. **(c)** The middle term in the expansion of

$(1+\alpha x)^4=T_3={}^4C_2(\alpha x)^2=6\alpha^2x^2$

The middle term in the expansion of

$(1-\alpha x)^6=T_4={}^6C_3(-\alpha x)^3=-20\alpha^3x^3$

According to the question

$$6\alpha^2=-20\alpha^3\Rightarrow\alpha=-\frac{3}{10}$$

32. **(a)** We have $({}^{21}C_1+{}^{21}C_2\ ......+{}^{21}C_{10})$

$-({}^{10}C_1+{}^{10}C_2\ .....\ {}^{10}C_{10})$

$$=\frac{1}{2}[({}^{21}C_1+....+{}^{21}C_{10})+({}^{21}C_{11}+....{}^{21}C_{20})]-(2^{10}-1)$$

$(\because {}^{10}C_1+{}^{10}C_2+....+{}^{10}C_{10}=2^{10}-1)$

$$=\frac{1}{2}[2^{21}-2]-(2^{10}-1)$$

$=(2^{20}-1)-(2^{10}-1)=2^{20}-2^{10}$

33. **(b)** Total number of terms $={}^{n+2}C_2=28$

$(n+2)(n+1)=56$

$x=6$

Sum of coefficients $=(1-2+4)^n=3^6=729$

34. **(c)** $(1-2\sqrt{x})^{50}={}^{50}C_0-{}^{50}C_1\,2\sqrt{x}+{}^{50}C_2\left(2\sqrt{x}\right)^2$ ...(1)

$(1+2\sqrt{x})^{50}={}^{50}C_0+{}^{50}C_1\,2\sqrt{x}-{}^{50}C_2(2\sqrt{x})^2$

$+...+{}^{50}C_3(2\sqrt{x})^3-{}^{50}C_4(2\sqrt{x})^4$ ...(2)

Adding equation (1) and (2)

$\left(1-2\sqrt{x}\right)^{50}+\left(1+2\sqrt{x}\right)^{50}$

$=2\left[{}^{50}C_0+{}^{50}C_2 2^2x+{}^{50}C_4 2^3x^2+...\right]$

Putting x = 1, we get above as $\frac{3^{50}+1}{2}$

35. (b) Given expansion $(1+x^n+x^{253})^{10}$

Let $x^{1012} = (1)^a\,(x^n)^b.\,(x^{253})^c$

Here a, b, c, n are all +ve integers and $a \le 10$, $b \le 10$, $c \le 4$, $n \le 22$, $a + b + c = 10$

Now $bn + 253c = 1012$

$\Rightarrow bn = 253\,(4 - c)$

For $c < 4$ and $n \le 22$; $b > 10$, which is not possible.

$\therefore c = 4,\ b = 0,\ a = 6$

$\therefore x^{1012} = (1)^6.\,(x^n)^0\,.\,(x^{253})^4$

Hence the coefficient of x^{1012}

$= \dfrac{10!}{6!0!4!}$

$= {}^{10}C_4$

36. (b) $S_2 = \sum_{j=1}^{10} j\ {}^{10}C_j = \sum_{j=1}^{10} 10\ {}^9C_{j-1}$

$= 10\left[{}^9C_0 + {}^9C_1 + {}^9C_2 + ... + {}^9C_9\right] = 10.2^9$

37. (a) The given situation in statement 1 is equivalent to find the non negative integral solutions of the equation $x_1+x_2+x_3+x_4+x_5=6$ which is coeff. of x^6 in the expansion of $(1+x+x^2+x^3+.....\infty)^5$= coeff. of x^6 in $(1-x)^{-5}$

$=$ coeff. of x^6 in $1+5x+\dfrac{5.6}{2!}x^2..........$

$= \dfrac{5\cdot6\cdot7\cdot8\cdot9\cdot10}{6!} = \dfrac{10!}{6!4!} = {}^{10}C_6$

$\therefore$ Statement 1 is wrong.

Number of ways of arranging $6A$'s and $4B$'s in a row

$= \dfrac{10!}{6!4!} = {}^{10}C_6$ which is same as the number of ways the child can buy six icecreams.

$\therefore$ Statement 2 is true.

38. (d) We know that, $(1+x)^{20} = {}^{20}C_0 + {}^{20}C_1x + {}^{20}C_2x^2 + ...\ {}^{20}C_{10}x^{10} + ...\ {}^{20}C_{20}x^{20}$

Put $x = -1$, $(0) = {}^{20}C_0 - {}^{20}C_1 + {}^{20}C_2 - {}^{20}C_3 + ...+ {}^{20}C_{10} - {}^{20}C_{11} .... + {}^{20}C_{20}$

$\Rightarrow 0 = 2[{}^{20}C_0 - {}^{20}C_1 + {}^{20}C_2 - {}^{20}C_3 + ... - {}^{20}C_9] + {}^{20}C_{10}$

$\Rightarrow {}^{20}C_{10} = 2[{}^{20}C_0 - {}^{20}C_1 + {}^{20}C_2 - {}^{20}C_3 + ... - {}^{20}C_9 + {}^{20}C_{10}]$

$\Rightarrow {}^{20}C_0 - {}^{20}C_1 + {}^{20}C_2 - {}^{20}C_3 + ... + {}^{20}C_{10} = \dfrac{1}{2}\,{}^{20}C_{10}$

39. (c) $\because$ x^3 and higher powers of x may be neglected

$$\therefore \frac{(1+x)^{\frac{3}{2}} - \left(1+\frac{x}{2}\right)^3}{\left(1-x\right)^{\frac{1}{2}}}$$

$$= (1-x)^{\frac{-1}{2}}\left[\left(1+\frac{3}{2}x+\frac{\frac{3}{2}\cdot\frac{1}{2}}{2!}x^2\right) - \left(1+\frac{3x}{2}+\frac{3.2}{2!}\frac{x^2}{4}\right)\right]$$

$$= \left[1+\frac{x}{2}+\frac{\frac{1}{2}\cdot\frac{3}{2}}{2!}x^2\right]\left[\frac{-3}{8}x^2\right] = \frac{-3}{8}x^2$$

(as x^3 and higher powers of x can be neglected)

40. (d) $T_{r+1} = \dfrac{n(n-1)(n-2).........(n-r+1)}{r!}(x)^r$

For first negative term,

$n - r + 1 < 0 \Rightarrow r > n + 1$

$\Rightarrow r > \dfrac{32}{5}\ \therefore r = 7.\ \left(\because n = \dfrac{27}{5}\right)$

Therefore, first negative term is T_8.

41. (d) $(1+0.0001)^{10000} = \left(1+\dfrac{1}{n}\right)^n,\ n = 10000$

$= 1 + n.\dfrac{1}{n} + \dfrac{n(n-1)}{2!}\dfrac{1}{n^2} + \dfrac{n(n-1)(n-2)}{3!}\dfrac{1}{n^3} + ...$

$= 1 + 1 + \dfrac{1}{2!}\left(1-\dfrac{1}{n}\right) + \dfrac{1}{3!}\left(1-\dfrac{1}{n}\right) + \left(1-\dfrac{2}{n}\right) + ...$

$< 1 + \dfrac{1}{1!} + \dfrac{1}{2!} + \dfrac{1}{3!} + ... + \dfrac{1}{(9999)!}$

$= 1 + \dfrac{1}{1!} + \dfrac{1}{2!} + ...\infty = e < 3$

42. (c) We have $2^n = 4096 = 2^{12} \Rightarrow n = 12$;

the greatest coeff= coeff of middle term.

So middle term

$= t_7$; $t_7 = t_{6+1}$

$\Rightarrow$ coeff of $t_7 = {}^{12}C_6 = \dfrac{12!}{6!6!} = 924.$

Sequences and Series

TOPIC-1 : Arithmetic Progression

1. For any three positive real numbers a, b and c, $9(25a^2+b^2)+25(c^2-3ac)=15b(3a+c)$. Then : **(2017)**
   (a) a, b and c are in G.P. (b) b, c and a are in G.P.
   (c) b, c and a are in A.P. (d) a, b and c are in A.P.

2. If three positive numbers *a*, *b* and *c* are in A.P. such that abc = 8, then the minimum possible value of *b* is : **[Online April 9, 2017]**
   (a) 2 (b) $4^{\frac{1}{3}}$
   (c) $4^{\frac{2}{3}}$ (d) 4

3. Let $a_1, a_2, a_3, \ldots, a_n$, be in A.P. If $a_3+a_7+a_{11}+a_{15}=72$, then the sum of its first 17 terms is equal to : **[Online April 10, 2016]**
   (a) 306 (b) 204
   (c) 153 (d) 612

4. Let α and β be the roots of equation $px^2+qx+r=0, p\neq 0$.
   If p, q, r are in A.P and $\frac{1}{\alpha}+\frac{1}{\beta}=4$, then the value of $|\alpha-\beta|$ is: **[2014]**
   (a) $\frac{\sqrt{34}}{9}$ (b) $\frac{2\sqrt{13}}{9}$
   (c) $\frac{\sqrt{61}}{9}$ (d) $\frac{2\sqrt{17}}{9}$

5. The sum of the first 20 terms common between the series 3 + 7 + 11 + 15 + ... and 1 + 6 + 11 + 16 + ..., is **[Online April 11, 2014]**
   (a) 4000 (b) 4020
   (c) 4200 (d) 4220

6. Given an A.P. whose terms are all positive integers. The sum of its first nine terms is greater than 200 and less than 220. If the second term in it is 12, then its 4th term is: **[Online April 9, 2014]**
   (a) 8 (b) 16
   (c) 20 (d) 24

7. If $a_1, a_2, a_3, \ldots, a_n, \ldots$ are in A.P. such that $a_4-a_7+a_{10}=m$, then the sum of first 13 terms of this A.P., is : **[Online April 23, 2013]**
   (a) 10m (b) 12m
   (c) 13m (d) 15m

8. Given sum of the first *n* terms of an A.P. is $2n+3n^2$. Another A.P. is formed with the same first term and double of the common difference, the sum of *n* terms of the new A.P. is : **[Online April 22, 2013]**
   (a) $n+4n^2$ (b) $6n^2-n$
   (c) n^2+4n (d) $3n+2n^2$

9. Let $a_1, a_2, a_3, \ldots$ be an A.P, such that
   $\frac{a_1+a_2+\ldots+a_p}{a_1+a_2+a_3+\ldots+a_q}=\frac{p^3}{q^3}; p\neq q$. Then $\frac{a_6}{a_{21}}$ is equal to: **[Online April 9, 2013]**
   (a) $\frac{41}{11}$ (b) $\frac{31}{121}$
   (c) $\frac{11}{41}$ (d) $\frac{121}{1861}$

10. If 100 times the 100th term of an AP with non zero common difference equals the 50 times its 50th term, then the 150th term of this AP is : **[2012]**
   (a) – 150 (b) 150 times its 50th term
   (c) 150 (d) Zero

11. If the A.M. between p^{th} and q^{th} terms of an A.P. is equal to the A.M. between r^{th} and s^{th} terms of the same A.P., then $p+q$ is equal to **[Online May 26, 2012]**
   (a) $r+s-1$ (b) $r+s-2$
   (c) $r+s+1$ (d) $r+s$

12. Suppose θ and φ (≠ 0) are such that sec (θ + φ), sec θ and sec (θ – φ) are in A.P. If $\cos\theta=k\cos\left(\frac{\phi}{2}\right)$ for some *k*, then *k* is equal to **[Online May 19, 2012]**
   (a) $\pm\sqrt{2}$ (b) ±1
   (c) $\pm\frac{1}{\sqrt{2}}$ (d) ±2

13. Let a_n be the nth term of an A.P. If $\sum_{r=1}^{100} a_{2r}=\alpha$ and $\sum_{r=1}^{100} a_{2r-1}=\beta$, then the common difference of the A.P. is

(a) $\alpha-\beta$ (b) $\frac{\alpha-\beta}{100}$ **[2011]**

(c) $\beta-\alpha$ (d) $\frac{\alpha-\beta}{200}$

14. A man saves ₹ 200 in each of the first three months of his service. In each of the subsequent months his saving increases by ₹ 40 more than the saving of immediately previous month. His total saving from the start of service will be ₹ 11040 after **[2011]**

(a) 19 months (b) 20 months
(c) 21 months (d) 18 months

15. A person is to count 4500 currency notes. Let a_n denote the number of notes he counts in the nth minute. If $a_1 = a_2 = ... = a_{10} = 150$ and $a_{10}, a_{11}, ...$ are in an AP with common difference –2, then the time taken by him to count all notes is **[2010]**

(a) 34 minutes (b) 125 minutes
(c) 135 minutes (d) 24 minutes

16. Let a_1, a_2, a_3........... be terms on A.P. If

$\frac{a_1+a_2+.........a_p}{a_1+a_2+.........+a_q}=\frac{p^2}{q^2}$, $p \neq q$, then $\frac{a_6}{a_{21}}$ equals **[2006]**

(a) $\frac{41}{11}$ (b) $\frac{7}{2}$

(c) $\frac{2}{7}$ (d) $\frac{11}{41}$

17. If the coefficients of rth, $(r+1)$th, and $(r+2)$th terms in the binomial expansion of $(1+y)^m$ are in A.P., then m and r satisfy the equation **[2005]**

(a) $m^2-m(4r-1)+4r^2-2=0$

(b) $m^2-m(4r+1)+4r^2+2=0$

(c) $m^2-m(4r+1)+4r^2-2=0$

(d) $m^2-m(4r-1)+4r^2+2=0$

18. Let T_r be the rth term of an A.P. whose first term is a and common difference is d. If for some positive integers $m, n, m \neq n, T_m=\frac{1}{n}$ and $T_n=\frac{1}{m}$, then $a-d$ equals **[2004]**

(a) $\frac{1}{m}+\frac{1}{n}$ (b) 1

(c) $\frac{1}{mn}$ (d) 0

19. If 1, $\log_9(3^{1-x}+2)$, $\log_3(4.3^x-1)$ are in A.P. then x equals **[2002]**

(a) $\log_3 4$ (b) $1-\log_3 4$
(c) $1-\log_4 3$ (d) $\log_4 3$

TOPIC-2 : Geometric Progression

20. If the 2nd, 5th and 9th terms of a non-constant A.P. are in G.P., then the common ratio of this G.P. is : **(2016)**

(a) 1 (b) $\frac{7}{4}$

(c) $\frac{8}{5}$ (d) $\frac{4}{3}$

21. Let $z=1+ai$ be a complex number, $a>0$, such that z^3 is a real number. Then the sum $1+z+z^2+....+z^{11}$ is equal to : **(Online April 10, 2016)**

(a) $1365\sqrt{3}i$ (b) $-1365\sqrt{3}i$
(c) $-1250\sqrt{3}i$ (d) $1250\sqrt{3}i$

22. If m is the A.M. of two distinct real numbers l and $n(l, n>1)$ and G_1, G_2 and G_3 are three geometric means between l and n, then $G_1^4+2G_2^4+G_3^4$ equals. **(2015)**

(a) $4lmn^2$ (b) $4l^2m^2n^2$
(c) $4l^2mn$ (d) $4lm^2n$

23. The sum of the 3rd and the 4th terms of a G.P. is 60 and the product of its first three terms is 1000. If the first term of this G.P. is positive, then its 7th term is : **(Online April 11, 2015)**

(a) 7290 (b) 640
(c) 2430 (d) 320

24. Three positive numbers form an increasing G. P. If the middle term in this G.P. is doubled, the new numbers are in A.P. then the common ratio of the G.P. is: **[2014]**

(a) $2-\sqrt{3}$ (b) $2+\sqrt{3}$
(c) $\sqrt{2}+\sqrt{3}$ (d) $3+\sqrt{2}$

25. The least positive integer n such that

$1-\frac{2}{3}-\frac{2}{3^2}-....-\frac{2}{3^{n-1}}<\frac{1}{100}$, is: **[Online April 12, 2014]**

(a) 4 (b) 5
(c) 6 (d) 7

26. In a geometric progression, if the ratio of the sum of first 5 terms to the sum of their reciprocals is 49, and the sum of the first and the third term is 35. Then the first term of this geometric progression is: **[Online April 11, 2014]**

(a) 7 (b) 21
(c) 28 (d) 42

27. The coefficient of x^{50} in the binomial expansion of $(1+x)^{1000}+x(1+x)^{999}+x^2(1+x)^{998}+....+x^{1000}$ is: **[Online April 11, 2014]**

(a) $\frac{(1000)!}{(50)!(950)!}$ (b) $\frac{(1000)!}{(49)!(951)!}$

(c) $\frac{(1001)!}{(51)!(950)!}$ (d) $\frac{(1001)!}{(50)!(951)!}$

28. Given a sequence of 4 numbers, first three of which are in G.P. and the last three are in A.P. with common difference six. If first and last terms of this sequence are equal, then the last term is : **[Online April 25, 2013]**

(a) 16 (b) 8
(c) 4 (d) 2

29. If a, b, c, d and p are distinct real numbers such that $(a^2+b^2+c^2)p^2-2p(ab+bc+cd)+(b^2+c^2+d^2)\leq 0$, then **[Online May 12, 2012]**

(a) a, b, c, d are in A.P.
(b) $ab = cd$
(c) $ac = bd$
(d) a, b, c, d are in G.P.

30. The difference between the fourth term and the first term of a Geometrical Progresssion is 52. If the sum of its first three terms is 26, then the sum of the first six terms of the progression is **[Online May 7, 2012]**

(a) 63 (b) 189
(c) 728 (d) 364

31. The first two terms of a geometric progression add up to 12. the sum of the third and the fourth terms is 48. If the terms of the geometric progression are alternately positive and negative, then the first term is **[2008]**

(a) –4 (b) –12
(c) 12 (d) 4

32. In a geometric progression consisting of positive terms, each term equals the sum of the next two terms. Then the common ratio of its progression is equals **[2007]**

(a) $\sqrt{5}$ (b) $\frac{1}{2}(\sqrt{5}-1)$
(c) $\frac{1}{2}(1-\sqrt{5})$ (d) $\frac{1}{2}\sqrt{5}$

33. The value of $\sum_{k=1}^{10}\left(\sin\frac{2k\pi}{11}+i\cos\frac{2k\pi}{11}\right)$ is **[2006]**

(a) i (b) 1
(c) -1 (d) $-i$

34. If the expansion in powers of x of the function $\frac{1}{(1-ax)(1-bx)}$ is $a_0+a_1x+a_2x^2+a_3x^3$...... then a_n is **[2006]**

(a) $\frac{b^n-a^n}{b-a}$ (b) $\frac{a^n-b^n}{b-a}$
(c) $\frac{a^{n+1}-b^{n+1}}{b-a}$ (d) $\frac{b^{n+1}-a^{n+1}}{b-a}$

35. Let two numbers have arithmetic mean 9 and geometric mean 4. Then these numbers are the roots of the quadratic equation **[2004]**

(a) $x^2-18x-16=0$ (b) $x^2-18x+16=0$
(c) $x^2+18x-16=0$ (d) $x^2+18x+16=0$

36. Sum of infinite number of terms of GP is 20 and sum of their square is 100. The common ratio of GP is **[2002]**

(a) 5 (b) 3/5
(c) 8/5 (d) 1/5

37. Fifth term of a GP is 2, then the product of its 9 terms is **[2002]**

(a) 256 (b) 512
(c) 1024 (d) none of these

TOPIC-3 : Harmonic Progression, Relation Between A. M., G. M. and H.M. of two Positive Numbers

38. If the arithmetic mean of two numbers a and b, $a > b > 0$, is five times their geometric mean, then $\frac{a+b}{a-b}$ is equal to : **[Online April 8, 2017]**

(a) $\frac{\sqrt{6}}{2}$ (b) $\frac{3\sqrt{2}}{4}$
(c) $\frac{7\sqrt{3}}{12}$ (d) $\frac{5\sqrt{6}}{12}$

39. If $A > 0$, $B > 0$ and $A + B = \frac{\pi}{6}$, then the minimum value of $\tan A + \tan B$ is : **[Online April 10, 2016]**

(a) $\sqrt{3}-\sqrt{2}$ (b) $4-2\sqrt{3}$
(c) $\frac{2}{\sqrt{3}}$ (d) $2-\sqrt{3}$

40. Let x, y, z be positive real numbers such that $x + y + z = 12$ and $x^3y^4z^5 = (0.1)(600)^3$. Then $x^3 + y^3 + z^3$ is equal to : **[Online April 9, 2016]**

(a) 342 (b) 216
(c) 258 (d) 270

41. Let G be the geometric mean of two positive numbers a and b, and M be the arithmetic mean of $\frac{1}{a}$ and $\frac{1}{b}$. If $\frac{1}{M}:G$ is 4 : 5, then a : b can be: **[Online April 12, 2014]**

(a) 1 : 4 (b) 1 : 2
(c) 2 : 3 (d) 3 : 4

42. If $a_1, a_2, \ldots\ldots\ldots, a_n$ are in H.P., then the expression $a_1a_2+a_2a_3+\ldots\ldots\ldots+a_{n-1}a_n$ is equal to **[2006]**

(a) $n(a_1-a_n)$ (b) $(n-1)(a_1-a_n)$
(c) na_1a_n (d) $(n-1)a_1a_n$

43. If $x=\sum_{n=0}^{\infty}a^n$, $y=\sum_{n=0}^{\infty}b^n$, $z=\sum_{n=0}^{\infty}c^n$ where a, b, c are in A.P and $|a|<1$, $|b|<1$, $|c|<1$ then x, y, z are in **[2005]**

(a) G.P.
(b) A.P.
(c) Arithmetic - Geometric Progression
(d) H.P.

44. If the sum of the roots of the quadratic equation $ax^2+bx+c=0$ is equal to the sum of the squares of their reciprocals, then $\frac{a}{c}, \frac{b}{a}$ and $\frac{c}{b}$ are in **[2003]**

(a) Arithmetic - Geometric Progression
(b) Arithmetic Progression
(c) Geometric Progression
(d) Harmonic Progression.

TOPIC-4 : Arithmetic-Geometric Sequence (A.G.S.), Some Special Sequences

45. Let a, b, c $\in$ R. If $f(x)=ax^2+bx+c$ is such that $a+b+c=3$ and $f(x+y)=f(x)+f(y)+xy, \forall x, y \in R$, then $\sum_{n=1}^{10} f(n)$ is equal to: **[2017]**

(a) 255 (b) 330
(c) 165 (d) 190

46. Let

$$S_n=\frac{1}{1^3}+\frac{1+2}{1^3+2^3}+\frac{1+2+3}{1^3+2^3+3^3}+\ldots\ldots+\frac{1+2+\ldots\ldots+n}{1^3+2^3+\ldots\ldots+n^3},$$

If 100 $S_n=n$, then n is equal to : **[Online April 9, 2017]**

(a) 199 (b) 99
(c) 200 (d) 19

47. If the sum of the first n terms of the series $\sqrt{3}+\sqrt{75}+\sqrt{243}+\sqrt{507}+\ldots\ldots$ is $435\sqrt{3}$, then n equals : **[Online April 8, 2017]**

(a) 18 (b) 15
(c) 13 (d) 29

48. If the sum of the first ten terms of the series $\left(1\frac{3}{5}\right)^2+\left(2\frac{2}{5}\right)^2+\left(3\frac{1}{5}\right)^2+4^2+\left(4\frac{4}{5}\right)^2+\ldots\ldots$, is $\frac{16}{5}$m, then m is equal to : **[2016]**

(a) 100 (b) 99
(c) 102 (d) 101

49. For $x \in R, x \neq -1$, if $(1+x)^{2016}+x(1+x)^{2015}+x^2(1+x)^{2014}+\ldots+x^{2016}=\sum_{i=0}^{2016} a_i x^i$, then a_{17} is equal to : **[Online April 9, 2016]**

(a) $\frac{2017!}{17!2000!}$ (b) $\frac{2016!}{17!\,1999!}$

(c) $\frac{2016!}{16!}$ (d) $\frac{2017!}{2000!}$

50. The sum of first 9 terms of the series. **[2015]**

$$\frac{1^3}{1}+\frac{1^3+2^3}{1+3}+\frac{1^3+2^3+3^3}{1+3+5}+\ldots$$

(a) 142 (b) 192
(c) 71 (d) 96

51. If $\sum_{n=1}^{5}\frac{1}{n(n+1)(n+2)(n+3)}=\frac{k}{3}$, then k is equal to **[Online April 11, 2015]**

(a) $\frac{1}{6}$ (b) $\frac{17}{105}$

(c) $\frac{55}{336}$ (d) $\frac{19}{112}$

52. The value of $\sum_{r=16}^{30}(r+2)(r-3)$ is equal to : **[Online April 10, 2015]**

(a) 7770 (b) 7785
(c) 7775 (d) 7780

53. If $(10)^9+2(11)^1(10^8)+3(11)^2(10)^7+\ldots\ldots+10(11)^9=k(10)^9$, then k is equal to: **[2014]**

(a) 100 (b) 110

(c) $\frac{121}{10}$ (d) $\frac{441}{100}$

54. The number of terms in an A.P. is even; the sum of the odd terms in it is 24 and that the even terms is 30. If the last term exceeds the first term by $10\frac{1}{2}$, then the number of terms in the A.P. is: **[Online April 19, 2014]**

(a) 4 (b) 8
(c) 12 (d) 16

55. If the sum

$$\frac{3}{1^2}+\frac{5}{1^2+2^2}+\frac{7}{1^2+2^2+3^2}+\ldots\ldots+$$ up to 20 terms is equal to $\frac{k}{21}$, then k is equal to: **[Online April 9, 2014]**

(a) 120 (b) 180
(c) 240 (d) 60

56. The sum of first 20 terms of the sequence 0.7, 0.77, 0.777,....., is **[2013]**

(a) $\frac{7}{81}(179-10^{-20})$ (b) $\frac{7}{9}(99-10^{-20})$

(c) $\frac{7}{81}(179+10^{-20})$ (d) $\frac{7}{9}(99+10^{-20})$

57. The value of $1^2+3^2+5^2+$ .... $+25^2$ is : **[Online April 25, 2013]**

(a) 2925 (b) 1469
(c) 1728 (d) 1456

58. The sum of the series :
$(2)^2+2(4)^2+3(6)^2+$ ... upto 10 terms is : **[Online April 23, 2013]**

(a) 11300 (b) 11200
(c) 12100 (d) 12300

59. The sum $\frac{3}{1^2}+\frac{5}{1^2+2^2}+\frac{7}{1^2+2^2+3^2}+\ldots$ upto 11-terms is: **[Online April 22, 2013]**

(a) $\frac{7}{2}$ (b) $\frac{11}{4}$
(c) $\frac{11}{2}$ (d) $\frac{60}{11}$

60. The sum of the series : **[Online April 9, 2013]**

$1+\frac{1}{1+2}+\frac{1}{1+2+3}+\ldots\ldots$ upto 10 terms, is :

(a) $\frac{18}{11}$ (b) $\frac{22}{13}$
(c) $\frac{20}{11}$ (d) $\frac{16}{9}$

61. **Statement-1:** The sum of the series $1+(1+2+4)+(4+6+9)+(9+12+16)+\ldots+(361+380+400)$ is 8000.

Statement-2: $\sum_{k=1}^{n}\left(k^3-(k-1)^3\right)=n^3$, for any natural number n. **[2012]**

(a) Statement-1 is false, Statement-2 is true.
(b) Statement-1 is true, statement-2 is true; statement-2 is a correct explanation for Statement-1.
(c) Statement-1 is true, statement-2 is true; statement-2 is **not** a correct explanation for Statement-1.
(d) Statement-1 is true, statement-2 is false.

62. If the sum of the series $1^2+2.2^2+3^2+2.4^2+5^2+\ldots 2.6^2+\ldots$ upto n terms, when n is even, is $\frac{n(n+1)^2}{2}$, then the sum of the series, when n is odd, is **[Online May 26, 2012]**

(a) $n^2(n+1)$ (b) $\frac{n^2(n-1)}{2}$
(c) $\frac{n^2(n+1)}{2}$ (d) $n^2(n-1)$

63. The sum of the series $1+\frac{4}{3}+\frac{10}{9}+\frac{28}{27}+\ldots$ upto n terms is **[Online May 19, 2012]**

(a) $\frac{7}{6}n+\frac{1}{6}-\frac{2}{3.2^{n-1}}$ (b) $\frac{5}{3}n-\frac{7}{6}+\frac{1}{2.3^{n-1}}$
(c) $n+\frac{1}{2}-\frac{1}{2.3^n}$ (d) $n-\frac{1}{3}-\frac{1}{3.2^{n-1}}$

64. The sum of the series

$\frac{1}{1+\sqrt{2}}+\frac{1}{\sqrt{2}+\sqrt{3}}+\frac{1}{\sqrt{3}+\sqrt{4}}+\ldots$

upto 15 terms is **[Online May 12, 2012]**

(a) 1 (b) 2
(c) 3 (d) 4

65. The sum of the series
$1^2+2.2^2+3^2+2.4^2+5^2+2.6^2+\ldots+2(2m)^2$ is **[Online May 7, 2012]**

(a) $m(2m+1)^2$ (b) $m^2(m+2)$
(c) $m^2(2m+1)$ (d) $m(m+2)^2$

66. The sum to infinite term of the series

$1+\frac{2}{3}+\frac{6}{3^2}+\frac{10}{3^3}+\frac{14}{3^4}+\ldots$ is **[2009]**

(a) 3 (b) 4
(c) 6 (d) 2

67. The sum of series $\frac{1}{2!}-\frac{1}{3!}+\frac{1}{4!}-\ldots\ldots$ upto infinity is **[2007]**

(a) $e^{-\frac{1}{2}}$ (b) $e^{+\frac{1}{2}}$
(c) e^{-2} (d) e^{-1}

68. The sum of the series

$1+\frac{1}{4.2!}+\frac{1}{16.4!}+\frac{1}{64.6!}+\ldots\ldots\ldots\ldots$ ad inf. is **[2005]**

(a) $\frac{e-1}{\sqrt{e}}$ (b) $\frac{e+1}{\sqrt{e}}$
(c) $\frac{e-1}{2\sqrt{e}}$ (d) $\frac{e+1}{2\sqrt{e}}$

69. The sum of series $\frac{1}{2!}+\frac{1}{4!}+\frac{1}{6!}+\ldots$ is **[2004]**

(a) $\frac{(e^2-2)}{e}$ (b) $\frac{(e-1)^2}{2e}$
(c) $\frac{(e^2-1)}{2e}$ (d) $\frac{(e^2-1)}{2}$

70. The sum of the first n terms of the series

$1^2 + 2.2^2 + 3^2 + 2.4^2 + 5^2 + 2.6^2 + ...$

is $\frac{n(n+1)^2}{2}$ when n is even. When n is odd the sum is **[2004]**

(a) $\left[\frac{n(n+1)}{2}\right]^2$ (b) $\frac{n^2(n+1)}{2}$

(c) $\frac{n(n+1)^2}{4}$ (d) $\frac{3n(n+1)}{2}$

71. If $S_n = \sum_{r=0}^{n} \frac{1}{{}^nC_r}$ and $t_n = \sum_{r=0}^{n} \frac{r}{{}^nC_r}$, then $\frac{t_n}{S_n}$ is equal to **[2004]**

(a) $\frac{2n-1}{2}$ (b) $\frac{1}{2}n-1$

(c) $n-1$ (d) $\frac{1}{2}n$

72. The sum of the series **[2003]**

$\frac{1}{1.2} - \frac{1}{2.3} + \frac{1}{3.4}$.......... up to ∞ is equal to

(a) $\log_e\left(\frac{4}{e}\right)$ (b) $2\log_e 2$

(c) $\log_e 2 - 1$ (d) $\log_e 2$

73. $1^3 - 2^3 + 3^3 - 4^3 + ... + 9^3 =$ **[2002]**

(a) 425 (b) –425

(c) 475 (d) –475

74. The value of $2^{1/4} . 4^{1/8} . 8^{1/16}$ ... ∞ is **[2002]**

(a) 1 (b) 2

(c) 3/2 (d) 4

Hints & Solutions

1. (c) We have
$9(25a^2+b^2)+25(c^2-3ac)=15b(3a+c)$
$\Rightarrow 225a^2+9b^2+25c^2-75ac=45ab+15bc$
$\Rightarrow (15a)^2+(3b)^2+(5c)^2-75ac-45ab-15bc=0$
$\frac{1}{2}[(15a-3b)^2+(3b-5c)^2+(5c-15a)^2]=0$
it is possible when $15a-3b=0$, $3b-5c=0$ and $5c-15a=0$
$\Rightarrow 15a=3b=5$
$\Rightarrow b=\frac{5c}{3}, a=\frac{c}{3}$
$\Rightarrow a+b=\frac{c}{3}+\frac{5c}{3}=\frac{6c}{3}$
$\Rightarrow a+b=2c$
$\Rightarrow$ b, c, a are in A.P.

2. (a) **By Arithmetic Mean:**
$a+c=2b$
Consider $a=b=c=2$
$\Rightarrow$ $abc=8$
$\Rightarrow$ $a+b=2b$
$\therefore$ minimum possible value of $b=2$

3. (a) $a_3+a_7+a_{11}+a_{15}=72$
$(a_3+a_{15})+(a_7+a_{11})=72$
$a_3+a_{15}+a_7+a_{11}=2(a_1+a_{17})$
$a_1+a_{17}=36$
$S_{17}=\frac{17}{2}[a_1+a_{17}]=17\times 18=306$

4. (b) Let p, q, r are in AP
$\Rightarrow 2q=p+r$ ...(i)
Given $\frac{1}{\alpha}+\frac{1}{\beta}=4$
$\Rightarrow \frac{\alpha+\beta}{\alpha\beta}=4$
We have $\alpha+\beta=-q/p$ and $\alpha\beta=\frac{r}{p}$
$\Rightarrow \frac{-\frac{q}{p}}{\frac{r}{p}}=4 \Rightarrow q=-4r$ ....(ii)
From (i), we have
$2(-4r)=p+r$
$p=-9r$
$q=-4r$
$r=r$
Now $|\alpha-\beta|=\sqrt{(\alpha+\beta)^2-4\alpha\beta}$
$=\sqrt{\left(\frac{-q}{p}\right)^2-\frac{4r}{p}}=\frac{\sqrt{q^2-4pr}}{|p|}$
$=\frac{\sqrt{16r^2+36r^2}}{|-9r|}=\frac{2\sqrt{13}}{9}$

5. (b) Given n = 20; S_{20} = ?
Series(1) $\rightarrow$ 3, 7, 11, 15, 19, 23, 27, 31, 35, 39, 43, 47, 51, 55, 59...
Series (2) $\rightarrow$ 1, 6, 11, 16, 21, 26, 31, 36, 41, 46, 51, 56, 61, 66, 71.
The common terms between both the series are 11, 31, 51, 71...
Above series forms an Arithmetic progression (A.P).
Therefore, first term (a) = 11 and
common difference (d) = 20
Now, $S_n=\frac{n}{2}[2a+(n-1)d]$
$S_{20}=\frac{20}{2}[2\times 11+(20-1)20]$
$S_{20}=10[22+19\times 20]$
$S_{20}=10\times 402=4020$
$\therefore S_{20}=4020$

6. (c) Let a be the first term and d be the common difference of given A.P.
Second term, $a+d=12$ ...(1)
Sum of first nine terms,
$S_9=\frac{9}{2}(2a+8d)=9(a+4d)$
Given that S_9 is more than 200 and less than 220
$\Rightarrow 200<S_9<220$
$\Rightarrow 200<9(a+4d)<220$
$\Rightarrow 200<9(a+d+3d)<220$
Putting value of $(a+d)$ from equation (1)
$200<9(12+3d)<220$
$\Rightarrow 200<108+27d<220$
$\Rightarrow 200-108<108+27d-108<220-108$
$\Rightarrow 92<27d<112$
Possible value of d is 4
$27\times 4=108$

Thus, $92 < 108 < 112$

Putting value of d in equation (1)

$a + d = 12$

$a = 12 - 4 = 8$

4th term $= a + 3d = 8 + 3 \times 4 = 20$

7. (c) If d be the common difference, then

$m = a_4 - a_7 + a_{10} = a_4 - a_7 + a_7 + 3d = a_7$

$$S_{13} = \frac{13}{2}[a_1 + a_{13}] = \frac{13}{2}[a_1 + a_7 + 6d]$$

$$= \frac{13}{2}[2a_7] = 13a_7 = 13\text{ m}$$

8. (b) Given $S_n = 2n + 3n^2$

Now, first term $= 2 + 3 = 5$

second term $= 2(2) + 3(4) = 16$

third term $= 2(3) + 3(9) = 33$

Now, sum given in option (b) only has the same first term and difference between 2nd and 1st term is double also.

9. (b) $$\frac{a_1 + a_2 + a_3 + ... + a_p}{a_1 + a_2 + a_3 + ... + a_q} = \frac{p^3}{q^3}$$

$$\Rightarrow \frac{a_1 + a_2}{a_1} = \frac{8}{1} \Rightarrow a_1 + (a_1 + d) = 8a_1$$

$\Rightarrow d = 6a_1$

Now $$\frac{a_6}{a_{21}} = \frac{a_1 + 5d}{a_1 + 20d}$$

$$= \frac{a_1 + 5 \times 6a_1}{a_1 + 20 \times 6a_1} = \frac{1 + 30}{1 + 120} = \frac{31}{121}$$

10. (d) Let 100th term of an AP is $a + (100 - 1)\,d$ $= a + 99d$ where 'a' is the first term of $A.P$ and 'd' is the common difference of $A.P.$

Similarly, 50th term $= a + (50 - 1)\,d$

$= a + 49d$

Now, According to the question

$100\,(a + 99d) = 50\,(a + 49d)$

$\Rightarrow 2a + 198\,d = a + 49d \Rightarrow a + 149\,d = 0$

This is the 150th term of an $A.P.$

Hence, $T_{150} = a + 149\,d = 0$

11. (d) Given : $$\frac{a_p + a_q}{2} = \frac{a_r + a_s}{2}$$

$\Rightarrow a + (p - 1)\,d + a + (q - 1)d$

$= a + (r - 1)d + a + (s - 1)d$

$\Rightarrow 2a + (p + q)d - 2d = 2a + (r + s)\,d - 2d$

$\Rightarrow (p + q)d = (r + s)d \Rightarrow p + q = r + s.$

12. (a) Since, $\sec(\theta - \phi)$, $\sec\theta$ and $\sec(\theta + \phi)$ are in A.P.,

$\therefore 2\sec\theta = \sec(\theta - \phi) + \sec(\theta + \phi)$

$$\Rightarrow \frac{2}{\cos\theta} = \frac{\cos(\theta + \phi) + \cos(\theta - \phi)}{\cos(\theta - \phi)\cos(\theta + \phi)}$$

$$\Rightarrow 2\left(\cos^2\theta - \sin^2\phi\right) = \cos\theta[2\cos\theta\cos\phi]$$

$$\Rightarrow \cos^2\theta(1 - \cos\phi) = \sin^2\phi = 1 - \cos^2\phi$$

$$\Rightarrow \quad \cos^2\theta = 1 + \cos\phi = 2\cos^2\frac{\phi}{2}$$

$$\therefore \quad \cos\theta = \sqrt{2}\cos\frac{\phi}{2}$$

But given $\cos\theta = k\cos\frac{\phi}{2}$

$\therefore \quad k = \sqrt{2}$

13. (b) Let A.P. be $a, a + d, a + 2d, ...$

$a_2 + a_4 + ... + a_{200} = \alpha$

$$\Rightarrow \frac{100}{2}\left[2(a + d) + (100 - 1)d\right] = \alpha \text{ ....(i)}$$

and $a_1 + a_3 + a_5 + ... + a_{199} = \beta$

$$\Rightarrow \frac{100}{2}[2a + (100 - 1)\,d] = \beta \text{ ....(ii)}$$

On solving (i) and (ii), we get

$$d = \frac{\alpha - \beta}{100}$$

14. (c) Let required number of months $=$ n

$\therefore 200 \times 3 + (240 + 280 + 320 + ... + (\text{n} - 3)^{\text{th}} \text{ term})$ $= 11040$

$$\Rightarrow \frac{n - 3}{2}[2 \times 240 + (n - 4) \times 40] = 11040 - 600$$

$\Rightarrow (n - 3)[240 + 20n - 80] = 10440$

$\Rightarrow (n - 3)(20n + 160) = 10440$

$\Rightarrow (n - 3)(n + 8) = 522$

$\Rightarrow n^2 + 5n - 546 = 0$

$\Rightarrow (n + 26)\,(n - 21) = 0$

$\therefore n = 21$

15. (a) Till 10th minute number of counted notes $= 1500$

$$3000 = \frac{n}{2}[2 \times 148 + (n - 1)(-2)] = n[148 - n + 1]$$

$n^2 - 149n + 3000 = 0$

$\Rightarrow n = 125, 24$

But $n = 125$ is not possible

$\therefore$ total time $= 24 + 10 = 34$ minutes.

16. (d) $$\frac{\frac{p}{2}[2a_1+(p-1)d]}{\frac{q}{2}[2a_1+(q-1)d]}=\frac{p^2}{q^2}$$

$$\Rightarrow \frac{2a_1+(p-1)d}{2a_1+(q-1)d}=\frac{p}{q}$$

$$\frac{a_1+\left(\frac{p-1}{2}\right)d}{a_1+\left(\frac{q-1}{2}\right)d}=\frac{p}{q}$$

For $\frac{a_6}{a_{21}}$, $p=11, q=41 \Rightarrow \frac{a_6}{a_{21}}=\frac{11}{41}$

17. (c) Given ${}^mC_{r-1}$, ${}^mC_r$, ${}^mC_{r+1}$ are in A.P.

$$2\,{}^mC_r={}^mC_{r-1}+{}^mC_{r+1}$$

$$\Rightarrow 2=\frac{{}^mC_{r-1}}{{}^mC_r}+\frac{{}^mC_{r+1}}{{}^mC_r}=\frac{r}{m-r+1}+\frac{m-r}{r+1}$$

$$\Rightarrow m^2-m(4r+1)+4r^2-2=0.$$

18. (d) $T_m=a+(m-1)d=\frac{1}{n}$ .....(1)

$T_n=a+(n-1)d=\frac{1}{m}$ .....(2)

$(1)-(2)\Rightarrow (m-n)d=\frac{1}{n}-\frac{1}{m}\Rightarrow d=\frac{1}{mn}$

From (1) $a=\frac{1}{mn}\Rightarrow a-d=0$

19. (b) $1, \log_9(3^{1-x}+2), \log_3(4.3^x-1)$ are in A.P.

$\Rightarrow 2\log_9(3^{1-x}+2)=1+\log_3(4.3^x-1)$

$\Rightarrow \log_3(3^{1-x}+2)=\log_3 3+\log_3(4.3^x-1)$

$\Rightarrow \log_3(3^{1-x}+2)=\log_3[3(4.3^x-1)]$

$\Rightarrow 3^{1-x}+2=3(4.3^x-1)$

$\Rightarrow 3.3^{-x}+2=12.3^x-3.$

Put $3^x=t$

$\Rightarrow \frac{3}{t}+2=12t-3$ or $12t^2-5t-3=0;$

Hence $t=-\frac{1}{3},\frac{3}{4}$

$\Rightarrow 3^x=\frac{3}{4}$ (as $3^x\neq -ve$)

$\Rightarrow x=\log_3\left(\frac{3}{4}\right)$ or $x=\log_3 3-\log_3 4$

$\Rightarrow x=1-\log_3 4$

20. (d) Let the GP be a, ar and ar^2 then $a=A+d$; $ar=A+4d$; $ar^2=A+8d$

$$\Rightarrow \frac{ar^2-ar}{ar-a}=\frac{(A+8d)-(A+4d)}{(A+4d)-(A+d)}$$

$$r=\frac{4}{3}$$

21. (b) $z=1+ai$

$z^2=1-a^2+2ai$

$z^2.z=\{(1-a^2)+2ai\}\ \{1+ai\}$

$=(1-a^2)+2ai+(1-a^2)\quad ai-2a^2$

$\because$ z^3 is real $\Rightarrow 2a+(1-a^2)a=0$

$a(3-a^2)=0\Rightarrow a=\sqrt{3}\ (a>0)$

$$1+z+z^2\,.........\,z^{11}=\frac{z^{12}-1}{z-1}=\frac{(1+\sqrt{3}i)^{12}-1}{1+\sqrt{3}i-1}$$

$$=\frac{(1+\sqrt{3}i)^{12}-1}{\sqrt{3}i}$$

$$(1+\sqrt{3}i)^{12}=2^{12}\left(\frac{1}{2}+\frac{\sqrt{3}}{2}i\right)^{12}$$

$$=2^{12}\left(\cos\frac{\pi}{3}+i\sin\frac{\pi}{3}\right)^{12}=2^{12}(\cos 4\pi+i\sin 4\pi)=2^{12}$$

$$\Rightarrow \frac{2^{12}-1}{\sqrt{3}i}=\frac{4095}{\sqrt{3}i}=-\frac{4095}{3}\sqrt{3}i=-1365\sqrt{3}i$$

22. (d) $m=\frac{l+n}{2}$ and common ratio of G.P. $=r=\left(\frac{n}{l}\right)^{\frac{1}{4}}$

$\therefore$ $G_1=l^{3/4}n^{1/4}, G_2=l^{1/2}n^{1/2}, G_3=l^{1/4}n^{3/4}$

$G_1^4+2G^4+G_3^4=l^3n+2l^2n^2+ln^3$

$=ln(l+n)^2$

$=ln\times 2m^2$

$=4lm^2n$

23. (d) Let a, ar and ar^2 be the first three terms of G.P

According to the question

$a(ar)(ar^2)=1000\Rightarrow (ar)^3=1000\Rightarrow ar=10$

and $ar^2+ar^3=60\Rightarrow ar(r+r^2)=60$

$\Rightarrow r^2+r-6=0$

$\Rightarrow r=2,-3$

$a=5, a=-\frac{10}{3}$ (reject)

Hence, $T_7=ar^6=5(2)^6=5\times 64=320.$

24. (b) Let a, ar, ar^2 are in G.P.

According to the question

$a, 2ar, ar^2$ are in A.P.

$\Rightarrow\ 2\times 2ar=a+ar^2$

$\Rightarrow \quad 4r = 1 + r^2 \Rightarrow r^2 - 4r + 1 = 0$

$$r = \frac{4 \pm \sqrt{16-4}}{2} = 2 \pm \sqrt{3}$$

Since $r > 1$

$\therefore \quad r = 2 - \sqrt{3}$ is rejected

Hence, $r = 2 + \sqrt{3}$

25. (b) $1 - \frac{2}{3} - \frac{2}{3^2} .... \frac{2}{3^{n-1}} < \frac{1}{100}$

$$\Rightarrow 1 - \frac{2}{3}\left[\frac{1}{3} + \frac{1}{3^2} + \frac{1}{3^3} + ... \frac{1}{3^{n-1}}\right] < \frac{1}{100}$$

$$\Rightarrow \frac{1 - 2\left[\frac{1}{3}\left(\frac{1}{3^n} - 1\right)\right]}{\frac{1}{3} - 1} < \frac{1}{100}$$

$$\Rightarrow 1 - 2\left[\frac{3^n - 1}{2.3^n}\right] < \frac{1}{100}$$

$$\Rightarrow 1 - \left[\frac{3^n - 1}{3^n}\right] < \frac{1}{100}$$

$$\Rightarrow 1 - 1 + \frac{1}{3^n} < \frac{1}{100}$$

$\Rightarrow 100 < 3^n$

Thus, least value of n is 5

26. (c) According to Question

$\Rightarrow \frac{S_5}{S_5'} = 49$ {here, S_5 = Sum of first 5 terms and S_5 = Sum of their reciprocals)

$$\Rightarrow \frac{\frac{a(r^5 - 1)}{(r-1)}}{\frac{a^{-1}(r^{-5} - 1)}{(r^{-1} - 1)}} = 49$$

$$\Rightarrow \frac{a(r^5 - 1) \times (r^{-1} - 1)}{a^{-1}(r^{-5} - 1) \times (r - 1)} = 49$$

or $$\frac{a^2(1-r^5) \times (1-r) \times r^5}{(1-r^5) \times (1-r) \times r} = 49$$

$\Rightarrow a^2r^4 = 49 \Rightarrow a^2r^4 = 7^2$

$\Rightarrow \boxed{ar^2 = 7}$ ...(1)

Also, given, $S_1 + S_3 = 35$

$a + ar^2 = 35$ ...(2)

Now substituting the value of eq. (1) in eq. (2)

$a + 7 = 35$

$\boxed{a = 28}$

27. (d) Let given expansion be

$S = (1 + x)^{1000} + x(1 + x)^{999} + x^2(1 + x)^{998} + ... + ... + x^{1000}$

Put $1 + x = t$

$S = t^{1000} + xt^{999} + x^2 (t)^{998} + ... + x^{1000}$

This is a G.P with common ratio $\frac{x}{t}$

$$S = \frac{t^{1000}\left[1 - \left(\frac{x}{t}\right)^{1001}\right]}{1 - \frac{x}{t}}$$

$$= \frac{(1+x)^{1000}\left[1 - \left(\frac{x}{1+x}\right)^{1001}\right]}{1 - \frac{x}{1+x}}$$

$$= \frac{(1+x)^{1001}\left[(1+x)^{1001} - x^{1001}\right]}{(1+x)^{1001}}$$

$= [(1+x)^{1001} - x^{1001}]$

Now coeff of x^{50} in above expansion is equal to coeff of x^{50} in $(1 + x)^{1001}$ which is ${}^{1001}C_{50}$

$$= \frac{(1001)!}{50!(951)!}$$

28. (b) Let a, b, c, d be four numbers of the sequence.

Now, according to the question $b^2 = ac$ and $c - b = 6$ and $a - c = 6$

Also, given $\boxed{a = d}$

$\therefore b^2 = ac \Rightarrow b^2 = a\left[\frac{a+b}{2}\right]$ $\quad (\because 2c = a + b)$

$\Rightarrow a^2 - 2b^2 + ab = 0$

Now, $c - b = 6$ and $a - c = 6$,

gives $a - b = 12$

$\Rightarrow b = a - 12$

$\therefore a^2 - 2b^2 + ab = 0$

$\Rightarrow a^2 - 2(a - 12)^2 + a(a - 12) = 0$

$\Rightarrow a^2 - 2a^2 - 288 + 48a + a^2 - 12a = 0$

$\Rightarrow 36a = 288 \Rightarrow a = 8$

Hence, last term is $d = a = 8$.

29. (d) The given relation can be written as

$$(a^2p^2 - 2abp + b^2) + (b^2p^2 + c^2 - 2bpc) + (c^2p^2 + d^2 - 2pcd) \le 0$$

or $(ap - b)^2 + (bp - c)^2 + (cp - d)^2 \le 0$ ...(1)

Since a, b, c, d and p are all real, the inequality (1) is possible only when each of factor is zero.

i.e., $ap - b = 0$, $bp - c = 0$ and $cp - d = 0$

or $p = \frac{b}{a} = \frac{c}{b} = \frac{d}{c}$

or a, b, c, d are in G.P.

30. (c) Let $a, ar, ar^2, ar^3, ar^4, ar^5$ be six terms of a G.P. where 'a' is first term and r is common ratio.

According to given conditions, we have

$ar^3 - a = 5 \Rightarrow a(r^3 - 1) = 52$ ...(1)

and $a + ar + ar^2 = 26$

$\Rightarrow a(1 + r + r^2) = 26$ ...(2)

To find: $a(1 + r + r^2 + r^3 + r^4 + r^5)$

Consider

$a[1 + r + r^2 + r^3 + r^4 + r^5]$

$= a[1 + r + r^2 + r^3(1 + r + r^2)]$

$= a[1 + r + r^2][1 + r^3]$ ...(3)

Divide (1) by (2), we get

$$\frac{r^3 - 1}{1 + r + r^2} = 2,$$

we know $r^3 - 1 = (r - 1)(1 + r + r^2)$

$\therefore r - 1 = 2 \Rightarrow r = 3$ and $a = 2$

$\therefore a(1 + r + r^2 + r^3 + r^4 + r^5)$

$= a(1 + r + r^2)(1 + r^3)$

$= 2(1 + 3 + 9)(1 + 27)$

$= 26 \times 28 = 728$

31. (b) As per question,

$a + ar = 12$ ...(1)

$ar^2 + ar^3 = 48$ ...(2)

$$\Rightarrow \frac{ar^2(1 + r)}{a(1 + r)} = \frac{48}{12} \Rightarrow r^2 = 4, \Rightarrow r = -2$$

($\because$ terms are = + ve and –ve alternately)

$\Rightarrow a = -12$

32. (b) Let the series a, ar, ar^2, ... are in geometric progression.

given, $a = ar + ar^2$

$\Rightarrow 1 = r + r^2 \quad \Rightarrow r^2 + r - 1 = 0$

$$\Rightarrow r = \frac{-1 \pm \sqrt{1 - 4 \times -1}}{2}$$

$$\Rightarrow r = \frac{-1 \pm \sqrt{5}}{2}$$

$$\Rightarrow r = \frac{\sqrt{5} - 1}{2}$$ [$\because$ terms of G.P. are positive

$\therefore$ r should be positive]

33. (d) $\sum_{k=1}^{10}\left(\sin\frac{2k\pi}{11} + i\cos\frac{2k\pi}{11}\right)$

$$= i\sum_{k=1}^{10}\left(\cos\frac{2k\pi}{11} - i\sin\frac{2k\pi}{11}\right)$$

$$= i\sum_{k=1}^{10} e^{-\frac{2k\pi}{11}i} = i\left\{\sum_{k=0}^{10} e^{-\frac{2k\pi}{11}i} - 1\right\}$$

$$= i\left[1 + e^{-\frac{2\pi}{11}i} + e^{-\frac{4\pi}{11}i} + \text{....11 terms}\right] - i$$

$$= i\left[\frac{1 - \left(e^{-\frac{2\pi}{11}i}\right)^{11}}{1 - e^{-\frac{2\pi}{11}i}}\right] - i = i\left[\frac{1 - e^{-2\pi i}}{1 - e^{-\frac{2\pi}{11}i}}\right] - i$$

$= i \times 0 - i \qquad [\because e^{-2\pi i} = 1]$

$= -i$

34. (d) $(1 - ax)^{-1}(1 - bx)^{-1}$

$= (1 + ax + a^2x^2 + ...)(1 + bx + b^2x^2 + ...)$

$\therefore$ Coefficient of x^n

$$x^n = b^n + ab^{n-1} + a^2b^{n-2} + ... + a^{n-1}b + a^n$$

{which is a G.P. with $r = \frac{a}{b}$

$$\therefore \text{Its sum is} = \frac{b^n\left[1 - \left(\frac{a}{b}\right)^{n+1}\right]}{1 - \frac{a}{b}}\}$$

$$= \frac{b^{n+1} - a^{n+1}}{b - a} \qquad \therefore a_n = \frac{b^{n+1} - a^{n+1}}{b - a}$$

35. (b) Let two numbers be a and b then $\frac{a + b}{2} = 9$ and $\sqrt{ab} = 4$

$\therefore$ Equation with roots a and b is

$x^2 - (a + b)x + ab = 0 \Rightarrow x^2 - 18x + 16 = 0$

36. (b) Let a = first term of G.P. and r = common ratio of G.P.; Then G.P. is a, ar, ar^2

Given $S_\infty = 20 \Rightarrow \frac{a}{1 - r} = 20$

$\Rightarrow a = 20(1 - r)$... (i)

Also $a^2 + a^2r^2 + a^2r^4 + ...$ to $\infty = 100$

$\Rightarrow \quad \dfrac{a^2}{1-r^2}=100$

$\Rightarrow a^2=100(1-r)(1+r)$... (ii)

From (i), $a^2=400(1-r)^2$;

From (ii), we get $100(1-r)(1+r)=400(1-r)^2$

$\Rightarrow \quad 1+r=4-4r \Rightarrow 5r=3 \Rightarrow r=3/5$.

37. **(b)** $ar^4=2$

$a\times ar\times ar^2\times ar^3\times ar^4\times ar^5\times ar^6\times ar^7\times ar^8$

$=a^9 r^{36}=(ar^4)^9=2^9=512$

38. **(d)**

A.T.Q.,

A.M. = 5 G.M.

$\dfrac{a+b}{2}=5\sqrt{ab}$

$\dfrac{a+b}{\sqrt{ab}}=10$

$\therefore \quad \dfrac{a}{b}=\dfrac{10+\sqrt{96}}{10-\sqrt{96}}=\dfrac{10+4\sqrt{6}}{10-4\sqrt{6}}$

Use Componendo and Dividendo

$\dfrac{a+b}{a-b}=\dfrac{20}{8\sqrt{6}}=\dfrac{5}{2\sqrt{6}}=\dfrac{5\sqrt{6}}{12}$

39. **(b)** $\tan(A+B)=\dfrac{\tan A+\tan B}{1-\tan A\tan B}$

$\Rightarrow \quad \dfrac{1}{\sqrt{3}}=\dfrac{y}{1-\tan A\tan B}$ where $y=\tan A+\tan B$

$\Rightarrow \quad \tan A\tan B=1-\sqrt{3}y$

Also AM $\geq$ GM

$\Rightarrow \quad \dfrac{\tan A+\tan B}{2}\geq\sqrt{\tan A\tan B}$

$\Rightarrow \quad y\geq 2\sqrt{1-\sqrt{3}y}$

$\Rightarrow \quad y^2\geq 4-4\sqrt{3}y$

$\Rightarrow \quad y^2+4\sqrt{3}y-4\geq 0$

$\Rightarrow \quad y\leq -2\sqrt{3}-4$ or $y\geq -2\sqrt{3}+4$

($y\leq -2\sqrt{3}-4$ is not possible as $\tan A\tan B>0$)

40. **(b)** $x+y+z=12$

AM $\geq$ GM

$$\frac{3\left(\frac{x}{3}\right)+4\left(\frac{y}{4}\right)+5\left(\frac{z}{5}\right)}{12}\geq\sqrt[12]{\left(\frac{x}{3}\right)^3\left(\frac{y}{4}\right)^4\left(\frac{z}{5}\right)^5}$$

$\dfrac{x^3y^4z^5}{3^3 4^4 5^5}\leq 1$

$x^3y^4z^5\leq 3^3.4^4.5^5$

$x^3y^4z^5\leq(0.1)(600)^3$

But, given $x^3y^4z^5=(0.1)(600)^3$

$\therefore$ all the number are equal

$\therefore \quad \dfrac{x}{3}=\dfrac{y}{4}=\dfrac{z}{5}\ (=k)$

$x=3k;\ y=4k;\ z=5k$

$x+y+z=12$

$3k+4k+5k=12$

$k=1$

$\therefore \quad x=3;\ y=4;\ z=5$

$\therefore \quad x^3+y^3+z^3=216$

41. **(a)** $G=\sqrt{ab}$

$M=\dfrac{\frac{1}{a}+\frac{1}{b}}{2}$

$M=\dfrac{a+b}{2ab}$

Given that $\dfrac{1}{M}:G=4:5$

$\dfrac{2ab}{(a+b)\sqrt{ab}}=\dfrac{4}{5}$

$\Rightarrow \quad \dfrac{a+b}{2\sqrt{ab}}=\dfrac{5}{4}$

$\Rightarrow \quad \dfrac{a+b+2\sqrt{ab}}{a+b-2\sqrt{ab}}=\dfrac{5+4}{5-4}$

{Using Componendo & Dividendo}

$\Rightarrow \quad \dfrac{(\sqrt{a})^2+(\sqrt{b})^2+2\sqrt{ab}}{(\sqrt{a})^2+(\sqrt{b})^2-2\sqrt{ab}}=\dfrac{9}{1}$

$\Rightarrow\left(\dfrac{\sqrt{b}+\sqrt{a}}{\sqrt{b}-\sqrt{a}}\right)^2=\dfrac{9}{1}\Rightarrow\dfrac{\sqrt{b}+\sqrt{a}}{\sqrt{b}-\sqrt{a}}=\dfrac{3}{1}$

$\Rightarrow \quad \dfrac{\sqrt{b}+\sqrt{a}+\sqrt{b}-\sqrt{a}}{\sqrt{b}+\sqrt{a}-\sqrt{b}+\sqrt{a}}=\dfrac{3+1}{3-1}$

{Using Componendo & Dividendo}

$\sqrt{\dfrac{b}{a}}=\dfrac{4}{2}=2$

$\dfrac{b}{a}=\dfrac{4}{1}$

$\dfrac{a}{b}=\dfrac{1}{4}\Rightarrow a:b=1:4$

42. (d) $\dfrac{1}{a_2}-\dfrac{1}{a_1}=\dfrac{1}{a_3}-\dfrac{1}{a_2}=.........=\dfrac{1}{a_n}-\dfrac{1}{a_{n-1}}=d$ (say)

Then $a_1a_2=\dfrac{a_1-a_2}{d}$, $a_2a_3=\dfrac{a_2-a_3}{d}$,

$.........., a_{n-1}a_n=\dfrac{a_{n-1}-a_n}{d}$

$\therefore \quad a_1a_2+a_2a_3+........+a_{n-1}a_n$

$=\dfrac{a_1-a_2}{d}+\dfrac{a_2-a_3}{d}+....+\dfrac{a_{n-1}-a_n}{d}$

$=\dfrac{1}{d}[a_1-a_2+a_2-a_3+....+a_{n-1}-a_n]=\dfrac{a_1-a_n}{d}$

Also, $\dfrac{1}{a_n}=\dfrac{1}{a_1}+(n-1)d$

$\Rightarrow \dfrac{a_1-a_n}{a_1a_n}=(n-1)d$

$\Rightarrow \dfrac{a_1-a_n}{d}=(n-1)a_1a_n$

Which is the required result.

43. (d) $x=\sum_{n=0}^{\infty}a^n=\dfrac{1}{1-a} \qquad a=1-\dfrac{1}{x}$

$y=\sum_{n=0}^{\infty}b^n=\dfrac{1}{1-b} \qquad b=1-\dfrac{1}{y}$

$z=\sum_{n=0}^{\infty}c^n=\dfrac{1}{1-c} \qquad c=1-\dfrac{1}{z}$

a, b, c are in A.P. OR $2b=a+c$

$2\left(1-\dfrac{1}{y}\right)=1-\dfrac{1}{x}+1-\dfrac{1}{y}$

$\dfrac{2}{y}=\dfrac{1}{x}+\dfrac{1}{z} \Rightarrow x, y, z$ are in H.P.

44. (d) $ax^2+bx+c=0,\ \alpha+\beta=\dfrac{-b}{a},\ \alpha\beta=\dfrac{c}{a}$

As for given condition, $\alpha+\beta=\dfrac{1}{\alpha^2}+\dfrac{1}{\beta^2}$

$$\alpha+\beta=\frac{\alpha^2+\beta^2}{\alpha^2\beta^2}-\frac{b}{a}=\frac{\frac{b^2}{a^2}-\frac{2c}{a}}{\frac{c^2}{a^2}}$$

On simplification $2a^2c=ab^2+bc^2$

$\Rightarrow \dfrac{2a}{b}=\dfrac{c}{a}+\dfrac{b}{c} \quad \Rightarrow \dfrac{c}{a}, \dfrac{a}{b}, \dfrac{b}{c}$ are in A.P.

$\therefore \dfrac{a}{c}, \dfrac{b}{a}, \& \dfrac{c}{b}$ are in H.P.

45. (b) $f(x)=ax^2+bx+c$

$f(1)=a+b+c=3 \Rightarrow f(a)=3$

Now $f(x+y)=f(x)+f(y)+xy$ ...(a)

Put $x=y=1$ in eqn (a)

$f(2)=f(1)+f(1)+1$

$=2f(1)+1$

$f(2)=7$

$\Rightarrow f(3)=12$

Now, $S_n=3+7+12+........t_n$ ...(a)

$S_n=\ 3+7+........t_{n-1}+t_n$ ...(b)

Subtract (b) from (a)

$t_n=3+4+5+....$ upto n terms

$t_n=\dfrac{(n^2+5n)}{2}$

$S_n=\sum t_n=\sum\dfrac{(n^2+5n)}{2}$

$S_n=\dfrac{1}{2}\left[\dfrac{n(n+1)(2n+1)}{6}+\dfrac{5n(n+1)}{2}\right]=\dfrac{n(n+1)(n+8)}{6}$

$S_{10}=\dfrac{10\times11\times18}{6}=330$

46. (a) $T_n=\dfrac{\frac{n(n+1)}{2}}{\left(\frac{n(n+1)}{2}\right)^2}$

$\Rightarrow T_n=\dfrac{2}{n(n+1)}$

$\Rightarrow S_n=\sum T_n=2\sum_{n=1}^{n}\left(\dfrac{1}{n}-\dfrac{1}{n+1}\right)$

$=2\left\{1-\dfrac{1}{n+1}\right\}$

$\Rightarrow \boxed{S_n=\dfrac{2n}{n+1}}$

$\because \quad 100\,S_n=n$

$\Rightarrow 100\times\dfrac{2n}{n+1}=n$

$\Rightarrow n+1=200$

$\Rightarrow n=199$

47. **(b)**

$\because \quad \sqrt{3}\left[1+\sqrt{25}+\sqrt{81}+\sqrt{69}+......\right]=435\sqrt{3}$

$\Rightarrow \quad \sqrt{3}\ [1+5+9+13+.....+T_n]=435\sqrt{3}$

$\Rightarrow \quad \sqrt{3}\times\frac{n}{2}\left[2+(n-1)_4\right]=435\sqrt{3}$

$\Rightarrow \quad 2n+4n^2-4n=870$

$\Rightarrow \quad 4n^2-2n-870=0$

$\Rightarrow \quad 2n^2-n-435=0$

$$n=\frac{1\pm\sqrt{1+4\times2\times435}}{4}=\frac{1\pm59}{4}$$

$$\therefore \quad n=\frac{1+59}{4}=15;\text{ or } n=\frac{1-59}{4}=14.5$$

48. **(d)** $\left(\frac{8}{5}\right)^2+\left(\frac{12}{5}\right)^2+\left(\frac{16}{5}\right)^2+\left(\frac{20}{5}\right)^2 ...+\left(\frac{44}{5}\right)^2$

$$S=\frac{16}{25}\left(2^2+3^2+4^2+...+11^2\right)$$

$$=\frac{16}{25}\left(\frac{11(11+1)(22+1)}{6}-1\right)$$

$$=\frac{16}{25}\times505=\frac{16}{5}\times101$$

$$\Rightarrow\frac{16}{5}m=\frac{16}{5}\times101$$

$\Rightarrow m=101.$

49. **(a)** $S=(1+x)^{2016}+x(1+x)^{2015}+x^2(1+x)^{2014}+.....+x^{2015}(1+x)+x^{2016}$ ...(i)

$$\left(\frac{x}{1+x}\right)S=x(1+x)^{2015}+x^2(1+x)^{2014}+.....+x^{2016}+\frac{x^{2017}}{1+x} \quad ...(ii)$$

Subtracting (i) from (ii)

$$\frac{S}{1+x}=(1+x)^{2016}-\frac{x^{2017}}{1+x}$$

$\therefore \quad S=(1+x)^{2017}-x^{2017}$

$$a_{17}=\text{coefficient of } x^{17}={}^{2017}C_{17}=\frac{2017!}{17!2000!}$$

50. **(d)** n^{th} term of series $=\dfrac{\left[\frac{n(n+1)}{2}\right]^2}{n^2}=\frac{1}{4}(n+1)^2$

Sum of n term $=\Sigma\frac{1}{4}(n+1)^2$

$$=\frac{1}{4}\left[\Sigma n^2+2\Sigma n+n\right]$$

$$=\frac{1}{4}\left[\frac{n(n+1)(2n+1)}{6}+\frac{2n(n+1)}{2}+n\right]$$

Sum of 9 terms

$$=\frac{1}{4}\left[\frac{9\times10\times19}{6}+\frac{18\times10}{2}+9\right]=\frac{384}{4}=96$$

51. **(c)** General term of given expression can be written as

$$T_r=\frac{1}{3}\left[\frac{1}{n(n+1)(n+2)}-\frac{1}{(n+1)(n+2)(n+3)}\right]$$

on taking summation both the side, we get

$$\sum_{r=1}^{5}T_r=\frac{1}{3}\left[\frac{1}{6}-\frac{1}{6.7.8}\right]=\frac{k}{3}$$

$$\Rightarrow\frac{1}{3}\times\frac{1}{6}\left(1-\frac{1}{56}\right)=\frac{k}{3}\Rightarrow\frac{1}{3}\times\frac{1}{6}\times\frac{55}{56}=\frac{k}{3}$$

$$\Rightarrow k=\frac{55}{336}$$

52. **(d)** $\sum_{r=16}^{20}\left(r^2-r-6\right)=7780$

53. **(a)** Let $10^9+2.(11)(10)^8+3(11)^2(10)^7+...+10(11)^9=k(10)^9$

Let $x=10^9+2.(11)(10)^8+3(11)^2(10)^7+...+10(11)^9$

Multiplied by $\frac{11}{10}$ on both the sides

$$\frac{11}{10}x=11.10^8+2.(11)^2.(10)^7+...+9(11)^9+11^{10}$$

$$x\left(1-\frac{11}{10}\right)=10^9+11(10)^8+11^2\times(10)^7+...+11^9-11^{10}$$

$$\Rightarrow\quad -\frac{x}{10}=10^9\left[\frac{\left(\frac{11}{10}\right)^{10}-1}{\frac{11}{10}-1}\right]-11^{10}$$

$$\Rightarrow\quad -\frac{x}{10}=(11^{10}-10^{10})-11^{10}=-10^{10}$$

$\Rightarrow\quad x=10^{11}=k.10^9$ Given

$\Rightarrow\quad k=100$

54. **(b)** Let a, d and $2n$ be the first term, common difference and total number of terms of an A.P. respectively i.e. $a+(a+d)+(a+2d)+...+(a+(2n-1)d)$

No. of even terms = n, No. of odd terms = n

Sum of odd terms :

$$S_o = \frac{n}{2}[2a+(n-1)(2d)] = 24$$

$\Rightarrow n\,[a + (n-1)d] = 24$ ...(1)

Sum of even terms :

$$S_e = \frac{n}{2}\left[2(a+d)+(n-1)2d\right] = 30$$

$\Rightarrow n\,[a + d + (n-1)\,d] = 30$ ...(2)

Subtracting equation (1) from (2), we get

$nd = 6$ ...(3)

Also, given that last term exceeds the first term by $\frac{21}{2}$

$$a + (2n-1)\,d = a + \frac{21}{2}$$

$$2nd - d = \frac{21}{2}$$

$$\Rightarrow 2\times 6 - \frac{21}{2} = d \qquad (\because nd = 6)$$

$$d = \frac{3}{2}$$

Putting value of d in equation (3)

$$n = \frac{6\times 2}{3} = 4$$

Total no. of terms = $2n = 2 \times 4 = 8$

55. (a) n^{th} term of given series is

$$\frac{2n+1}{\frac{n(n+1)(2n+1)}{6}} = \frac{6}{n(n+1)}$$

Let n^{th} term, $a_n = 6\left[\frac{1}{n} - \frac{1}{n+1}\right]$

Sum of 20 terms, $S_{20} = a_1 + a_2 + a_3 + ... + a_{20}$

$$S_{20} = 6\left(\frac{1}{1}-\frac{1}{2}\right)+6\left(\frac{1}{2}-\frac{1}{3}\right)+6\left(\frac{1}{3}-\frac{1}{4}\right)+\ldots$$
$$+6\left(\frac{1}{18}-\frac{1}{19}\right)+6\left(\frac{1}{19}-\frac{1}{20}\right)+6\left(\frac{1}{20}-\frac{1}{21}\right)$$

$$S_{20} = \left[\left(1-\frac{1}{2}\right)+\left(\frac{1}{2}-\frac{1}{3}\right)+\left(\frac{1}{3}-\frac{1}{4}\right)+\ldots\right.$$
$$\left.+\left(\frac{1}{18}-\frac{1}{19}\right)+\left(\frac{1}{19}-\frac{1}{20}\right)+\left(\frac{1}{20}-\frac{1}{21}\right)\right]$$

$$S_{20} = 6\left(1-\frac{1}{21}\right) = \frac{120}{21} \quad .....(1)$$

Given that $S_{20} = \frac{k}{21}$ .....(2)

On comparing (1) and (2), we get

$k = 120$

56. (c) Given sequence can be written as

$$\frac{7}{10}+\frac{77}{100}+\frac{777}{10^3}+\ldots\ldots+ \text{ up to 20 terms}$$

$$= 7\left[\frac{1}{10}+\frac{11}{100}+\frac{111}{10^3}+\ldots\ldots+\text{up to 20 terms}\right]$$

Multiply and divide by 9

$$= \frac{7}{9}\left[\frac{9}{10}+\frac{99}{100}+\frac{999}{1000}+\ldots\ldots\text{up to 20 terms}\right]$$

$$= \frac{7}{9}\left[\left(1-\frac{1}{10}\right)+\left(1-\frac{1}{10^2}\right)+\left(1-\frac{1}{10^3}\right) +\ldots\ldots\text{up to 20 terms}\right]$$

$$= \frac{7}{9}\left[20 - \frac{\frac{1}{10}\left(1-\left(\frac{1}{10}\right)^{20}\right)}{1-\frac{1}{10}}\right]$$

$$= \frac{7}{9}\left[\frac{179}{9}+\frac{1}{9}\left(\frac{1}{10}\right)^{20}\right]$$

$$= \frac{7}{81}\,[179+(10)^{-20}]$$

57. (a) Consider $1^2+3^2+5^2+\ldots\ldots+25^2$

n^{th} term $T_n = (2n-1)^2$, $n = 1, \ldots\ldots 13$

Now, $S_n = \sum_{n=1}^{13} T_n = \sum_{n=1}^{13} (2n-1)^2$

$$= \sum_{n=1}^{13} 4n^2 + \sum_{n=1}^{13} 1 - \sum_{n=1}^{13} 4n$$

$$= 4\sum n^2 + 13 - 4\sum n$$

$$= 4\left[\frac{n(n+1)(2n+1)}{6}\right] + 13 - 4\,\frac{n(n+1)}{2}$$

Put $n = 13$, we get

$S_n = 26 \times 14 \times 9 + 13 - 26 \times 14$

$= 3276 + 13 - 364$

$= 2925.$

58. (c) $2^2 + 2(4)^2 + 3(6)^2 + \ldots\ldots$ upto 10 terms

$= 2^2\,[1^3 + 2^3 + 3^3 + \ldots\ldots$ upto 10 terms]

$$= 4.\left(\frac{10\times 11}{2}\right)^2 = 12100$$

59. **(c)** Given sum is

$$\frac{3}{12}+\frac{5}{1^2+2^2}+\frac{7}{1^2+2^2+3^2}+.....$$

nth term $= T_n$

$$=\frac{2n+1}{\frac{n(n+1)(2n+1)}{6}}=\frac{6}{n(n+1)}$$

or $T_n = 6\left[\frac{1}{n}-\frac{1}{n+1}\right]$

$$\therefore\quad S_n=\sum T_n=6\sum\frac{1}{n}-6\sum\frac{1}{n+1}=\frac{6n}{n}-\frac{6}{n+1}$$

$$=6-\frac{6}{n+1}=\frac{6n}{n+1}$$

So, sum upto 11 terms means

$$S_{11}=\frac{6\times 11}{11+1}=\frac{66}{12}=\frac{33}{6}=\frac{11}{2}$$

60. **(c)** $T_r=\frac{1}{1+2+3+...+r}=\frac{2}{r(r+1)}$

$$S_{10}=2\sum_{r=1}^{10}\frac{1}{r(r+1)}=2\sum_{r=1}^{10}\left[\frac{r+1}{r(r+1)}-\frac{r}{r(r+1)}\right]$$

$$=2\sum_{r=1}^{10}\left(\frac{1}{r}-\frac{1}{r+1}\right)$$

$$=2\left[\left(\frac{1}{1}-\frac{1}{2}\right)+\left(\frac{1}{2}-\frac{1}{3}\right)+\left(\frac{1}{3}-\frac{1}{4}\right)+...+\left(\frac{1}{10}-\frac{1}{11}\right)\right]$$

$$=2\left[1-\frac{1}{11}\right]=2\times\frac{10}{11}=\frac{20}{11}$$

61. **(b)** nth term of the given series

$$=T_n=(n-1)^2+(n-1)n+n^2$$

$$=\frac{\left((n-1)^3-n^3\right)}{(n-1)-n}=n^3-(n-1)^3$$

$$\Rightarrow S_n=\sum_{k=1}^{n}\left[k^3-(k-1)^3\right]\Rightarrow 8000=n^3$$

$\Rightarrow$ $n=20$ which is a natural number.

Now, put $n=1,2,3,....20$

$T_1=1^3-0^3$

$T_2=2^3-1^3$

$\vdots$

$T_{20}=20^3-19^3$

Now, $T_1+T_2+---+T_{20}=S_{20}$

$\Rightarrow$ $S_{20}=20^3-0^3=8000$

Hence, both the given statement is true.

62. **(c)** If n is odd, the required sum is

$1^2+2.2^2+3^2+2.4^2+.....+2(n-1)^2+n^2$

$$=\frac{(n-1)(n-1+1)^2}{2}+n^2\quad(\because n-1\text{ is even})$$

$$=\left(\frac{n-1}{2}+1\right)n^2=\frac{n^2(n+1)}{2}$$

63. **(c)** Given series is

$$1+\frac{4}{3}+\frac{10}{9}+\frac{28}{27}+....\ n\text{ terms}$$

$$=1+\left(1+\frac{1}{3}\right)+\left(1+\frac{1}{9}\right)+\left(1+\frac{1}{27}\right)+....\ n\text{ terms}$$

$= (1 + 1 + 1 + ... + n$ terms)

$$+\left(\frac{1}{3}+\frac{1}{9}+\frac{1}{27}+....n\text{ terms}\right)$$

$$=n+\frac{\frac{1}{3}\left(1-\frac{1}{3^n}\right)}{1-\frac{1}{3}}=n+\frac{1}{3}\times\frac{3}{2}[1-3^{-n}]$$

$$=n+\frac{1}{2}[1-3^{-n}]=n+\frac{1}{2}-\frac{1}{2.3^n}$$

64. **(c)** Given series is

$$\frac{1}{1+\sqrt{2}}+\frac{1}{\sqrt{2}+\sqrt{3}}+\frac{1}{\sqrt{3}+\sqrt{4}}+.....$$

$$n^{\text{th}}\text{ term}=\frac{1}{\sqrt{n}+\sqrt{n+1}}$$

$$\therefore\ 15^{\text{th}}\text{ term}=\frac{1}{\sqrt{15}+\sqrt{16}}$$

Thus, given series upto 15 terms is

$$\frac{1}{1+\sqrt{2}}+\frac{1}{\sqrt{2}+\sqrt{3}}+\frac{1}{\sqrt{3}+\sqrt{4}}+......+\frac{1}{\sqrt{15}+\sqrt{16}}$$

This can be re-written as

$$\frac{1-\sqrt{2}}{-1}+\frac{\sqrt{2}-\sqrt{3}}{-1}+\frac{\sqrt{3}-\sqrt{4}}{-1}+......+\frac{\sqrt{15}-\sqrt{16}}{-1}$$

(By rationalization)

$$=-1+\sqrt{2}-\sqrt{2}+\sqrt{3}-\sqrt{3}+\sqrt{4}+.....-\sqrt{14}+\sqrt{15}-\sqrt{15}+\sqrt{16}$$

$$=-1+\sqrt{16}=-1+4=3$$

Hence, the required sum $= 3$

65. **(a)** The sum of the given series $1^2+2.2^2+3^2+2.4^2+5^2+2.6^2+........+2(2m)^2$ is $\frac{2m(2m+1)^2}{2}=m(2m+1)^2$

66. **(a)** We have

$$S=1+\frac{2}{3}+\frac{6}{3^2}+\frac{10}{3^3}+\frac{14}{3^4}+.......\infty\qquad....(1)$$

Multiplying both sides by $\frac{1}{3}$ we get

$$\frac{1}{3}S = \frac{1}{3} + \frac{2}{3^2} + \frac{6}{3^3} + \frac{10}{3^4} + ...\infty \quad ....(2)$$

Subtracting eqn. (2) from eqn. (1) we get

$$\frac{2}{3}S = 1 + \frac{1}{3} + \frac{4}{3^2} + \frac{4}{3^3} + \frac{4}{3^4} + ...\infty$$

$$\Rightarrow \frac{2}{3}S = \frac{4}{3} + \frac{4}{3^2} + \frac{4}{3^3} + \frac{4}{3^4} + ...\infty$$

$$\Rightarrow \frac{2}{3}S = \frac{\frac{4}{3}}{1-\frac{1}{3}} = \frac{4}{3} \times \frac{3}{2} \Rightarrow S = 3$$

67. **(d)** We know that $e^x = 1 + x + \frac{x^2}{2!} + \frac{x^3}{3!} + ...\infty$

Put $x = -1$

$$\therefore \quad e^{-1} = 1 - 1 + \frac{1}{2!} - \frac{1}{3!} + \frac{1}{4!} ....\infty$$

$$\therefore \quad e^{-1} = \frac{1}{2!} - \frac{1}{3!} + \frac{1}{4!} - \frac{1}{5!} ....\infty$$

68. **(d)** $\frac{e^x + e^{-x}}{2} = 1 + \frac{x^2}{2!} + \frac{x^4}{4!} + \frac{x^6}{6!} ....$

Putting $x = \frac{1}{2}$ we get

$$1 + \frac{1}{4.2!} + \frac{1}{16.4!} + \frac{1}{64.6!} + ...$$

$$\infty = \frac{e^{\frac{1}{2}} + e^{\frac{-1}{2}}}{2} = \frac{\sqrt{e} + \frac{1}{\sqrt{e}}}{2} = \frac{e+1}{2\sqrt{e}}$$

69. **(b)** We know that $e = 1 + \frac{1}{1!} + \frac{1}{2!} + \frac{1}{3!} + ...$

and $e^{-1} = 1 - \frac{1}{1!} + \frac{1}{2!} - \frac{1}{3!} + ...$

$$\therefore e + e^{-1} = 2\left[1 + \frac{1}{2!} + \frac{1}{4!} + ...\right]$$

$$\therefore \frac{1}{2!} + \frac{1}{4!} + \frac{1}{6!} + ... = \frac{e + e^{-1}}{2} - 1$$

$$= \frac{e^2 + 1 - 2e}{2e} = \frac{(e-1)^2}{2e}$$

70. **(b)** If n is odd, the required sum is

$$1^2 + 2.2^2 + 3^2 + 2.4^2 + ... + 2.(n-1)^2 + n^2$$

$$= \frac{(n-1)(n-1+1)^2}{2} + n^2$$

[$\because$ $(n-1)$ is even

$\therefore$ using given formula for the sum of $(n-1)$ terms.]

$$= \left(\frac{n-1}{2} + 1\right)n^2 = \frac{n^2(n+1)}{2}$$

71. **(d)** $S_n = \frac{1}{{}^nC_0} + \frac{1}{{}^nC_1} + \frac{1}{{}^nC_2} + ... + \frac{1}{{}^nC_n}$

$$t_n = \frac{0}{{}^nC_0} + \frac{1}{{}^nC_1} + \frac{2}{{}^nC_2} + ... + \frac{n}{{}^nC_n}$$

$$t_n = \frac{n}{{}^nC_n} + \frac{n-1}{{}^nC_{n-1}} + \frac{n-2}{{}^nC_{n-2}} + ... + \frac{0}{{}^nC_0}$$

Add, $2t_n = (n)\left[\frac{1}{{}^nC_0} + \frac{1}{{}^nC_1} + ... \frac{1}{{}^nC_n}\right] = nS_n$

$$\therefore \frac{t_n}{S_n} = \frac{n}{2}$$

72. **(a)** $\frac{1}{1.2} - \frac{1}{2.3} + \frac{1}{3.4} ....\infty$

$$|T_n| = \frac{1}{n(n+1)} = \left(\frac{1}{n} - \frac{1}{n+1}\right)$$

$$S = T_1 - T_2 + T_3 - T_4 + T_5 ....\infty$$

$$= \left(\frac{1}{1} - \frac{1}{2}\right) - \left(\frac{1}{2} - \frac{1}{3}\right) + \left(\frac{1}{3} - \frac{1}{4}\right) - \left(\frac{1}{4} - \frac{1}{5}\right) ....$$

$$= 1 - 2\left[\frac{1}{2} - \frac{1}{3} + \frac{1}{4} - \frac{1}{5} ....\infty\right]$$

$$= 1 - 2[-\log(1+1) + 1] = 2\log 2 - 1 = \log\left(\frac{4}{e}\right).$$

73. **(a)** $1^3 - 2^3 + 3^3 - 4^3 + ... + 9^3$

$$= 1^3 + 2^3 + 3^3 + ... + 9^3 - 2(2^3 + 4^3 + 6^3 + 8^3)$$

$$= \left[\frac{9 \times 10}{2}\right]^2 - 2.2^3\left[1^3 + 2^3 + 3^3 + 4^3\right]$$

$$= (45)^2 - 16.\left[\frac{4 \times 5}{2}\right]^2 = 2025 - 1600 = 425$$

74. **(b)** The product is $P = 2^{1/4}.2^{2/8}.2^{3/16}.........$

$$= 2^{1/4 + 2/8 + 3/16 + ...\infty}$$

Now let $S = \frac{1}{4} + \frac{2}{8} + \frac{3}{16} + ...\infty \quad ......(1)$

$$\frac{1}{2}S = \frac{1}{8} + \frac{2}{16} + ...\infty \quad ......(2)$$

Subtracting (2) from (1)

$$\Rightarrow \frac{1}{2}S = \frac{1}{4} + \frac{1}{8} + \frac{1}{16} + ...\infty$$

or $\frac{1}{2}S = \frac{1/4}{1 - 1/2} = \frac{1}{2} \Rightarrow S = 1$

$$\therefore P = 2^S = 2$$

Chapter 10 Straight Lines and Pair of Straight Lines

TOPIC-1 : Distance Formula, Section Formula, Results of Triangle, Locus, Equation of Locus, Slope of a Straight Line, Slope of a line joining two points, Parallel and Perpendicular Lines

1. A square, of each side 2, lies above the x-axis and has one vertex at the origin. If one of the sides passing through the origin makes an angle 30° with the positive direction of the x-axis, then the sum of the x-coordinates of the vertices of the square is : **[Online April 9, 2017]**

   (a) $2\sqrt{3}-1$ (b) $2\sqrt{3}-2$
   (c) $\sqrt{3}-2$ (d) $\sqrt{3}-1$

2. A ray of light is incident along a line which meets another line, $7x-y+1=0$, at the point (0, 1). The ray is then reflected from this point along the line, $y+2x=1$. Then the equation of the line of incidence of the ray of light is : **[Online April 10, 2016]**

   (a) $41x-25y+25=0$ (b) $41x+25y-25=0$
   (c) $41x-38y+38=0$ (d) $41x+38y-38=0$

3. Let L be the line passing through the point P(1, 2) such that its intercepted segment between the co-ordinate axes is bisected at P. If L_1 is the line perpendicular to L and passing through the point (–2, 1), then the point of intersection of L and L_1 is : **[Online April 10, 2015]**

   (a) $\left(\frac{4}{5},\frac{12}{5}\right)$ (b) $\left(\frac{3}{5},\frac{23}{10}\right)$
   (c) $\left(\frac{11}{20},\frac{29}{10}\right)$ (d) $\left(\frac{3}{10},\frac{17}{5}\right)$

4. The points $\left(0,\frac{8}{3}\right)$, (1, 3) and (82, 30) : **[Online April 10, 2015]**

   (a) form an acute angled triangle.
   (b) form a right angled triangle.
   (c) lie on a straight line.
   (d) form an obtuse angled triangle.

5. The x-coordinate of the incentre of the triangle that has the coordinates of mid points of its sides as (0, 1) (1, 1) and (1, 0) is : **[2013]**

   (a) $2+\sqrt{2}$ (b) $2-\sqrt{2}$
   (c) $1+\sqrt{2}$ (d) $1-\sqrt{2}$

6. A light ray emerging from the point source placed at P(1, 3) is reflected at a point Q in the axis of x. If the reflected ray passes through the point R (6, 7), then the abscissa of Q is: **[Online April 9, 2013]**

   (a) 1 (b) 3
   (c) $\frac{7}{2}$ (d) $\frac{5}{2}$

7. Let A (h, k), B(1, 1) and C (2, 1) be the vertices of a right angled triangle with AC as its hypotenuse. If the area of the triangle is 1 square unit, then the set of values which 'k' can take is given by **[2007]**

   (a) $\{-1,3\}$ (b) $\{-3,-2\}$
   (c) $\{1,3\}$ (d) $\{0,2\}$

8. If a vertex of a triangle is (1, 1) and the mid points of two sides through this vertex are (–1, 2) and (3, 2) then the centroid of the triangle is **[2005]**

   (a) $\left(-1,\frac{7}{3}\right)$ (b) $\left(\frac{-1}{3},\frac{7}{3}\right)$
   (c) $\left(1,\frac{7}{3}\right)$ (d) $\left(\frac{1}{3},\frac{7}{3}\right)$

9. If the equation of the locus of a point equidistant from the point (a_1, b_1) and (a_2, b_2) is $(a_1-b_2)x+(a_1-b_2)y+c=0$, then the value of 'c' is **[2003]**

   (a) $\sqrt{a_1^2+b_1^2-a_2^2-b_2^2}$ (b) $\frac{1}{2}a_2^2+b_2^2-a_1^2-b_1^2$
   (c) $a_1^2-a_2^2+b_1^2-b_2^2$ (d) $\frac{1}{2}(a_1^2+a_2^2+b_1^2+b_2^2)$

10. Locus of centroid of the triangle whose vertices are $(a\cos t, a\sin t), (b\sin t, -b\cos t)$ and (1, 0), where t is a parameter, is **[2003]**

    (a) $(3x+1)^2+(3y)^2=a^2-b^2$
    (b) $(3x-1)^2+(3y)^2=a^2-b^2$
    (c) $(3x-1)^2+(3y)^2=a^2+b^2$
    (d) $(3x+1)^2+(3y)^2=a^2+b^2$

11. A triangle with vertices (4, 0), (–1, –1), (3, 5) is **[2002]**
(a) isosceles and right angled
(b) isosceles but not right angled
(c) right angled but not isosceles
(d) neither right angled nor isosceles

TOPIC -2 : Various Forms of Equation of a Line

12. Two sides of a rhombus are along the lines, $x - y + 1 = 0$ and $7x - y - 5 = 0$. If its diagonals intersect at (–1, –2), then which one of the following is a vertex of this rhombus? **[2016]**
(a) $\left(\frac{1}{3}, -\frac{8}{3}\right)$ (b) $\left(-\frac{10}{3}, -\frac{7}{3}\right)$
(c) (–3, –9) (d) (–3, –8)

13. A straight line through origin O meets the lines $3y = 10 - 4x$ and $8x + 6y + 5 = 0$ at points A and B respectively. Then O divides the segment AB in the ratio : **[Online April 10, 2016]**
(a) 2 : 3 (b) 1 : 2
(c) 4 : 1 (d) 3 : 4

14. If a variable line drawn through the intersection of the lines $\frac{x}{3}+\frac{y}{4} = 1$ and $\frac{x}{4}+\frac{y}{3} = 1$, meets the coordinate axes at A and B, $(A \neq B)$, then the locus of the midpoint of AB is :
(a) $7xy = 6(x + y)$ **[Online April 9, 2016]**
(b) $4(x + y)^2 - 28(x + y) + 49 = 0$
(c) $6xy = 7(x + y)$
(d) $14(x + y)^2 - 97(x + y) + 168 = 0$

15. The point (2, 1) is translated parallel to the line L : $x - y = 4$ by $2\sqrt{3}$ units. If the new points Q lies in the third quadrant, then the equation of the line passing through Q and perpendicular to L is : **[Online April 9, 2016]**
(a) $x + y = 2 - \sqrt{6}$ (b) $2x + 2y = 1 - \sqrt{6}$
(c) $x + y = 3 - 3\sqrt{6}$ (d) $x + y = 3 - 2\sqrt{6}$

16. A straight line L through the point (3, – 2) is inclined at an angle of 60° to the line $\sqrt{3}x + y = 1$. If L also intersects the x-axis, then the equation of L is : **[Online April 11, 2015]**
(a) $y + \sqrt{3}x + 2 - 3\sqrt{3} = 0$
(b) $\sqrt{3}y + x - 3 + 2\sqrt{3} = 0$
(c) $y - \sqrt{3}x + 2 + 3\sqrt{3} = 0$
(d) $\sqrt{3}y - x + 3 + 2\sqrt{3} = 0$

17. The circumcentre of a triangle lies at the origin and its centroid is the mid point of the line segment joining the points $(a^2 + 1, a^2 + 1)$ and $(2a, -2a)$, $a \neq 0$. Then for any a, the orthocentre of this triangle lies on the line:
(a) $y - 2ax = 0$ **[Online April 19, 2014]**
(b) $y - (a^2 + 1)x = 0$
(c) $y + x = 0$
(d) $(a - 1)^2x - (a + 1)^2y = 0$

18. If a line intercepted between the coordinate axes is trisected at a point A(4, 3), which is nearer to x-axis, then its equation is: **[Online April 12, 2014]**
(a) $4x - 3y = 7$ (b) $3x + 2y = 18$
(c) $3x + 8y = 36$ (d) $x + 3y = 13$

19. Given three points P, Q, R with P(5, 3) and R lies on the x-axis. If equation of RQ is $x - 2y = 2$ and PQ is parallel to the x-axis, then the centroid of ΔPQR lies on the line: **[Online April 9, 2014]**
(a) $2x + y - 9 = 0$ (b) $x - 2y + 1 = 0$
(c) $5x - 2y = 0$ (d) $2x - 5y = 0$

20. A ray of light along $x + \sqrt{3}y = \sqrt{3}$ gets reflected upon reaching x-axis, the equation of the reflected ray is **[2013]**
(a) $y = x + \sqrt{3}$ (b) $\sqrt{3}y = x - \sqrt{3}$
(c) $y = \sqrt{3}x - \sqrt{3}$ (d) $\sqrt{3}y = x - 1$

21. Let A (–3, 2) and B (–2, 1) be the vertices of a triangle ABC. If the centroid of this triangle lies on the line $3x + 4y + 2 = 0$, then the vertex C lies on the line : **[Online April 25, 2013]**
(a) $4x + 3y + 5 = 0$ (b) $3x + 4y + 3 = 0$
(c) $4x + 3y + 3 = 0$ (d) $3x + 4y + 5 = 0$

22. If the extremities of the base of an isosceles triangle are the points $(2a, 0)$ and $(0, a)$ and the equation of one of the sides is $x = 2a$, then the area of the triangle, in square units, is : **[Online April 23, 2013]**
(a) $\frac{5}{4}a^2$ (b) $\frac{5}{2}a^2$
(c) $\frac{25a^2}{4}$ (d) $5a^2$

23. If the x-intercept of some line L is double as that of the line, $3x + 4y = 12$ and the y-intercept of L is half as that of the same line, then the slope of L is : **[Online April 22, 2013]**
(a) –3 (b) –3/8
(c) –3/2 (d) –3/16

24. If the line $2x + y = k$ passes through the point which divides the line segment joining the points (1,1) and (2,4) in the ratio 3 :2, then k equals : **[2012]**
(a) $\frac{29}{5}$ (b) 5
(c) 6 (d) $\frac{11}{5}$

25. The line parallel to x-axis and passing through the point of intersection of lines $ax + 2by + 3b = 0$ and $bx - 2ay - 3a = 0$, where $(a, b) \neq (0, 0)$ is **[Online May 26, 2012]**
(a) above x-axis at a distance 2/3 from it
(b) above x-axis at a distance 3/2 from it
(c) below x-axis at a distance 3/2 from it
(d) below x-axis at a distance 2/3 from it

26. If the point (1, a) lies between the straight lines $x+y=1$ and $2(x+y)=3$ then a lies in interval [Online May 12, 2012]

(a) $\left(\frac{3}{2},\infty\right)$ (b) $\left(1,\frac{3}{2}\right)$

(c) $(-\infty,0)$ (d) $\left(0,\frac{1}{2}\right)$

27. If the straight lines $x+3y=4$, $3x+y=4$ and $x+y=0$ form a triangle, then the triangle is [Online May 7, 2012]

(a) scalene
(b) equilateral triangle
(c) isosceles
(d) right angled isosceles

28. If A (2, – 3) and B (– 2, 1) are two vertices of a triangle and third vertex moves on the line $2x+3y=9$, then the locus of the centroid of the triangle is : [2011RS]

(a) $x-y=1$ (b) $2x+3y=1$

(c) $2x+3y=3$ (d) $2x-3y=1$

29. If (a,a^2) falls inside the angle made by the lines $y=\frac{x}{2}$, $x>0$ and $y=3x$, $x>0$, then a belong to [2006]

(a) $\left(0,\frac{1}{2}\right)$ (b) $(3,\infty)$

(c) $\left(\frac{1}{2},3\right)$ (d) $\left(-3,-\frac{1}{2}\right)$

30. A straight line through the point A (3, 4) is such that its intercept between the axes is bisected at A. Its equation is [2006]

(a) $x+y=7$ (b) $3x-4y+7=0$

(c) $4x+3y=24$ (d) $3x+4y=25$

31. The line parallel to the x- axis and passing through the intersection of the lines $ax + 2by + 3b = 0$ and $bx-2ay-3a=0$, where $(a, b) \neq (0, 0)$ is [2005]

(a) below the x - axis at a distance of $\frac{3}{2}$ from it

(b) below the x - axis at a distance of $\frac{2}{3}$ from it

(c) above the x - axis at a distance of $\frac{3}{2}$ from it

(d) above the x - axis at a distance of $\frac{2}{3}$ from it

32. The equation of the straight line passing through the point (4, 3) and making intercepts on the co-ordinate axes whose sum is –1 is [2004]

(a) $\frac{x}{2}-\frac{y}{3}=1$ and $\frac{x}{-2}+\frac{y}{1}=1$

(b) $\frac{x}{2}-\frac{y}{3}=-1$ and $\frac{x}{-2}+\frac{y}{1}=-1$

(c) $\frac{x}{2}+\frac{y}{3}=1$ and $\frac{x}{2}+\frac{y}{1}=1$

(d) $\frac{x}{2}+\frac{y}{3}=-1$ and $\frac{x}{-2}+\frac{y}{1}=-1$

33. Let $A(2,-3)$ and $B(-2,3)$ be vertices of a triangle ABC. If the centroid of this triangle moves on the line $2x+3y=1$, then the locus of the vertex C is the line

(a) $3x-2y=3$ (b) $2x-3y=7$ [2004]

(c) $3x+2y=5$ (d) $2x+3y=9$

34. Locus of mid point of the portion between the axes of $x\cos\alpha + y\sin\alpha = p$ whre p is constant is [2002]

(a) $x^2+y^2=\frac{4}{p^2}$ (b) $x^2+y^2=4p^2$

(c) $\frac{1}{x^2}+\frac{1}{y^2}=\frac{2}{p^2}$ (d) $\frac{1}{x^2}+\frac{1}{y^2}=\frac{4}{p^2}$

TOPIC-3 : Distance Between two Lines, Angle Between two Lines and Bisector of the Angle Between the two Lines, Perpendicular Distance of a Point from a Line, Foot of the Perpendicular, Position of a Point with Respect to a Line, Pedal Points, Condition for Concurrency of Three Lines

35. Let a, b, c and d be non-zero numbers. If the point of intersection of the lines $4ax+2ay+c=0$ and $5bx+2by+d=0$ lies in the fourth quadrant and is equidistant from the two axes then [2014]

(a) $3bc-2ad=0$ (b) $3bc+2ad=0$

(c) $2bc-3ad=0$ (d) $2bc+3ad=0$

36. Let PS be the median of the triangle vertices $P(2, 2)$, $Q(6,-1)$ and $R(7, 3)$. The equation of the line passing through $(1,-1)$ and parallel to PS is: [2014]

(a) $4x+7y+3=0$ (b) $2x-9y-11=0$

(c) $4x-7y-11=0$ (d) $2x+9y+7=0$

37. If a line L is perpendicular to the line $5x-y=1$, and the area of the triangle formed by the line L and the coordinate axes is 5, then the distance of line L from the line $x+5y=0$ is: [Online April 19, 2014]

(a) $\frac{7}{\sqrt{5}}$ (b) $\frac{5}{\sqrt{13}}$

(c) $\frac{7}{\sqrt{13}}$ (d) $\frac{5}{\sqrt{7}}$

38. If the three distinct lines $x + 2ay + a = 0$, $x + 3by + b = 0$ and $x + 4ay + a = 0$ are concurrent, then the point (a, b) lies on a: **[Online April 12, 2014]**

(a) circle (b) hyperbola
(c) straight line (d) parabola

39. The base of an equilateral triangle is along the line given by $3x + 4y = 9$. If a vertex of the triangle is (1, 2), then the length of a side of the triangle is: **[Online April 11, 2014]**

(a) $\frac{2\sqrt{3}}{15}$ (b) $\frac{4\sqrt{3}}{15}$
(c) $\frac{4\sqrt{3}}{5}$ (d) $\frac{2\sqrt{3}}{5}$

40. If the image of point P(2, 3) in a line L is Q(4, 5), then the image of point R(0, 0) in the same line is: **[Online April 25, 2013]**

(a) (2,2) (b) (4,5)
(c) (3,4) (d) (7,7)

41. Let θ_1 be the angle between two lines $2x + 3y + c_1 = 0$ and $-x + 5y + c_2 = 0$ and θ_2 be the angle between two lines $2x + 3y + c_1 = 0$ and $-x + 5y + c_3 = 0$, where c_1, c_2, c_3 are any real numbers :

Statement-1: If c_2 and c_3 are proportional, then $\theta_1 = \theta_2$.
Statement-2: $\theta_1 = \theta_2$ for all c_2 and c_3. **[Online April 23, 2013]**

(a) Statement-1 is true, Statement-2 is true; Statement-2 is a correct explanation of Statement-1.
(b) Statement-1 is true, Statement-2 is true; Statement-2 is **not** a correct explanation of Statement-1.
(c) Statement-1 is false; Statement-2 is true.
(d) Statement-1 is true; Statement-2 is false.

42. If the three lines $x - 3y = p$, $ax + 2y = q$ and $ax + y = r$ form a right-angled triangle then : **[Online April 9, 2013]**

(a) $a^2 - 9a + 18 = 0$ (b) $a^2 - 6a - 12 = 0$
(c) $a^2 - 6a - 18 = 0$ (d) $a^2 - 9a + 12 = 0$

43. Consider the straight lines
$L_1 : x - y = 1$
$L_2 : x + y = 1$
$L_3 : 2x + 2y = 5$
$L_4 : 2x - 2y = 7$
The correct statement is **[Online May 26, 2012]**

(a) $L_1 \parallel L_4$, $L_2 \parallel L_3$, L_1 intersect L_4.
(b) $L_1 \perp L_2$, $L_1 \parallel L_3$, L_1 intersect L_2.
(c) $L_1 \perp L_2$, $L_2 \parallel L_3$, L_1 intersect L_4.
(d) $L_1 \perp L_2$, $L_1 \perp L_3$, L_2 intersect L_4.

44. If $a, b, c \in$ R and 1 is a root of equation $ax^2 + bx + c = 0$, then the curve $y = 4ax^2 + 3bx + 2c$, $a \neq 0$ intersect x-axis at **[Online May 26, 2012]**

(a) two distinct points whose coordinates are always rational numbers
(b) no point
(c) exactly two distinct points
(d) exactly one point

45. Let L be the line $y = 2x$, in the two dimensional plane. **[Online May 19, 2012]**

Statement 1: The image of the point (0, 1) in L is the point $\left(\frac{4}{5}, \frac{3}{5}\right)$.

Statement 2: The points (0, 1) and $\left(\frac{4}{5}, \frac{3}{5}\right)$ lie on opposite sides of the line L and are at equal distance from it.

(a) Statement 1 is true, Statement 2 is false.
(b) Statement 1 is true, Statement 2 is true, Statement 2 is not a correct explanation for Statement 1.
(c) Statement 1 is true, Statement 2 is true, Statement 2 is a correct explanation for Statement 1.
(d) Statement 1 is false, Statement 2 is true.

46. If two vertices of a triangle are (5, –1) and (–2, 3) and its orthocentre is at (0, 0), then the third vertex is **[Online May 12, 2012]**

(a) (4, –7) (b) (–4, –7)
(c) (–4, 7) (d) (4, 7)

47. If two vertical poles 20 m and 80 m high stand apart on a horizontal plane, then the height (in m) of the point of intersection of the lines joining the top of each pole to the foot of other is **[Online May 7, 2012]**

(a) 16 (b) 18
(c) 50 (d) 15

48. The point of intersection of the lines
$(a^3 + 3)x + ay + a - 3 = 0$ and
$(a^5 + 2)x + (a + 2)y + 2a + 3 = 0$ (a real) lies on the y-axis for **[Online May 7, 2012]**

(a) no value of a
(b) more than two values of a
(c) exactly one value of a
(d) exactly two values of a

49. The lines $x + y = |a|$ and $ax - y = 1$ intersect each other in the first quadrant. Then the set of all possible values of a in the interval : **[2011RS]**

(a) $(0, \infty)$ (b) $[1, \infty)$
(c) $(-1, \infty)$ (d) $(-1, 1)$

50. The lines $L_1 : y - x = 0$ and $L_2 : 2x + y = 0$ intersect the line $L_3 : y + 2 = 0$ at P and Q respectively. The bisector of the acute angle between L_1 and L_2 intersects L_3 at R. **[2011]**

Statement-1: The ratio $PR : RQ$ equals $2\sqrt{2} : \sqrt{5}$

Statement-2: In any triangle, bisector of an angle divides the triangle into two similar triangles.

(a) Statement-1 is true, Statement-2 is true; Statement-2 is **not** a correct explanation for Statement-1.
(b) Statement-1 is true, Statement-2 is false.
(c) Statement-1 is false, Statement-2 is true.
(d) Statement-1 is true, Statement-2 is true; Statement-2 is a correct explanation for Statement-1.

51. The lines $p(p^2+1)x-y+q=0$ and $(p^2+1)^2x+(p^2+1)y+2q=0$ are perpendicular to a common line for : [2009]
(a) exactly one values of p
(b) exactly two values of p
(c) more than two values of p
(d) no value of p

52. The shortest distance between the line $y-x=1$ and the curve $x=y^2$ is : [2009]
(a) $\frac{2\sqrt{3}}{8}$ (b) $\frac{3\sqrt{2}}{5}$
(c) $\frac{\sqrt{3}}{4}$ (d) $\frac{3\sqrt{2}}{8}$

53. The perpendicular bisector of the line segment joining P (1, 4) and Q(k, 3) has y-intercept –4. Then a possible value of k is [2008]
(a) 1 (b) 2
(c) –2 (d) – 4

54. Let P = (–1, 0), Q = (0, 0) and R = $(3, 3\sqrt{3})$ be three point. The equation of the bisector of the angle PQR is [2007]
(a) $\frac{\sqrt{3}}{2}x+y=0$ (b) $x+\sqrt{3}y=0$
(c) $\sqrt{3}x+y=0$ (d) $x+\frac{\sqrt{3}}{2}y=0$

55. If x_1, x_2, x_3 and y_1, y_2, y_3 are both in G.P. with the same common ratio, then the points $(x_1, y_1), (x_2, y_2)$ and (x_3, y_3) [2003]
(a) are vertices of a triangle
(b) lie on a straight line
(c) lie on an ellipse
(d) lie on a circle.

56. A square of side a lies above the x-axis and has one vertex at the origin. The side passing through the origin makes an angle $\alpha\left(0<\alpha<\frac{\pi}{4}\right)$ with the positive direction of x-axis. The equation of its diagonal not passing through the origin is [2003]
(a) $y(\cos\alpha+\sin\alpha)+x(\cos\alpha-\sin\alpha)=a$
(b) $y(\cos\alpha-\sin\alpha)-x(\sin\alpha-\cos\alpha)=a$
(c) $y(\cos\alpha+\sin\alpha)+x(\sin\alpha-\cos\alpha)=a$
(d) $y(\cos\alpha+\sin\alpha)+x(\sin\alpha+\cos\alpha)=a$.

TOPIC-4 : Pair of Straight Lines

57. If one of the lines of $my^2+(1-m^2)xy-mx^2=0$ is a bisector of the angle between the lines $xy=0$, then m is [2007]
(a) 1 (b) 2
(c) –1/2 (d) –2

58. If one of the lines given by
$6x^2-xy+4cy^2=0$ is $3x+4y=0$, then c equals [2004]
(a) –3 (b) 1
(c) 3 (d) 1

59. If the sum of the slopes of the lines given by $x^2-2cxy-7y^2=0$ is four times their product c has the value [2004]
(a) –2 (b) –1
(c) 2 (d) 1

60. If the pair of straight lines $x^2-2pxy-y^2=0$ and $x^2-2qxy-y^2=0$ be such that each pair bisects the angle between the other pair, then [2003]
(a) $pq=-1$ (b) $p=q$
(c) $p=-q$ (d) $pq=1$.

61. The pair of lines represented by
$3ax^2+5xy+(a^2-2)y^2=0$
are perpendicular to each other for [2002]
(a) two values of a (b) $\forall\, a$
(c) for one value of a (d) for no values of a

62. If the pair of lines $ax^2+2hxy+by^2+2gx+2fy+c=0$ intersect on the y-axis then [2002]
(a) $2fgh=bg^2+ch^2$ (b) $bg^2\neq ch^2$
(c) $abc=2fgh$ (d) none of these

Hints & Solutions

1. **(b)**

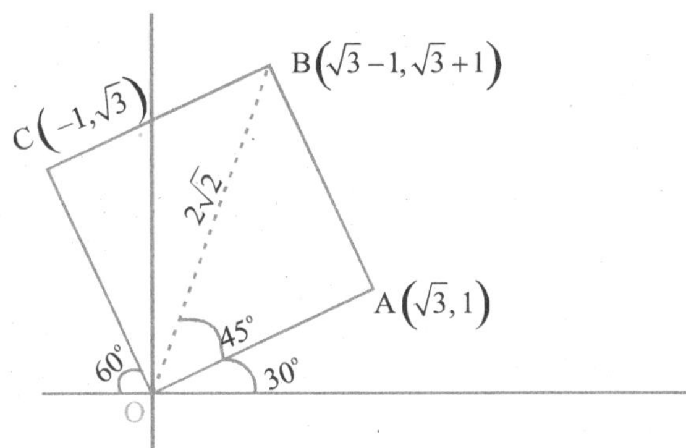

For A;

$$\frac{x}{\cos 30^\circ} = \frac{y}{\sin 30^\circ} = 2$$

$\Rightarrow x = \sqrt{3}$

and $y = 1$

For C,

$$\frac{x}{\cos 120^\circ} = \frac{y}{\sin 120^\circ} = 2$$

$\Rightarrow x = -1, y = \sqrt{3}$

For B,

$$\frac{x}{\cos 75^\circ} = \frac{y}{\sin 75^\circ} = 2\sqrt{2}$$

$\Rightarrow x = \sqrt{3} - 1$

and $y = \sqrt{3} + 1$

$\therefore$ Sum $= 2\sqrt{3} - 2$

2. **(c)** Let slope of incident ray be m.

$\therefore$ angle of incidence = angle of reflection

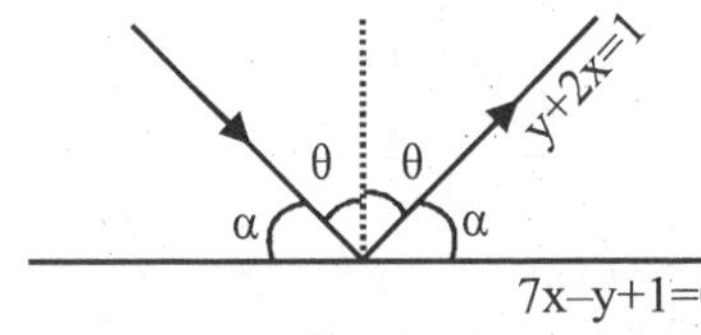

$$\therefore \left|\frac{m-7}{1+7m}\right| = \left|\frac{-2-7}{1-14}\right| = \frac{9}{13}$$

$\Rightarrow \frac{m-7}{1+7m} = \frac{9}{13}$ or $\frac{m-7}{1+7m} = -\frac{9}{13}$

$\Rightarrow 13m - 91 = 9 + 63m$ or $13m - 91 = -9 - 63m$

$\Rightarrow 50m = -100$ or $76m = 82$

$\Rightarrow m = -\frac{1}{2}$ or $m = \frac{41}{38}$

$\Rightarrow y - 1 = -\frac{1}{2}(x - 0)$ or $y - 1 = \frac{41}{38}(x - 0)$

i.e $x + 2y - 2 = 0$ or $38y - 38 - 41x = 0$

$\Rightarrow 41x - 38y + 38 = 0$

3. **(a)** Equation of line L

$$\frac{x}{2} + \frac{y}{4} = 1$$

$2x + y = 4$ ...(1)

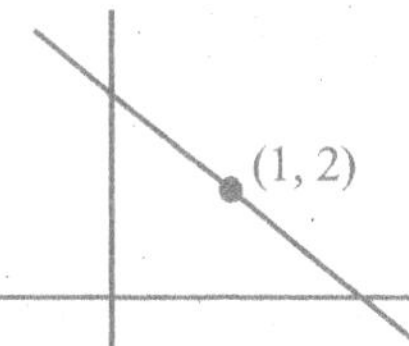

For line

$x - 2y = -4$ ...(2)

solving equation (1) and (2); we get point of intersection

$$\left(4/5, \frac{12}{5}\right)$$

4. **(c)** $A\left(0, \frac{8}{3}\right) B(1, 3) C(89, 30)$

Slope of AB $= \frac{1}{3}$

Slope of BC $= \frac{1}{3}$

So, lies on same line

5. **(b)** From the figure, we have

$a = 2, b = 2\sqrt{2}, c = 2$

$x_1 = 0, x_2 = 0, x_3 = 2$

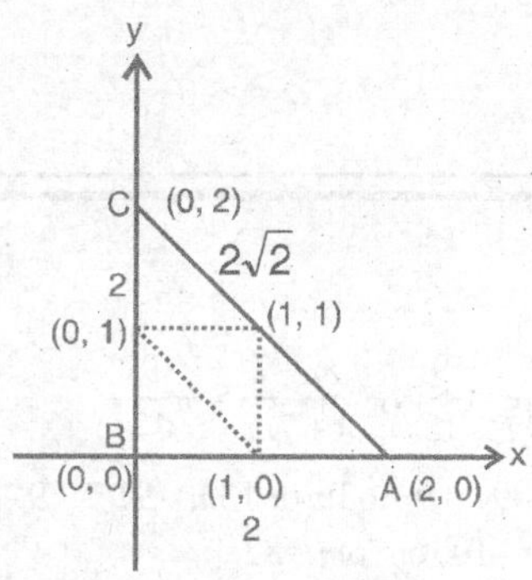

Now, x-co-ordinate of incentre is given as

$$\frac{ax_1 + bx_2 + cx_3}{a+b+c}$$

$\Rightarrow$ x-coordinate of incentre

$$= \frac{2 \times 0 + 2\sqrt{2}.0 + 2.2}{2 + 2 + 2\sqrt{2}}$$

$$= \frac{2}{2+\sqrt{2}} = 2 - \sqrt{2}$$

6. **(d)** Let abcissa of Q $= x$

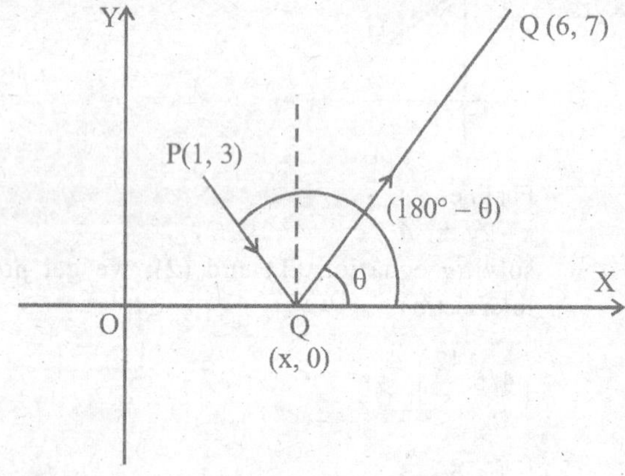

$\therefore$ Q $= (x, 0)$

$$\tan\theta = \frac{0-7}{x-6}, \tan(180° - \theta) = \frac{0-3}{x-1}$$

Now, $\tan(180° - \theta) = -\tan\theta$

$$\therefore \quad \frac{-3}{x-1} = \frac{-7}{x-6} \Rightarrow x = \frac{5}{2}$$

7. **(a)** **Given :** The vertices of a right angled triangle A(1, k), B(1, 1) and C(2, 1) and Area of $\Delta ABC = 1$ square unit

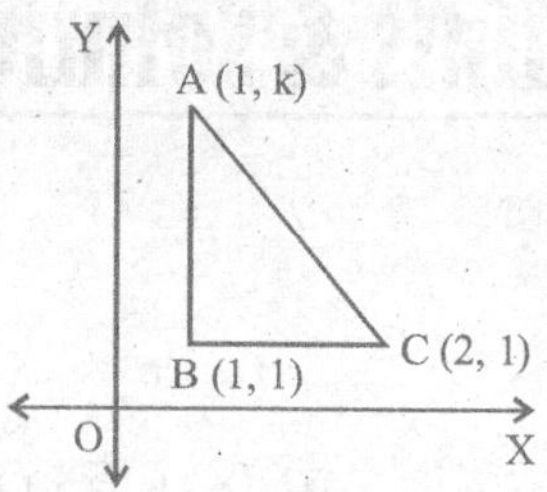

We know that, area of right angled triangle

$$= \frac{1}{2} \times BC \times AB = 1 = \frac{1}{2}(1)\,|(k-1)|$$

$$\Rightarrow \pm(k-1) = 2 \Rightarrow k = -1, 3$$

8. **(c)** Vertex of triangle is (1, 1) and midpoint of sides through this vertex is (– 1, 2) and (3, 2)

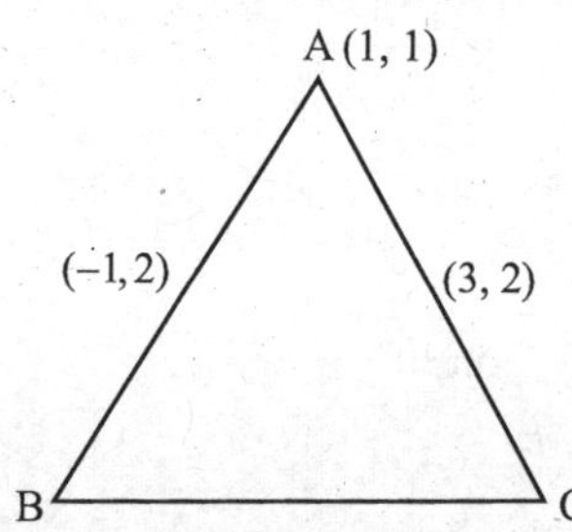

$\Rightarrow$ vertex B and C come out to be (– 3, 3) and (5, 3)

$$\therefore \text{ Centroid is } \frac{1-3+5}{3}, \frac{1+3+5}{3}$$

$$\Rightarrow \left(1, \frac{7}{3}\right)$$

9. **(b)** $(x-a_1)^2 + (y-b_1)^2 = (x-a_2)^2 + (y-b_2)^2$

$$(a_1 - a_2)x + (b_1 - b_2)y + \frac{1}{2}(a_2{}^2 + b_2{}^2 - a_1{}^2 - b_1{}^2) = 0$$

$$c = \frac{1}{2}(a_2{}^2 + b_2{}^2 - a_1{}^2 - b_1{}^2)$$

10. **(c)** $x = \dfrac{a\cos t + b\sin t + 1}{3}$

$\Rightarrow a\cos t + b\sin t = 3x - 1$

$$y = \frac{a\sin t - b\cos t}{3}$$

$\Rightarrow a\sin t - b\cos t = 3y$

Squaring and adding,

$$(3x-1)^2 + (3y)^2 = a^2 + b^2$$

11. (a) $AB = \sqrt{(4+1)^2 + (0+1)^2} = \sqrt{26}$;

$BC = \sqrt{(3+1)^2 + (5+1)^2} = \sqrt{52}$

$CA = \sqrt{(4-3)^2 + (0-5)^2} = \sqrt{26}$;

In isosceles triangle side $AB = CA$

For right angled triangle, $BC^2 = AB^2 + AC^2$

So, here $BC = \sqrt{52}$ or $BC^2 = 52$

or $(\sqrt{26})^2 + (\sqrt{26})^2 = 52$

So, the given triangle is right angled and also isosceles

12. (a)

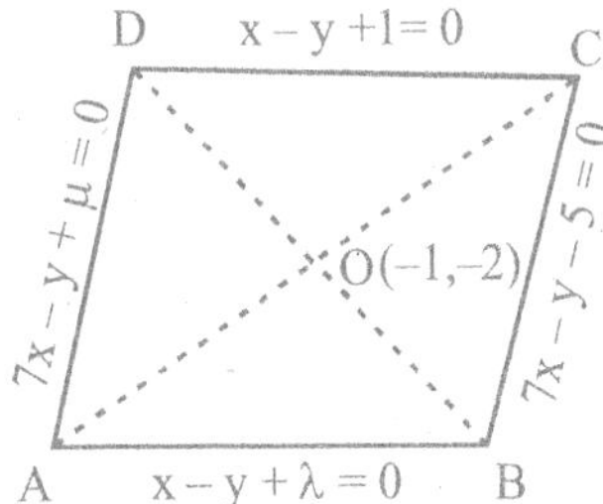

Let other two sides of rhombus are

$x - y + \lambda = 0$

and $7x - y + \mu = 0$

then O is equidistant from AB and DC and from AD and BC

$\therefore |-1+2+1| = |-1+2+\lambda| \Rightarrow \lambda = -3$

and $|-7+2-5| = |-7+2+\mu| \Rightarrow \mu = 15$

$\therefore$ Other two sides are $x - y - 3 = 0$ and $7x - y + 15 = 0$

On solving the eqⁿs of sides pairwise, we get

the vertices as $\left(\frac{1}{3}, \frac{-8}{3}\right), (1, 2), \left(\frac{-7}{3}, \frac{-4}{3}\right), (-3, -6)$

13. (c) Length of $\perp$ to $4x + 3y = 10$ from origin (0, 0)

$P_1 = \frac{10}{5} = 2$

Length of $\perp$ to $8x + 6y + 5 = 0$ from origin (0, 0)

$P_2 = \frac{5}{10} = \frac{1}{2}$

$\because$ Lines are parallel to each other $\Rightarrow$ ratio will be 4 : 1 or 1 : 4

14. (a) $L_1 : 4x + 3y - 12 = 0$

$L_2 : 3x + 4y - 12 = 0$

$L_1 + \lambda L_2 = 0$

$(4x + 3y - 12) + \lambda(3x + 4y - 12) = 0$

$x(4 + 3\lambda) + y(3 + 4\lambda) - 12(1 + \lambda) = 0$

Point A $\left(\frac{12(1+\lambda)}{4+3\lambda}, 0\right)$

Point B $\left(0, \frac{12(1+\lambda)}{3+4\lambda}\right)$

mid point $\Rightarrow h = \frac{6(1+\lambda)}{4+3\lambda}$ ..... (i)

$k = \frac{6(1+\lambda)}{3+4\lambda}$ ..... (ii)

Eliminate λ from (i) and (ii), then

$6(h + k) = 7hk$

$6(x + y) = 7xy$

15. (d) $x - y = 4$

To find equation of R

slope of L = 0 is 1

$\Rightarrow$ slope of QR = – 1

Let QR is $y = mx + c$

$y = -x + c$

$x + y - c = 0$

distance of QR from (2, 1) is $2\sqrt{3}$

$2\sqrt{3} = \frac{|2+1-c|}{\sqrt{2}}$

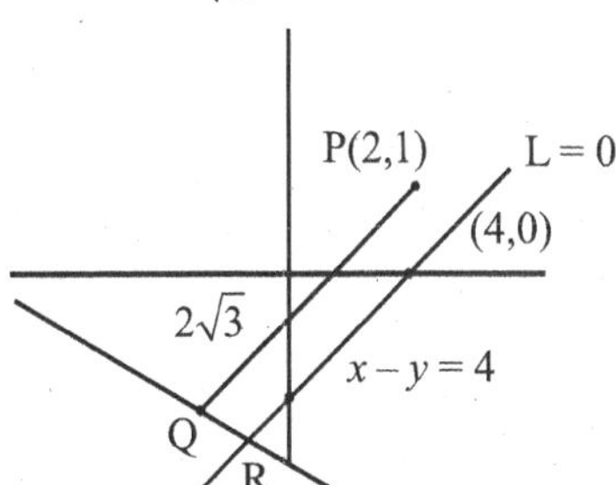

$2\sqrt{6} = |3 - c|$

$c - 3 = \pm 2\sqrt{6}$ $c = 3 \pm 2\sqrt{6}$

Line can be $x + y = 3 \pm 2\sqrt{6}$

$x + y = 3 - 2\sqrt{6}$

16. (c) Given eqn of line is $y + \sqrt{3}x - 1 = 0$

$\Rightarrow y = -\sqrt{3}x + 1$

$\Rightarrow$ (slope) $m_2 = -\sqrt{3}$

Let the other slope be m_1

$\therefore \tan 60° = \left|\frac{m_1 - (-\sqrt{3})}{1 + (-\sqrt{3}m_1)}\right|$

$\Rightarrow m_1 = 0, m_2 = \sqrt{3}$

Since line L is passing through (3, –2)

$\therefore y - (-2) = +\sqrt{3}(x - 3)$

$\Rightarrow y + 2 = \sqrt{3}(x - 3)$

$y - \sqrt{3}x + 2 + 3\sqrt{3} = 0$

17. (d) Circumcentre = (0, 0)

$$\text{Centroid} = \left(\frac{(a+1)^2}{2}, \frac{(a-1)^2}{2}\right)$$

We know the circumcentre (O), Centroid (G) and orthocentre (H) of a triangle lie on the line joining the O and G.

$$\text{Also, } \frac{HG}{GO} = \frac{2}{1}$$

$$\Rightarrow \text{Coordinate of orthocentre} = \frac{3(a+1)^2}{2}, \frac{3(a-1)^2}{2}$$

Now, these coordinates satisfies eqn given in option (d)

Hence, required eqn of line is

$(a-1)^2 x - (a+1)^2 y = 0$

18. (b)

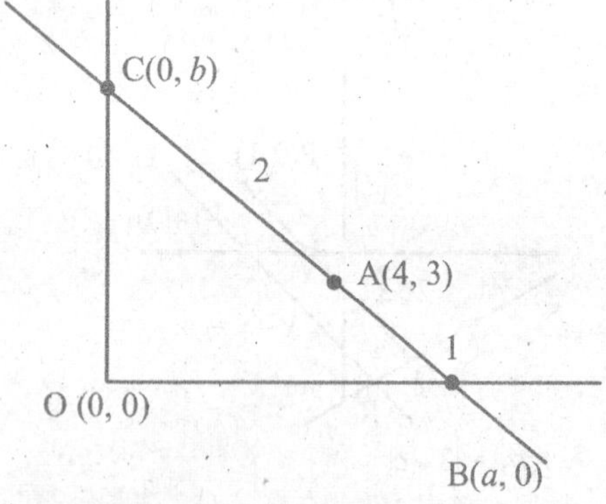

A divides CB in 2 : 1

$$\Rightarrow 4 = \left(\frac{1\times 0 + 2\times a}{1+2}\right) = \frac{2a}{3}$$

$\Rightarrow a = 6 \Rightarrow$ coordinate of B is B (6, 0)

$$3 = \left(\frac{1\times b + 2\times 0}{1+2}\right) = \frac{b}{3}$$

$\Rightarrow b = 9$ and C (0, 9)

Slope of line passing through (6, 0), (0, 9)

$$\text{slope, m} = \frac{9}{-6} = -\frac{3}{2}$$

$$\text{Equation of line } y - 0 = \frac{-3}{2}(x-6)$$

$2y = -3x + 18$

$3x + 2y = 18$

19. (d)

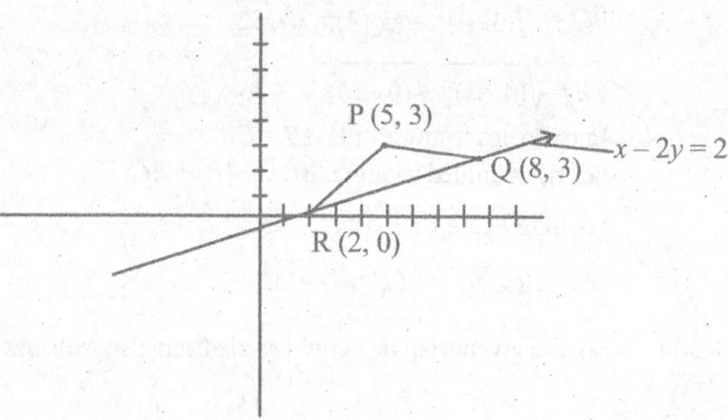

Equation of RQ is $x - 2y = 2$ ...(1)

at $y = 0$, $x = 2$ [R (2, 0)]

as PQ is parallel to x, y-coordinates of Q is also 3

Putting value of y in equation (1), we get

Q (8, 3)

$$\text{Centroid of } \Delta PQR = \left(\frac{8+5+2}{3}, \frac{3+3}{3}\right) = (5, 2)$$

Only $(2x - 5y = 0)$ satisfy the given co-ordinates.

20. (b) Suppose B(0, 1) be any point on given line and co-ordinate of A is $(\sqrt{3}, 0)$. So, equation of

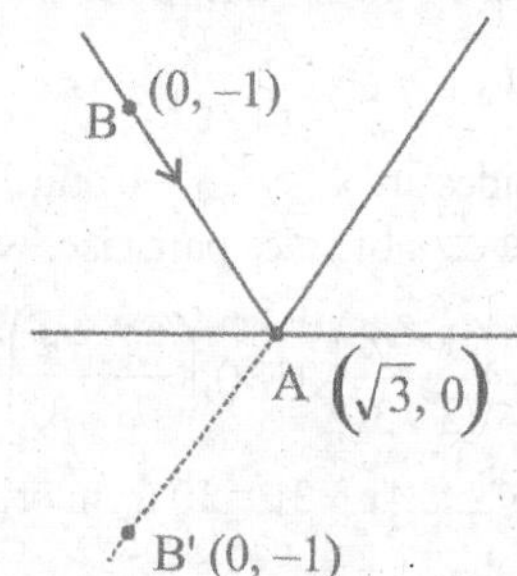

$$\text{Reflected Ray is } \frac{-1-0}{0-\sqrt{3}} = \frac{y-0}{x-\sqrt{3}}$$

$$\Rightarrow \sqrt{3}y = x - \sqrt{3}$$

21. (b) Let $C = (x_1, y_1)$

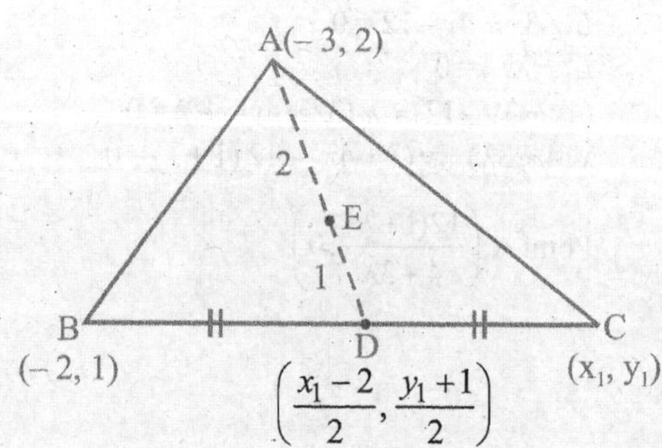

Centroid, $E = \left(\frac{x_1 - 5}{3}, \frac{y_1 + 3}{3} \right)$

Since centroid lies on the line

$3x + 4y + 2 = 0$

$\therefore \quad 3\left(\frac{x_1 - 5}{3}\right) + 4\left(\frac{y_1 + 3}{3}\right) + 2 = 0$

$\Rightarrow \quad 3x_1 + 4y_1 + 3 = 0$

Hence vertex (x_1, y_1) lies on the line

$3x + 4y + 3 = 0$

22. (b) Let y-coordinate of C = b

$\therefore$ C = $(2a, b)$

AB = $\sqrt{4a^2 + a^2} = \sqrt{5}a$

Now, AC = BC $\Rightarrow b = \sqrt{4a^2 + (b-a)^2}$

$\Rightarrow b^2 = 4a^2 + b^2 + a^2 - 2ab$

$\Rightarrow 2ab = 5a^2 \Rightarrow b = \frac{5a}{2}$

$\therefore$ C = $\left(2a, \frac{5a}{2}\right)$

Hence area of the triangle

$$= \frac{1}{2}\begin{vmatrix} 2a & 0 & 1 \\ 0 & a & 1 \\ 2a & \frac{5a}{2} & 1 \end{vmatrix} = \frac{1}{2}\begin{vmatrix} 2a & 0 & 1 \\ 0 & a & 1 \\ 0 & \frac{5a}{2} & 0 \end{vmatrix}$$

$$= \frac{1}{2} \times 2a\left(-\frac{5a}{2}\right) = -\frac{5a^2}{2}$$

Since area is always +ve, hence area

$= \frac{5a^2}{2}$ sq. unit

23. (d) Given line $3x + 4y = 12$ can be rewritten as

$\frac{3x}{12} + \frac{4y}{12} = 1 \Rightarrow \frac{x}{4} + \frac{y}{3} = 1$

$\Rightarrow$ x-intercept = 4 and y-intercept = 3

Let the required line be

L: $\frac{x}{a} + \frac{y}{b} = 1$ where

a = x-intercept and b = y-intercept

According to the question

$a = 4 \times 2 = 8$ and $b = 3/2$

$\therefore$ Required line is $\frac{x}{8} + \frac{2y}{3} = 1$

$\Rightarrow 3x + 16y = 24$

$\Rightarrow y = \frac{-3}{16}x + \frac{24}{16}$

Hence, required slope = $\frac{-3}{16}$.

24. (c) Let the joining points be A (1,1) and B (2,4).

Let point C divides line AB in the ratio 3 : 2.

So, by section formula we have

$C = \left(\frac{3 \times 2 + 2 \times 1}{3+2}, \frac{3 \times 4 + 2 \times 1}{3+2}\right) = \left(\frac{8}{5}, \frac{14}{5}\right)$

Since Line $2x + y = k$ passes through $C\left(\frac{8}{5}, \frac{14}{5}\right)$

$\therefore$ C satisfies the equation $2x + y = k$.

$\Rightarrow \quad \frac{2+8}{5} + \frac{14}{5} = k \Rightarrow k = 6$

25. (c) Given lines are

$ax + 2by + 3b = 0$ and $bx - 2ay - 3a = 0$

Since, required line is || to x-axis

$\therefore x = 0$

We put $x = 0$ in given equation, we get

$2by = -3b \Rightarrow y = -\frac{3}{2}$

This shows that the required line is below x-axis at a distance of $\frac{3}{2}$ from it.

26. (d)

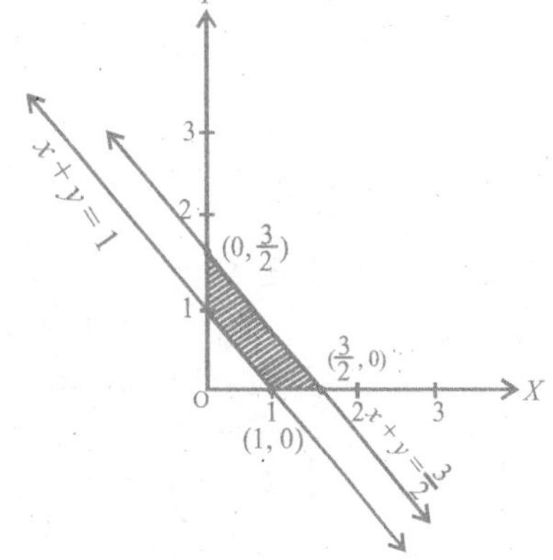

Since, $(1, a)$ lies between $x+y=1$
and $2(x+y)=3$
$\therefore$ Put $x=1$ in $2(x+y)=3$.
We get the range of y. Thus,

$$2(1+y)=3 \Rightarrow y=\frac{3}{2}-1=\frac{1}{2}$$

Thus 'a' lies in $\left(0, \frac{1}{2}\right)$

27. (c) Let equation of $AB: x+3y=4$
Let equation of $BC: 3x+y=4$
Let equation of $CA: x+y=0$
Now, By solving these equations we get
$A=(-2, 2), B=(1, 1)$ and $C=(2,-2)$
Now, $AB=\sqrt{9+1}=\sqrt{10}$,
$BC=\sqrt{1+9}=\sqrt{10}$
and $CA=\sqrt{16+16}=\sqrt{32}$
Since, length of AB and BC are same therefore triangle is isosceles.

28. (b)

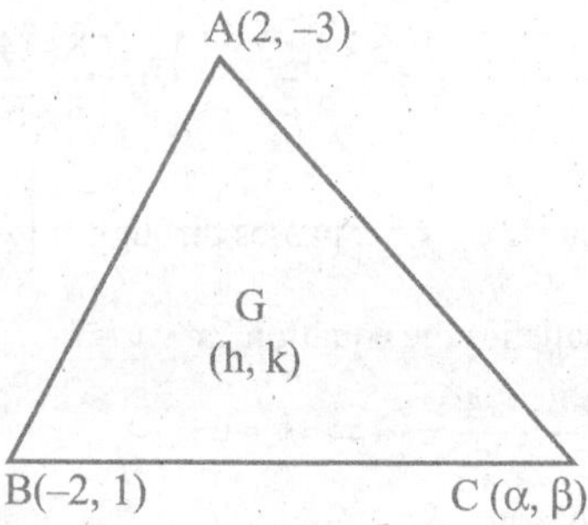

$\alpha=3h$
$\beta-2=3k$
$\beta=3k+2$

Third vertex (α, β) lies on the line
$2x+3y=9$
$2\alpha+3\beta=9$
$2(3h)+3(3k+2)=9$
$2h+3k=1$
$2x+3y=1$

29. (c) Clearly for point P,

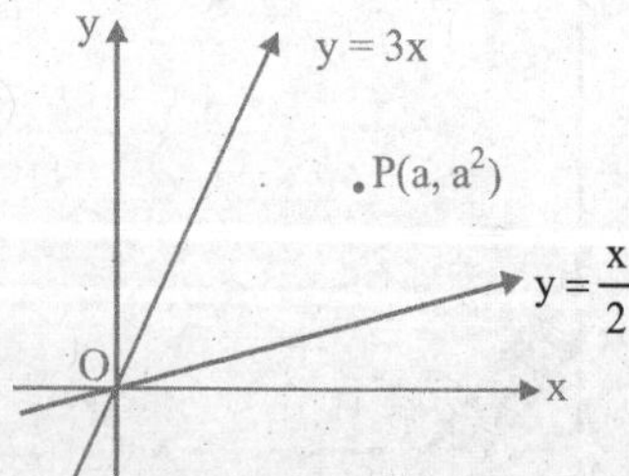

$a^2-3a<0$ and $a^2-\frac{a}{2}>0 \Rightarrow \frac{1}{2}<a<3$

30. (c)

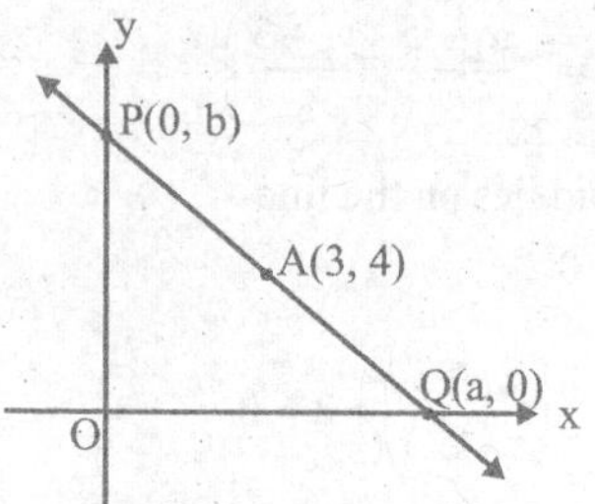

$\because A$ is the mid point of PQ, therefore

$$\frac{a+0}{2}=3, \quad \frac{0+b}{2}=4 \Rightarrow a=6, b=8$$

$\therefore$ Equation of line is $\frac{x}{6}+\frac{y}{8}=1$

or $4x+3y=24$

31. (a) The line passing through the intersection of lines $ax+2by=3b=0$ and $bx-2ay-3a=0$ is

$ax+2by+3b+\lambda(bx-2ay-3a)=0$

$\Rightarrow (a+b\lambda)x+(2b-2a\lambda)y+3b-3\lambda a=0$

As this line is parallel to x-axis.

$\therefore a+b\lambda=0 \Rightarrow \lambda=-a/b$

$\Rightarrow ax+2by+3b-\frac{a}{b}(bx-2ay-3a)=0$

$\Rightarrow ax+2by+3b-ax+\frac{2a^2}{b}y+\frac{3a^2}{b}=0$

$y\left(2b+\frac{2a^2}{b}\right)+3b+\frac{3a^2}{b}=0$

$y\left(\frac{2b^2+2a^2}{b}\right)=-\left(\frac{3b^2+3a^2}{b}\right)$

$y=\frac{-3(a^2+b^2)}{2(b^2+a^2)}=\frac{-3}{2}$

So it is 3/2 units below x-axis.

32. (a) Let the required line be $\frac{x}{a}+\frac{y}{b}=1$ ....(1)

then $a+b=-1$ ....(2)

(1) passes through $(4, 3)$, $\Rightarrow \frac{4}{a}+\frac{3}{b}=1$

$\Rightarrow 4b+3a=ab$ ....(3)

Eliminating b from (2) and (3), we get

$a^2-4=0 \Rightarrow a=\pm 2 \Rightarrow b=-3$ or 1

$\therefore$ Equations of straight lines are

$\frac{x}{2}+\frac{y}{-3}=1$ or $\frac{x}{-2}+\frac{y}{1}=1$

33. **(d)** Let the vertex C be (h, k), then the centroid of ΔABC is $\left(\frac{2-2+h}{3}, \frac{-3+1+k}{3}\right)$

or $\left(\frac{h}{3}, \frac{-2+k}{3}\right)$. It lies on $2x + 3y = 1$

$\Rightarrow \frac{2h}{3} - 2 + k = 1 \Rightarrow 2h + 3k = 9$

$\Rightarrow$ Locus of C is $2x + 3y = 9$

34. **(d)** Equation of AB is

$x\cos\alpha + y\sin\alpha = p$;

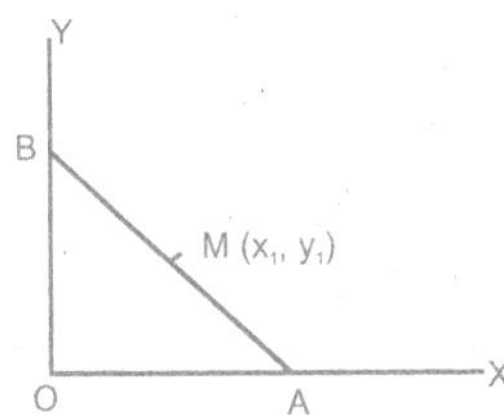

$\Rightarrow \frac{x\cos\alpha}{p} + \frac{y\sin\alpha}{p} = 1$;

$\Rightarrow \frac{x}{p/\cos\alpha} + \frac{y}{p/\sin\alpha} = 1$

So co-ordinates of A and B are

$\left(\frac{p}{\cos\alpha}, 0\right)$ and $\left(0, \frac{p}{\sin\alpha}\right)$;

So coordinates of midpoint of AB are

$\left(\frac{p}{2\cos\alpha}, \frac{p}{2\sin\alpha}\right) = (x_1, y_1)(let)$;

$x_1 = \frac{p}{2\cos\alpha}$ & $y_1 = \frac{p}{2\sin\alpha}$;

$\Rightarrow \cos\alpha = p/2x_1$ and $\sin\alpha = p/2y_1$;

$\cos^2\alpha + \sin^2\alpha = 1 \Rightarrow \frac{p^2}{4}\left(\frac{1}{x_1^2} + \frac{1}{y_1^2}\right) = 1$

Locus of (x_1, y_1) is $\frac{1}{x^2} + \frac{1}{y^2} = \frac{4}{p^2}$.

35. **(a)** Given lines are

$4ax + 2ay + c = 0$

$5bx + 2by + d = 0$

The point of intersection will be

$$\frac{x}{2ad - 2bc} = \frac{-y}{4ad - 5bc} = \frac{1}{8ab - 10ab}$$

$\Rightarrow \quad x = \frac{2(ad - bc)}{-2ab} = \frac{bc - ad}{ab}$

$\Rightarrow \quad y = \frac{5bc - 4ad}{-2ab} = \frac{4ad - 5bc}{2ab}$

$\because$ Point of intersection is in fourth quadrant so x is positive and y is negative.

Also distance from axes is same

So $x = -y$ ($\because$ distance from x-axis is $-y$ as y is negative)

$\frac{bc - ad}{ab} = \frac{5bc - 4ad}{2ab} \Rightarrow 3bc - 2ad = 0$

36. **(d)** Let P, Q, R, be the vertices of ΔPQR

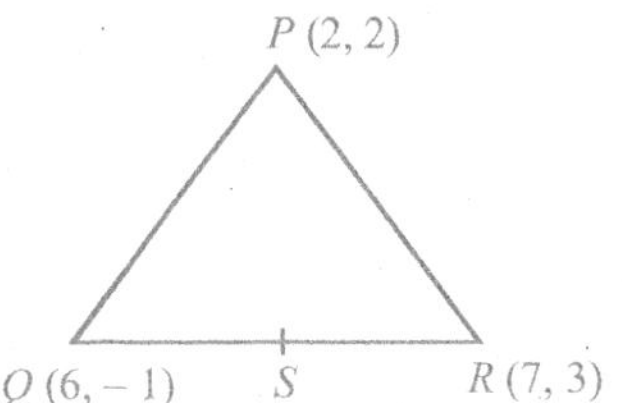

Since PS is the median

S is mid-point of QR

So, $S = \left(\frac{7+6}{2}, \frac{3-1}{2}\right) = \left(\frac{13}{2}, 1\right)$

Now, slope of $PS = \frac{2-1}{2-\frac{13}{2}} = -\frac{2}{9}$

Since, required line is parallel to PS therefore

slope of required line = slope of PS

Now, eqn of line passing through $(1, -1)$ and having slope $-\frac{2}{9}$ is

$y - (-1) = -\frac{2}{9}(x - 1)$

$9y + 9 = -2x + 2 \Rightarrow 2x + 9y + 7 = 0$

37. **(b)** Let equation of line L, perpendicular to $5x - y = 1$ be $x + 5y = c$

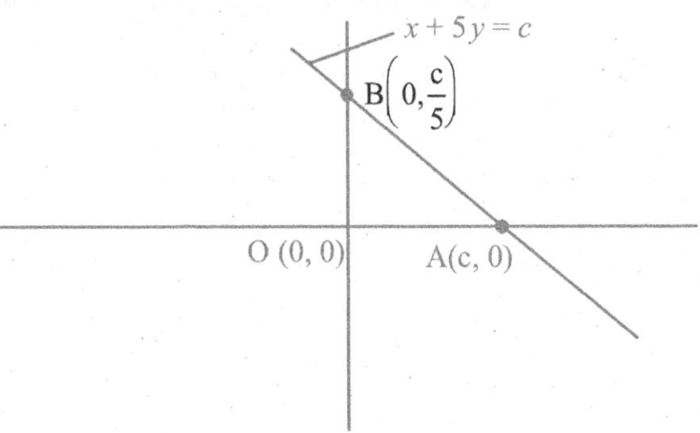

Given that area of ΔAOB is 5.

We know

$\left\{\text{area, } A = \frac{1}{2}[x_1(y_2 - y_3) + x_2(y_3 - y_1) + x_3(y_1 - y_2)]\right\}$

$\Rightarrow 5 = \frac{1}{2}\left[c\left(\frac{c}{5}\right)\right]$

$$\left(\begin{array}{l}\because (x_1, y_1) = (10, 0), (x_3, y_3) = \left(0, \frac{c}{5}\right) \\ (x_2, y_2) = (c, 0)\end{array}\right)$$

$\Rightarrow c = \pm\sqrt{50}$

$\therefore$ Equation of line L is $x + 5y = \pm\sqrt{50}$

Distance between L and line $x + 5y = 0$ is

$$d = \left|\frac{\pm\sqrt{50} - 0}{\sqrt{1^2 + 5^2}}\right| = \frac{\sqrt{50}}{\sqrt{26}} = \frac{5}{\sqrt{13}}$$

38. (c) $x + 2ay + a = 0$ ...(1)

$x + 3by + b = 0$ ...(2)

$x + 4ay + a = 0$ ...(3)

Subtracting equation (3) from (1)

$-2ay = 0$

$ay = 0 \Rightarrow y = 0$

Putting value of y in equation (1), we get

$x + 0 + a = 0$

$x = -a$

Putting value of x and y in equation (2), we get

$-a + b = 0$

$a = b$

Thus, (a, b) lies on a straight line

39. (b)

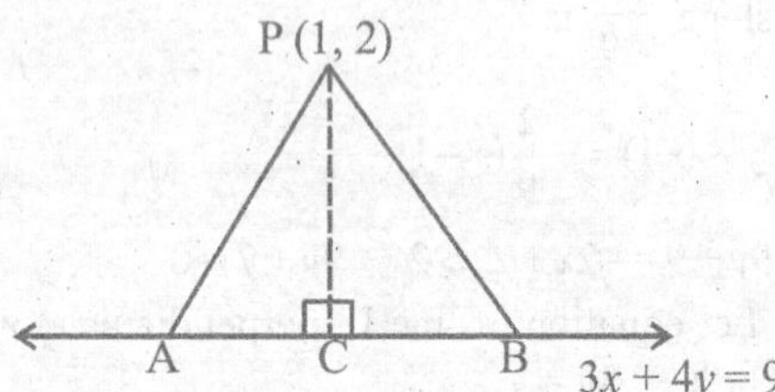

Shortest distance of a point (x_1, y_1) from line

$ax + by = c$ is $d = \left|\frac{ax_1 + by_1 - c}{\sqrt{a^2 + b^2}}\right|$

Now shortest distance of P (1, 2) from $3x + 4y = 9$ is

$$PC = d = \left|\frac{3(1) + 4(2) - 9}{\sqrt{3^2 + 4^2}}\right| = \frac{2}{5}$$

Given that ΔAPB is an equilateral triangle

Let 'a' be its side

then PB = a, CB = $\frac{a}{2}$

Now, In ΔPCB, $(PB)^2 = (PC)^2 + (CB)^2$

(By Pythagoras theoresm)

$$a^2 = \left(\frac{2}{5}\right)^2 + \frac{a^2}{4}$$

$$a^2 - \frac{a^4}{4} = \frac{4}{25} \Rightarrow \frac{3a^2}{4} = \frac{4}{25}$$

$$a^2 = \frac{16}{75} \Rightarrow a = \sqrt{\frac{16}{75}} = \frac{4}{5\sqrt{3}} \times \frac{\sqrt{3}}{\sqrt{3}} = \frac{4\sqrt{3}}{15}$$

$\therefore$ Length of Equilateral triangle $(a) = \frac{4\sqrt{3}}{15}$

40. (d) Mid-point of P(2, 3) and Q(4, 5) = (3, 4)

Slope of PQ = 1

Slope of the line L = – 1

Mid-point (3, 4) lies on the line L.

Equation of line L,

$y - 4 = -1(x - 3) \Rightarrow x + y - 7 = 0$ ...(i)

Let image of point R(0, 0) be $S(x_1, y_1)$

Mid-point of RS = $\left(\frac{x_1}{2}, \frac{y_1}{2}\right)$

Mid-point $\left(\frac{x_1}{2}, \frac{y_1}{2}\right)$ lies on the line (i)

$\therefore \quad x_1 + y_1 = 14$ ...(ii)

Slope of RS = $\frac{y_1}{x_1}$

Since RS $\perp$ line L

$\therefore \quad \frac{y_1}{x_1} \times (-1) = -1$

$\therefore \quad x_1 = y_1$ ...(iii)

From (ii) and (iii),

$x_1 = y_1 = 7$

Hence the image of R = (7, 7)

41. (a) Two lines $-x + 5y + c_2 = 0$ and $-x + 5y + c_3 = 0$ are parallel to each other. Hence statement-1 is true, statement-2 is true and statement-2 is the correct explanation of statement-1.

42. (a) Since three lines $x - 3y = p$, $ax + 2y = q$ and $ax + y = r$ form a right angled triangle

$\therefore$ product of slopes of any two lines = –1

Suppose $ax + 2y = q$ and $x - 3y = p$ are $\perp$ to each other.

$\therefore \quad \frac{-a}{2} \times \frac{1}{3} = -1 \Rightarrow a = 6$

Now, consider option one by one

$a = 6$ satisfies only option (a)

$\therefore$ Required answer is $a^2 - 9a + 18 = 0$

43. (d) Consider the lines
$L_1 : x - y = 1$
$L_2 : x + y = 1$
$L_3 : 2x + 2y = 5$
$L_4 : 2x - 2y = 7$
$L_1 \perp L_2$ is correct statement
($\because$ Product of their slopes = – 1)
$L_1 \perp L_3$ is also correct statement
($\because$ Product of their slopes = – 1)
Now, $L_2 : x + y = 1$
$L_4 : 2x - 2y = 7$
$\Rightarrow 2x - 2(1 - x) = 7$
$\Rightarrow 2x - 2 + 2x = 7$

$$\Rightarrow x = \frac{9}{4} \text{ and } y = \frac{-5}{4}$$

Hence, L_2 intersects L_4.

44. (d) Given $ax^2 + bx + c = 0$
$\Rightarrow ax^2 = -bx - c$
Now, consider
$y = 4ax^2 + 3bx + 2c$
$= 4[-bx - c] + 3bx + 2c$
$= -4bx - 4c + 3bx + 2c$
$= -bx - 2c$
Since, this curve intersects x-axis
$\therefore$ put $y = 0$, we get
$-bx - 2c = 0 \Rightarrow -bx = 2c$

$$\Rightarrow x = \frac{-2c}{b}$$

Thus, given curve intersects x-axis at exactly one point.

45. (c) Statement - 1
Let $P'(x_1, y_1)$ be the image of (0, 1) with respect to the line $2x - y = 0$ then

$$\frac{x_1}{2} = \frac{y_1 - 1}{-1} = \frac{-4(0) + 2(1)}{5}$$

$$\Rightarrow x_1 = \frac{4}{5}, y_1 = \frac{3}{5}$$

Thus, statement-1 is true.
Also, statement-2 is true and correct explanation for statement-1.

46. (b)

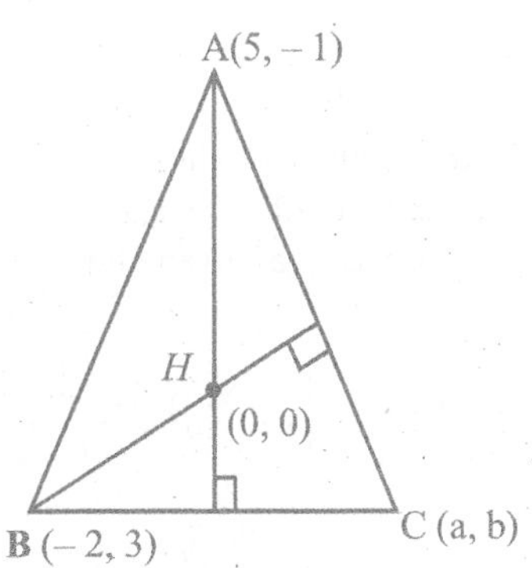

Let the third vertex of ΔABC be (a, b).
Orthocentre = $H(0, 0)$
Let A (5, – 1) and B (– 2, 3) be other two vertices of ΔABC.
Now, (Slope of AH) × (Slope of BC) = – 1

$$\Rightarrow \left(\frac{-1-0}{5-0}\right)\left(\frac{b-3}{a+2}\right) = -1$$

$$\Rightarrow b - 3 = 5(a + 2) \quad ...(1)$$

Similarly,
(Slope of BH) × (Slope of AC) = – 1

$$\Rightarrow -\left(\frac{3}{2}\right) \times \left(\frac{b+1}{a-5}\right) = -1$$

$$\Rightarrow 3b + 3 = 2a - 10$$

$$\Rightarrow 3b - 2a + 13 = 0 \quad ...(2)$$

On solving equation (1) and (2) we get
$a = -4, b = -7$
Hence, third vertex is (– 4, – 7).

47. (a)

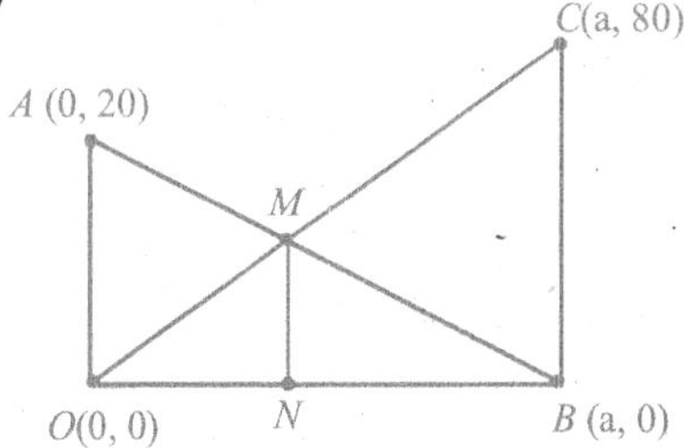

We put one pole at origin.
$BC = 80$ m, $OA = 20$ m
Line OC and AB intersect at M.
To find: Length of MN.

$$\text{Eqn of } OC: y = \left(\frac{80-0}{a-0}\right)x$$

$$\Rightarrow y = \frac{80}{a}x \quad ...(1)$$

$$\text{Eqn of } AB: y = \left(\frac{20-0}{0-a}\right)(x - a)$$

$$\Rightarrow y = \frac{-20}{a}(x - a) \quad ...(2)$$

At M: (1) = (2)

$$\Rightarrow \frac{80}{a}x = \frac{-20}{a}(x - a)$$

$$\Rightarrow \frac{80}{a}x = \frac{-20}{a}x + 20 \Rightarrow x = \frac{a}{5}$$

$$\therefore \quad y = \frac{80}{a} \times \frac{a}{5} = 16$$

48. (a) Given equation of lines are
$(a^3+3)x+ay+a-3=0$ and
$(a^5+2)x+(a+2)y+2a+3=0$ (a real)
Since point of intersection of lines lies on y-axis.
$\therefore$ Put $x=0$ in each equation, we get
$ay+a-3=0$ and
$(a+2)y+2a+3=0$
On solving these we get
$(a+2)(a-3)-a(2a+3)=0$
$\Rightarrow a^2-a-6-2a^2-3a=0$
$\Rightarrow -a^2-4a-6=0 \Rightarrow a^2+4a+6=0$

$$\Rightarrow a=\frac{-4\pm\sqrt{16-24}}{2}=\frac{-4\pm\sqrt{-8}}{2}$$

(not real)

This shows that the point of intersection of the lines lies on the y-axis for no value of 'a'.

49. (b) $x+y=|a|$

and $ax-y=1$

Case I : If $a>0$

$x+y=a$ ....(1)

$ax-y=1$ ....(2)

On adding equation (1) and (2), we get

$x(1+a)=1+a \Rightarrow x=1$

$y=a-1$

It is in first quadrant

so $a-1\geq 0$

$\Rightarrow a\geq 1$

$\Rightarrow a\in[1,\infty)$

Case II : If $a<0$

$x+y=-a$ ....(3)

$ax-y=1$ ....(4)

On adding equation (3) and (4), we get

$x(1+a)=1-a$

$$x=\frac{1-a}{1+a}>0 \Rightarrow \frac{a-1}{a+1}<0$$

Since $a-1<0$

$\therefore a+1>0$

$\Rightarrow a>-1$ ....(5)

$$y=-a-\frac{1-a}{1+a}>0=\frac{-a-a^2-1+a}{1+a}>0$$

$$\Rightarrow -\left(\frac{a^2+1}{a+1}\right)>0 \Rightarrow \frac{a^2+1}{a+1}<0$$

Since $a^2+1>0$

$\therefore a+1<0$

$\Rightarrow a<-1$ ....(6)

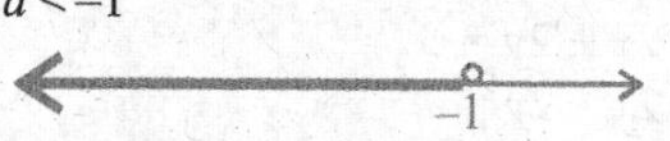

From (5) and (6), $a\in\phi$
Hence Case-II is not possible.
So, correct answer is $a\in[1,\infty)$

50. (b)

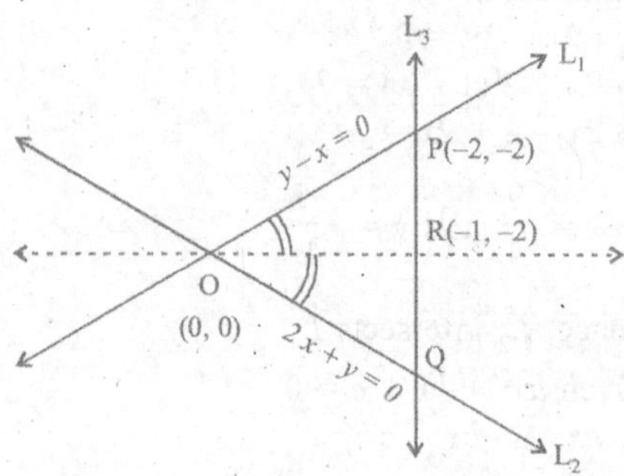

$L_1: y-x=0$
$L_2: 2x+y=0$
$L_3: y+2=0$
On solving the equation of line L_1 and L_2 we get their point of intersection (0, 0) i.e., origin O.
On solving the equation of line L_1 and L_3, we get $P=(-2,-2)$.
Similarly, we get $Q=(-1,-2)$
We know that bisector of an angle of a triangle, divide the opposite side the triangle in the ratio of the sides including the angle [Angle Bisector Theorem of a Triangle]

$$\therefore \frac{PR}{RQ}=\frac{OP}{OQ}=\frac{\sqrt{(-2)^2+(-2)^2}}{\sqrt{(-1)^2+(-2)^2}}=\frac{2\sqrt{2}}{\sqrt{5}}$$

51. (a) If the lines $p(p^2+1)x-y+q=0$
and $(p^2+1)^2x+(p^2+1)y+2q=0$
are perpendicular to a common line then these lines must be parallel to each other,

$$\therefore m_1=m_2 \Rightarrow -\frac{p(p^2+1)}{-1}=-\frac{(p^2+1)^2}{p^2+1}$$

$\Rightarrow (p^2+1)(p+1)=0$
$\Rightarrow p=-1$
$\therefore p$ can have exactly one value.

52. (d) Let (a^2, a) be the point of shortest distance on $x=y^2$
Then distance between (a^2, a) and line $x-y+1=0$ is given by

$$D=\frac{a^2-a+1}{\sqrt{2}}=\frac{1}{\sqrt{2}}\left[(a-\frac{1}{2})^2+\frac{3}{4}\right]$$

It is min when $a = \frac{1}{2}$ and D_{min}

$= \frac{3}{4\sqrt{2}} = \frac{3\sqrt{2}}{8}$

53. (d) Slope of $PQ = \frac{3-4}{k-1} = \frac{-1}{k-1}$

$\therefore$ Slope of perpendicular bisector of PQ = (k – 1)

Also mid point of PQ $\left(\frac{k+1}{2}, \frac{7}{2}\right)$.

$\therefore$ Equation of perpendicular bisector is

$$y - \frac{7}{2} = (k-1)\left(x - \frac{k+1}{2}\right)$$

$\Rightarrow \quad 2y - 7 = 2(k-1)x - (k^2 - 1)$

$\Rightarrow \quad 2(k-1)x - 2y + (8 - k^2) = 0$

$\therefore \quad$ y-intercept $= -\frac{8-k^2}{-2} = -4$

$\Rightarrow \quad 8 - k^2 = -8$ or $k^2 = 16 \Rightarrow k = \pm 4$

54. (c) Given : The coordinates of points P, Q, R are (–1, 0), (0, 0), $(3, 3\sqrt{3})$ respectively.

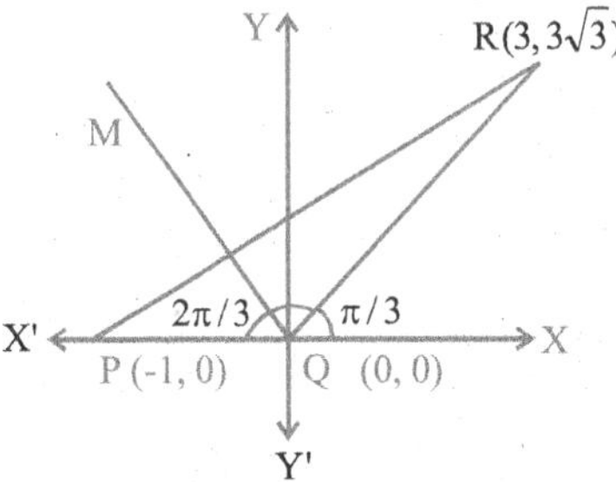

Slope of QR $= \frac{y_2 - y_1}{x_2 - x_1} = \frac{3\sqrt{3}}{3}$

$\Rightarrow \quad \tan\theta = \sqrt{3} \Rightarrow \theta = \frac{\pi}{3}$

$\Rightarrow \quad \angle RQX = \frac{\pi}{3}$

$\therefore \quad \angle RQP = \pi - \frac{\pi}{3} = \frac{2\pi}{3}$

Let QM bisects the $\angle PQR$,

$\therefore$ Slope of the line QM $= \tan\frac{2\pi}{3} = -\sqrt{3}$

$\therefore$ Equation of line QM is $(y - 0) = -\sqrt{3}(x - 0)$

$\Rightarrow \quad y = -\sqrt{3}x \Rightarrow \sqrt{3}x + y = 0$

55. (b) Taking co-ordinates as

$\left(\frac{x}{r}, \frac{y}{r}\right); (x, y) \,\&\, (xr, yr)$.

Then slope of line joining

$$\left(\frac{x}{r}, \frac{y}{r}\right), (x, y) = \frac{y\left(1 - \frac{1}{r}\right)}{x\left(1 - \frac{1}{r}\right)} = \frac{y}{x}$$

and slope of line joining (x, y) and (xr, yr)

$$= \frac{y(r-1)}{x(r-1)} = \frac{y}{x}$$

$\therefore m_1 = m_2$

$\Rightarrow$ Points lie on the straight line.

56. (a) Co-ordinates of $A = (a\cos\alpha, a\sin\alpha)$

Equation of OB,

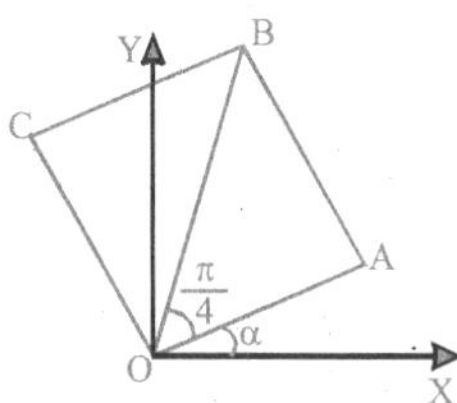

$$y = \tan\left(\frac{\pi}{4} + \alpha\right)x$$

CA $\perp^r$ to OB

$\therefore$ slope of CA $= -\cot\left(\frac{\pi}{4} + \alpha\right)$

Equation of CA

$$y - a\sin\alpha = -\cot\left(\frac{\pi}{4} + \alpha\right)(x - a\cos\alpha)$$

$$\Rightarrow (y - a\sin\alpha)\left(\tan\left(\frac{\pi}{4} + \alpha\right)\right) = (a\cos\alpha - x).$$

$$\Rightarrow (y - a\sin\alpha)\left(\frac{\tan\frac{\pi}{4} + \tan\alpha}{1 - \tan\frac{\pi}{4}\tan\alpha}\right)(a\cos\alpha - x)$$

$$\Rightarrow (y - a\sin\alpha)(1 + \tan\alpha) = (a\cos\alpha - x)(1 - \tan\alpha)$$

$$\Rightarrow (y - a\sin\alpha)(\cos\alpha + \sin\alpha) = (a\cos\alpha - x)(\cos\alpha - \sin\alpha)$$

$$\Rightarrow y(\cos + \sin\alpha) - a\sin\alpha\cos\alpha - a\sin^2\alpha$$

$$= a\cos^2\alpha - a\cos\alpha\sin\alpha - x(\cos\alpha - \sin\alpha)$$

$$\Rightarrow y(\cos\alpha + \sin\alpha) + x(\cos\alpha - \sin\alpha) = a$$

$$y(\sin\alpha + \cos\alpha) + x(\cos\alpha - \sin\alpha) = a.$$

57. **(a)** Equation of bisectors of lines, xy = 0 are y = ± x

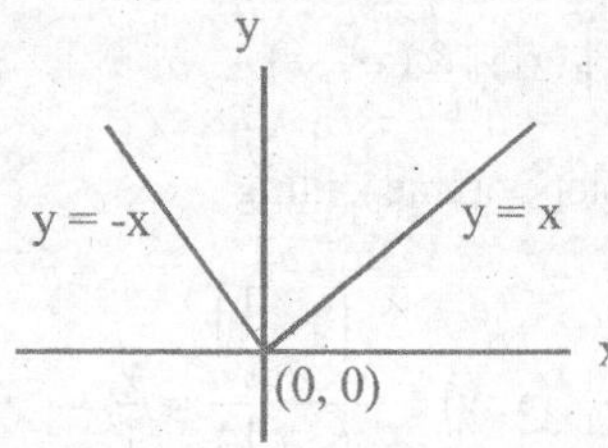

$\therefore$ Put y = ± x in the given equation
$my^2 + (1 - m^2)xy - mx^2 = 0$
$\therefore$ $mx^2 + (1 - m^2)x^2 - mx^2 = 0$
$\Rightarrow$ $1 - m^2 = 0 \Rightarrow m = \pm 1$

58. **(a)** $3x + 4y = 0$ is one of the lines of the pair

$6x^2 - xy + 4cy^2 = 0$, Put $y = -\frac{3}{4}x$,

we get $6x^2 + \frac{3}{4}x^2 + 4c\left(-\frac{3}{4}x\right)^2 = 0$

$\Rightarrow 6 + \frac{3}{4} + \frac{9c}{4} = 0 \Rightarrow c = -3$

59. **(c)** Let the lines be $y = m_1x$ and $y = m_2x$ then

$m_1 + m_2 = -\frac{2c}{7}$ and $m_1m_2 = -\frac{1}{7}$

Given $m_1 + m_2 = 4\ m_1m_2$

$\Rightarrow \frac{2c}{7} = -\frac{4}{7} \Rightarrow c = 2$

60. **(a)** Equation of bisectors of second pair of straight lines is,

$qx^2 + 2xy - qy^2 = 0$ ....(1)

It must be identical to the first pair

$x^2 - 2pxy - y^2 = 0$ ....(2)

from (1) and (2)

$\frac{q}{1} = \frac{2}{-2p} = \frac{-q}{-1} \Rightarrow pq = -1$.

61. **(a)** $3a + a^2 - 2 = 0 \Rightarrow a^2 + 3a - 2 = 0$.;

$\Rightarrow a = \frac{-3 \pm \sqrt{9+8}}{2} = \frac{-3 \pm \sqrt{17}}{2}$

62. **(a)** Put $x = 0$ in the given equation
$\Rightarrow by^2 + 2fy + c = 0$.
For unique point of intersection $f^2 - bc = 0$
$\Rightarrow af^2 - abc = 0$.
Since $abc + 2fgh - af^2 - bg^2 - ch^2 = 0$
$\Rightarrow 2fgh - bg^2 - ch^2 = 0$

Conic Sections

TOPIC-1 : Circles

1. The radius of a circle, having minimum area, which touches the curve $y = 4 - x^2$ and the lines, $y = |x|$ is : **[2017]**
   (a) $4(\sqrt{2}+1)$ (b) $2(\sqrt{2}+1)$
   (c) $2(\sqrt{2}-1)$ (d) $4(\sqrt{2}-1)$

2. The equation
   $\text{Im}\left(\frac{iz-2}{z-i}\right)+1=0, z \in C, z \neq i$ represents a part of a circle having radius equal to : **[Online April 9, 2017]**
   (a) 2 (b) 1
   (c) $\frac{3}{4}$ (d) $\frac{1}{2}$

3. A line drawn through the point P(4, 7) cuts the circle $x^2 + y^2 = 9$ at the points A and B. Then PA·PB is equal to : **[Online April 9, 2017]**
   (a) 53 (b) 56
   (c) 74 (d) 65

4. The two adjacent sides of a cyclic quadrilateral are 2 and 5 and the angle between them is 60°. If the area of the quadrilateral is $4\sqrt{3}$, then the perimeter of the quadrilateral is : **[Online April 9, 2017]**
   (a) 12.5 (b) 13.2
   (c) 12 (d) 13

5. Let $z \in C$, the set of complex numbers. Then the equation, $2|z+3i| - |z-i| = 0$ represents : **[Online April 8, 2017]**
   (a) a circle with radius $\frac{8}{3}$.
   (b) a circle with diameter $\frac{10}{3}$.
   (c) an ellipse with length of major axis $\frac{16}{3}$.
   (d) an ellipse with length of minor axis $\frac{16}{9}$

6. If a point P has co–ordinates (0, –2) and Q is any point on the circle, $x^2 + y^2 - 5x - y + 5 = 0$, then the maximum value of $(PQ)^2$ is : **[Online April 8, 2017]**
   (a) $\frac{25+\sqrt{6}}{2}$ (b) $14+5\sqrt{3}$
   (c) $\frac{47+10\sqrt{6}}{2}$ (d) $8+5\sqrt{3}$

7. If two parallel chords of a circle, having diameter 4 units, lie on the opposite sides of the centre and subtend angles $\cos^{-1}\left(\frac{1}{7}\right)$ and $\sec^{-1}(7)$ at the centre respectively, then the distance between these chords, is : **[Online April 8, 2017]**
   (a) $\frac{4}{\sqrt{7}}$ (b) $\frac{8}{\sqrt{7}}$
   (c) $\frac{8}{7}$ (d) $\frac{16}{7}$

8. If one of the diameters of the circle, given by the equation, $x^2 + y^2 - 4x + 6y - 12 = 0$, is a chord of a circle S, whose centre is at (–3, 2), then the radius of S is: **[2016]**
   (a) 5 (b) 10
   (c) $5\sqrt{2}$ (d) $5\sqrt{3}$

9. Equation of the tangent to the circle, at the point (1, –1) whose centre is the point of intersection of the straight lines $x - y = 1$ and $2x + y = 3$ is : **[Online April 10, 2016]**
   (a) $x + 4y + 3 = 0$ (b) $3x - y - 4 = 0$
   (c) $x - 3y - 4 = 0$ (d) $4x + y - 3 = 0$

10. A circle passes through (–2, 4) and touches the y-axis at (0, 2). Which one of the following equations can represent a diameter of this circle ? **[Online April 9, 2016]**
    (a) $2x - 3y + 10 = 0$ (b) $3x + 4y - 3 = 0$
    (c) $4x + 5y - 6 = 0$ (d) $5x + 2y + 4 = 0$

11. Locus of the image of the point (2, 3) in the line $(2x - 3y + 4) + k(x - 2y + 3) = 0$, $k \in \mathbf{R}$, is a : **[2015]**
    (a) circle of radius $\sqrt{2}$.
    (b) circle of radius $\sqrt{3}$.
    (c) straight line parallel to x-axis
    (d) straight line parallel to y-axis

12. The number of common tangents to the circles $x^2 + y^2 - 4x - 6x - 12 = 0$ and $x^2 + y^2 + 6x + 18y + 26 = 0$, is : **[2015]**
    (a) 3 (b) 4
    (c) 1 (d) 2

13. If the incentre of an equilateral triangle is (1, 1) and the equation of its one side is $3x + 4y + 3 = 0$, then the equation of the circumcircle of this triangle is : **[Online April 11, 2015]**

(a) $x^2 + y^2 - 2x - 2y - 14 = 0$
(b) $x^2 + y^2 - 2x - 2y - 2 = 0$
(c) $x^2 + y^2 - 2x - 2y + 2 = 0$
(d) $x^2 + y^2 - 2x - 2y - 7 = 0$

14. If a circle passing through the point (–1, 0) touches y-axis at (0, 2), then the length of the chord of the circle along the x-axis is : **[Online April 11, 2015]**

(a) $\frac{3}{2}$ (b) 3
(c) $\frac{5}{2}$ (d) 5

15. Let the tangents drawn to the circle, $x^2 + y^2 = 16$ from the point P(0, h) meet the x-axis at point A and B. If the area of ΔAPB is minimum, then h is equal to : **[Online April 10, 2015]**

(a) $4\sqrt{2}$ (b) $3\sqrt{3}$
(c) $3\sqrt{2}$ (d) $4\sqrt{3}$

16. If $y + 3x = 0$ is the equation of a chord of the circle, $x^2 + y^2 - 30x = 0$, then the equation of the circle with this chord as diameter is : **[Online April 10, 2015]**

(a) $x^2+y^2+3x+9y=0$ (b) $x^2+y^2+3x-9y=0$
(c) $x^2+y^2-3x-9y=0$ (d) $x^2+y^2-3x+9y=0$

17. The largest value of r for which the region represented by the set $\{\omega \in C|\omega - 4 - i| \le r\}$ is contained in the region represented by the set $(z \in c / |z-1| \le |z+i|)$, is equal to: **[Online April 10, 2015]**

(a) $\frac{5}{2}\sqrt{2}$ (b) $2\sqrt{2}$
(c) $\frac{3}{2}\sqrt{2}$ (d) $\sqrt{17}$

18. Let C be the circle with centre at (1, 1) and radius = 1. If T is the circle centred at (0, y), passing through origin and touching the circle C externally, then the radius of T is equal to **[2014]**

(a) $\frac{1}{2}$ (b) $\frac{1}{4}$
(c) $\frac{\sqrt{3}}{\sqrt{2}}$ (d) $\frac{\sqrt{3}}{2}$

19. The equation of circle described on the chord $3x+y+5=0$ of the circle $x^2+y^2=16$ as diameter is: **[Online April 19, 2014]**

(a) $x^2+y^2+3x+y-11=0$
(b) $x^2+y^2+3x+y+1=0$
(c) $x^2+y^2+3x+y-2=0$
(d) $x^2+y^2+3x+y-22=0$

20. For the two circles $x^2+y^2=16$ and $x^2+y^2-2y=0$, there is/are **[Online April 12, 2014]**

(a) one pair of common tangents
(b) two pair of common tangents
(c) three pair of common tangents
(d) no common tangent

21. The set of all real values of λ for which exactly two common tangents can be drawn to the circles $x^2+y^2-4x-4y+6=0$ and $x^2+y^2-10x-10y+\lambda=0$ is the interval: **[Online April 11, 2014]**

(a) (12,32) (b) (18,42)
(c) (12,24) (d) (18,48)

22. If the point (1, 4) lies inside the circle $x^2+y^2-6x-10y+P=0$ and the circle does not touch or intersect the coordinate axes, then the set of all possible values of P is the interval: **[Online April 9, 2014]**

(a) (0,25) (b) (25,39)
(c) (9,25) (d) (25,29)

23. Let a and b be any two numbers satisfying $\frac{1}{a^2}+\frac{1}{b^2}=\frac{1}{4}$. Then, the foot of perpendicular from the origin on the variable line, $\frac{x}{a}+\frac{y}{b}=1$, lies on: **[Online April 9, 2014]**

(a) a hyperbola with each semi-axis = $\sqrt{2}$
(b) a hyperbola with each semi-axis = 2
(c) a circle of radius = 2
(d) a circle of radius = $\sqrt{2}$

24. The circle passing through (1, –2) and touching the axis of x at (3, 0) also passes through the point **[2013]**

(a) (–5, 2) (b) (2, –5)
(c) (5, –2) (d) (–2, 5)

25. If a circle of unit radius is divided into two parts by an arc of another circle subtending an angle 60° on the circumference of the first circle, then the radius of the arc is: **[Online April 25, 2013]**

(a) $\sqrt{3}$ (b) $\frac{1}{2}$
(c) 1 (d) $\sqrt{2}$

26. **Statement 1**: The only circle having radius $\sqrt{10}$ and a diameter along line $2x+y=5$ is $x^2+y^2-6x+2y=0$.
Statement 2 : $2x + y = 5$ is a normal to the circle $x^2+y^2-6x+2y=0$. **[Online April 25, 2013]**

(a) Statement 1 is false; Statement 2 is true.
(b) Statement 1 is true; Statement 2 is true, Statement 2 is a correct explanation for Statement 1.
(c) Statement 1 is true; Statement 2 is false.
(d) Statement 1 is true; Statement 2 is true; Statement 2 is not a correct explanation for Statement 1.

27. If the circle $x^2+y^2-6x-8y+(25-a^2)=0$ touches the axis of x, then a equals. **[Online April 23, 2013]**

(a) 0 (b) ± 4

(c) ± 2 (d) ± 3

28. If a circle C passing through (4, 0) touches the circle $x^2 + y^2 + 4x - 6y - 12 = 0$ externally at a point $(1, -1)$, then the radius of the circle C is : **[Online April 22, 2013]**

(a) 5 (b) $2\sqrt{5}$

(c) 4 (d) $\sqrt{57}$

29. If two vertices of an equilateral triangle are $A(-a, 0)$ and $B(a, 0)$, $a > 0$, and the third vertex C lies above x-axis then the equation of the circumcircle of ΔABC is : **[Online April 22, 2013]**

(a) $3x^2 + 3y^2 - 2\sqrt{3}ay = 3a^2$

(b) $3x^2 + 3y^2 - 2ay = 3a^2$

(c) $x^2 + y^2 - 2ay = a^2$

(d) $x^2 + y^2 - \sqrt{3}ay = a^2$

30. If each of the lines $5x + 8y = 13$ and $4x - y = 3$ contains a diameter of the circle $x^2 + y^2 - 2(a^2 - 7a + 11)x - 2(a^2 - 6a + 6)y + b^3 + 1 = 0$, then **[Online April 9, 2013]**

(a) $a = 5$ and $b \notin (-1, 1)$ (b) $a = 1$ and $b \notin (-1, 1)$

(c) $a = 2$ and $b \notin (-\infty, 1)$ (d) $a = 5$ and $b \in (-\infty, 1)$

31. The length of the diameter of the circle which touches the x-axis at the point (1,0) and passes through the point (2,3) is: **[2012]**

(a) $\frac{10}{3}$ (b) $\frac{3}{5}$

(c) $\frac{6}{5}$ (d) $\frac{5}{3}$

32. The number of common tangents of the circles given by $x^2 + y^2 - 8x - 2y + 1 = 0$ and $x^2 + y^2 + 6x + 8y = 0$ is **[Online May 26, 2012]**

(a) one (b) four

(c) two (d) three

33. If the line $y = mx + 1$ meets the circle $x^2 + y^2 + 3x = 0$ in two points equidistant from and on opposite sides of x-axis, then **[Online May 19, 2012]**

(a) $3m + 2 = 0$ (b) $3m - 2 = 0$

(c) $2m + 3 = 0$ (d) $2m - 3 = 0$

34. If three distinct points A, B, C are given in the 2-dimensional coordinate plane such that the ratio of the distance of each one of them from the point (1, 0) to the distance from (– 1, 0) is equal to $\frac{1}{2}$, then the circumcentre of the triangle ABC is at the point **[Online May 19, 2012]**

(a) $\left(\frac{5}{3}, 0\right)$ (b) (0, 0)

(c) $\left(\frac{1}{3}, 0\right)$ (d) (3, 0)

35. The equation of the circle passing through the point (1, 2) and through the points of intersection of $x^2 + y^2 - 4x - 6y - 21 = 0$ and $3x + 4y + 5 = 0$ is given by **[Online May 7, 2012]**

(a) $x^2 + y^2 + 2x + 2y + 11 = 0$

(b) $x^2 + y^2 - 2x + 2y - 7 = 0$

(c) $x^2 + y^2 + 2x - 2y - 3 = 0$

(d) $x^2 + y^2 + 2x + 2y - 11 = 0$

36. The equation of the circle passing through the point (1, 0) and (0, 1) and having the smallest radius is - **[2011 RS]**

(a) $x^2 + y^2 - 2x - 2y + 1 = 0$

(b) $x^2 + y^2 - x - y = 0$

(c) $x^2 + y^2 + 2x + 2y - 7 = 0$

(d) $x^2 + y^2 + x + y - 2 = 0$

37. The two circles $x^2 + y^2 = ax$ and $x^2 + y^2 = c^2$ $(c > 0)$ touch each other if **[2011]**

(a) $|a| = c$ (b) $a = 2c$

(c) $|a| = 2c$ (d) $2|a| = c$

38. The circle $x^2 + y^2 = 4x + 8y + 5$ intersects the line $3x - 4y = m$ at two distinct points if **[2010]**

(a) $-35 < m < 15$ (b) $15 < m < 65$

(c) $35 < m < 85$ (d) $-85 < m < -35$

39. If P and Q are the points of intersection of the circles $x^2 + y^2 + 3x + 7y + 2p - 5 = 0$ and $x^2 + y^2 + 2x + 2y - p^2 = 0$ then there is a circle passing through P, Q and (1, 1) for: **[2009]**

(a) all except one value of p

(b) all except two values of p

(c) exactly one value of p

(d) all values of p

40. Three distinct points A, B and C are given in the 2-dimensional coordinates plane such that the ratio of the distance of any one of them from the point (1, 0) to the distance from the point (–1, 0) is equal to $\frac{1}{3}$. Then the circumcentre of the triangle ABC is at the point: **[2009]**

(a) $\left(\frac{5}{4}, 0\right)$ (b) $\left(\frac{5}{2}, 0\right)$

(c) $\left(\frac{5}{3}, 0\right)$ (d) (0, 0)

41. The point diametrically opposite to the point $P(1, 0)$ on the circle $x^2 + y^2 + 2x + 4y - 3 = 0$ is **[2008]**

(a) $(3, -4)$ (b) $(-3, 4)$

(c) $(-3, -4)$ (d) $(3, 4)$

42. Consider a family of circles which are passing through the point (– 1, 1) and are tangent to x-axis. If (h, k) are the coordinate of the centre of the circles, then the set of values of k is given by the interval **[2007]**

(a) $-\frac{1}{2} \le k \le \frac{1}{2}$ (b) $k \le \frac{1}{2}$

(c) $0 \le k \le \frac{1}{2}$ (d) $k \ge \frac{1}{2}$

43. Let C be the circle with centre (0, 0) and radius 3 units. The equation of the locus of the mid points of the chords of the circle C that subtend an angle of $\frac{2\pi}{3}$ at its center is

(a) $x^2 + y^2 = \frac{3}{2}$ (b) $x^2 + y^2 = 1$ **[2006]**

(c) $x^2 + y^2 = \frac{27}{4}$ (d) $x^2 + y^2 = \frac{9}{4}$

44. If the lines $3x - 4y - 7 = 0$ and $2x - 3y - 5 = 0$ are two diameters of a circle of area 49π square units, the equation of the circle is **[2006]**

(a) $x^2 + y^2 + 2x - 2y - 47 = 0$

(b) $x^2 + y^2 + 2x - 2y - 62 = 0$

(c) $x^2 + y^2 - 2x + 2y - 62 = 0$

(d) $x^2 + y^2 - 2x + 2y - 47 = 0$

45. If a circle passes through the point (a, b) and cuts the circle $x^2 + y^2 = p^2$ orthogonally, then the equation of the locus of its centre is **[2005]**

(a) $x^2 + y^2 - 3ax - 4by + (a^2 + b^2 - p^2) = 0$

(b) $2ax + 2by - (a^2 - b^2 + p^2) = 0$

(c) $x^2 + y^2 - 2ax - 3by + (a^2 - b^2 - p^2) = 0$

(d) $2ax + 2by - (a^2 + b^2 + p^2) = 0$

46. If the pair of lines $ax^2 + 2(a + b)xy + by^2 = 0$ lie along diameters of a circle and divide the circle into four sectors such that the area of one of the sectors is thrice the area of another sector then **[2005]**

(a) $3a^2 - 10ab + 3b^2 = 0$

(b) $3a^2 - 2ab + 3b^2 = 0$

(c) $3a^2 + 10ab + 3b^2 = 0$

(d) $3a^2 + 2ab + 3b^2 = 0$

47. If the circles $x^2 + y^2 + 2ax + cy + a = 0$ and $x^2 + y^2 - 3ax + dy - 1 = 0$ intersect in two distinct points P and Q then the line $5x + by - a = 0$ passes through P and Q for **[2005]**

(a) exactly one value of a

(b) no value of a

(c) infinitely many values of a

(d) exactly two values of a

48. If a circle passes through the point (a, b) and cuts the circle $x^2 + y^2 = 4$ orthogonally, then the locus of its centre is **[2004]**

(a) $2ax - 2by - (a^2 + b^2 + 4) = 0$

(b) $2ax + 2by - (a^2 + b^2 + 4) = 0$

(c) $2ax - 2by + (a^2 + b^2 + 4) = 0$

(d) $2ax + 2by + (a^2 + b^2 + 4) = 0$

49. A variable circle passes through the fixed point $A(p, q)$ and touches x-axis. The locus of the other end of the diameter through A is **[2004]**

(a) $(y - q)^2 = 4px$ (b) $(x - q)^2 = 4py$

(c) $(y - p)^2 = 4qx$ (d) $(x - p)^2 = 4qy$

50. If the lines $2x + 3y + 1 = 0$ and $3x - y - 4 = 0$ lie along diameter of a circle of circumference 10π, then the equation of the circle is **[2004]**

(a) $x^2 + y^2 + 2x - 2y - 23 = 0$

(b) $x^2 + y^2 - 2x - 2y - 23 = 0$

(c) $x^2 + y^2 + 2x + 2y - 23 = 0$

(d) $x^2 + y^2 - 2x + 2y - 23 = 0$

51. Intercept on the line $y = x$ by the circle $x^2 + y^2 - 2x = 0$ is AB. Equation of the circle on AB as a diameter is **[2004]**

(a) $x^2 + y^2 + x - y = 0$ (b) $x^2 + y^2 - x + y = 0$

(c) $x^2 + y^2 + x + y = 0$ (d) $x^2 + y^2 - x - y = 0$

52. If the two circles $(x - 1)^2 + (y - 3)^2 = r^2$ and $x^2 + y^2 - 8x + 2y + 8 = 0$ intersect in two distinct point, then **[2003]**

(a) $r > 2$ (b) $2 < r < 8$

(c) $r < 2$ (d) $r = 2$.

53. The lines $2x - 3y = 5$ and $3x - 4y = 7$ are diameters of a circle having area as 154 sq.units. Then the equation of the circle is **[2003]**

(a) $x^2 + y^2 - 2x + 2y = 62$ (b) $x^2 + y^2 + 2x - 2y = 62$

(c) $x^2 + y^2 + 2x - 2y = 47$ (d) $x^2 + y^2 - 2x + 2y = 47$.

54. If the chord $y = mx + 1$ of the circle $x^2+y^2=1$ subtends an angle of measure 45° at the major segment of the circle then value of m is **[2002]**

(a) $2 \pm \sqrt{2}$ (b) $-2 \pm \sqrt{2}$

(c) $-1 \pm \sqrt{2}$ (d) none of these

55. The centres of a set of circles, each of radius 3, lie on the circle $x^2+y^2=25$. The locus of any point in the set is **[2002]**

(a) $4 \le x^2+y^2 \le 64$ (b) $x^2+y^2 \le 25$

(c) $x^2+y^2 \ge 25$ (d) $3 \le x^2+y^2 \le 9$

56. The centre of the circle passing through (0, 0) and (1, 0) and touching the circle $x^2+y^2=9$ is **[2002]**

(a) $\left(\frac{1}{2},\frac{1}{2}\right)$ (b) $\left(\frac{1}{2},-\sqrt{2}\right)$

(c) $\left(\frac{3}{2},\frac{1}{2}\right)$ (d) $\left(\frac{1}{2},\frac{3}{2}\right)$

57. The equation of a circle with origin as a centre and passing through equilateral triangle whose median is of length $3a$ is **[2002]**

(a) $x^2+y^2=9a^2$ (b) $x^2+y^2=16a^2$

(c) $x^2+y^2=4a^2$ (d) $x^2+y^2=a^2$

TOPIC-2 : Parabola

58. If $y = mx + c$ is the normal at a point on the parabola $y^2 = 8x$ whose focal distance is 8 units, then |c| is equal to : **[Online April 9, 2017]**

(a) $2\sqrt{3}$ (b) $8\sqrt{3}$

(c) $10\sqrt{3}$ (d) $16\sqrt{3}$

59. If the common tangents to the parabola, $x^2 = 4y$ and the circle, $x^2 + y^2 = 4$ intersect at the point P, then the distance of P from the origin, is : **[Online April 8, 2017]**

(a) $\sqrt{2}+1$ (b) $2(3+2\sqrt{2})$

(c) $2(\sqrt{2}+1)$ (d) $3+2\sqrt{2}$

60. Let P be the point on the parabola, $y^2 = 8x$ which is at a minimum distance from the centre C of the circle, $x^2 + (y + 6)^2 = 1$. Then the equation of the circle, passing through C and having its centre at P is: **[2016]**

(a) $x^2+y^2-\frac{x}{4}+2y-24=0$

(b) $x^2+y^2-4x+9y+18=0$

(c) $x^2+y^2-4x+8y+12=0$

(d) $x^2+y^2-x+4y-12=0$

61. P and Q are two distinct points on the parabola, $y^2 = 4x$, with parameters t and t_1 respectively. If the normal at P passes through Q, then the minimum value of t_1^2 is : **[Online April 10, 2016]**

(a) 8 (b) 4

(c) 6 (d) 2

62. Let O be the vertex and Q be any point on the parabola, $x^2 = 8y$. If the point P divides the line segment OQ internally in the ratio 1 : 3, then locus of P is : **[2015]**

(a) $y^2 = 2x$ (b) $x^2 = 2y$

(c) $x^2 = y$ (d) $y^2 = x$

63. Let PQ be a double ordinate of the parabola, $y^2 = -4x$, where P lies in the second quadrant. If R divides PQ in the ratio 2 : 1 then the locus of R is : **[Online April 11, 2015]**

(a) $3y^2 = -2x$ (b) $3y^2 = 2x$

(c) $9y^2 = 4x$ (d) $9y^2 = -4x$

64. The slope of the line touching both the parabolas $y^2 = 4x$ and $x^2 = -32y$ is **[2014]**

(a) $\frac{1}{8}$ (b) $\frac{2}{3}$

(c) $\frac{1}{2}$ (d) $\frac{3}{2}$

65. A chord is drawn through the focus of the parabola $y^2 = 6x$ such that its distance from the vertex of this parabola is $\frac{\sqrt{5}}{2}$, then its slope can be: **[Online April 19, 2014]**

(a) $\frac{\sqrt{5}}{2}$ (b) $\frac{\sqrt{3}}{2}$

(c) $\frac{2}{\sqrt{5}}$ (d) $\frac{2}{\sqrt{3}}$

66. Two tangents are drawn from a point (– 2, – 1) to the curve, $y^2 = 4x$. If α is the angle between them, then |tan α| is equal to: **[Online April 12, 2014]**

(a) $\frac{1}{3}$ (b) $\frac{1}{\sqrt{3}}$

(c) $\sqrt{3}$ (d) 3

67. Let L_1 be the length of the common chord of the curves $x^2 + y^2 = 9$ and $y^2 = 8x$, and L_2 be the length of the latus rectum of $y^2 = 8x$, then: **[Online April 11, 2014]**

(a) $L_1 > L_2$ (b) $L_1 = L_2$

(c) $L_1 < L_2$ (d) $\frac{L_1}{L_2} = \sqrt{2}$

68. **Given :** A circle, $2x^2 + 2y^2 = 5$ and a parabola, $y^2 = 4\sqrt{5}x$.

Statement-1 : An equation of a common tangent to these curves is $y = x + \sqrt{5}$.

Statement-2 : If the line, $y = mx + \frac{\sqrt{5}}{m}$ $(m \ne 0)$ is their common tangent, then m satisfies $m^4 - 3m^2 + 2 = 0$. **[2013]**

(a) Statement-1 is true; Statement-2 is true; Statement-2 is a correct explanation for Statement-1.
(b) Statement-1 is true; Statement-2 is true; Statement-2 is not a correct explanation for Statement-1.
(c) Statement-1 is true; Statement-2 is false.
(d) Statement-1 is false; Statement-2 is true.

69. The point of intersection of the normals to the parabola $y^2 = 4x$ at the ends of its latus rectum is : **[Online April 23, 2013]**
(a) $(0,2)$ (b) $(3,0)$
(c) $(0,3)$ (d) $(2,0)$

70. **Statement-1:** The line $x - 2y = 2$ meets the parabola, $y^2 + 2x = 0$ only at the point $(-2, -2)$.

Statement-2: The line $y = mx - \frac{1}{2m} (m \neq 0)$ is tangent to the parabola, $y^2 = -2x$ at the point $\left(-\frac{1}{2m^2}, -\frac{1}{m}\right)$.
[Online April 22, 2013]
(a) Statement-1 is true; Statement-2 is false.
(b) Statement-1 is true; Statement-2 is true; Statement-2 is a correct explanation for statement-1.
(c) Statement-1 is false; Statement-2 is true.
(d) Statement-1 a true; Statement-2 is true; Statement-2 is **not** a correct explanation for statement-1.

71. The normal at $\left(2, \frac{3}{2}\right)$ to the ellipse, $\frac{x^2}{16} + \frac{y^2}{3} = 1$ touches a parabola, whose equation is **[Online May 26, 2012]**
(a) $y^2 = -104x$ (b) $y^2 = 14x$
(c) $y^2 = 26x$ (d) $y^2 = -14x$

72. The chord PQ of the parabola $y^2 = x$, where one end P of the chord is at point $(4, -2)$, is perpendicular to the axis of the parabola. Then the slope of the normal at Q is **[Online May 26, 2012]**
(a) -4 (b) $-\frac{1}{4}$
(c) 4 (d) $\frac{1}{4}$

73. **Statement 1:** $y = mx - \frac{1}{m}$ is always a tangent to the parabola, $y^2 = -4x$ for all non-zero values of m.
Statement 2: Every tangent to the parabola, $y^2 = -4x$ will meet its axis at a point whose abscissa is non-negative.
[Online May 7, 2012]
(a) Statement 1 is true, Statement 2 is true; Statement 2 is a correct explanation of Statement 1.
(b) Statement 1 is false, Statement 2 is true.
(c) Statement 1 is true, Statement 2 is false.
(d) Statement 1 is true, Statement 2 is true, Statement 2 is not a correct explanation of Statement 1.

74. The shortest distance between line $y - x = 1$ and curve $x = y^2$ is **[2011]**
(a) $\frac{3\sqrt{2}}{8}$ (b) $\frac{8}{3\sqrt{2}}$
(c) $\frac{4}{\sqrt{3}}$ (d) $\frac{\sqrt{3}}{4}$

75. If two tangents drawn from a point P to the parabola $y^2 = 4x$ are at right angles, then the locus of P is **[2010]**
(a) $2x + 1 = 0$ (b) $x = -1$
(c) $2x - 1 = 0$ (d) $x = 1$

76. A parabola has the origin as its focus and the line $x = 2$ as the directrix. Then the vertex of the parabola is at **[2008]**
(a) $(0,2)$ (b) $(1,0)$
(c) $(0,1)$ (d) $(2,0)$

77. The equation of a tangent to the parabola $y^2 = 8x$ is $y = x + 2$. The point on this line from which the other tangent to the parabola is perpendicular to the given tangent is **[2007]**
(a) $(2,4)$ (b) $(-2,0)$
(c) $(-1,1)$ (d) $(0,2)$

78. The locus of the vertices of the family of parabolas $y = \frac{a^3x^2}{3} + \frac{a^2x}{2} - 2a$ is **[2006]**
(a) $xy = \frac{105}{64}$ (b) $xy = \frac{3}{4}$
(c) $xy = \frac{35}{16}$ (d) $xy = \frac{64}{105}$

79. Let P be the point $(1, 0)$ and Q a point on the locus $y^2 = 8x$. The locus of mid point of PQ is **[2005]**
(a) $y^2 - 4x + 2 = 0$ (b) $y^2 + 4x + 2 = 0$
(c) $x^2 + 4y + 2 = 0$ (d) $x^2 - 4y + 2 = 0$

80. A circle touches the x- axis and also touches the circle with centre at (0,3) and radius 2. The locus of the centre of the circle is **[2005]**
(a) an ellipse (b) a circle
(c) a hyperbola (d) a parabola

81. If $a \neq 0$ and the line $2bx + 3cy + 4d = 0$ passes through the points of intersection of the parabolas $y^2 = 4ax$ and $x^2 = 4ay$, then **[2004]**
(a) $d^2 + (3b - 2c)^2 = 0$ (b) $d^2 + (3b + 2c)^2 = 0$
(c) $d^2 + (2b - 3c)^2 = 0$ (d) $d^2 + (2b + 3c)^2 = 0$

82. The normal at the point $(bt_1^2, 2bt_1)$ on a parabola meets the parabola again in the point $(bt_2^2, 2bt_2)$, then **[2003]**
(a) $t_2 = t_1 + \frac{2}{t_1}$ (b) $t_2 = -t_1 - \frac{2}{t_1}$
(c) $t_2 = -t_1 + \frac{2}{t_1}$ (d) $t_2 = t_1 - \frac{2}{t_1}$

83. Two common tangents to the circle $x^2+y^2=2a^2$ and parabola $y^2=8ax$ are [2002]

(a) $x=\pm(y+2a)$ (b) $y=\pm(x+2a)$

(c) $x=\pm(y+a)$ (d) $y=\pm(x+a)$

TOPIC-3 : Ellipse

84. The eccentricity of an ellipse having centre at the origin, axes along the co-ordinate axes and passing through the points (4, –1) and (–2, 2) is : [Online April 9, 2017]

(a) $\frac{1}{2}$ (b) $\frac{2}{\sqrt{5}}$

(c) $\frac{\sqrt{3}}{2}$ (d) $\frac{\sqrt{3}}{4}$

85. Consider an ellipse, whose centre is at the origin and its major axis is along the x–axis. If its eccentricity is $\frac{3}{5}$ and the distance between its foci is 6, then the area (in sq. units) of the quadrilateral inscribed in the ellipse, with the vertices as the vertices of the ellipse, is : [Online April 8, 2017]

(a) 8 (b) 32

(c) 80 (d) 40

86. If the tangent at a point on the ellipse $\frac{x^2}{27}+\frac{y^2}{3}=1$ meets the coordinate axes at A and B, and O is the origin, then the minimum area (in sq. units) of the triangle OAB is : [Online April 9, 2016]

(a) $3\sqrt{3}$ (b) $\frac{9}{2}$

(c) 9 (d) $\frac{9}{\sqrt{3}}$

87. The area (in sq. units) of the quadrilateral formed by the tangents at the end points of the latera recta to the ellipse $\frac{x^2}{9}+\frac{y^2}{5}=1$, is : (2015)

(a) $\frac{27}{2}$ (b) 27

(c) $\frac{27}{4}$ (d) 18

88. If the distance between the foci of an ellipse is half the length of its latus rectum, then the eccentricity of the ellipse is: [Online April 11, 2015]

(a) $\frac{2\sqrt{2}-1}{2}$ (b) $\sqrt{2}-1$

(c) $\frac{1}{2}$ (d) $\frac{\sqrt{2}-1}{2}$

89. The locus of the foot of perpendicular drawn from the centre of the ellipse $x^2+3y^2=6$ on any tangent to it is [2014]

(a) $\left(x^2+y^2\right)^2=6x^2+2y^2$

(b) $\left(x^2+y^2\right)^2=6x^2-2y^2$

(c) $\left(x^2-y^2\right)^2=6x^2+2y^2$

(d) $\left(x^2-y^2\right)^2=6x^2-2y^2$

90. A stair-case of length l rests against a vertical wall and a floor of a room. Let P be a point on the stair-case, nearer to its end on the wall, that divides its length in the ratio 1 : 2. If the stair-case begins to slide on the floor, then the locus of P is: [Online April 11, 2014]

(a) an ellipse of eccentricity $\frac{1}{2}$

(b) an ellipse of eccentricity $\frac{\sqrt{3}}{2}$

(c) a circle of radius $\frac{1}{2}$

(d) a circle of radius $\frac{\sqrt{3}}{2}l$

91. If OB is the semi-minor axis of an ellipse, F_1 and F_2 are its foci and the angle between F_1B and F_2B is a right angle, then the square of the eccentricity of the ellipse is: [Online April 9, 2014]

(a) $\frac{1}{2}$ (b) $\frac{1}{\sqrt{2}}$

(c) $\frac{1}{2\sqrt{2}}$ (d) $\frac{1}{4}$

92. The equation of the circle passing through the foci of the ellipse $\frac{x^2}{16}+\frac{y^2}{9}=1$, and having centre at (0, 3) is [2013]

(a) $x^2+y^2-6y-7=0$

(b) $x^2+y^2-6y+7=0$

(c) $x^2+y^2-6y-5=0$

(d) $x^2+y^2-6y+5=0$

93. A point on the ellipse, $4x^2+9y^2=36$, where the normal is parallel to the line, $4x-2y-5=0$, is : [Online April 25, 2013]

(a) $\left(\frac{9}{5},\frac{8}{5}\right)$ (b) $\left(\frac{8}{5},-\frac{9}{5}\right)$

(c) $\left(-\frac{9}{5},\frac{8}{5}\right)$ (d) $\left(\frac{8}{5},\frac{9}{5}\right)$

94. Let the equations of two ellipses be

$$E_1 : \frac{x^2}{3} + \frac{y^2}{2} = 1 \text{ and } E_2 : \frac{x^2}{16} + \frac{y^2}{b^2} = 1,$$

If the product of their eccentricities is $\frac{1}{2}$, then the length of the minor axis of ellipse E_2 is : **[Online April 22, 2013]**

(a) 8 (b) 9
(c) 4 (d) 2

95. Equation of the line passing through the points of intersection of the parabola $x^2 = 8y$ and the ellipse $\frac{x^2}{3} + y^2 = 1$ is : **[Online April 9, 2013]**

(a) $y - 3 = 0$ (b) $y + 3 = 0$
(c) $3y + 1 = 0$ (d) $3y - 1 = 0$

96. If P_1 and P_2 are two points on the ellipse $\frac{x^2}{4} + y^2 = 1$ at which the tangents are parallel to the chord joining the points (0, 1) and (2, 0), then the distance between P_1 and P_2 is **[Online May 12, 2012]**

(a) $2\sqrt{2}$ (b) $\sqrt{5}$
(c) $2\sqrt{3}$ (d) $\sqrt{10}$

97. Equation of the ellipse whose axes are the axes of coordinates and which passes through the point (–3, 1) and has eccentricity $\sqrt{\frac{2}{5}}$ is **[2011]**

(a) $5x^2 + 3y^2 - 48 = 0$ (b) $3x^2 + 5y^2 - 15 = 0$
(c) $5x^2 + 3y^2 - 32 = 0$ (d) $3x^2 + 5y^2 - 32 = 0$

98. The ellipse $x^2 + 4y^2 = 4$ is inscribed in a rectangle aligned with the coordinate axes, which in turn is inscribed in another ellipse that passes through the point (4, 0). Then the equation of the ellipse is : **[2009]**

(a) $x^2 + 12y^2 = 16$ (b) $4x^2 + 48y^2 = 48$
(c) $4x^2 + 64y^2 = 48$ (d) $x^2 + 16y^2 = 16$

99. A focus of an ellipse is at the origin. The directrix is the line $x = 4$ and the eccentricity is $\frac{1}{2}$. Then the length of the semi-major axis is **[2008]**

(a) $\frac{8}{3}$ (b) $\frac{2}{3}$ (c) $\frac{4}{3}$ (d) $\frac{5}{3}$

100. In an ellipse, the distance between its foci is 6 and minor axis is 8. Then its eccentricity is **[2006]**

(a) $\frac{3}{5}$ (b) $\frac{1}{2}$
(c) $\frac{4}{5}$ (d) $\frac{1}{\sqrt{5}}$

101. An ellipse has OB as semi minor axis, F and F' its focii and the angle FBF' is a right angle. Then the eccentricity of the ellipse is **[2005]**

(a) $\frac{1}{\sqrt{2}}$ (b) $\frac{1}{2}$
(c) $\frac{1}{4}$ (d) $\frac{1}{\sqrt{3}}$

102. The eccentricity of an ellipse, with its centre at the origin, is $\frac{1}{2}$. If one of the directrices is $x = 4$, then the equation of the ellipse is: **[2004]**

(a) $4x^2 + 3y^2 = 1$ (b) $3x^2 + 4y^2 = 12$
(c) $4x^2 + 3y^2 = 12$ (d) $3x^2 + 4y^2 = 1$

TOPIC-4 : Hyperbola

103. A hyperbola passes through the point $P(\sqrt{2}, \sqrt{3})$ and has foci at (± 2, 0). Then the tangent to this hyperbola at P also passes through the point : **[2017]**

(a) $(-\sqrt{2}, -\sqrt{3})$ (b) $(3\sqrt{2}, 2\sqrt{3})$
(c) $(2\sqrt{2}, 3\sqrt{3})$ (d) $(\sqrt{3}, \sqrt{2})$

104. The locus of the point of intersection of the straight lines,
$tx - 2y - 3t = 0$
$x - 2ty + 3 = 0$ ($t \in R$), is : **[Online April 8, 2017]**

(a) an ellipse with eccentricity $\frac{2}{\sqrt{5}}$
(b) an ellipse with the length of major axis 6
(c) a hyperbola with eccentricity $\sqrt{5}$
(d) a hyperbola with the length of conjugate axis 3

105. The eccentricity of the hyperbola whose length of the latus rectum is equal to 8 and the length of its conjugate axis is equal to half of the distance between its foci, is : **[2016]**

(a) $\frac{2}{\sqrt{3}}$ (b) $\sqrt{3}$
(c) $\frac{4}{3}$ (d) $\frac{4}{\sqrt{3}}$

106. A hyperbola whose transverse axis is along the major axis of the conic, $\frac{x^2}{3} + \frac{y^2}{4} = 4$ and has vertices at the foci of this conic. If the eccentricity of the hyperbola is $\frac{3}{2}$, then which of the following points does NOT lie on it ? **[Online April 10, 2016]**

(a) $(\sqrt{5}, 2\sqrt{2})$ (b) (0, 2)
(c) $(5, 2\sqrt{3})$ (d) $(\sqrt{10}, 2\sqrt{3})$

107. Let a aand b respectively be the semitransverse and semi-conjugate axes of a hyperbola whose eccentricity satisfies the equation $9e^2 - 18e + 5 = 0$. If S(5, 0) is a focus and $5x = 9$ is the corresponding directrix of this hyperbola, then $a^2 - b^2$ is equal to : **[Online April 9, 2016]**

(a) –7 (b) –5
(c) 5 (d) 7

108. An ellipse passes through the foci of the hyperbola, $9x^2 - 4y^2 = 36$ and its major and minor axes lie along the transverse and conjugate axes of the hyperbola respectively. If the product of eccentricities of the two conics is $\frac{1}{2}$, then which of the following points **does not** lie on the ellipse? **[Online April 10, 2015]**

(a) $\left(\sqrt{\frac{13}{2}}, \sqrt{6}\right)$ (b) $\left(\frac{\sqrt{39}}{2}, \sqrt{3}\right)$

(c) $\left(\frac{1}{2}\sqrt{13}, \frac{\sqrt{3}}{2}\right)$ (d) $\left(\sqrt{13}, 0\right)$

109. The tangent at an extremity (in the first quadrant) of latus rectum of the hyperbola $\frac{x^2}{4} - \frac{y^2}{5} = 1$, meet x-axis and y-axis at A and B respectively. Then $(OA)^2 - (OB)^2$, where O is the origin, equals: **[Online April 19, 2014]**

(a) $-\frac{20}{9}$ (b) $\frac{16}{9}$

(c) 4 (d) $-\frac{4}{3}$

110. Let P (3 sec θ, 2 tan θ) and Q (3 sec ϕ, 2 tan ϕ) where $\theta + \phi = \frac{\pi}{2}$, be two distinct points on the hyperbola $\frac{x^2}{9} - \frac{y^2}{4} = 1$. Then the ordinate of the point of intersection of the normals at P and Q is: **[Online April 11, 2014]**

(a) $\frac{11}{3}$ (b) $-\frac{11}{3}$

(c) $\frac{13}{2}$ (d) $-\frac{13}{2}$

111. A common tangent to the conics $x^2 = 6y$ and $2x^2 - 4y^2 = 9$ is: **[Online April 25, 2013]**

(a) $x - y = \frac{3}{2}$ (b) $x + y = 1$

(c) $x + y = \frac{9}{2}$ (d) $x - y = 1$

112. A tangent to the hyperbola $\frac{x^2}{4} - \frac{y^2}{2} = 1$ meets x-axis at P and y-axis at Q. Lines PR and QR are drawn such that OPRQ is a rectangle (where O is the origin). Then R lies on : **[Online April 23, 2013]**

(a) $\frac{4}{x^2} + \frac{2}{y^2} = 1$ (b) $\frac{2}{x^2} - \frac{4}{y^2} = 1$

(c) $\frac{2}{x^2} + \frac{4}{y^2} = 1$ (d) $\frac{4}{x^2} - \frac{2}{y^2} = 1$

113. If the foci of the ellipse $\frac{x^2}{16} + \frac{y^2}{b^2} = 1$ coincide with the foci of the hyperbola $\frac{x^2}{144} - \frac{y^2}{81} = \frac{1}{25}$, then b^2 is equal to **[Online May 19, 2012]**

(a) 8 (b) 10
(c) 7 (d) 9

114. If the eccentricity of a hyperbola $\frac{x^2}{9} - \frac{y^2}{b^2} = 1$, which passes through $(k, 2)$, is $\frac{\sqrt{13}}{3}$, then the value of k^2 is **[Online May 7, 2012]**

(a) 18 (b) 8
(c) 1 (d) 2

115. The equation of the hyperbola whose foci are (– 2, 0) and (2, 0) and eccentricity is 2 is given by : **[2011RS]**

(a) $x^2 - 3y^2 = 3$ (b) $3x^2 - y^2 = 3$
(c) $-x^2 + 3y^2 = 3$ (d) $-3x^2 + y^2 = 3$

116. For the Hyperbola $\frac{x^2}{\cos^2\alpha} - \frac{y^2}{\sin^2\alpha} = 1$, which of the following remains constant when α varies = ? **[2007]**

(a) abscissae of vertices (b) abscissae of foci
(c) eccentricity (d) directrix.

117. The locus of a point $P(\alpha, \beta)$ moving under the condition that the line $y = \alpha x + \beta$ is a tangent to the hyperbola $\frac{x^2}{a^2} - \frac{y^2}{b^2} = 1$ is **[2005]**

(a) an ellipse (b) a circle
(c) a parabola (d) a hyperbola

118. The foci of the ellipse $\frac{x^2}{16} + \frac{y^2}{b^2} = 1$ and the hyperbola $\frac{x^2}{144} - \frac{y^2}{81} = \frac{1}{25}$ coincide. Then the value of b^2 is **[2003]**

(a) 9 (b) 1
(c) 5 (d) 7

Hints & Solutions

1. **(None)**

(Let the equation of circle be

$x^2 + (y-k)^2 = r^2$

It touches $x - y = 0$

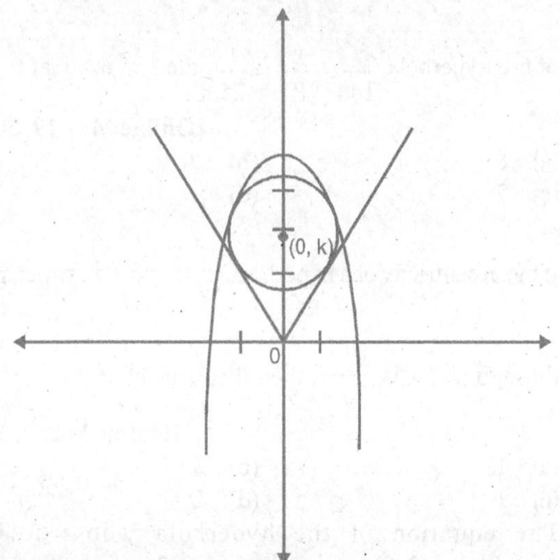

$\Rightarrow \left|\frac{0-k}{\sqrt{2}}\right| = r$

$\Rightarrow k = r\sqrt{2}$

$\therefore$ Equation of circle becomes

$x^2 + (y-k)^2 = \frac{k^2}{2}$ ...(i)

It touches $y = 4 - x^2$ as well

$\therefore$ Solving the two equations

$\Rightarrow 4 - y + (y-k)^2 = \frac{k^2}{2}$

$\Rightarrow y^2 - y(2k+1) + \frac{k^2}{2} + 4 = 0$

It will give equal roots $\therefore D = 0$

$\Rightarrow (2k+1)^2 = 4\left(\frac{k^2}{2} + 4\right)$

$\Rightarrow 2k^2 + 4k - 15 = 0$

$\Rightarrow k = \frac{-2+\sqrt{34}}{2}$

$\therefore r = \frac{k}{\sqrt{2}} = \frac{-2+\sqrt{34}}{2\sqrt{2}}$

Which is not matching with any of the option given here.

2. **(c)** Let $z = x + y$

$\text{Im}\left[\left(\frac{ix-y-2}{x+(y-1)i}\right)\left(\frac{x-(y-1)i}{x-(y-1)i}\right)\right] + 1 = 0$

On solving, we get:

$2x^2 + 2y^2 - y - 1 = 0$

$\Rightarrow x^2 + y^2 - 1/2y - 1/2 = 0$

$\Rightarrow x^2 + \left(y - \frac{1}{4}\right)^2 = \frac{9}{16}$

$\Rightarrow r = \frac{3}{4}$

3. **(b)** P (4, 7). Here, $x = 4$, $y = 7$

$x - y = -3$

$\therefore PA \times PB = PT^2$

Also; $PT = \sqrt{x^2 + y^2 - (x-y)^2}$

$\Rightarrow PT = \sqrt{16+49-9} = \sqrt{56}$

$\Rightarrow PT^2 = 56 \therefore PA \times PB = 56$

4. **(c)**

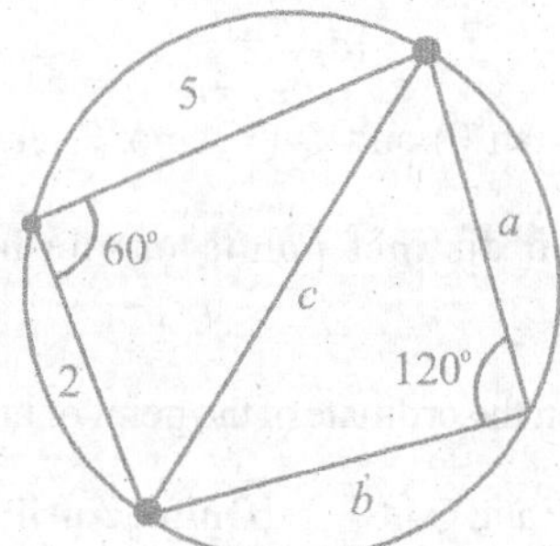

Here; $\cos\theta = \frac{a^2+b^2-c^2}{2ab}$

and $\theta = 60^\circ$

$\Rightarrow \cos 60^\circ = \frac{4+25-c^2}{2.2.5}$

$\Rightarrow 10 = 29 - c^2$

$\Rightarrow c^2 = 19$

$\Rightarrow \boxed{c = \sqrt{19}}$

also; $\cos\theta = \frac{a^2+b^2-c^2}{2ab}$

and $\theta = 120^\circ$

$\Rightarrow -\frac{1}{2} = \frac{a^2+b^2-19}{2ab}$

$\Rightarrow a^2 + b^2 - 19 = -ab$

$\Rightarrow a^2 + b^2 + ab = 19$

$\therefore$ Area $= \frac{1}{2} \times 2 \times 5 \sin 60 + \frac{1}{2} ab \sin 120^\circ = 4\sqrt{3}$

$\Rightarrow \frac{5\sqrt{3}}{2} + \frac{ab\sqrt{3}}{4} = 4\sqrt{3}$

$\Rightarrow \frac{ab}{4} = 4 - \frac{5}{2} = \frac{3}{2}$

$\Rightarrow \boxed{ab = 6}$

$\therefore a^2 + b^2 = 13$

$\Rightarrow a = 2, b = 3$

Perimeter = Sum of all sides

$= 2 + 5 + 2 + 3 = 12$

5. **(a)** Let $z = x + iy$

$\Rightarrow 2|x + i(y+3)| = |x + i(y-1)|$

$\Rightarrow 2\sqrt{x^2+(y+3)^2} = \sqrt{x^2+(y-1)^2}$

$\Rightarrow 4x^2 + 4(y+3)^2 = x^2 + (y-1)^2$

$\Rightarrow 3x^2 = y^2 - 2y + 1 - 4y^2 - 24y - 36$

$\Rightarrow 3x^2 + 3y^2 + 26y + 35 = 0$ (which is a circle)

$\Rightarrow x^2 + y^2 + \frac{26}{3}y + \frac{35}{3} = 0$

$\Rightarrow r = \sqrt{0 + \frac{169}{9} - \frac{35}{3}}$

$\Rightarrow r = \sqrt{\frac{64}{9}} = \frac{8}{3}$

6. **(b)**

Given that $x^2 + y^2 - 5x - y + 5 = 0$

$\Rightarrow (x - 5/2)^2 - \frac{25}{4} + (y - 1/2)^2 - 1/4 = 0$

$\Rightarrow (x - 5/2)^2 + (y - 1/2)^2 = 3/2$

on circle $\left[Q \equiv \left(5/2 + \sqrt{3/2}\cos Q, \frac{1}{2} + \sqrt{3/2}\sin Q\right)\right]$

$\Rightarrow PQ^2 = \left(\frac{5}{2} + \sqrt{3/2}\cos Q\right)^2 + \left(\frac{5}{2} + \sqrt{3/2}\sin Q\right)^2$

$\Rightarrow PQ^2 = \frac{25}{2} + \frac{3}{2} + 5\sqrt{3/2}(\cos Q + \sin Q)$

$= 14 + 5\sqrt{3/2}\ (\cos Q + \sin Q)$

$\therefore$ Maximum value of PQ^2

$= 14 + 5\sqrt{3/2} \times \sqrt{2} = 14 + 5\sqrt{3}$

7. **(b)**

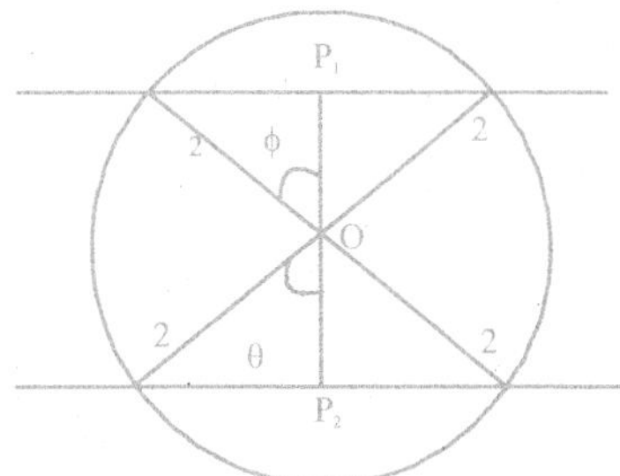

Since $\cos 2\theta = 1/7 \Rightarrow 2\cos^2 Q - 1 = 1/7$

$\Rightarrow 2\cos^2\theta = 8/7$

$\Rightarrow \cos^2\theta = 4/7$

$\Rightarrow \cos^2\theta = \frac{4}{7}$

$\Rightarrow \cos^2\phi = \frac{2}{\sqrt{7}}$

Also, $\sec^2\phi = 7 = \frac{1}{2\cos^2\phi - 1} = 7$

$= \cos^2\phi - 1 = \frac{1}{7}$

$= 2\cos^2\phi = \frac{8}{7}$

$= \cos\phi = \frac{2}{\sqrt{7}}$

$P_1P_2 = r\cos\theta + r\cos\phi$

$= \frac{4}{\sqrt{7}} + \frac{4}{\sqrt{7}} = \frac{8}{\sqrt{7}}$

8. **(d)**

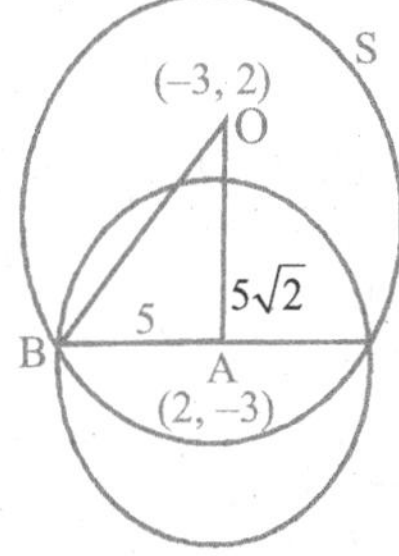

Centre of S : O (–3, 2) centre of given circle A(2, –3)

$\Rightarrow OA = 5\sqrt{2}$

Also AB = 5 ($\because$ AB = r of the given circle)

$\Rightarrow$ Using pythagoras theorem in ΔOAB

$r = 5\sqrt{3}$

9. **(a)** Point of intersection of lines

$x-y=1$ and $2x+y=3$ is $\left(\frac{4}{3},\frac{1}{3}\right)$

$$\text{Slope of OP} = \frac{\frac{1}{3}+1}{\frac{4}{3}-1} = \frac{\frac{4}{3}}{\frac{1}{3}} = 4$$

$$\text{Slope of tangent} = -\frac{1}{4}$$

Equation of tangent $y+1=-\frac{1}{4}(x-1)$

$4y+4=-x+1$

$x+4y+3=0$

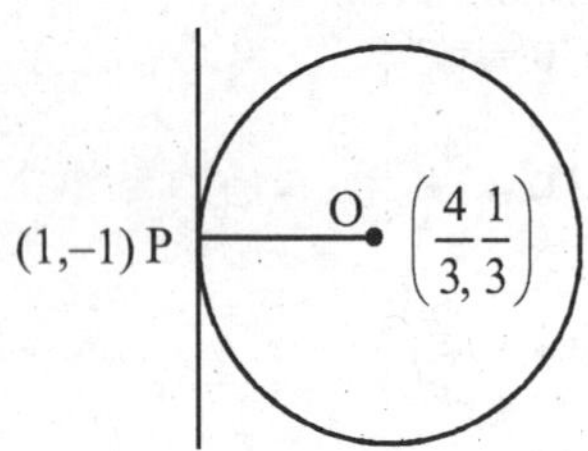

10. **(a)**

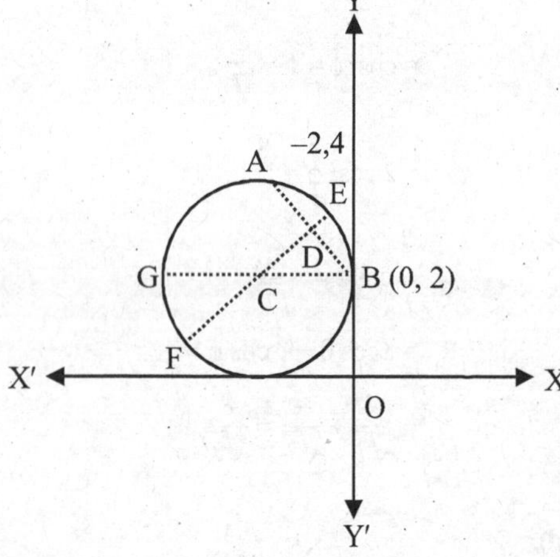

EF = perpendicular bisector of chord AB

BG = perpendicular to y-axis

Here C = centre of the circle

mid-point of chord AB, D = (– 1, 3)

$$\text{slope of AB} = \frac{4-2}{-2-0} = -1$$

$\because$ EF $\perp$ AB

$\therefore$ Slope of EF = 1

Equation of EF, $y-3=1(x+1)$

$\Rightarrow y=x+4$ ...(i)

Equation of BG

$y=2$ ...(ii)

From equations (i) and (ii)

$x=-2, y=2$

since C be the point of intersection of EF and BG, therefore centre, C = (–2, 2)

Now coordinates of centre C satisfy the equation $2x-3y+10=0$

Hence $2x-3y+10=0$ is the equation of the diameter

11. **(a)** Intersection point of $2x-3y+4=0$ and $x-2y+3=0$ is (1, 2)

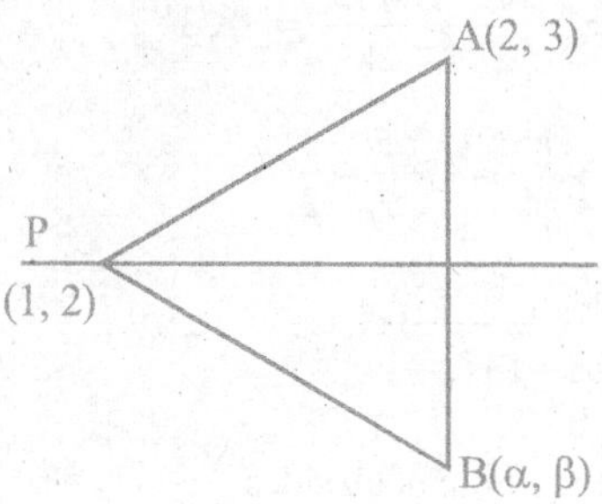

Since, P is the fixed point for given family of lines

So, PB = PA

$(\alpha-1)^2+(\beta-2)^2=(2-1)^2+(3-2)^2$

$(\alpha-1)^2+(\beta-2)^2=1+1=2$

$(x-1)^2+(y-2)^2=(\sqrt{2})^2$

$(x-a)^2+(y-b)^2=r^2$

Therefore, given locus is a circle with centre (1, 2) and radius $\sqrt{2}$.

12. **(a)** $x^2+y^2-4x-6y-12=0$ ...(i)

Centre, $C_1=(2,3)$

Radius, $r_1=5$ units

$x^2+y^2+6x+18y+26=0$ ...(ii)

Centre, $C_2=(-3,-9)$

Radius, $r_2=8$ units

$C_1C_2=\sqrt{(2+3)^2+(3+9)^2}=13$ units

$r_1+r_2=5+8=13$

$\therefore C_1C_2=r_1+r_2$

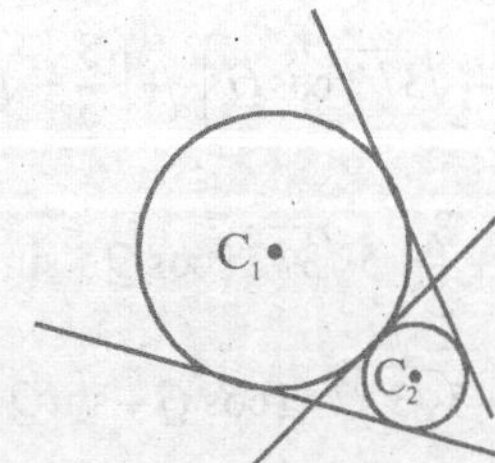

Therefore there are three common tangents.

13. (a) Let radius of circumcircle be
According to the question,

$$\frac{r}{2}=\frac{10}{5}\Rightarrow r=4$$

So equation of required circle is
$(x-1)^2+(y-1)^2=16$
$\Rightarrow x^2+y^2-2x-2y-14=0$

14. (b) Let 'h' be the radius of the circle and since circle touches y–axis at (0, 2) therefore centre = (h, 2)
Now, eqn of circle is
$(h+1)^2+2^2=h^2$
$\Rightarrow 2h+5=0$

$$h=-\frac{5}{2}$$

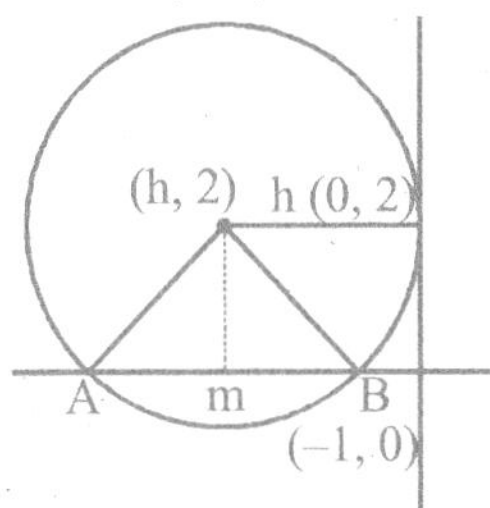

From the figure, it is clear that AB is the chord along x–axis

$$\therefore AB=2(AM)=2\sqrt{\frac{25}{4}-4}=2\left(\frac{3}{2}\right)=3$$

15. (a) $OP=\dfrac{4}{\sin\theta}$

$OB=\dfrac{4}{\cos\theta}$

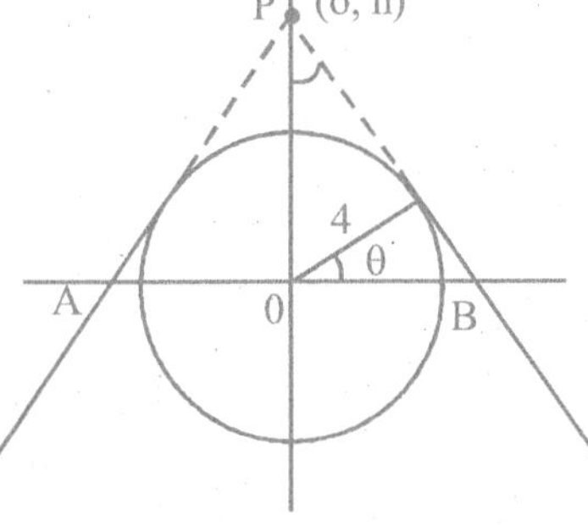

$$\text{Area}=OP\times OB=\frac{16}{\sin\theta\cos\theta}=\frac{32}{\sin 2\theta}$$

least value $\sin 2\theta=1;\ \theta=45°$

$$\text{So, } h=\frac{4}{\sin 45°}=4\sqrt{2}$$

16. (d) Given that $y+3x=0$ is the equation of a chord of the circle then
$y=-3x$ ....(i)
$(x^2)+(-3x)^2-30x=0$
$10x^2-30x=0$
$10x(x-3)=0$
$x=0, y=0$
so the equation of the circle is
$(x-3)(x-0)+(y+9)(y-0)=0$
$x^2-3x+y^2+9y=0$
$x^2+y^2-3x+9y=0$

17. (a) Radius

$$CP=\frac{4+1}{\sqrt{2}}$$

$$=\frac{5}{\sqrt{2}}=\frac{5}{2}\sqrt{2}$$

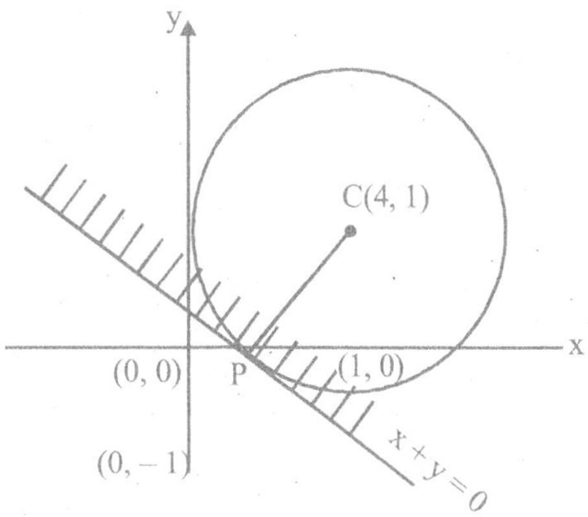

18. (b)

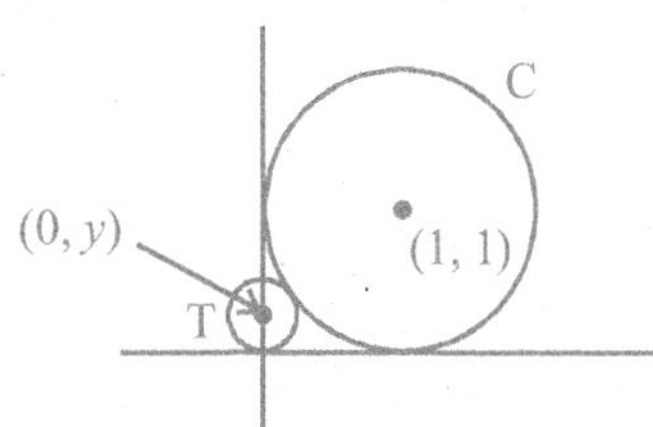

Equation of circle

$$C\equiv(x-1)^2+(y-1)^2=1$$

Radius of T = $|y|$
T touches C externally therefore,
Distance between the centres = sum of their radii

$\Rightarrow \sqrt{(0-1)^2+(y-1)^2}=1+|y|$
$\Rightarrow (0-1)^2+(y-1)^2=(1+|y|)^2$
$\Rightarrow 1+y^2+1-2y=1+y^2+2|y|$
$2|y|=1-2y$

If $y>0$ then $2y=1-2y\Rightarrow y=\dfrac{1}{4}$

If $y<0$ then $-2y=1-2y\Rightarrow 0=1$ (not possible)

$$\therefore\quad y=\frac{1}{4}$$

19. (a) Given circle is $x^2+y^2-16=0$
Eqn of chord say AB of given circle is
$3x+y+5=0$.
Equation of required circle is

$$x^2+y^2-16+\lambda(3x+y+5)=0$$

$$\Rightarrow x^2+y^2+(3\lambda)x+(\lambda)y+5\lambda-16=0 \quad ...(1)$$

$$\text{Centre } C=\left(\frac{-3\lambda}{2},\frac{-\lambda}{2}\right).$$

If line AB is the diameter of circle (1), then

$C\left(\frac{-3\lambda}{2}, \frac{-\lambda}{2}\right)$ will lie on line AB.

i.e. $3\left(\frac{-3\lambda}{2}\right)+\left(\frac{-\lambda}{2}\right)+5 = 0$

$\Rightarrow -\frac{9\lambda-\lambda}{2} + 5 = 0 \Rightarrow \lambda = 1$

Hence, required eqn of circle is

$x^2+y^2+3x+y+5-16 = 0$

$\Rightarrow x^2+y^2+3x+y-11 = 0$

20. (d) Let, $x^2 + y^2 = 16$ or $x^2 + y^2 = 4^2$
radius of circle $r_1 = 4$, centre C_1 (0, 0)
we have, $x^2 + y^2 - 2y = 0$
$\Rightarrow x^2 + (y^2 - 2y + 1) - 1 = 0$ or $x^2 + (y-1)^2 = 1^2$
Radius 1, centre C_2 (0, 1)
$|C_1C_2| = 1$
$|r_2 - r_1| = |4 - 1| = 3$
$|C_1C_2| < |r_2 - r_1|$

21. (b) The equations of the circles are

$x^2+y^2-10x-10y+\lambda = 0$ ...(1)

and $x^2+y^2-4x-4y+6 = 0$ ...(2)

C_1 = centre of (1) = (5, 5)

C_2 = centre of (2) = (2, 2)

d = distance between centres

$= C_1C_2 = \sqrt{9+9} = \sqrt{18}$

$r_1 = \sqrt{50-\lambda}$, $r_2 = \sqrt{2}$

For exactly two common tangents we have

$r_1 - r_2 < C_1C_2 < r_1 + r_2$

$\Rightarrow \sqrt{50-\lambda} - \sqrt{2} < 3\sqrt{2} < \sqrt{50-\lambda} + \sqrt{2}$

$\Rightarrow \sqrt{50-\lambda} - \sqrt{2} < 3\sqrt{2}$ or $3\sqrt{2} < \sqrt{50-\lambda} + \sqrt{2}$

$\Rightarrow \sqrt{50-\lambda} < 4\sqrt{2}$ or $2\sqrt{2} < \sqrt{50-\lambda}$

$\Rightarrow 50-\lambda < 32$ or $8 < 50-\lambda$

$\Rightarrow \lambda > 18$ or $\lambda < 42$

Required interval is (18, 42)

22. (d)

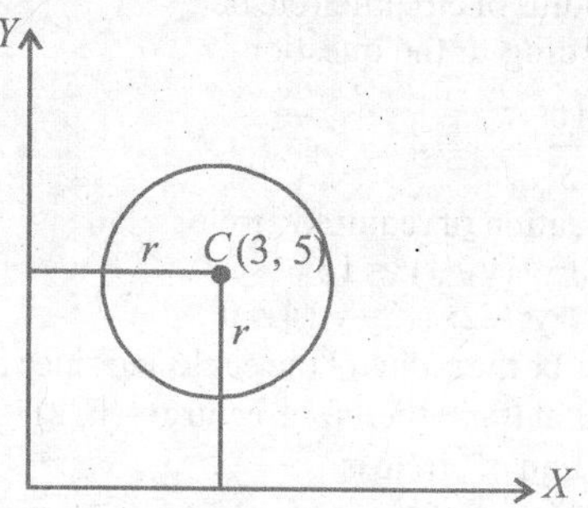

The equation of circle is

$x^2+y^2-6x-10y+P = 0$ ...(i)

$(x-3)^2+(y-5)^2 = (\sqrt{34-P})^2$

Centre (3, 5) and radius 'r' $= \sqrt{34-P}$
If circle does not touch or intersect the x-axis then radius $x < y$ - coordiante of centre C

or $\sqrt{34-P} < 5$
$\Rightarrow 34 - P < 25$
$\Rightarrow P > 9$ ...(ii)
Also if the circle does not touch or intersect x-axis the radius $r < x$-coordinate of centre C.

or $\sqrt{34-P} < 3 \Rightarrow 34-P < 9 \Rightarrow P > 25$ ... (iii)
If the point (1, 4) is inside the circle, then its distance from centre C < r.

or $\sqrt{[(3-1)^2+(5-4)^2]} < \sqrt{34-P}$
$\Rightarrow 5 < 34 - K$
$\Rightarrow P < 29$ ... (iv)
Now all the conditions (ii), (iii) and (iv) are satisfied if $25 < P < 29$ which is required value of P.

23. (c) Let the foot of the perpendicular from (0, 0) on the variable line $\frac{x}{a}+\frac{y}{b}=1$ is $(x_1 > y_1)$
Hence, perpendicular distance of the variable line $\frac{x}{a}+\frac{y}{b}=1$ from the point O (0, 0) = OA

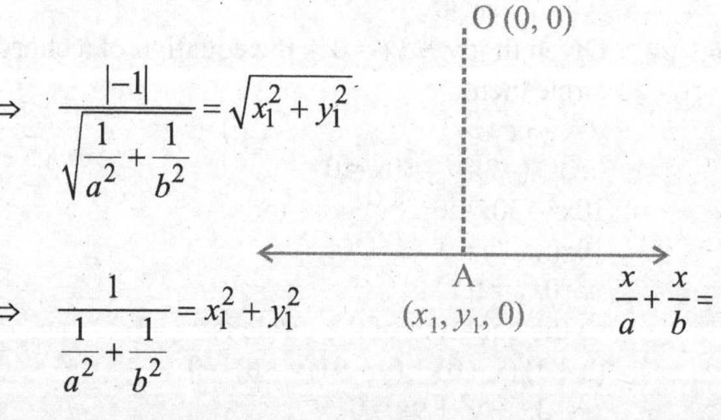

$\Rightarrow \frac{|-1|}{\sqrt{\frac{1}{a^2}+\frac{1}{b^2}}} = \sqrt{x_1^2+y_1^2}$

$\Rightarrow \frac{1}{\frac{1}{a^2}+\frac{1}{b^2}} = x_1^2+y_1^2$

$\Rightarrow 4 = x_1^2+y_1^2 \quad \left[\because \frac{1}{a^2}+\frac{1}{b^2}=\frac{1}{4}\right]$,

which is equation of a circle with radius 2.
Hence (x_1, y_1) i.e., the foot of the perpendicular from

the point (0, 0) to the variable line $\frac{x}{a}+\frac{x}{b}=1$ is lies on a circle with radius = 2

24. **(c)** Since circle touches x-axis at (3, 0)

$\therefore$ the equation of circle be

$(x-3)^2+(y-0)^2+\lambda y=0$

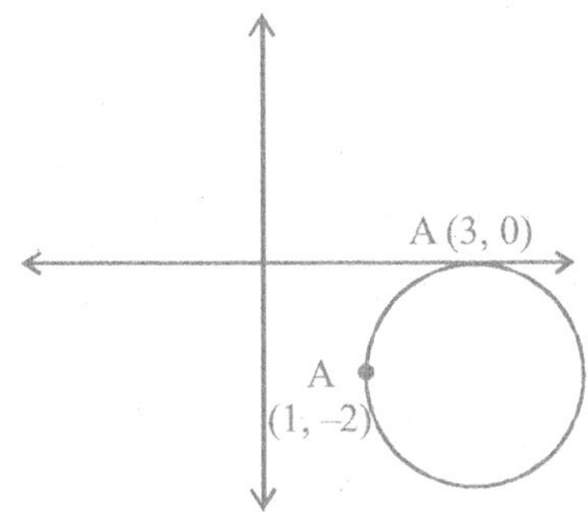

As it passes through (1, –2)

$\therefore$ Put $x=1, y=-2$

$\Rightarrow (1-3)^2+(-2)^2+\lambda(-2)=0$

$\Rightarrow \lambda=4$

$\therefore$ equation of circle is

$(x-3)^2+y^2-8=0$

Now, from the options (5, –2) satisfies equation of circle.

25. **(*)** Given information is incomplete in the question.

26. **(a)** Circle : $x^2+y^2-6x+2y=0$ ...(i)

Line : $2x+y=5$ ...(ii)

Centre = (3, – 1)

Now, $2\times 3-1=5$, hence centre lies on the given line. Therefore line passes through the centre. The given line is normal to the circle.

Thus statement-2 is true, but statement-1 is not true as there are infinite circle according to the given conditions.

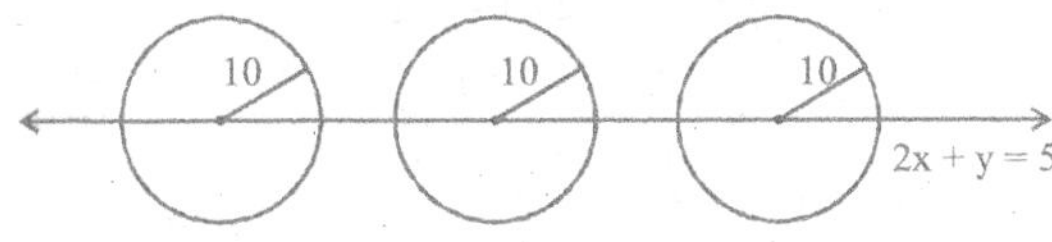

27. **(b)**

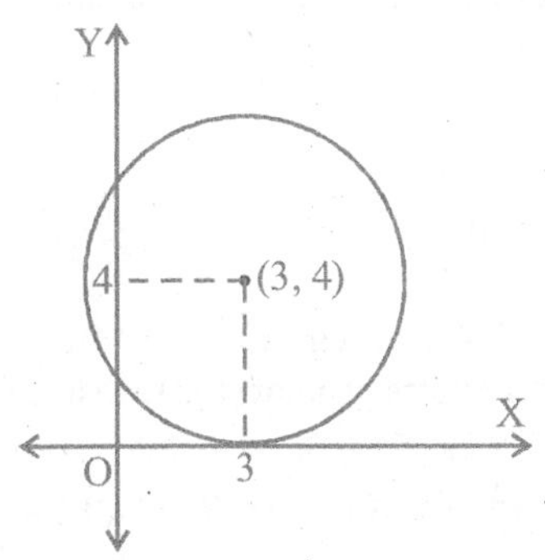

$x^2+y^2-6x-8y+(25-a^2)=0$

Radius = $4=\sqrt{9+16+(25-a^2)}$

$\Rightarrow a=\pm 4$

28. **(a)** Let A be the centre of given circle and B be the centre of circle C.

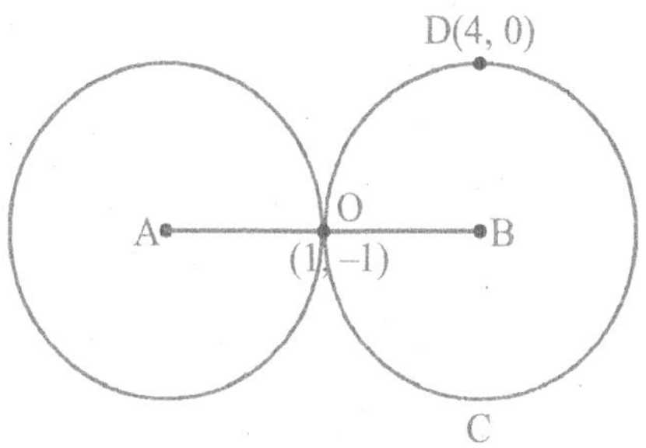

$x^2+y^2+4x-6y-12=0$

$\therefore$ A = (– 2, 3) and B = (g, f)

Now, from the figure, we have

$\frac{-2+g}{2}=1$ and $\frac{3+f}{2}=-1$

(By mid point formula)

$\Rightarrow g=4$ and $f=-5$

29. **(a)** Let C = (x, y)

Now, $CA^2=CB^2=AB^2$

$\Rightarrow (x+a)^2+y^2=(x-a)^2+y^2=(2a)^2$

$\Rightarrow x^2+2ax+a^2+y^2=4a^2$ ...(i)

and $x^2-2ax+a^2+y^2=4a^2$ ...(ii)

From (i) and (ii), $x=0$ and $y=\pm\sqrt{3}a$

Since point C(x, y) lies above the x-axis and $a>0$, hence $y=\sqrt{3}a$

$\therefore$ C = $(0, \sqrt{3}a)$

Let the equation of circumcircle be

$x^2+y^2+2gx+2fy+C=0$

Since points A$(-a, 0)$, B$(a, 0)$ and C$(0, \sqrt{3}a)$ lie on the circle, therefore

$a^2-2ga+C=0$ ...(iii)

$a^2+2ga+C=0$ ...(iv)

and $3a^2+2\sqrt{3}af+C=0$ ...(v)

From (iii), (iv), and (v)

$g=0, c=-a^2, f=-\frac{a}{\sqrt{3}}$

Hence equation of the circumcircle is

$x^2+y^2-\frac{2a}{\sqrt{3}}y-a^2=0$

$\Rightarrow x^2+y^2-\dfrac{2\sqrt{3}ay}{3}-a^2=0$

$\Rightarrow 3x^2+3y^2-2\sqrt{3}ay=3a^2$

30. **(d)** Point of intersection of two given lines is (1, 1). Since each of the two given lines contains a diameter of the given circle, therefore the point of intersection of the two given lines is the centre of the given circle.

Hence centre = (1, 1)

$\therefore\ a^2-7a+11=1 \Rightarrow a=2, 5$ ...(i)

and $a^2-6a+6=1 \Rightarrow a=1, 5$ ...(ii)

From both (i) and (ii), $a=5$

Now on replacing each of $(a^2-7a+11)$ and (a^2-6a+6) by 1, the equation of the given circle is

$x^2+y^2-2x-2y+b^3+1=0$

$\Rightarrow (x-1)^2+(y-1)^2+b^3=1$

$\Rightarrow b^3=1-[(x-1)^2+(y-1)^2]$

$\therefore\ b\in(-\infty, 1)$

31. **(a)** Let centre of the circle be (1,h)

[$\because$ circle touches x-axis at (1,0)]

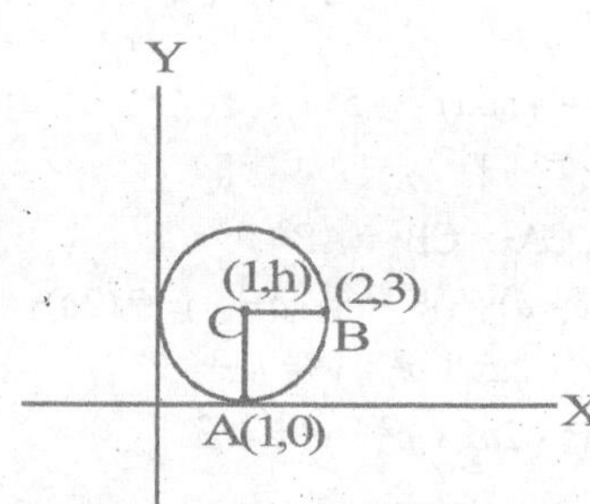

Let the circle passes through the point B (2,3)

$\therefore$ $CA=CB$ (radius)

$\Rightarrow$ $CA^2=CB^2$

$\Rightarrow$ $(1-1)^2+(h-0)^2=(1-2)^2+(h-3)^2$

$\Rightarrow$ $h^2=1+h^2+9-6h$

$\Rightarrow$ $h=\dfrac{10}{6}=\dfrac{5}{3}$

32. **(c)** Given circles are

$x^2+y^2-8x-2y+1=0$

and $x^2+y^2+6x+8y=0$

Their centres and radius are

$C_1(4, 1), r_1=\sqrt{16}=4$

$C_2(-3,-4), r_2=\sqrt{25}=5$

Now, $C_1C_2=\sqrt{49+25}=\sqrt{74}$

$r_1-r_2=-1, r_1+r_2=9$

Since, $r_1-r_2<C_1C_2<r_1+r_2$

$\therefore$ Number of common tangents = 2

33. **(b)** Circle : $x^2+y^2+3x=0$

Centre, $B=\left(-\dfrac{3}{2}, 0\right)$

Radius $=\dfrac{3}{2}$ units.

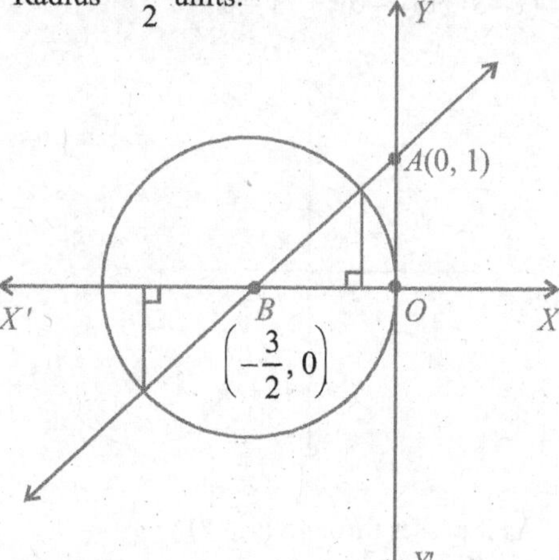

Line : $y=mx+1$

y-intercept of the line = 1

$\therefore$ A = (0, 1)

Slope of line, $m=\tan\theta=\dfrac{OA}{OB}$

$\Rightarrow m=\dfrac{1}{\frac{3}{2}}=\dfrac{2}{3}$

$\Rightarrow 3m-2=0$

34. **(a)** Let $P(1, 0)$ and $Q(-1, 0)$, $A(x, y)$

Given: $\dfrac{AP}{AQ}=\dfrac{BP}{BQ}=\dfrac{CP}{CQ}=\dfrac{1}{2}$

$\Rightarrow 2AP=AQ$

$\Rightarrow 4(AP)^2=AQ^2$

$\Rightarrow 4[(x-1)^2+y^2]=(x+1)^2+y^2$

$\Rightarrow 4(x^2+1-2x)+4y^2=x^2+1+2x+y^2$

$\Rightarrow 3x^2+3y^2-8x-2x+4-1=0$

$\Rightarrow 3x^2+3y^2-10x+3=0$

$\Rightarrow x^2+y^2-\dfrac{10}{3}x+1=0$ ...(1)

$\therefore$ A lies on the circle given by (1). As B and C also follow the same condition.

$\therefore$ Centre of circumcircle of ΔABC = centre of circle given by (1)

$=\left(\dfrac{5}{3}, 0\right)$.

35. **(d)** Point (1, 2) lies on the circle $x^2+y^2+2x+2y-11=0$, because coordinates of point (1, 2) satisfy the equation $x^2+y^2+2x+2y-11=0$

Now, $x^2+y^2-4x-6y-21=0$ ...(i)

$x^2+y^2+2x+2y-11=0$ ...(ii)

$3x+4y+5=0$ ...(iii)

From (i) and (iii),

$$x^2+\left(-\frac{3x+5}{4}\right)^2-4x-6\left(-\frac{3x+5}{4}\right)-21=0$$

$\Rightarrow$ $16x^2+9x^2+30x+25-64x+72x+120-336=0$

$\Rightarrow$ $25x^2+38x-191=0$ ...(iv)

From (ii) and (iii),

$$x^2+\left(-\frac{3x+5}{4}\right)^2+2x+2\left(-\frac{3x+5}{4}\right)-11=0$$

$\Rightarrow$ $16x^2+9x^2+30x+25+32x-24x-40-176=0$

$\Rightarrow$ $25x^2+38x-191=0$ ...(v)

Thus we get the same equation from (ii) and (iii) as we get from equation (i) and (iii). Hence the point of intersections of (ii) and (iii) will be same as the point of intersections of (i) and (iii). Therefore the circle (ii) passing through the point of intersection of circle(i) and point (1, 2) also as shown in the figure.

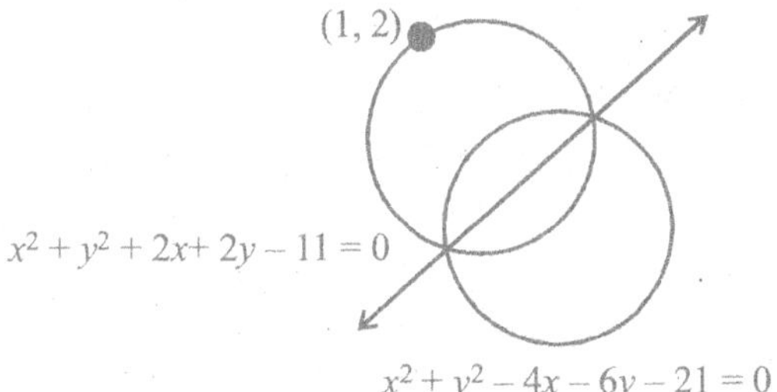

Hence equation(ii) i.e.

$x^2+y^2+2x+2y-11=0$ is the equation of required circle.

36. **(b)** Circle whose diametric end points are (1,0) and (0,1) will be of smallest radius. Equation of this smallest circle is

$(x-1)(x-0)+(y-0)(y-1)=0$

$\Rightarrow$ $x^2+y^2-x-y=0$

37. **(a)** If the two circles touch each other, then they must touch each other internally.

So, $\frac{|a|}{2}=c-\frac{|a|}{2} \Rightarrow |a|=c$

38. **(a)** Circle $x^2+y^2-4x-8y-5=0$

Centre = (2, 4), Radius = $\sqrt{4+16+5}=5$

If circle is intersecting line $3x-4y=m$, at two distinct points.

$\Rightarrow$ length of perpendicular from centre to the line < radius

$\Rightarrow \frac{|6-16-m|}{5}<5 \Rightarrow |10+m|<25$

$\Rightarrow -25<m+10<25 \Rightarrow -35<m<15$

39. **(a)** The given circles are

$S_1 \equiv x^2+y^2+3x+7y+2p-5=0$....(1)

$S_2 \equiv x^2+y^2+2x+2y-p^2=0$ ....(2)

$\therefore$ Equation of common chord PQ is

$S_1-S_2=0$

$\Rightarrow$ $L \equiv x+5y+p^2+2p-5=0$

$\Rightarrow$ Equation of circle passing through P and Q is

$S_1+\lambda L=0$

$\Rightarrow (x^2+y^2+3x+7y+2p-5)$
$+\lambda(x+5y+p^2+2p-5)=0$

As it passes through (1, 1), therefore

$(7+2p)+\lambda(2p+p^2+1)=0$

$\Rightarrow \lambda=-\frac{2p+7}{(p+1)^2}$

which does not exist for $p=-1$

40. **(a)** Given that $P(1,0), Q(-1,0)$

and $\frac{AP}{AQ}=\frac{BP}{BQ}=\frac{CP}{CQ}=\frac{1}{3}$

$\Rightarrow 3AP=AQ$

Let $A=(x,y)$ then

$3AP=AQ \Rightarrow 9AP^2=AQ^2$

$\Rightarrow 9(x-1)^2+9y^2=(x+1)^2+y^2$

$\Rightarrow 9x^2-18x+9+9y^2=x^2+2x+1+y^2$

$\Rightarrow 8x^2-20x+8y^2+8=0$

$\Rightarrow x^2+y^2-\frac{5}{3}x+1=0$ ....(1)

$\therefore$ A lies on the circle given by eq (1). As B and C also follow the same condition, they must lie on the same circle.

$\therefore$ Centre of circumcircle of ΔABC

= Centre of circle given by (1) = $\left(\frac{5}{4},0\right)$

41. **(c)** The given circle is $x^2+y^2+2x+4y-3=0$

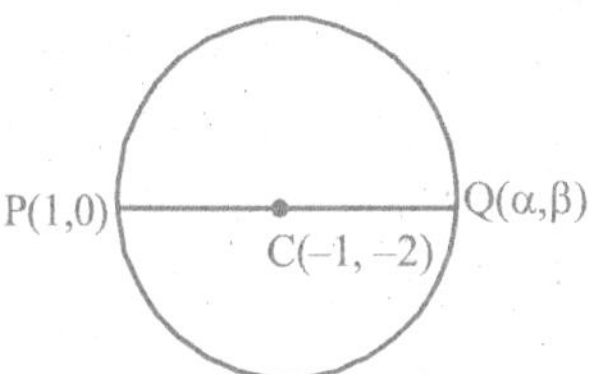

Centre (–1, –2)

Let $Q(\alpha,\beta)$ be the point diametrically opposite to the point $P(1,0)$,

then $\frac{1+\alpha}{2}=-1$ and $\frac{0+\beta}{2}=-2$

$\Rightarrow \alpha=-3, \beta=-4$

So, Q is (–3, –4)

42. (d) Equation of circle whose centre is (h, k)
i.e $(x-h)^2+(y-k)^2=k^2$

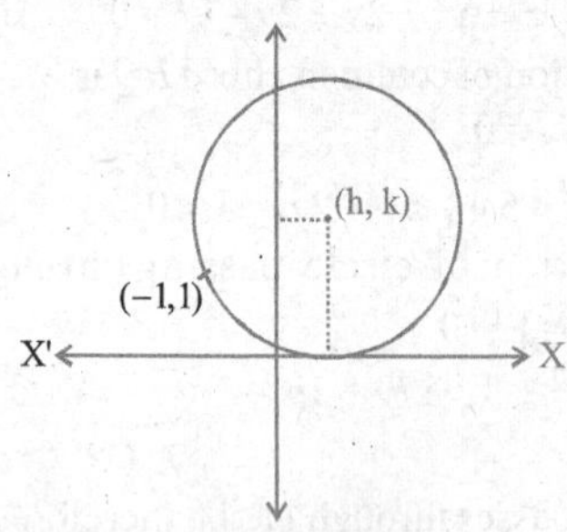

(radius of circle $= k$ because circle is tangent to x-axis)
Equation of circle passing through $(-1, +1)$

$\therefore (-1-h)^2+(1-k)^2=k^2$

$\Rightarrow 1+h^2+2h+1+k^2-2k=k^2$

$\Rightarrow h^2+2h-2k+2=0$

$D \geq 0$

$\therefore (2)^2-4\times 1.(-2k+2)\geq 0$

$\Rightarrow 4-4(-2k+2)\geq 0 \Rightarrow 1+2k-2\geq 0 \Rightarrow k\geq \frac{1}{2}$

43. (d) Let $M(h, k)$ be the mid point of chord AB where

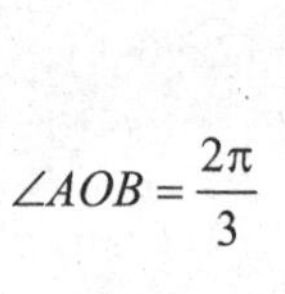

$\angle AOB = \frac{2\pi}{3}$

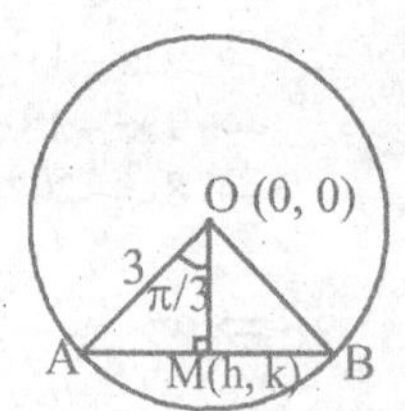

$\therefore \angle AOM = \frac{\pi}{3}$. Also $OM = 3\cos\frac{\pi}{3} = \frac{3}{2}$

$\Rightarrow \sqrt{h^2+k^2} = \frac{3}{2} \Rightarrow h^2+k^2 = \frac{9}{4}$

$\therefore$ Locus of (h, k) is $x^2+y^2=\frac{9}{4}$

44. (d) Point of intersection of $3x-4y-7=0$ and $2x-3y-5=0$ is $(1,-1)$ which is the centre of the circle and radius $= 7$

$\therefore$ Equation is $(x-1)^2+(y+1)^2=49$

$\Rightarrow x^2+y^2-2x+2y-47=0$

45. (d) Let the centre be (α, β)

$\because$ It cuts the circle $x^2+y^2=p^2$ orthogonally

$\therefore$ Using $2g_1g_2+2f_1f_2=c_1+c_2$, we get

$2(-\alpha)\times 0+2(-\beta)\times 0=c_1-p^2$

$c_1=p^2$

Let equation of circle is

$x^2+y^2-2\alpha x-2\beta y+p^2=0$

It passes through

$(a,b) \Rightarrow a^2+b^2-2\alpha a-2\beta b+p^2=0$

$\therefore$ Locus of (α, β) is

$\therefore 2ax+2by-(a^2+b^2+p^2)=0$.

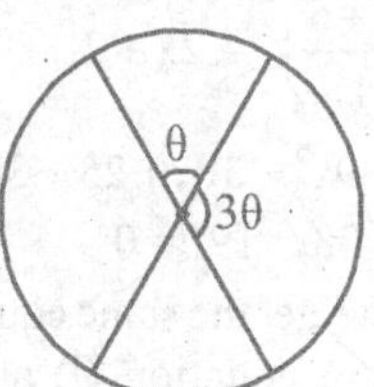

46. (d)

As per question area of one sector = 3 area of another sector

$\Rightarrow$ angle at centre by one sector $= 3\times$ angle at centre by another sector

Let one angle be θ then other $= 3\theta$

Clearly $\theta+3\theta=180 \Rightarrow \theta=45^\circ$

$\therefore$ Angle between the diameters represented by combined equation

$ax^2+2(a+b)xy+by^2=0$ *is* 45°

$\therefore$ Using $\tan\theta = \frac{2\sqrt{h^2-ab}}{a+b}$

we get $\tan 45^\circ = \frac{2\sqrt{(a+b)^2-ab}}{a+b}$

$\Rightarrow 1 = \frac{2\sqrt{a^2+b^2+ab}}{a+b}$

$\Rightarrow (a+b)^2 = 4(a^2+b^2+ab)$

$\Rightarrow a^2+b^2+2ab = 4a^2+4b^2+4ab$

$\Rightarrow 3a^2+3b^2+2ab=0$

47. (b) $s_1 = x^2+y^2+2ax+cy+a=0$

$s_2 = x^2+y^2-3ax+dy-1=0$.

Equation of common chord of circles s_1 and s_2 is given by $s_1-s_2=0$

$\Rightarrow 5ax+(c-d)y+a+1=0$

Given that $5x+by-a=0$ passes through P and Q

$\therefore$ The two equations should represent the same line

$\Rightarrow \frac{a}{1} = \frac{c-d}{b} = \frac{a+1}{-a} \Rightarrow a+1 = -a^2$

$a^2 + a + 1 = 0$

No real value of a.

48. **(b)** Let the variable circle is

$x^2 + y^2 + 2gx + 2fy + c = 0$ ......(1)

It passes through (a, b)

$\therefore a^2 + b^2 + 2ga + 2fb + c = 0$ ......(2)

(1) cuts $x^2 + y^2 = 4$ orthogonally

$\therefore 2(g \times 0 + f \times 0) = c - 4 \Rightarrow c = 4$

$\therefore$ from (2) $a^2 + b^2 + 2ga + 2fb + 4 = 0$

$\therefore$ Locus of centre $(-g, -f)$ is

$a^2 + b^2 - 2ax - 2by + 4 = 0$

or $2ax + 2by = a^2 + b^2 + 4$

49. **(d)** Let the variable circle be

$x^2 + y^2 + 2gx + 2fy + c = 0$ ....(1)

$\therefore p^2 + q^2 + 2gp + 2fq + c = 0$ ....(2)

Circle (1) touches x-axis,

$\therefore g^2 - c = 0 \Rightarrow c = g^2$. From (2)

$p^2 + q^2 + 2gp + 2fq + g^2 = 0$ ....(3)

Let the other end of diameter through (p, q) be (h, k), then

$\frac{h+p}{2} = -g$ and $\frac{k+q}{2} = -f$

Put in (3)

$$p^2 + q^2 + 2p\left(-\frac{h+p}{2}\right) + 2q\left(-\frac{k+q}{2}\right) + \left(\frac{h+p}{2}\right)^2 = 0$$

$\Rightarrow h^2 + p^2 - 2hp - 4kq = 0$

$\therefore$ locus of (h, k) is $x^2 + p^2 - 2xp - 4yq = 0$

$\Rightarrow (x-p)^2 = 4qy$

50. **(d)** Two diameters are along

$2x + 3y + 1 = 0$ and $3x - y - 4 = 0$

solving we get centre $(1, -1)$

circumference $= 2\pi r = 10\pi$

$\therefore r = 5$.

Required circle is, $(x-1)^2 + (y+1)^2 = 5^2$

$\Rightarrow x^2 + y^2 - 2x + 2y - 23 = 0$

51. **(d)** Solving $y = x$ and the circle

$x^2 + y^2 - 2x = 0$, we get

$x = 0, y = 0$ and $x = 1, y = 1$

$\therefore$ Extremities of diameter of the required circle are (0, 0) and (1, 1). Hence, the equation of circle is

$(x-0)(x-1) + (y-0)(y-1) = 0$

$\Rightarrow x^2 + y^2 - x - y = 0$

52. **(b)** $|r_1 - r_2| < C_1C_2$ for intersection

$\Rightarrow r - 3 < 5 \Rightarrow r < 8$ ...(1)

and $r_1 + r_2 > C_1C_2$, $r + 3 > 5 \Rightarrow r > 2$ ...(2)

From (1) and (2), $2 < r < 8$.

53. **(d)** $\pi r^2 = 154 \Rightarrow r = 7$

For centre on solving equation

$2x - 3y = 5 \,\&\, 3x - 4y = 7$ we get $x = 1, y = -1$

$\therefore$ centre $= (1, -1)$

Equation of circle, $(x-1)^2 + (y+1)^2 = 7^2$

$x^2 + y^2 - 2x + 2y = 47$

54. **(c)** Equation of circle $x^2 + y^2 = 1 = (1)^2$

$\Rightarrow x^2 + y^2 = (y - mx)^2$

$\Rightarrow x^2 = m^2x^2 - 2\,mxy;$

$\Rightarrow x^2(1 - m^2) + 2mxy = 0$. Which represents the pair of lines between which the angle is 45°.

$\tan 45 = \pm \frac{2\sqrt{m^2 - 0}}{1 - m^2} = \frac{\pm 2m}{1 - m^2};$

$\Rightarrow 1 - m^2 = \pm\, 2m \Rightarrow m^2 \pm 2m - 1 = 0$

$\Rightarrow m = \frac{-2 \pm \sqrt{4+4}}{2}$

$= \frac{-2 \pm 2\sqrt{2}}{2} = -1 \pm \sqrt{2}$.

55. **(a)** For any point P (x, y) in the given circle,

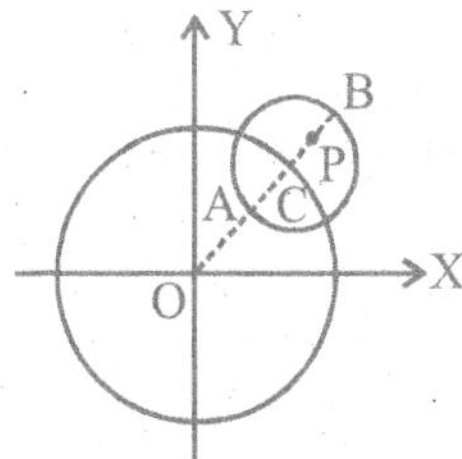

we should have

$OA \le OP \le OB$

$\Rightarrow (5-3) \le \sqrt{x^2+y^2} \le 5+3$

$\Rightarrow 4 \le x^2+y^2 \le 64$

56. (b) Let the required circle be

$x^2 + y^2 + 2gx + 2fy + c = 0$

Since it passes through (0, 0) and (1, 0)

$\Rightarrow c = 0$ and $g = -\frac{1}{2}$

Points (0, 0) and (1, 0) lie inside the circle $x^2 + y^2 = 9$, so two circles touch internally

$\Rightarrow c_1c_2 = r_1 - r_2$

$\therefore \sqrt{g^2+f^2} = 3 - \sqrt{g^2+f^2} \Rightarrow \sqrt{g^2+f^2} = \frac{3}{2}$

$\Rightarrow f^2 = \frac{9}{4} - \frac{1}{4} = 2 \qquad \therefore f = \pm\sqrt{2}$.

Hence, the centres of required circle are

$\left(\frac{1}{2}, \sqrt{2}\right)$ or $\left(\frac{1}{2}, -\sqrt{2}\right)$

57. (c) Let ABC be an equilateral triangle, whose median is AD.

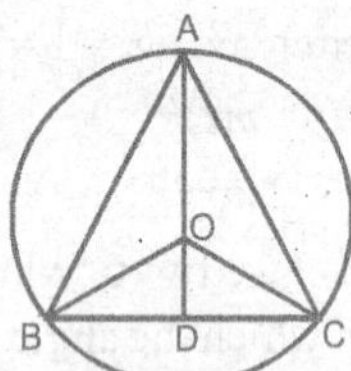

Given $AD = 3a$.

In ΔABD, $AB^2 = AD^2 + BD^2$;

$\Rightarrow x^2 = 9a^2 + (x^2/4)$ where $AB = BC = AC = x$.

$\frac{3}{4}x^2 = 9a^2 \Rightarrow x^2 = 12a^2$.

In ΔOBD, $OB^2 = OD^2 + BD^2$

$\Rightarrow r^2 = (3a - r)^2 + \frac{x^2}{4}$

$\Rightarrow r^2 = 9a^2 - 6ar + r^2 + 3a^2$; $\Rightarrow 6ar = 12a^2$

$\Rightarrow r = 2a$

So equation of circle is $x^2 + y^2 = 4a^2$

58. (c) $c = -29m - 9m^3$

$a = 2$

Given $(at^2 - a)^2 + 4a^2t^2 = 64$

$\Rightarrow (a(t^2+1)) = 8$

$\Rightarrow t^2 + 1 = 4 \Rightarrow t^2 = 3$

$\Rightarrow t = \sqrt{3}$

$\therefore c = 2at(2 + t^2)$

$= 2\sqrt{3}(5)$

$|c| = 10\sqrt{3}$.

59. (c)

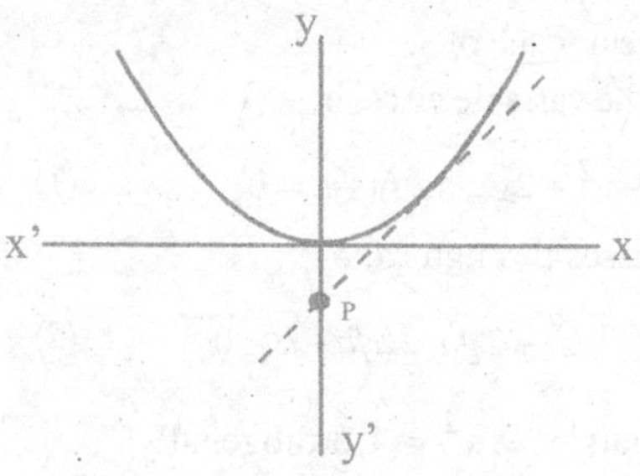

Tangent to $x^2 + y^2 = 4$ is

$y = mx \pm 2\sqrt{1+m^2}$

Also, $x^2 = 4y$

$x^2 = 4mx + 8\sqrt{1+m^2}$ or $x^2 = 4mx - 8\sqrt{1+m^2}$

For D = 0

we have; $16m^2 + 4.8\sqrt{1+m^2} = 0$

$\Rightarrow m^2 + 2\sqrt{1+m^2} = 0$

$\Rightarrow m^2 = -2\sqrt{1+m^2}$

$\Rightarrow m^4 = 4 + 4m^2$

$\Rightarrow m^4 - 4m^2 - 4 = 0$

$\Rightarrow m^2 = \frac{4 \pm \sqrt{16+16}}{2}$

$\Rightarrow m^2 = \frac{4 \pm 4\sqrt{2}}{2}$

$\Rightarrow m^2 = 2 + 2\sqrt{2}$

60. (c) Minimum distance $\Rightarrow$ perpendicular distance

Eq^n of normal at $p(2t^2, 4t)$

$y = -tx + 4t + 2t^3$

It passes through C(0, –6)

$\Rightarrow t^3 + 2t + 3 = 0 \Rightarrow t = -1$

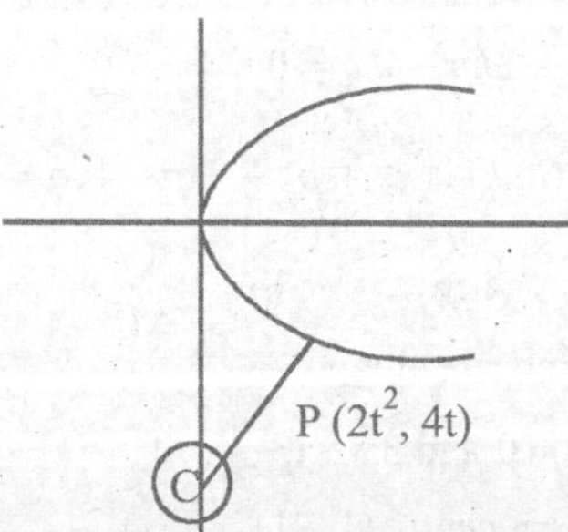

Centre of new circle = $P(2t^2, 4t)$

= P(2, – 4)

Radius = PC

$= \sqrt{(2-0)^2 + (-4+6)^2}$

$= 2\sqrt{2}$

$\therefore$ Equation of circle is :

$(x-2)^2 + (y+4) = \left(2\sqrt{2}\right)^2$

$\Rightarrow x^2 + y^2 - 4x + 8y + 12 = 0$

61. **(a)** $t_1 = -t - \frac{2}{t}$

$t_1^2 = t^2 + \frac{4}{t^2} + 4$

$t^2 + \frac{4}{t^2} \geq 2\sqrt{t^2 \cdot \frac{4}{t^2}} = 4$

Minimum value of $t_1^2 = 8$

62. **(b)** Let P(h, k) divides OQ in the ratio 1 : 3

Let any point Q on $x^2 = 8y$ is $(4t, 2t^2)$.

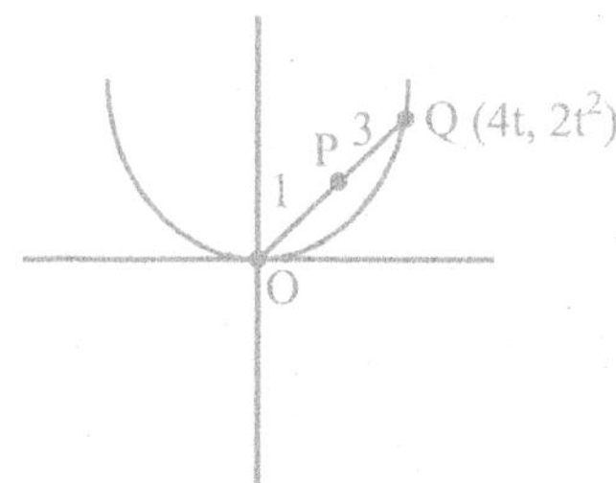

Then by section formula

$\Rightarrow k = \frac{t^2}{2}$ and $h = t$

$\Rightarrow 2k = h^2$

Required locus of P is $x^2 = 2y$

63. **(d)** Let P $(-at_1^2, 2at_1)$, Q$(-at_1^2, -2at_1)$ and R (h, k)

By using section formula, we have

$h = -at_1^2, k = \frac{-2at_1}{3}$

$k = -\frac{2at_1}{3}$

$\Rightarrow 3k = -2at_1$

$\Rightarrow 9k^2 = 4a^2 t_1^2 = 4a(-h)$

$\Rightarrow 9k^2 = -4ah$

$\Rightarrow 9k^2 = -4h \Rightarrow 9y^2 = -4x$

64. **(c)** Given parabolas are

$y^2 = 4x$ ...(i)

$x^2 = -32y$ ...(ii)

Let m be slope of common tangent

Equation of tangent of parabola (1)

$y = mx + \frac{1}{m}$ ...(i)

Equation of tangent of parabola (2)

$y = mx + 8m^2$ ...(ii)

(i) and (ii) are identical

$\Rightarrow \frac{1}{m} = 8m^2 \Rightarrow m^3 = \frac{1}{8} \Rightarrow \boxed{m = \frac{1}{2}}$

ALTERNATIVE METHOD:

Let tangent to $y^2 = 4x$ be $y = mx + \frac{1}{m}$

Since this is also tangent to $x^2 = -32y$

$\therefore \quad x^2 = -32\left(mx + \frac{1}{m}\right)$

$\Rightarrow x^2 + 32mx + \frac{32}{m} = 0$

Now, D = 0

$(32)^2 - 4\left(\frac{32}{m}\right) = 0$

$\Rightarrow m^3 = \frac{4}{32} \quad \Rightarrow m = \frac{1}{2}$

65. **(a)** Equation of parabola, $y^2 = 6x$

$\Rightarrow y^2 = 4 \times \frac{3}{2}x$

$\therefore$ Focus $= \left(\frac{3}{2}, 0\right)$

Let equation of chord passing through focus be

$ax + by + c = 0$ ...(1)

Since chord is passing through $\left(\frac{3}{2}, 0\right)$

$\therefore$ Put $x = \frac{3}{2}, y = 0$ in eqn (1), we get

$\frac{3}{2}a + c = 0$

$\Rightarrow c = -\frac{3}{2}a$ ...(2)

distance of chord from origin is $\frac{\sqrt{5}}{2}$

$\frac{\sqrt{5}}{2} = \left|\frac{a(0) + b(0) + c}{\sqrt{a^2 + b^2}}\right| = \frac{c}{\sqrt{a^2 + b^2}}$

Squaring both sides

$$\frac{5}{4} = \frac{c^2}{a^2+b^2}$$

$$\Rightarrow a^2 + b^2 = \frac{4}{5}c^2$$

Putting value of c from (2), we get

$$a^2 + b^2 = \frac{4}{5} \times \frac{9}{4}a^2$$

$$b^2 = \frac{9}{5}a^2 - a^2 = \frac{4}{5}a^2$$

$$\frac{a^2}{b^2} = \frac{5}{4}, \frac{a}{b} = \pm\frac{\sqrt{5}}{2}$$

Slope of chord, $\frac{dy}{dx} = -\frac{a}{b} = -\left(\frac{\pm\sqrt{5}}{2}\right) = \mp\frac{\sqrt{5}}{2}$

66. (d) The locus of the point of intersection of tangents to the parabola $y^2 = 4ax$ inclined at an angle α to each other is

$\tan^2\alpha\ (x + a)^2 = y^2 - 4ax$

Given equation of Parabola $y^2 = 4x$ $\{a = 1\}$

Point of intersection $(-2, -1)$

$\tan^2\alpha\ (-2 + 1)^2 = (-1)^2 - 4 \times 1 \times (-2)$

$\Rightarrow \tan^2\alpha = 9$

$\Rightarrow \tan\alpha = \pm 3$

$\Rightarrow |\tan\alpha| = 3$

67. (c)

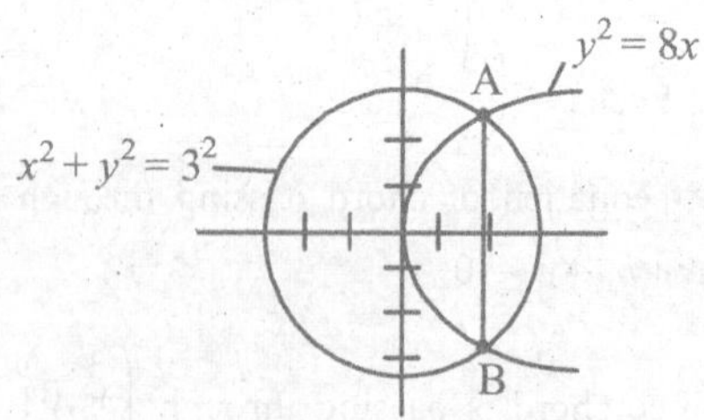

We have

$x^2 + (8x) = 9$

$x^2 + 9x - x - 9 = 0$

$x(x + 9) - 1(x + 9) = 0$

$(x + 9)(x - 1) = 0$

$x = -9, 1$

for $x = 1$, $y = \pm 2\sqrt{2x} = \pm 2\sqrt{2}$

L_1 = Length of AB

$$= \sqrt{(2\sqrt{2}+2\sqrt{2})^2 + (1-1)^2} = 4\sqrt{2}$$

L_2 = Length of latus rectum $= 4a = 4 \times 2 = 8$

$L_1 < L_2$

68. (b) Let common tangent be

$$y = mx + \frac{\sqrt{5}}{m}$$

Since, perpendicular distance from centre of the circle to the common tangent is equal to radius of the circle,

therefore $\dfrac{\frac{\sqrt{5}}{m}}{\sqrt{1+m^2}} = \sqrt{\dfrac{5}{2}}$

On squaring both the side, we get

$m^2(1+m^2) = 2$

$\Rightarrow m^4 + m^2 - 2 = 0$

$\Rightarrow (m^2+2)(m^2-1) = 0$

$\Rightarrow m = \pm 1 \qquad (\because m \neq \pm\sqrt{2})$

$y = \pm\left(x+\sqrt{5}\right)$, both statements are correct as $m = \pm 1$ satisfies the given equation of statement-2.

69. (b) We know that point of intersection of the normal to the parabola $y^2 = 4ax$ at the ends of its latus rectum is $(3a, 0)$

Hence required point of intersection $= (3, 0)$

70. (b) Both statements are true and statement-2 is the correct explanation of statement-1

$\therefore$ The straight line $y = mx + \frac{a}{m}$ is always a tangent to the parabola $y^2 = 4ax$ for any value of m.

The co-ordinates of point of contact $\left(\frac{a}{m^2}, \frac{2a}{m}\right)$

Now, required radius $= \text{OB} = \sqrt{9+16} = \sqrt{25} = 5$

71. (a) Ellipse is $\frac{x^2}{16} + \frac{y^2}{3} = 1$

Now, equation of normal at $(2, 3/2)$ is

$$\frac{16x}{2} - \frac{3y}{3/2} = 16 - 3$$

$\Rightarrow 8x - 2y = 13$

$\Rightarrow y = 4x - \frac{13}{2}$

Let $y = 4x - \frac{13}{2}$ touches a parabola

$y^2 = 4ax$.

We know, a straight line $y = mx + c$ touches a parabola $y^2 = 4ax$ if $a - mc = 0$

$\therefore a - (4)\left(-\frac{13}{2}\right) = 0 \Rightarrow a = -26$

Hence, required equation of parabola is

$y^2 = 4(-26)x = -104x$

72. **(a)** Point P is (4, –2) and $PQ \perp x$-axis
So, Q = (4, 2)

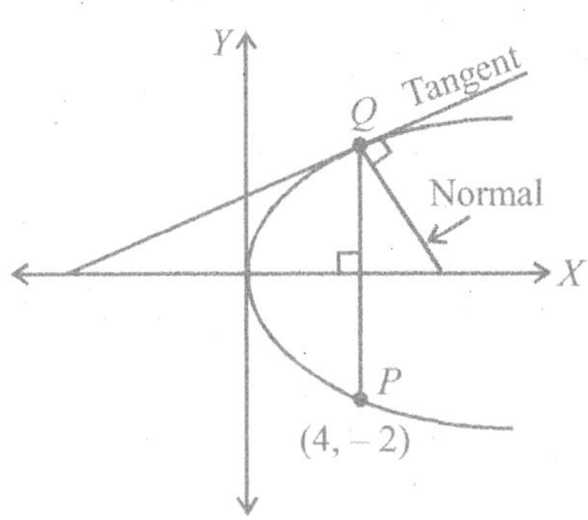

Equation of tangent at (4, 2) is

$$yy_1 = \frac{1}{2}(x + x_1)$$

$$\Rightarrow 2y = \frac{1}{2}(x+2) \Rightarrow 4y = x + 2$$

$$\Rightarrow y = \frac{x}{4} + \frac{1}{2}$$

So, slope of tangent = $\frac{1}{4}$

$\therefore$ Slope of normal = – 4

73. **(d)** Both the given statements are true.
Statement - 2 is not the correct explanation for statement - 1.

74. **(a)** Shortest distance between two curve occurred along the common normal, so $-2t = -1$.
$\Rightarrow t = 1/2$

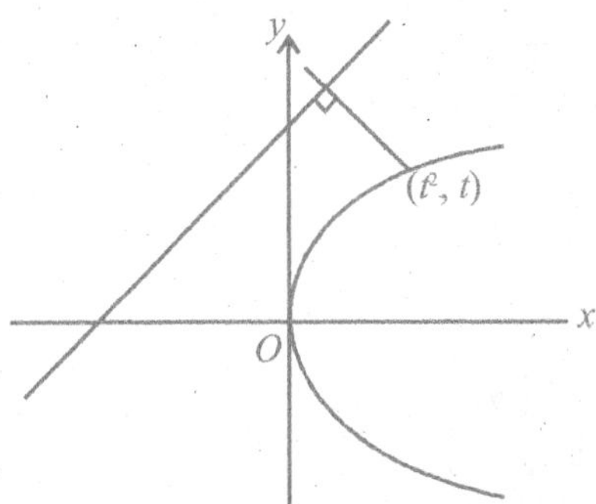

So shortest distance between them is $\frac{3\sqrt{2}}{8}$

75. **(b)** The locus of perpendicular tangents is directrix i.e.,
$x = -a; x = -1$

76. **(b)** Vertex of a parabola is the mid point of focus and the point

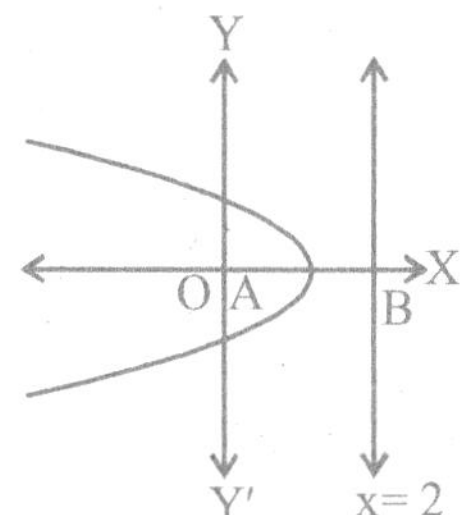

where directrix meets the axis of the parabola.
Here focus is $O(0, 0)$ and directrix meets the axis at $B(2,0)$
$\therefore$ Vertex of the parabola is (1, 0)

77. **(b)** Parabola $y^2 = 8x$

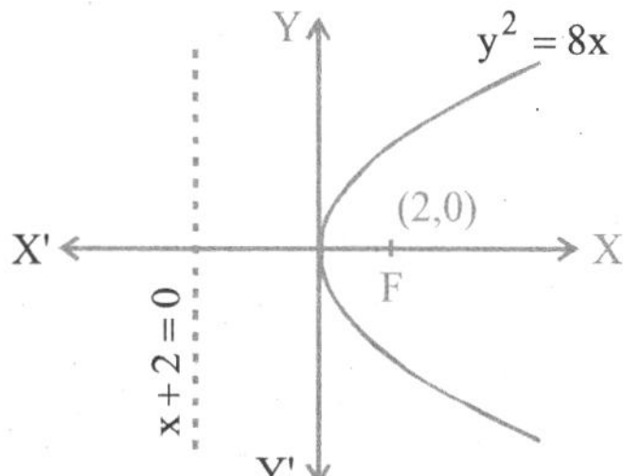

We know that the locus of point of intersection of two perpendicular tangents to a parabola is its directrix.
Point must be on the directrix of parabola
$\because$ equation of directrix $x + 2 = 0$
$\Rightarrow x = -2$
Hence the point is (–2, 0)

78. **(a)** Given parabola is $y = \frac{a^3x^2}{3} + \frac{a^2x}{2} - 2a$

$$\Rightarrow y = \frac{a^3}{3}\left(x^3 + \frac{3}{2a}x + \frac{9}{16a^2}\right) - \frac{3a}{16} - 2a$$

$$\Rightarrow y + \frac{35a}{16} = \frac{a^3}{\cdot 3}\left(x + \frac{3}{4a}\right)^2$$

$\therefore$ Vertex of parabola is $\left(\frac{-3}{4a}, \frac{-35a}{16}\right)$

To find locus of this vertex,

$$x = \frac{-3}{4a} \text{ and } y = \frac{-35a}{16}$$

$$\Rightarrow a = \frac{-3}{4x} \text{ and } a = -\frac{16y}{35}$$

$$\Rightarrow \frac{-3}{4x} = \frac{-16y}{35} \Rightarrow 64xy = 105$$

$$\Rightarrow xy = \frac{105}{64}$$ which is the required locus.

79. **(a)** $P=(1,0)$ $Q=(h,k)$ Such that $K^2=8h$

Let (α,β) be the midpoint of PQ

$\alpha=\frac{h+1}{2}$, $\beta=\frac{k+0}{2}$

$2\alpha-1=h$ $2\beta=k.$

$(2\beta)^2=8(2\alpha-1) \Rightarrow \beta^2=4\alpha-2$

$\Rightarrow y^2-4x+2=0.$

80. **(d)** Equation of circle with centre (0, 3) and radius 2 is $x^2+(y-3)^2=4$

Let locus of the variable circle is (α,β)

$\because$ It touches x - axis.

$\therefore$ It's equation is $(x-\alpha)^2+(y+\beta)^2=\beta^2$

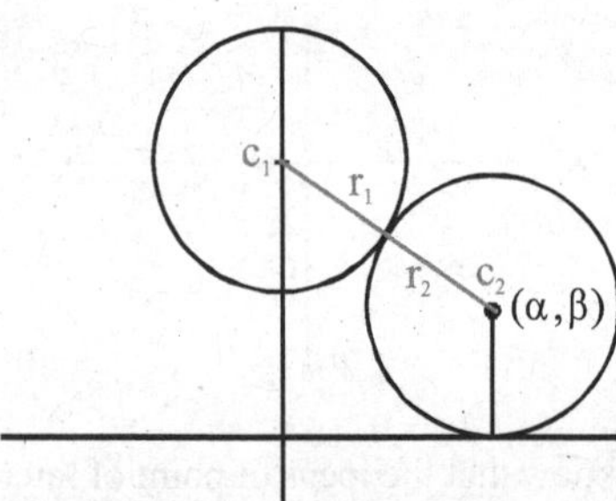

Circle touch externally $\Rightarrow c_1c_2=r_1+r_2$

$\therefore \sqrt{\alpha^2+(\beta-3)^2}=2+\beta$

$\alpha^2+(\beta-3)^2=\beta^2+4+4\beta$

$\Rightarrow \alpha^2=10(\beta-1/2)$

$\therefore$ Locus is $x^2=10\left(y-\frac{1}{2}\right)$

Which is parabola.

81. **(d)** Solving equations of parabolas

$y^2=4ax$ and $x^2=4ay$

we get (0, 0) and $(4a, 4a)$

Substituting in the given equation of line

$2bx+3cy+4d=0$,

we get $d=0$ and $2b+3c=0$

$\Rightarrow d^2+(2b+3c)^2=0$

82. **(b)** Equation of the normal to a parabola $y^2=4bx$ at point $\left(bt_1^2, 2bt_1\right)$ is $y=-t_1x+2bt_1+bt_1^3$

As given, it also passes through $\left(bt_2^2, 2bt_2\right)$ then

$2bt_2=-t_1bt_2^2+2bt_1+bt_1^3$

$2t_2-2t_1=-t_1\left(t_2^2-t_1^2\right)$

$=-t_1(t_2+t_1)(t_2-t_1)$

$\Rightarrow 2=-t_1(t_2+t_1) \Rightarrow t_2+t_1=-\frac{2}{t_1}$

$\Rightarrow t_2=-t_1-\frac{2}{t_1}$

83. **(b)** Any tangent to the parabola $y^2=8ax$ is

$y=mx+\frac{2a}{m}$ ...(i)

If (i) is a tangent to the circle, $x^2+y^2=2a^2$ then,

$\sqrt{2}a=\pm\frac{2a}{m\sqrt{m^2+1}}$

$\Rightarrow m^2(1+m^2)=2 \Rightarrow (m^2+2)(m^2-1)=0 \Rightarrow m=\pm 1.$

So from (i), $y=\pm(x+2a)$.

84. **(c)** Centre at (0, 0)

$\frac{x^2}{a^2}+\frac{y^2}{b^2}=1$

at point (4, –1)

$\frac{16}{a^2}+\frac{1}{b^2}=1$

$\Rightarrow 16b^2+a^2=a^2b^2$ ...(i)

at point (–2, 2)

$\frac{4}{a^2}+\frac{4}{b^2}=1$

$\Rightarrow 4b^2+4a^2=a^2b^2$ ...(ii)

$\Rightarrow 16b^2+a^2=4a^2+4b^2$

From equations (i) and (ii)

$\Rightarrow 3a^2=12b^2$

$\Rightarrow \boxed{a^2=4b^2}$

$b^2=a^2(1-e^2)$

$\Rightarrow e^2=\frac{3}{4}$

$\Rightarrow e=\frac{\sqrt{3}}{2}$

85. **(d)** $e=3/5$ & $2ae=6 \Rightarrow a=5$

$\because b^2=a^2(1-e^2)$

$\Rightarrow b^2=25(1-9/25)$

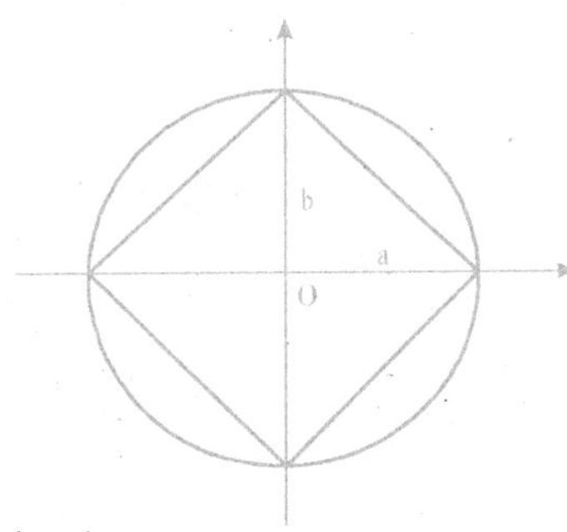

$\Rightarrow$ b = 4

$\therefore$ area of required quadrilateral = 4 (1/2 ab)
= 2ab = 40

86. (c) Equation of tangent to ellipse

$$\frac{x}{\sqrt{27}}\cos\theta + \frac{y}{\sqrt{3}}\sin\theta = 1$$

Area bounded by line and co-ordinate axis

$$\Delta = \frac{1}{2}.\frac{\sqrt{27}}{\cos\theta}.\frac{\sqrt{3}}{\sin\theta} = \frac{9}{\sin 2\theta}$$

Δ = will be minimum when $\sin 2\theta = 1$

$\Delta_{min} = 9$

87. (b) The end point of latus rectum of ellipse $\frac{x^2}{a^2}+\frac{y^2}{b^2}=1$ in first quadrant is $\left(ae, \frac{b^2}{a}\right)$ and the tangent at this point intersects x-axis at $\left(\frac{a}{e}, 0\right)$ and y-axis at (0, a).

The given ellipse is $\frac{x^2}{9}+\frac{y^2}{5}=1$

Then $a^2 = 9, b^2 = 5$

$$\Rightarrow \quad e = \sqrt{1-\frac{5}{9}} = \frac{2}{3}$$

$\therefore$ end point of latus rectum in first quadrant is $L(2, 5/3)$

Equation of tangent at L is $\frac{2x}{9}+\frac{y}{3}=1$

It meets x-axis at A (9/2, 0) and y-axis at B (0, 3)

$\therefore$ Area of ΔOAB $= \frac{1}{2}\times\frac{9}{2}\times 3 = \frac{27}{4}$

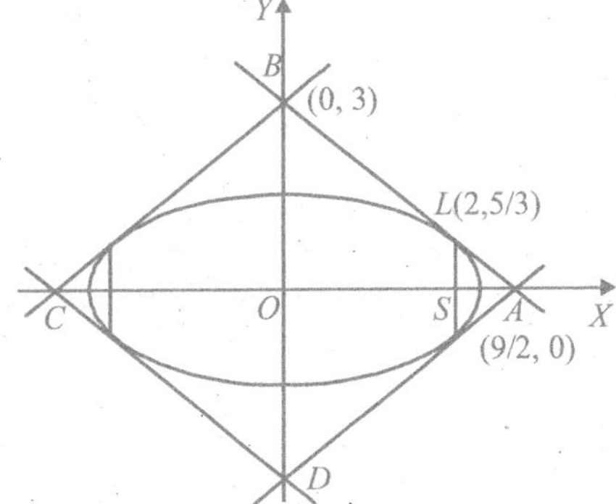

By symmetry area of quadrilateral

$$= 4 \times (\text{Area } \Delta OAB) = 4\times\frac{27}{4} = 27 \text{ sq. units.}$$

88. (b) Focus of an ellipse is given as (± ae, 0)

Distance between them = 2ae

According to the question, $2ae = \frac{b^2}{a}$

$\Rightarrow 2a^2e = b^2 = a^2(1-e^2)$

$\Rightarrow 2e = 1 - e^2 \Rightarrow (e+1)^2 = 2 \Rightarrow e = \sqrt{2}-1$

89. (a) Given equation of ellipse can be written as

$$\frac{x^2}{6}+\frac{y^2}{2}=1$$

$\Rightarrow \quad a^2 = 6, b^2 = 2$

Now, equation of any variable tangent is

$$y = mx \pm \sqrt{a^2m^2+b^2} \quad ...(i)$$

where m is slope of the tangent

So, equation of perpendicular line drawn from centre to tangent is

$$y = \frac{-x}{m} \quad ...(ii)$$

Eliminating *m*, we get

$$(x^4+y^4+2x^2y^2) = a^2x^2+b^2y^2$$

$$\Rightarrow \quad (x^2+y^2)^2 = a^2x^2+b^2y^2$$

$$\Rightarrow \quad \boxed{(x^2+y^2)^2 = 6x^2+2y^2}$$

90. (b) Let point A (a, 0) is on x-axis and B (0, b) is on y-axis.

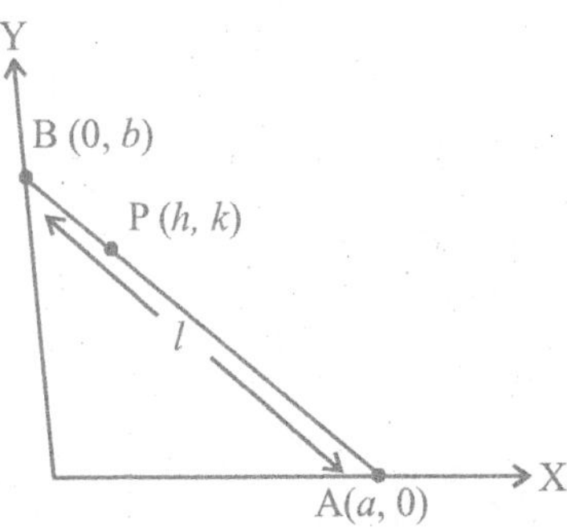

Let P (h, k) divides AB in the ratio 1 : 2.
So, by section formula

$$h = \frac{2(0)+1(a)}{1+2} = \frac{a}{3}$$

$$k = \frac{2(b)+1(0)}{3} = \frac{2b}{3}$$

$$\Rightarrow a = 3h \text{ and } b = \frac{3k}{2}$$

Now, $a^2 + b^2 = l^2$

$$\Rightarrow 9h^2 + \frac{9k^2}{4} = l^2$$

$$\Rightarrow \frac{h^2}{\left(\frac{l}{3}\right)^2} + \frac{k^2}{\left(\frac{2l}{3}\right)^2} = 1$$

$$\text{Now e} = \sqrt{1-\left(\frac{l^2}{9}\times\frac{9}{4l^2}\right)} = \sqrt{1-\frac{1}{4}} = \frac{\sqrt{3}}{2}$$

Thus, required locus of P is an ellipse with eccentricity $\frac{\sqrt{3}}{2}$.

91. **(a)** Let $\frac{x^2}{a^2}+\frac{y^2}{b^2}=1$ be the equation of ellipse.

Given that F_1B and F_2B are perpendicular to each other.

Slope of F_1B × slope of F_2B = – 1

$$\left(\frac{0-b}{-ae-0}\right)\times\left(\frac{0-b}{ae-0}\right) = -1$$

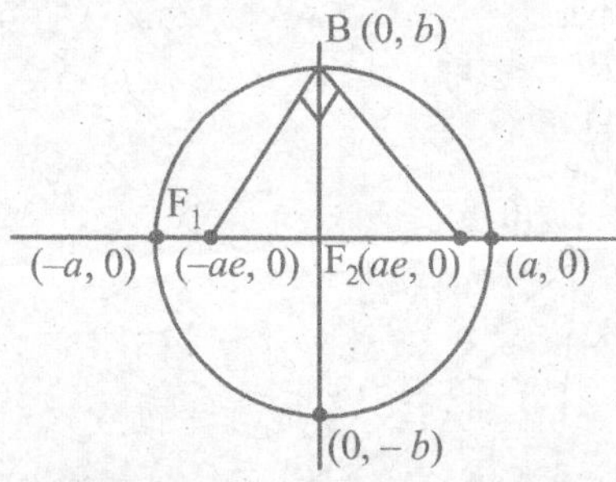

$$\left(\frac{b}{ae}\right)\times\left(\frac{-b}{ae}\right) = -1$$

$$b^2 = a^2e^2$$

$$e^2 = \frac{b^2}{a^2} \qquad \left\{\because e^2 = 1-\frac{b^2}{a^2}\right\}$$

$$1-\frac{b^2}{a^2} = \frac{b^2}{a^2}$$

$$1 = 2\frac{b^2}{a^2} \Rightarrow \frac{b^2}{a^2} = \frac{1}{2}$$

$$e^2 = 1-\frac{b^2}{a^2} = 1-\frac{1}{2} = \frac{1}{2}$$

$$e^2 = \frac{1}{2}$$

No common tangents for these two circles.

92. **(a)** From the given equation of ellipse, we have

$$a=4, b=3, e=\sqrt{1-\frac{9}{16}}$$

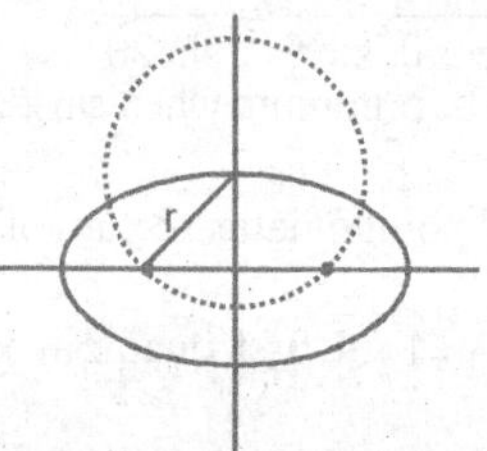

$$\Rightarrow e = \frac{\sqrt{7}}{4}$$

Now, radius of this circle $= a^2 = 16$

$\Rightarrow$ Focii $= (\pm\sqrt{7}, 0)$

Now equation of circle is $(x-0)^2+(y-3)^2=16$

$x^2+y^2-6y-7=0$

93. **(c)** Given ellipse is $4x^2+9y^2=36$

$$\Rightarrow \frac{x^2}{9}+\frac{y^2}{4}=1$$

Normal at the point is parallel to the line $4x-2y-5=0$

Slope of normal $= 2$

Slope of tangent $= \frac{-1}{2}$

Point of contact to ellipse $\frac{x^2}{a^2}+\frac{y^2}{b^2}=1$ and line is $\left(\frac{a^2m}{\sqrt{a^2m^2+b^2}}, \frac{b}{\sqrt{a^2m^2+b^2}}\right)$

Now, $a^2=9$, $b^2=4$

$$\therefore \text{ Point} = \left(\frac{-9}{5}, \frac{8}{5}\right)$$

94. **(c)** Given equations of ellipses

$$E_1 : \frac{x^2}{3}+\frac{y^2}{2}=1$$

$$\Rightarrow e_1=\sqrt{1-\frac{2}{3}}=\frac{1}{\sqrt{3}}$$

and $$E_2 : \frac{x^2}{16}+\frac{y^2}{b^2}=1$$

$$\Rightarrow e_2=\sqrt{\frac{1-b^2}{16}}=\sqrt{\frac{16-b^2}{4}}$$

Also, given $e_1 \times e_2=\frac{1}{2}$

$$\Rightarrow \frac{1}{\sqrt{3}}\times\sqrt{\frac{16-b^2}{4}}=\frac{1}{2} \Rightarrow 16-b^2=12$$

$\Rightarrow b^2=4$

$\therefore$ Length of minor axis of

$E_2=2b=2\times 2=4$

95. **(d)** $x^2=8y$ ...(i)

$$\frac{x^2}{3}+y^2=1 \quad ...(ii)$$

From (i) and (ii),

$$\frac{8y}{3}+y^2=1 \Rightarrow y=-3,\ \frac{1}{3}$$

When $y=-3$, then $x^2=-24$, which is not possible.

When $y=\frac{1}{3}$, then $x=\pm\frac{2\sqrt{6}}{3}$

Point of intersection are

$$\left(\frac{2\sqrt{6}}{3},\frac{1}{3}\right) \text{ and } \left(-\frac{2\sqrt{6}}{3},\frac{1}{3}\right)$$

Required equation of the line,

$$y-\frac{1}{3}=0 \Rightarrow 3y-1=0$$

96. **(d)** Any tangent on an ellipse $\frac{x^2}{a^2}+\frac{y^2}{b^2}=1$ is given by

$$y=mx\pm\sqrt{a^2m^2+b^2}$$

Here $a=2, b=1$

$$m=\frac{1-0}{0-2}=-\frac{1}{2}$$

$$c=\sqrt{4\left(-\frac{1}{2}\right)^2+1^2}=\sqrt{2}$$

So, $y=-\frac{1}{2}x\pm\sqrt{2}$

For ellipse : $\frac{x^2}{4}+\frac{y^2}{1}=1$

We put $y=-\frac{1}{2}x+\sqrt{2}$

$$\therefore \frac{x^2}{4}+\left(-\frac{x}{2}+\sqrt{2}\right)^2=1$$

$$\frac{x^2}{4}+\left(\frac{x^2}{4}-2\left(\frac{x}{2}\right)\sqrt{2}+2\right)=1$$

$$\Rightarrow x^2+2\sqrt{2}x+2=0$$

or $x^2-2\sqrt{2}x+2=0$

$$\Rightarrow x=\sqrt{2} \text{ or } -\sqrt{2}$$

If $x=\sqrt{2}, y=\frac{1}{\sqrt{2}}$ and $x=-\sqrt{2},\ y=-\frac{1}{\sqrt{2}}$

$\therefore$ Points are $\left(\sqrt{2},\frac{1}{\sqrt{2}}\right), \left(-\sqrt{2},-\frac{1}{\sqrt{2}}\right)$

$$\therefore P_1P_2=\sqrt{\left\{\frac{1}{\sqrt{2}}-\left(-\frac{1}{\sqrt{2}}\right)\right\}^2+\left\{\sqrt{2}-(-\sqrt{2})\right\}^2}$$

$$=\sqrt{\left(\frac{2}{\sqrt{2}}\right)^2+\left(2\sqrt{2}\right)^2}=\sqrt{2+8}=\sqrt{10}$$

97. **(d)** Let the ellipse be $\frac{x^2}{a^2}+\frac{y^2}{b^2}=1$

It passes through (–3, 1) so $\frac{9}{a^2}+\frac{1}{b^2}=1$ ..(i)

Also, $b^2=a^2(1-2/5)$

$\Rightarrow 5b^2=3a^2$ ...(ii)

Solving (i) and (ii) we get $a^2=\frac{32}{3}, b^2=\frac{32}{5}$

So, the equation of the ellipse is

$$3x^2+5y^2=32$$

98. (a) The given ellipse is $\frac{x^2}{4}+\frac{y^2}{1}=1$

So $A=(2, 0)$ and $B=(0, 1)$

If $PQRS$ is the rectangle in which it is inscribed, then $P=(2, 1)$.

Let $\frac{x^2}{a^2}+\frac{y^2}{b^2}=1$ be the ellipse circumscribing the rectangle $PQRS$.

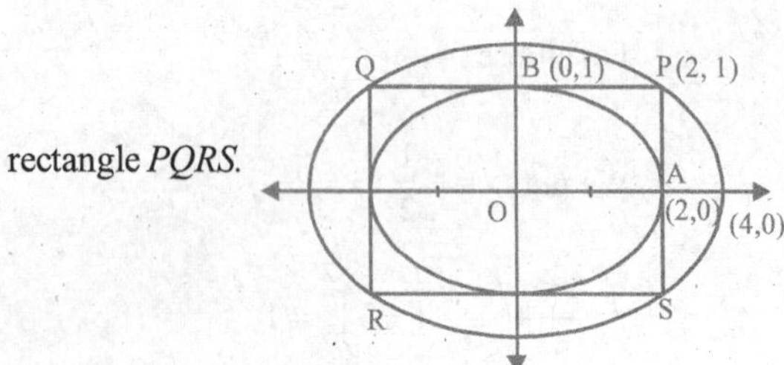

Then it passed through P (2,1)

$\therefore \frac{4}{a^2}+\frac{1}{b^2}=1$ ....(A)

Also, given that, it passes through (4, 0)

$\therefore \frac{16}{a^2}+0=1 \Rightarrow a^2=16$

$\Rightarrow b^2=4/3$ [substituting $a^2=16$ in eq^n (A)]

$\therefore$ The required ellipse is $\frac{x^2}{16}+\frac{y^2}{4/3}=1$

or $x^2+12y^2=16$

99. (a) Perpendicular distance of directrix from focus

$=\frac{a}{e}-ae=4$

$\Rightarrow a\left(2-\frac{1}{2}\right)=4$

$\Rightarrow a=\frac{8}{3}$

$\therefore$ Semi major axis $=8/3$

100. (a) $2ae=6 \Rightarrow ae=3$; $2b=8 \Rightarrow b=4$

$b^2=a^2(1-e^2)$; $16=a^2-a^2e^2$

$\Rightarrow a^2=16+9=25 \Rightarrow a=5$

$\therefore e=\frac{3}{a}=\frac{3}{5}$

101. (a) $\because \angle FBF'=90° \Rightarrow FB^2+F'B^2=FF'^2$

$\therefore \left(\sqrt{a^2e^2+b^2}\right)^2+\left(\sqrt{a^2e^2+b^2}\right)^2=(2ae)^2$

$\Rightarrow 2(a^2e^2+b^2)=4a^2e^2 \Rightarrow e^2=\frac{b^2}{a^2}$

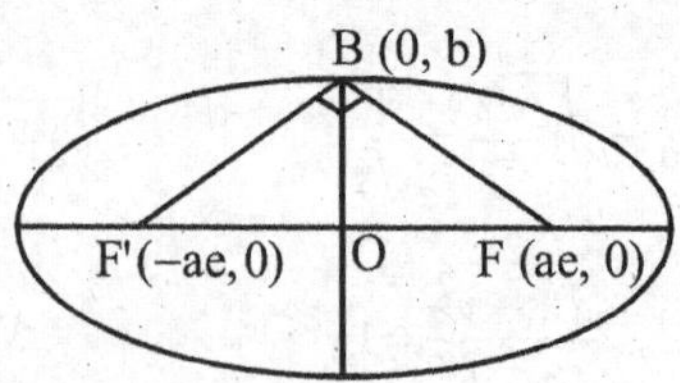

Also $e^2=1-b^2/a^2=1-e^2$

$\Rightarrow 2e^2=1,\ e=\frac{1}{\sqrt{2}}$.

102. (b) $e=\frac{1}{2}$. Directrix, $x=\frac{a}{e}=4$

$\therefore a=4\times\frac{1}{2}=2$ $\qquad \therefore b=2\sqrt{1-\frac{1}{4}}=\sqrt{3}$

Equation of ellipse is

$\frac{x^2}{4}+\frac{y^2}{3}=1 \Rightarrow 3x^2+4y^2=12$

103. (c) Equation of hyperbola is $\frac{x^2}{a^2}-\frac{y^2}{b^2}=1$

foci is $(\pm 2, 0) \Rightarrow ae=2 \Rightarrow a^2e^2=4$

Since $b^2=a^2(e^2-1)$

$b^2=a^2e^2-a^2$

$\therefore \quad a^2+b^2=4$ ...(a)

Hyperbola passes through $(\sqrt{2},\sqrt{3})$

$\therefore \frac{2}{a^2}-\frac{3}{b^2}=1$ ...(b)

$\frac{2}{4-b^2}\ \frac{-3}{b^2}=1$

$\Rightarrow b^4+b^2-12=0$

$\Rightarrow (b^2-3)(b^2+4)=0$

$\Rightarrow b^2=3$

$b^2=-4$ (Not possible)

For $b^2=3$

$\Rightarrow a^2=1$

$\therefore \frac{x^2}{1}-\frac{y^2}{3}=1$

Equation of tangent is $\frac{\sqrt{2}x}{1}-\frac{\sqrt{3}y}{3}=1$

Clearly $(2\sqrt{2},3\sqrt{3})$ satisfies it.

104. (d) Here, $tx-2y-3t=0$ & $x-2ty+3=0$

On solving, we get;

$y = \frac{6t}{2t^2-2} = \frac{3t}{t^2-1}$ & $x = \frac{3t^2+3}{t^2-1}$

Put $t = \tan\theta$

$\therefore$ $x = -3\sec 2\theta$ & $2y = 3(-\tan 2\theta)$

$\because$ $\sec^2 2\theta - \tan^2 2\theta = 1$

$\Rightarrow$ $\frac{x^2}{9} - \frac{y^2}{9/4} = 1$

which represents a hyperbola

$\therefore$ $a^2 = 9$ & $b^2 = 9/4$

$\lambda(\text{T.A.}) = 6;\ e^2 = 1 + \frac{9/4}{9} = 1 + \frac{1}{4} \Rightarrow e = \frac{\sqrt{5}}{2}$

105. (a) $\frac{2b^2}{a} = 8$ and $2b = \frac{1}{2}(2ae)$

$\Rightarrow 4b^2 = a^2e^2 \Rightarrow 4a^2(e^2-1) = a^2e^2$

$\Rightarrow 3e^2 = 4 \Rightarrow e = \frac{2}{\sqrt{3}}$

106. (c) $\frac{x^2}{12} + \frac{y^2}{16} = 1$

$e = \sqrt{1 - \frac{12}{16}} = \frac{1}{2}$

Foci (0, 2) & (0, – 2)

So, transverse axis of hyperbola = $2b = 4 \Rightarrow b = 2$

& $a^2 = 1^2(e^2 - 1)$

$\Rightarrow$ $a^2 = 4\left(\frac{9}{4} - 1\right)$

$\Rightarrow$ $a^2 = 5$

$\therefore$ It's equation is $\frac{x^2}{5} - \frac{y^2}{4} = -1$

The point $(5, 2\sqrt{3})$ does not satisfy the above equation.

107. (a) $S(5, 0)$ is focus $\Rightarrow ae = 5$ (focus) ——— (a)

$x = \frac{a}{5} \Rightarrow \frac{a}{e} = \frac{9}{5}$ (directrix) ——— (b)

(a) & (b) $\Rightarrow a^2 = 9$

(a) $\Rightarrow (e) = \frac{5}{3}$

$b^2 = a^2(e^2 - 1) \Rightarrow b^2 = 16$

$a^2 - b^2 = 9 - 16 = -7$

108. (c) Equation of hyperbola is

$\frac{x^2}{4} - \frac{y^2}{9} = 1$

Its Foci = $(\pm\sqrt{13}, 0)$

$e = \frac{\sqrt{13}}{2}$

If e, be the eccentricity of the ellipse, then

$e_1 \times \frac{\sqrt{13}}{2} = \frac{1}{2} \Rightarrow e_1 = \frac{1}{\sqrt{13}}$

Equation of ellipse is

$\frac{x^2}{a^2} + \frac{y^2}{b^2} = 1$

Since ellipse passes through the foci $(\pm\sqrt{13}, 0)$ of the hyperbola, therefore

$a^2 = 13$

Now $\sqrt{a^2 - b^2} = ae_1$

$\therefore 13 - b^2 = 1$

$\Rightarrow b^2 = 12$

Hence, equation of ellipse is

$\frac{x^2}{13} + \frac{y^2}{12} = 1$

Now putting the coordinate of the point $\left(\frac{\sqrt{13}}{2}, \frac{\sqrt{3}}{2}\right)$ in the equation of the ellipse, we get

$\frac{13}{4\times 13} + \frac{3}{4\times 12} = 1$

$\Rightarrow \frac{1}{4} + \frac{1}{16} = 1$, which is not true,

Hence the point $\left(\frac{\sqrt{13}}{2}, \frac{\sqrt{3}}{2}\right)$ does not lie on the ellipse.

109. (a)

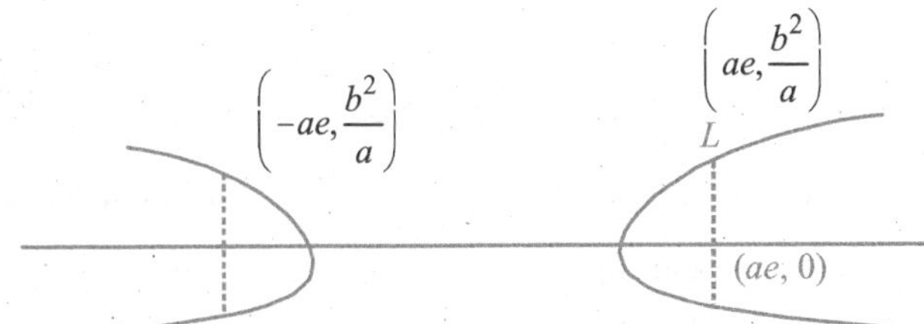

Given $\frac{x^2}{4} - \frac{y^2}{5} = 1$

$\Rightarrow$ $a^2 = 4,\ b^2 = 5$

$e = \sqrt{\frac{a^2+b^2}{a^2}} = \sqrt{\frac{4+5}{4}} = \frac{3}{2}$

$L = \left(2\times\frac{3}{2}, \frac{5}{2}\right) = \left(3, \frac{5}{2}\right)$

Equation of tangent at (x_1, y_1) is

$\frac{xx_1}{a^2} - \frac{yy_1}{b^2} = 1$

Here $x_1 = 3, y_1 = \frac{5}{2}$

$$\Rightarrow \frac{3x}{4} - \frac{y}{2} = 1 \Rightarrow \frac{x}{\frac{4}{3}} + \frac{y}{-2} = 1$$

x-intercept of the tangent, OA $= \frac{4}{3}$

y-intercept of the tangent, OB $= -2$

$$OA^2 - OB^2 = \frac{16}{9} - 4 = -\frac{20}{9}$$

110. (d) Let the coordinate at point of intersection of normals at P and Q be (h, k)

Since, equation of normals to the hyperbola

$\frac{x^2}{a^2} - \frac{y^2}{b^2} = 1$ At point (x_1, y_1) is $\frac{a^2x}{x_1} + \frac{b^2y}{y_1} = a^2 + b^2$

therefore equation of normal to the hyperbola

$\frac{x^2}{3^2} - \frac{y^2}{2^2} = 1$ at point P $(3\sec\theta, 2\tan\theta)$ is

$$\frac{3^2x}{3\sec\theta} + \frac{2^2y}{2\tan\theta} = 3^2 + 2^2$$

$$\Rightarrow \boxed{3x\cos\theta + 2y\cot\theta = 3^2 + 2^2} \quad ...(1)$$

Similarly, Equation of normal to the hyperbola

$\frac{x^2}{3^2} - \frac{y^2}{2^2}$ at point Q $(3\sec\phi, 2\tan\phi)$ is

$$\frac{3^2x}{3\sec\phi} + \frac{2^2y}{2\tan\phi} = 3^2 + 2^2$$

$$\Rightarrow \boxed{3x\cos\phi + 2y\cot\phi = 3^2 + 2^2} \quad ...(2)$$

Given $\theta + \phi = \frac{\pi}{2} \Rightarrow \phi = \frac{\pi}{2} - \theta$ and these passes through (h, k)

$\therefore$ From eq. (2)

$$3x\cos\left(\frac{\pi}{2} - \theta\right) + 2y\cot\left(\frac{\pi}{2} - \theta\right) = 3^2 + 2^2$$

$$\Rightarrow \boxed{3h\sin\theta + 2k\tan\theta = 3^2 + 2^2} \quad ...(3)$$

and $\boxed{3h\cos\theta + 2k\cot\theta = 3^2 + 2^2}$ ...(4)

Comparing equation (3) & (4), we get

$$3h\cos\theta + 2k\cot\theta = 3h\sin\theta + 2k\tan\theta$$

$$3h\cos\theta - 3h\sin\theta = 2k\tan\theta - 2k\cot\theta$$

$$3h(\cos\theta - \sin\theta) = 2k(\tan\theta - \cot\theta)$$

$$3h(\cos\theta - \sin\theta) = 2k\frac{(\sin\theta - \cos\theta)(\sin\theta + \cos\theta)}{\sin\theta\cos\theta}$$

$$\text{or, } 3h = \frac{-2k(\sin\theta + \cos\theta)}{\sin\theta\cos\theta} \quad ...(5)$$

Now, putting the value of equation (5) in eq. (3)

$$\frac{-2k(\sin\theta + \cos\theta)\sin\theta}{\sin\theta\cos\theta} + 2k\tan\theta = 3^2 + 2^2$$

$$\Rightarrow 2k\tan\theta - 2k + 2k\tan\theta = 13$$

$$-2k = 13 \Rightarrow k = \frac{-13}{2}$$

Hence, ordinate of point of intersection of normals at P and Q is $\frac{-13}{2}$

111. (a) $x^2 - 6y$ ...(i)

$2x^2 - 4y^2 = 9$ ...(ii)

Consider the line,

$$x - y = \frac{3}{2} \quad ...(iii)$$

On solving (i) and (iii), we get only

$$x = 3, y = \frac{3}{2}$$

Hence $\left(3, \frac{3}{2}\right)$ is the point of contact of conic (i), and line (iii)

On solving (ii) and (iii), we get only $x = 3,\ y = \frac{3}{2}$

Hence $\left(3, \frac{3}{2}\right)$ is also the point of contact of conic (ii) and line (iii).

Hence line (iii) is the common tangent to both the given conics.

112. (d) Equation of the tangent at the point 'θ' is

$$\frac{x\sec\theta}{a} - \frac{y\tan\theta}{b} = 1$$

$$\Rightarrow P = (a\cos\theta, 0) \text{ and } Q = (0, -b\cot\theta)$$

Let R be (h, k) $\Rightarrow h = a\cos\theta,\ k = -b\cot\theta$

$$\Rightarrow \frac{k}{h} = \frac{-b}{a\sin\theta} \Rightarrow \sin\theta = \frac{-bh}{ak} \text{ and } \cos\theta = \frac{h}{a}$$

By squaring and adding,

$$\frac{b^2h^2}{a^2k^2} + \frac{h^2}{a^2} = 1$$

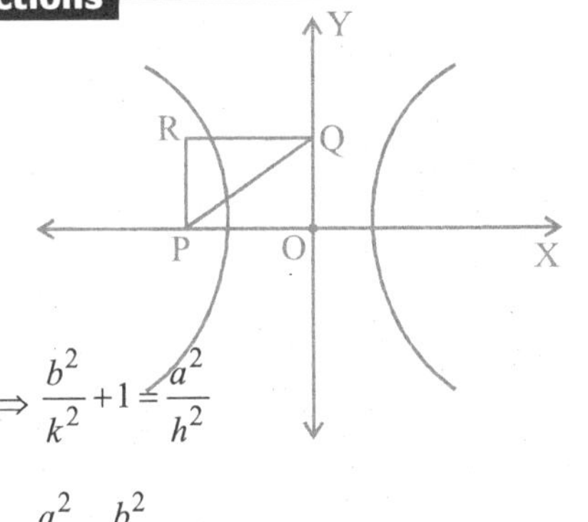

$\Rightarrow \frac{b^2}{k^2}+1=\frac{a^2}{h^2}$

$\Rightarrow \frac{a^2}{h^2}-\frac{b^2}{k^2}=1$

Now, given eq^n of hyperbola is $\frac{x^2}{4}-\frac{y^2}{2}=1$

$\Rightarrow a^2=4, b^2=2$

$\therefore$ R lies on $\frac{a^2}{x^2}-\frac{b^2}{y^2}=1$ i.e., $\frac{4}{x^2}-\frac{2}{y^2}=1$

113. (c) Given equation of ellipse is

$\frac{x^2}{16}+\frac{y^2}{b^2}=1$

eccentricity $= e=\sqrt{1-\frac{b^2}{16}}$

foci: $\pm ae=\pm 4\sqrt{1-\frac{b^2}{16}}$

Equation of hyperbola is $\frac{x^2}{144}-\frac{y^2}{81}=\frac{1}{25}$

$\Rightarrow \frac{x^2}{\frac{144}{25}}-\frac{y^2}{\frac{81}{25}}=1$

eccentricity $= e=\sqrt{1+\frac{81}{25}\times\frac{25}{144}}=\sqrt{1+\frac{81}{144}}$

$=\sqrt{\frac{225}{144}}=\frac{15}{12}$

foci: $\pm ae=\pm\frac{12}{5}\times\frac{15}{12}=\pm 3$

Since, foci of ellipse and hyperbola coincide

$\therefore \ \pm 4\sqrt{1-\frac{b^2}{16}}=\pm 3 \Rightarrow b^2=7$

$\frac{K^2}{9}-\frac{4}{4}=1 \qquad (\because b=\pm 2)$

$\Rightarrow \ K^2=18$

114. (a) Given hyperbola is

$\frac{x^2}{9}-\frac{y^2}{b^2}=1$

Since this passes through $(K, 2)$, therefore

$\frac{K^2}{9}-\frac{4}{b^2}=1 \qquad \text{...(1)}$

Also, given $e=\sqrt{1+\frac{b^2}{a^2}}=\frac{\sqrt{13}}{3}$

$\Rightarrow \ \sqrt{1+\frac{b^2}{9}}=\frac{\sqrt{13}}{3} \Rightarrow 9+b^2=13$

$\Rightarrow b=\pm 2$

Now, from eq^n (1), we have

$\frac{K^2}{9}-\frac{4}{4}=1 \qquad (\because b=\pm 2)$

$\Rightarrow \ K^2=18$

115. (b) $ae=2$

$e=2$

$\therefore \quad a=1$

$b^2=a^2\left(e^2-1\right)$

$b^2=1(4-1)$

$b^2=3$

Equation of hyperbola, $\frac{x^2}{a^2}-\frac{y^2}{b^2}=1$

$\Rightarrow \ \frac{x^2}{1}-\frac{y^2}{3}=1$

$3x^2-y^2=3$

116. (b) Given, equation of hyperbola is

$\frac{x^2}{\cos^2\alpha}-\frac{y^2}{\sin^2\alpha}=1$

We know that the equation of hyperbola is

$\frac{x^2}{a^2}-\frac{y^2}{b^2}=1$ Here, $a^2=\cos^2\alpha$ and

$b^2=\sin^2\alpha$

We know that, $b^2=a^2(e^2-1)$

$\Rightarrow \ \sin^2\alpha=\cos^2\alpha(e^2-1)$

$\Rightarrow \ \sin^2\alpha+\cos^2\alpha=\cos^2\alpha.e^2$

$\Rightarrow e^2=1+\tan^2\alpha=\sec^2\alpha$

$\Rightarrow e=\sec\alpha$

$\therefore \quad ae = \cos\alpha \cdot \frac{1}{\cos\alpha} = 1$

Co-ordinates of foci are $(\pm ae, 0)$

i.e. $(\pm 1, 0)$
Hence, abscissae of foci remain constant when α varies.

117. (d) Tangent to the hyperbola $\frac{x^2}{a^2} - \frac{y^2}{b^2} = 1$ is

$y = mx \pm \sqrt{a^2m^2 - b^2}$

Given that $y = \alpha x + \beta$ is the tangent of hyperbola

$\Rightarrow \quad m = \alpha$ and $a^2m^2 - b^2 = \beta^2$

$\therefore \quad a^2\alpha^2 - b^2 = \beta^2$

Locus is $a^2x^2 - y^2 = b^2$ which is hyperbola.

118. (d) $\frac{x^2}{144} - \frac{y^2}{81} = \frac{1}{25}$

$a = \sqrt{\frac{144}{25}}, b = \sqrt{\frac{81}{25}}, \quad e = \sqrt{1 + \frac{81}{144}} = \frac{15}{12} = \frac{5}{4}$

$\because \quad$ Foci $= (\pm 3, 0)$

$\therefore \quad$ foci of ellipse = foci of hyperbola

$\therefore \quad$ for ellipse $ae = 3$ but $a = 4$,

$\therefore \quad e = \frac{3}{4}$

Then $b^2 = a^2(1 - e^2)$

$\Rightarrow b^2 = 16\left(1 - \frac{9}{16}\right) = 7$

Limits and Derivatives

TOPIC-1 : Limit of a Function, Left Hand & Right Hand limits, Existance of Limits, Sandwitch Theorem, Evaluation of Limits when X→ ∞, Limits by Factorisation, Substitution & Rationalisation

1. $\lim_{x\to\frac{\pi}{2}} \frac{\cot x - \cos x}{(\pi - 2x)^3}$ equals : **[2017]**

(a) $\frac{1}{4}$ (b) $\frac{1}{24}$

(c) $\frac{1}{16}$ (d) $\frac{1}{8}$

2. $\lim_{x\to 3} \frac{\sqrt{3x}-3}{\sqrt{2x-4}-\sqrt{2}}$ is equal to : **[Online April 8, 2017]**

(a) $\sqrt{3}$ (b) $\frac{1}{\sqrt{2}}$

(c) $\frac{\sqrt{3}}{2}$ (d) $\frac{1}{2\sqrt{2}}$

3. $\lim_{x\to 0} \frac{(1-\cos 2x)(3+\cos x)}{x \tan 4x}$ is equal to : **[2015]**

(a) 2 (b) $\frac{1}{2}$

(c) 4 (d) 3

4. $\lim_{x\to 0} \frac{e^{x^2} - \cos x}{\sin^2 x}$ is equal to : **[Online April 10, 2015]**

(a) 2 (b) 3

(c) $\frac{3}{2}$ (d) $\frac{5}{4}$

5. $\lim_{x\to 0} \frac{\sin\left(\pi \cos^2 x\right)}{x^2}$ is equal to: **[2014]**

(a) $-\pi$ (b) π

(c) $\frac{\pi}{2}$ (d) 1

6. If

$$\lim_{x\to 2} \frac{\tan(x-2)\left\{x^2+(k-2)x-2k\right\}}{x^2-4x+4} = 5,$$

then k is equal to: **[Online April 11, 2014]**

(a) 0 (b) 1

(c) 2 (d) 3

7. $\lim_{x\to 0} \frac{(1-\cos 2x)(3+\cos x)}{x \tan 4x}$ is equal to **[2013]**

(a) $-\frac{1}{4}$ (b) $\frac{1}{2}$

(c) 1 (d) 2

8. $\lim_{x\to 0} \frac{\sin\left(\pi \cos^2 x\right)}{x^2}$ equals **[Online May 26, 2012]**

(a) $-\pi$ (b) 1

(c) -1 (d) π

9. $\lim_{x\to 0} \left(\frac{x - \sin x}{x}\right) \sin\left(\frac{1}{x}\right)$ **[Online May 7, 2012]**

(a) equals 1 (b) equals 0

(c) does not exist (d) equals – 1

10. Let $f : R \to [0,\infty)$ be such that $\lim_{x\to 5} f(x)$ exists and

$$\lim_{x\to 5} \frac{(f(x))^2 - 9}{\sqrt{|x-5|}} = 0$$ **[2011RS]**

Then $\lim_{x\to 5} f(x)$ equals :

(a) 0 (b) 1

(c) 2 (d) 3

11. $\lim_{x\to 2} \left(\frac{\sqrt{1-\cos\{2(x-2)\}}}{x-2}\right)$ **[2011]**

(a) equals $\sqrt{2}$ (b) equals $-\sqrt{2}$

(c) equals $\frac{1}{\sqrt{2}}$ (d) does not exist

12. Let f : R → R be a positive increasing function with

$\lim_{x\to\infty} \frac{f(3x)}{f(x)} = 1$ then $\lim_{x\to\infty} \frac{f(2x)}{f(x)} =$ **[2010]**

(a) $\frac{2}{3}$ (b) $\frac{3}{2}$

(c) 3 (d) 1

13. Let α and β be the distinct roots of $ax^2+bx+c=0$, then $\lim_{x\to\alpha}\frac{1-\cos(ax^2+bx+c)}{(x-\alpha)^2}$ is equal to **[2005]**

(a) $\frac{a^2}{2}(\alpha-\beta)^2$ (b) 0

(c) $\frac{-a^2}{2}(\alpha-\beta)^2$ (d) $\frac{1}{2}(\alpha-\beta)^2$

14. $\lim_{x\to\frac{\pi}{2}}\frac{\left[1-\tan\left(\frac{x}{2}\right)\right][1-\sin x]}{\left[1+\tan\left(\frac{x}{2}\right)\right][\pi-2x]^3}$ is **[2003]**

(a) ∞ (b) $\frac{1}{8}$

(c) 0 (d) $\frac{1}{32}$

15. $\lim_{x\to 0}\frac{\log x^n-[x]}{[x]}, n\in N$, ([x] denotes greatest integer less than or equal to x) **[2002]**

(a) has value -1 (b) has value 0

(c) has value 1 (d) does not exist

16. $\lim_{x\to\infty}\left(\frac{x^2+5x+3}{x^2+x+2}\right)^x$ **[2002]**

(a) e^4 (b) e^2

(c) e^3 (d) 1

17. $\lim_{x\to 0}\frac{\sqrt{1-\cos 2x}}{\sqrt{2}x}$ is **[2002]**

(a) 1 (b) –1

(c) zero (d) does not exist

TOPIC-2 : Limits Using L-hospital's Rule, Evaluation of Limits of the form 1^∞, Limits by Expansion Method

18. Let $p=\lim_{x\to 0^+}\left(1+\tan^2\sqrt{x}\right)^{\frac{1}{2x}}$ then log p is equal to : **[2016]**

(a) $\frac{1}{2}$ (b) $\frac{1}{4}$

(c) 2 (d) 1

19. $\lim_{x\to 0}\frac{(1-\cos 2x)^2}{2x\tan x-x\tan 2x}$ is : **[Online April 10, 2016]**

(a) 2 (b) $-\frac{1}{2}$

(c) –2 (d) $\frac{1}{2}$

20. If $\lim_{x\to\infty}\left(1+\frac{a}{x}-\frac{4}{x^2}\right)^{2x}=e^3$, then 'a' is equal to : **[Online April 9, 2016]**

(a) 2 (b) $\frac{3}{2}$

(c) $\frac{1}{2}$ (d) $\frac{2}{3}$

21. If $\lim_{x\to\infty}\left(1+\frac{a}{x}+\frac{b}{x^2}\right)^{2x}=e^2$, then the values of a and b, are **[2004]**

(a) $a=1$ and $b=2$ (b) $a=1, b\in R$

(c) $a\in R, b=2$ (d) $a\in R, b\in R$

22. Let $f(x)=4$ and $f'(x)=4$. Then $\lim_{x\to 2}\frac{xf(2)-2f(x)}{x-2}$ is given by **[2002]**

(a) 2 (b) –2

(c) –4 (d) 3

TOPIC-3 : Derivatives of Polynomial & Trigonometric Functions, Derivative of Sum, Difference, Product & Quotient of two functions

23. Let f(x) be a polynomial of degree four having extreme values at x = 1 and x = 2. If $\lim_{x\to 0}\left[1+\frac{f(x)}{x^2}\right]=3$, then f(2) is equal to : **[2015]**

(a) 0 (b) 4

(c) –8 (d) –4

24. Let $f(1)=-2$ and $f'(x)\geq 4.2$ for $1\leq x\leq 6$. The possible value of $f(6)$ lies in the interval : **[April 25, 2013]**

(a) [15, 19) (b) $(-\infty, 12)$

(c) [12, 15) (d) $[19, \infty)$

25. If $f(x)=3x^{10}-7x^8+5x^6-21x^3+3x^2-7$, then $\lim_{\alpha\to 0}\frac{f(1-\alpha)-f(1)}{\alpha^3+3\alpha}$ is **[Online May 19, 2012]**

(a) $-\frac{53}{3}$ (b) $\frac{53}{3}$

(c) $-\frac{55}{3}$ (d) $\frac{55}{3}$

Hints & Solutions

1. (c) $\lim\limits_{x\to\frac{\pi}{2}} \dfrac{\cot x(1-\sin x)}{-8\left(x-\frac{\pi}{2}\right)^3} = \lim\limits_{x\to\frac{\pi}{2}} \dfrac{\cot x(1-\sin x)}{8\left(\frac{\pi}{2}-x\right)^3}$

Put $\frac{\pi}{2}-x=t \Rightarrow$ as $x\to\frac{\pi}{2} \Rightarrow t\to 0$

$= \lim\limits_{t\to 0} \dfrac{\cot\left(\frac{\pi}{2}-t\right)\left(1-\sin\left(\frac{\pi}{2}-t\right)\right)}{8t^3}$

$= \lim\limits_{t\to 0} \dfrac{\tan t(1-\cos t)}{8t^3}$

$= \lim\limits_{t\to 0} \dfrac{\tan t}{8t}.\dfrac{1-\cos t}{t^2}$

$= \dfrac{1}{8}.1.\dfrac{1}{2} = \dfrac{1}{16}$

2. (b) Let $A = \lim\limits_{x\to 3} \dfrac{\sqrt{3x}-3}{\sqrt{2x-4}-\sqrt{2}}$

Rationalise

$\Rightarrow A = \lim\limits_{x\to 3} \dfrac{(3x-9)\times\left(2x-4+\sqrt{2}\right)}{\{(2x-4)-2\}\times\left(\sqrt{3x}+3\right)}$

$= \lim\limits_{x\to 3} \dfrac{3(x-3)}{2(x-3)} \times \dfrac{\sqrt{2x-4}+\sqrt{2}}{\left(\sqrt{3x}+3\right)}$

$= \dfrac{3}{2}\times\dfrac{2\sqrt{2}}{6} = \dfrac{1}{\sqrt{2}}$

3. (a) Multiply and divide by x in the given expression, we get

$\lim\limits_{x\to 0} \dfrac{(1-\cos 2x)}{x^2} \dfrac{(3+\cos x)}{1} \cdot \dfrac{x}{\tan 4x}$

$= \lim\limits_{x\to 0} \dfrac{2\sin^2 x}{x^2} \cdot \dfrac{3+\cos x}{1} \cdot \dfrac{x}{\tan 4x}$

$= 2\lim\limits_{x\to 0} \dfrac{\sin^2 x}{x^2} \cdot \lim\limits_{x\to 0} 3+\cos x \cdot \lim\limits_{x\to 0} \dfrac{x}{\tan 4x}$

$= 2.4\,\dfrac{1}{4} \lim\limits_{x\to 0} \dfrac{4x}{\tan 4x} = 2.4.\dfrac{1}{4} = 2$

4. (c) $\lim\limits_{x\to 0} \dfrac{2xe^{x^2}+\sin x}{2\sin x\cos x}$

$\lim\limits_{x\to 0} \left(\dfrac{x}{\sin x} e^{x^2} + \dfrac{1}{2}\right) \dfrac{1}{\cos x} = 1+\dfrac{1}{2} = \dfrac{3}{2}$

5. (b) Consider $\lim\limits_{x\to 0} \dfrac{\sin(\pi\cos^2 x)}{x^2}$

$= \lim\limits_{x\to 0} \dfrac{\sin\left[\pi(1-\sin^2 x)\right]}{x^2}$

$= \lim\limits_{x\to 0} \sin\dfrac{(\pi-\pi\sin^2 x)}{x^2}$ $[\because \sin(\pi-\theta)=\sin\theta]$

$= \lim\limits_{x\to 0} \sin\dfrac{(\pi\sin^2 x)}{\pi\sin^2 x} \times \dfrac{\pi\sin^2 x}{x^2}$

$= \lim\limits_{x\to 0} 1\times\pi\left(\dfrac{\sin x}{x}\right)^2 = \pi$

6. (d) $\lim\limits_{x\to 2} \dfrac{\tan(x-2)\{x^2+(k-2)x-2k\}}{x^2-4x+4} = 5$

$\Rightarrow \lim\limits_{x\to 2} \dfrac{\tan(x-2)\{x^2+kx-2x-2k\}}{(x-2)^2} = 5$

$\Rightarrow \lim\limits_{x\to 2} \dfrac{\tan(x-2)\{x(x-2)+k(x-2)\}}{(x-2)\times(x-2)} = 5$

$\Rightarrow \lim\limits_{x\to 2} \left(\dfrac{\tan(x-2)}{(x-2)}\right) \times \lim\limits_{x\to 2} \left(\dfrac{(k+x)\cancel{(x-2)}}{\cancel{(x-2)}}\right) = 5$

$\Rightarrow 1\times \lim\limits_{x\to 2}(k+x) = 5$ $\left\{\because \lim\limits_{h\to 0} \dfrac{\tan h}{h} = 1\right\}$

or $k+2=5$

$\Rightarrow \boxed{k=3}$

7. (d) Multiply and divide by x in the given expression, we get

$\lim\limits_{x\to 0} \dfrac{(1-\cos 2x)}{x^2} \dfrac{(3+\cos x)}{1} \cdot \dfrac{x}{\tan 4x}$

$= \lim\limits_{x\to 0} \dfrac{2\sin^2 x}{x^2} \cdot \dfrac{3+\cos x}{1} \cdot \dfrac{x}{\tan 4x}$

$= 2\lim\limits_{x\to 0} \dfrac{\sin^2 x}{x^2} \cdot \lim\limits_{x\to 0} 3+\cos x \cdot \lim\limits_{x\to 0} \dfrac{x}{\tan 4x}$

$= 2.4\,\dfrac{1}{4} \lim\limits_{x\to 0} \dfrac{4x}{\tan 4x} = 2.4.\dfrac{1}{4} = 2$

8. **(d)** Consider

$$\lim_{x\to 0}\frac{\sin\left(\pi\cos^2 x\right)}{x^2}$$

$$=\lim_{x\to 0}\frac{\sin\left(\pi-\pi\sin^2 x\right)}{x^2}\quad\left[\because \sin(\pi-\theta)=\sin\theta\right]$$

$$=\lim_{x\to 0}\frac{\sin\left(\pi\sin^2 x\right)}{\pi\sin^2 x}\times\frac{\left(\pi\sin^2 x\right)}{x^2}=\pi$$

9. **(b)** Consider $\lim_{x\to 0}\left(\frac{x-\sin x}{x}\right)\sin\left(\frac{1}{x}\right)$

$$=\lim_{x\to 0}\left[\frac{x\left(1-\frac{\sin x}{x}\right)}{x}\right]\times\lim_{x\to 0}\sin\left(\frac{1}{x}\right)$$

$$=\lim_{x\to 0}\left[1-\frac{\sin x}{x}\right]\times\lim_{x\to 0}\sin\left(\frac{1}{x}\right)$$

$$=\left[1-\lim_{x\to 0}\frac{\sin x}{x}\right]\times\lim_{x\to 0}\sin\left(\frac{1}{x}\right)$$

$$=0\times\lim_{x\to 0}\sin\left(\frac{1}{x}\right)=0$$

10. **(d)** $\lim_{x\to 5}\frac{(f(x))^2-9}{\sqrt{|x-5|}}=0$

$\lim_{x\to 5}[(f(x))^2-9]=0\Rightarrow\lim_{x\to 5}f(x)=3$

11. **(d)** $\lim_{x\to 2}\frac{\sqrt{1-\cos\{2(x-2)\}}}{x-2}$

$$=\lim_{x\to 2}\frac{\sqrt{2}\,|\sin(x-2)|}{x-2}$$

$$\underset{(\text{at } x=2)}{\text{L.H.L}}=-\lim_{x\to 2}\frac{\sqrt{2}\sin(x-2)}{(x-2)}=-1$$

$$\underset{(\text{at } x=2)}{\text{R.H.L}}=\lim_{x\to 2}\frac{\sqrt{2}\sin(x-2)}{(x-2)}=1$$

Thus $\underset{(\text{at } x=2)}{\text{L.H.L}}\neq\underset{(\text{at } x=2)}{\text{R.H.L}}$

Hence, $\lim_{x\to 2}\frac{\sqrt{1-\cos\{2(x-2)\}}}{x-2}$ does not exist.

12. **(d)** f(x) is a positive increasing function.

$\therefore\ 0<f(x)<f(2x)<f(3x)$

$$\Rightarrow 0<1<\frac{f(2x)}{f(x)}<\frac{f(3x)}{f(x)}$$

$$\Rightarrow\lim_{x\to\infty}1\le\lim_{x\to\infty}\frac{f(2x)}{f(x)}\le\lim_{x\to\infty}\frac{f(3x)}{f(x)}$$

By Sandwich Theorem.

$$\Rightarrow\lim_{x\to\infty}\frac{f(2x)}{f(x)}=1$$

13. **(a)** Given limit $=\lim_{x\to\alpha}\frac{1-\cos a(x-\alpha)(x-\beta)}{(x-\alpha)^2}$

$$=\lim_{x\to\alpha}\frac{2\sin^2\left(a\frac{(x-\alpha)(x-\beta)}{2}\right)}{(x-\alpha)^2}$$

$$=\lim_{x\to\alpha}\frac{2}{(x-\alpha)^2}\times\frac{\sin^2\left(a\frac{(x-\alpha)(x-\beta)}{2}\right)}{\frac{a^2(x-\alpha)^2(x-\beta)^2}{4}}\times\frac{a^2(x-\alpha)^2(x-\beta)^2}{4}$$

$$=\frac{a^2(\alpha-\beta)^2}{2}.$$

14. **(d)** $\lim_{x\to\frac{\pi}{2}}\frac{\tan\left(\frac{\pi}{4}-\frac{x}{2}\right).(1-\sin x)}{(\pi-2x)^3}$

Let $x=\frac{\pi}{2}+y;\ y\to 0$

$$=\lim_{y\to 0}\frac{\tan\left(-\frac{y}{2}\right).(1-\cos y)}{(-2y)^3}$$

$$=\lim_{y\to 0}\frac{-\tan\frac{y}{2}2\sin^2\frac{y}{2}}{(-8).\frac{y^3}{8}.8}$$

$$=\lim_{y\to 0}\frac{1}{32}\frac{\tan\frac{y}{2}}{\left(\frac{y}{2}\right)}.\left[\frac{\sin y/2}{y/2}\right]^2=\frac{1}{32}$$

15. **(d)** Since $\lim_{x\to 0}[x]$ does not exist, hence the required limit does not exist.

16. **(a)** $\lim_{x\to\infty}\left(\frac{x^2+5x+3}{x^2+x+2}\right)^x$

$$=\lim_{x\to\infty}\left(1+\frac{4x+1}{x^2+x+2}\right)^x$$

$$=\lim_{x\to\infty}\left[\left(1+\frac{4x+1}{x^2+x+2}\right)^{\frac{x^2+x+2}{4x+1}}\right]^{\frac{(4x+1)x}{x^2+x+2}}$$

$$= e^{\lim_{x\to\infty}\frac{4x^2+x}{x^2+x+2}}\left[\because \lim_{x\to\infty}(1+\lambda x)^{\frac{1}{x}} = e^{\lambda}\right]$$

$$= e^{\lim_{x\to\infty}\frac{4+\frac{1}{x}}{1+\frac{1}{x}+\frac{2}{x^2}}} = e^4$$

17. (d) $\lim \frac{\sqrt{1-\cos 2x}}{\sqrt{2}x} \Rightarrow \lim \frac{\sqrt{1-(1-2\sin^2 x)}}{\sqrt{2}x}$;

$$\lim_{x\to 0}\frac{\sqrt{2\sin^2 x}}{\sqrt{2}x} \Rightarrow \lim_{x\to 0}\frac{|\sin x|}{x}$$

The limit of above does not exist as

LHS = –1 ≠ RHL = 1

18. (a) $\ln p = \lim_{x\to 0^+}\frac{1}{2x}\ln(1+\tan^2\sqrt{x})$

$$\lim_{x\to 0^+}\frac{1}{x}\ln\left(\sec\sqrt{x}\right)$$

Applying L hospital's rule :

$$= \lim_{x\to 0^+}\frac{\sec\sqrt{x}\tan\sqrt{x}}{\sec\sqrt{x}\cdot 2\sqrt{x}}$$

$$= \lim_{x\to 0^+}\frac{\tan\sqrt{x}}{2\sqrt{x}} = \frac{1}{2}$$

19. (c) $\lim_{x\to 0}\frac{(1-\cos 2x)^2}{2x\tan x - x\tan 2x}$

$$= \lim_{x\to 0}\frac{(2\sin^2 x)^2}{2x\left(x+\frac{x^3}{3}+\frac{2x^5}{15}+.....\right)-x\left(2x+\frac{2^3x^3}{3}+2\frac{2^5x^5}{15}+.....\right)}$$

$$= \lim_{x\to 0}\frac{4\left(x-\frac{x^3}{3!}+\frac{x^5}{5!}-.....\right)^4}{x^4\left(\frac{2}{3}-\frac{8}{5}\right)+x^6\left(\frac{4}{15}-\frac{64}{15}\right)}$$

$$= \lim_{x\to 0}\frac{4\left(1-\frac{x^2}{3!}+\frac{x^4}{5!}-.....\right)^4}{-2+x^2\left(-\frac{60}{15}\right)+.....}$$

(dividing numerator & denominator by x^4)

= –2

20. (b) $\lim_{x\to\infty}\left(1+\frac{a}{x}-\frac{4}{x^2}\right)^{2x}$ (1^∞ form)

$$= e\left[\lim_{x\to\infty}\left(1+\frac{a}{x}-\frac{4}{x^2}-1\right)2x\right]$$

$$= e\lim_{x\to\infty}\left(2a-\frac{8}{x}\right) = e^{2a}$$

$\therefore\ 2a = 3 \Rightarrow a = 3/2$

21. (b) We know that $\lim_{x\to\infty}(1+x)^{\frac{1}{x}} = e$

$$\therefore \lim_{x\to\infty}\left(1+\frac{a}{x}+\frac{b}{x^2}\right)^{2x} = e^2$$

$$\Rightarrow \lim_{x\to\infty}\left[\left(1+\frac{a}{x}+\frac{b}{x^2}\right)^{\left(\frac{1}{\frac{a}{x}+\frac{b}{x^2}}\right)}\right]^{2x\left(\frac{a}{x}+\frac{b}{x^2}\right)} = e^2$$

$$\Rightarrow e^{\lim_{x\to\infty}2\left[a+\frac{b}{x}\right]} = e^2 \Rightarrow e^{2a} = e^2$$

$\Rightarrow a = 1$ and $b \in R$

ALTERNATE SOLUTION

$$\lim_{x\to\infty}\left(1+\frac{a}{x}+\frac{b}{x^2}\right)^{2x} = e^2 \Rightarrow e^{\lim_{x\to\infty}\left(1+\frac{a}{x}+\frac{b}{x^2}-1\right)2x} = e^2$$

$$\Rightarrow \lim_{x\to\infty}\left(2a+\frac{2b}{x}\right) = 2$$

$\Rightarrow 2a+0 = 2, b \in R \Rightarrow a = 1, b \in R$

22. (c) Apply L H Rule

We have, $\lim_{x\to 2}\frac{xf(2)-2f(x)}{x-2}\ \left(\frac{0}{0}\right)$

$$= \lim_{x\to 2} f(2)-2f'(x) = f(2)-2f'(2)$$

= 4 – 2 × 4 = –4.

23. (a) $\lim_{x\to 0}\left[1+\frac{f(x)}{x^2}\right] = 3$

$$\Rightarrow \lim_{x\to 0}\frac{f(x)}{x^2} = 2$$

So, f(x) contain terms in x^2, x^3 and x^4.

Let $f(x) = a_1x^2 + a_2x^3 + a_3x^4$

Since $\lim_{x\to 0}\frac{f(x)}{x^2} = 2 \Rightarrow a_1 = 2$

Hence, $f(x) = 2x^2 + a_2x^3 + a_3x^4$

$f'(x) = 4x + 3a_2x^2 + 4a_3x^3$

As given : $f'(1) = 0$ adn $f'(2) = 0$

Hence, $4 + 3a_2 + 4a_3 = 0$ ...(a)

and $8 + 12a_2 + 32a_3 = 0$ ...(2)

By 4x(eq1) – eq(2), we get

$16 + 12a_2 + 16a_3 - (8 + 12a_2 + 32a_3) = 0$

$\Rightarrow 8 - 16a_3 = 0 \Rightarrow a_3 = 1/2$

and by eqn. (a), $4 + 3a_2 + 4/2 = 0 \Rightarrow a_2 = -2$

$\Rightarrow f(x) = 2x^2 - 2x^3 + \frac{1}{2}x^4$

$f(2) = 2 \times 4 - 2 \times 8 + \frac{1}{2} \times 16 = 0$

24. **(d)** Given $f(1) = -2$ and $f'(x) \geq 4.2$ for $1 \leq x \leq 6$

Consider $f'(x) = \dfrac{f(x+h) - f(x)}{h}$

$\Rightarrow f(x+h) - f(x) = f'(x) \,.\, h \geq (4.2)h$

So, $f(x+h) \geq f(x) + (4.2)\,h$

put $x = 1$ and $h = 5$, we get

$f(6) \geq f(1) + 5(4.2) \Rightarrow f(6) \geq 19$

Hence $f(6)$ lies in $[19, \infty)$

25. **(b)** Let $f(x) = 3x^{10} - 7x^8 + 5x^6 - 21x^3 + 3x^2 - 7$

$f'(x) = 30x^9 - 56x^7 + 30x^5 - 63x^2 + 6x$

$f'(1) = 30 - 56 + 30 - 63 + 6$

$= 66 - 63 - 56 = -53$

Consider $\lim\limits_{\alpha \to 0} \dfrac{f(1-\alpha) - f(1)}{\alpha^3 + 3\alpha}$

$= \lim\limits_{\alpha \to 0} \dfrac{f'(1-\alpha)(-1) - 0}{3\alpha^2 + 3}$ (By using L'hospital rule)

$= \dfrac{f'(1-0)(-1)}{3(0)^2 + 3} = \dfrac{-f'(1)}{3} = \dfrac{53}{3}$

Chapter 13 Mathematical Reasoning

TOPIC-1 : Statement, Truth value of a statement, Logical Connectives, Truth Table, Logical Equivalance, Tautology & Contradiction, Duality

1. The following statement $(p \to q) \to [(\sim p \to q) \to q]$ is : **[2017]**
   (a) a fallacy (b) a tautology
   (c) equivalent to $\sim p \to q$ (d) equivalent to $p \to \sim q$

2. The proposition $(\sim p) \vee (p \wedge \sim q)$ **[Online April 8, 2017]**
   (a) $P \to \sim q$ (b) $P \wedge (\sim q)$
   (c) $q \to p$ (d) $p \vee (\sim q)$

3. The Boolean Expression $(p \wedge \sim q) \vee q \vee (\sim p \wedge q)$ is equivalent to: **[2016]**
   (a) $p \vee q$ (b) $p \vee \sim q$
   (c) $\sim p \wedge q$ (d) $p \wedge q$

4. The negation of $\sim s \vee (\sim r \wedge s)$ is equivalent to : **[2015]**
   (a) $s \vee (r \vee \sim s)$ (b) $s \wedge r$
   (c) $s \wedge \sim r$ (d) $s \wedge (r \wedge \sim s)$

5. The statement $\sim (p \leftrightarrow \sim q)$ is: **[2014]**
   (a) a tautology
   (b) a fallacy
   (c) eqivalent to $p \leftrightarrow q$
   (d) equivalent to $\sim p \leftrightarrow q$

6. Let p, q, r denote arbitrary statements. Then the logically equivalent of the statement $p \Rightarrow (q \vee r)$ is: **[Online April 12, 2014]**
   (a) $(p \vee q) \Rightarrow r$
   (b) $(p \Rightarrow q) \vee (p \Rightarrow r)$
   (c) $(p \Rightarrow \sim q) \wedge (p \Rightarrow r)$
   (d) $(p \Rightarrow q) \wedge (p \Rightarrow \sim r)$

7. The proposition $\sim (p \vee \sim q) \vee \sim (p \vee q)$ is logically equivalent to: **[Online April 11, 2014]**
   (a) p (b) q
   (c) $\sim p$ (d) $\sim q$

8. Consider
   Statement-1 : $(p \wedge \sim q) \wedge (\sim p \wedge q)$ is a fallacy.
   Statement-2 : $(p \to q) \leftrightarrow (\sim q \to \sim p)$ is a tautology. **[2013]**
   (a) Statement-1 is true; Statement-2 is true; Statement-2 is a correct explanation for Statement-1.
   (b) Statement-1 is true; Statement-2 is true; Statement-2 is not a correct explanation for Statement-1.
   (c) Statement-1 is true; Statement-2 is false.
   (d) Statement-1 is false; Statement-2 is true.

9. Let p and q be any two logical statements and $r : p \to (\sim p \vee q)$. If r has a truth value F, then the truth values of p and q are respectively : **[Online April 25, 2013]**
   (a) F, F (b) T, T
   (c) T, F (d) F, T

10. For integers m and n, both greater than 1, consider the following three statements :
    P : m divides n
    Q : m divides n^2
    R : m is prime,
    then **[Online April 23, 2013]**
    (a) $Q \wedge R \to P$ (b) $P \wedge Q \to R$
    (c) $Q \to R$ (d) $Q \to P$

11. The statement $p \to (q \to p)$ is equivalent to : **[Online April 22, 2013]**
    (a) $p \to q$ (b) $p \to (p \vee q)$
    (c) $p \to (p \to q)$ (d) $p \to (p \wedge q)$

12. **Statement-1:** The statement $A \to (B \to A)$ is equivalent to $A \to (A \vee B)$.
    Statement-2: The statement $\sim [(A \wedge B) \to (\sim A \vee B)]$ is a Tautology. **[Online April 9, 2013]**
    (a) Statement-1 is false; Statement-2 is true.
    (b) Statement-1 is true; Statement-2 is true; Statement- 2 is **not** correct explanation for Statement-1.
    (c) Statement-1 is true; Statement-2 is false.
    (d) Statement-1 is true; Statement-2 is true; Statement- 2 is the correct explanation for Statement-1.

13. Let p and q be two Statements. Amongst the following, the Statement that is equivalent to $p \to q$ is **[Online May 19, 2012]**
(a) $p \wedge \sim q$ (b) $\sim p \vee q$
(c) $\sim p \wedge q$ (d) $p \vee \sim q$

14. The logically equivalent preposition of $p \Leftrightarrow q$ is **[Online May 12, 2012]**
(a) $(p \Rightarrow q) \wedge (q \Rightarrow p)$ (b) $p \wedge q$
(c) $(p \wedge q) \vee (q \Rightarrow p)$ (d) $(p \wedge q) \Rightarrow (q \vee p)$

15. The only statement among the following that is a tautology is **[2011RS]**
(a) $A \wedge (A \vee B)$
(b) $A \vee (A \wedge B)$
(c) $[A \wedge (A \to B)] \to B$
(d) $B \to [A \wedge (A \to B)]$

16. **Statement-1 :** $\sim (p \leftrightarrow \sim q)$ is equivalent to $p \leftrightarrow q$.
Statement-2 : $\sim (p \leftrightarrow \sim q)$ is a tantology **[2009]**
(a) Statement-1 is true, Statement-2 is true; Statement-2 is not a correct explanation for Statement-1.
(b) Statement-1 is true, Statement-2 is false.
(c) Statement-1 is false, Statement-2 is true.
(d) Statement-1 is true, Statement-2 is true, Statement-2 is a correct explanation for statement -1

17. The statement $p \to (q \to p)$ is equivalent to **[2008]**
(a) $p \to (p \to q)$ (b) $p \to (p \vee q)$
(c) $p \to (p \wedge q)$ (d) $p \to (p \leftrightarrow q)$

18. Let p be the statement "x is an irrational number", q be the statement "y is a transcendental number", and r be the statement "x is a rational number iff y is a transcendental number". **[2008]**
Statement-1 : r is equivalent to either q or p
Statement-2 : r is equivalent to $\sim(p \leftrightarrow \sim q)$.
(a) Statement -1 is false, Statement-2 is true
(b) Statement -1 is true, Statement-2 is true; Statement -2 is a correct explanation for Statement-1
(c) Statement -1 is true, Statement-2 is true; Statement -2 is not a correct explanation for Statement-1
(d) Statement -1 is true, Statement-2 is false

TOPIC-2 : Converse, Inverse & Contrapositive of the Conditional Statement, Negative of a Compound Statement, Algebra of Statement

19. Contrapositive of the statement
'If two numbers are not equal, then their squares are not equal', is : **[Online April 9, 2017]**
(a) If the squares of two numbers are equal, then the numbers are equal.
(b) If the squares of two numbers are equal, then the numbers are not equal.
(c) If the squares of two numbers are not equal, then the numbers are not equal.
(d) If the squares of two numbers are not equal, then the numbers are equal.

20. The contrapositive of the following statement,
"If the side of a square doubles, then its area increases four times", is : **[Online April 10, 2016]**
(a) If the area of a square increases four times, then its side is not doubled.
(b) If the area of a square increases four times, then its side is doubled.
(c) If the area of a square does not increases four times, then its side is not doubled.
(d) If the side of a square is not doubled, then its area does not increase four times.

21. Consider the following two statements :
P : If 7 is an odd number, then 7 is divisible by 2.
Q : If 7 is a prime number, then 7 is an odd number.
If V_1 is the truth value of the contrapositive of P and V_2 is the truth value of contrapositive of Q, then the ordered pair (V_1, V_2) equals: **[Online April 9, 2016]**
(a) (F, F) (b) (F, T)
(c) (T, F) (d) (T, T)

22. Consider the following statements :
P : Suman is brilliant
Q : Suman is rich.
R : Suman is honest
the negation of the statement
"Suman is brilliant and dishonest if and only if suman is rich" can be equivalently expressed as : **[Online April 11, 2015]**
(a) $\sim Q \leftrightarrow \sim P \vee R$ (b) $\sim Q \leftrightarrow \sim P \wedge R$
(c) $\sim Q \leftrightarrow P \vee \sim R$ (d) $\sim Q \leftrightarrow P \wedge \sim R$

23. The contrapositive of the statement "If it is raining, then I will not come", is : **[Online April 10, 2015]**
(a) If I will not come, then it is raining.
(b) If I will not come, then it is not raining.
(c) If I will come, then it is raining.
(d) If I will come, then it is not raining.

24. The contrapositive of the statement "if I am not feeling well, then I will go to the doctor" is **[Online April 19, 2014]**
(a) If I am feeling well, then I will not go to the doctor
(b) If I will go to the doctor, then I am feeling well
(c) If I will not go to the doctor, then I am feeling well
(d) If I will go to the doctor, then I am not feeling well.

25. The contrapositive of the statement "I go to school if it does not rain" is **[Online April 9, 2014]**
(a) If it rains, I do not go to school.

(b) If I do not go to school, it rains.
(c) If it rains, I go to school.
(d) If I go to school, it rains.

26. The negation of the statement
"If I become a teacher, then I will open a school", is : **[2012]**
(a) I will become a teacher and I will not open a school.
(b) Either I will not become a teacher or I will not open a school.
(c) Neither I will become a teacher nor I will open a school.
(d) I will not become a teacher or I will open a school.

27. Let p and q denote the following statements
p : The sun is shining
q: I shall play tennis in the afternoon
The negation of the statement "If the sun is shining then I shall play tennis in the afternoon", is **[Online May 26, 2012]**
(a) $q \Rightarrow \sim p$ (b) $q \wedge \sim p$
(c) $p \wedge \sim q$ (d) $\sim q \Rightarrow \sim p$

28. The Statement that is TRUE among the following is **[Online May 7, 2012]**
(a) The contrapositive of $3x+2=8 \Rightarrow x=2$ is $x \neq 2 \Rightarrow 3x+2 \neq 8$.
(b) The converse of $\tan x = 0 \Rightarrow x = 0$ is $x \neq 0 \Rightarrow \tan x = 0$.
(c) $p \Rightarrow q$ is equivalent to $p \vee \sim q$.
(d) $p \vee q$ and $p \wedge q$ have the same truth table.

29. Let S be a non-empty subset of R. Consider the following statement :
P : There is a rational number $x \in$ S such that $x > 0$.
Which of the following statements is the negation of the statement P ? **[2010]**
(a) There is no rational number $x \in$ S such than $x \leq 0$.
(b) Every rational number $x \in$ S satisfies $x \leq 0$.
(c) $x \in$ S and $x \leq 0 \Rightarrow x$ is not rational.
(d) There is a rational number $x \in$ S such that $x \leq 0$.

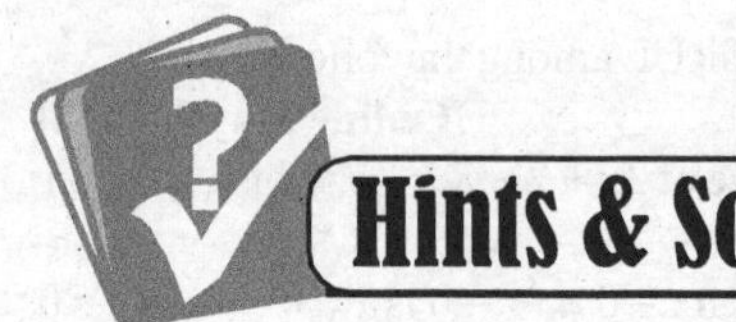

Hints & Solutions

1. (b) We have

p	q	~ p	p → q	~ p → q	(~ p → q) → q	(p → q) → ((~p→q)→ q)
T	F	F	F	T	F	T
T	T	F	T	T	T	T
F	F	T	T	F	T	T
F	T	T	T	T	T	T

$\therefore$ It is tautology.

2. (b) $(\sim p) \vee (p \wedge \sim q)$

P	q	~ p	~ q	p∧ ~ q	(~ p)∨(p ∧ ~ q)
T	T	F	F	F	F
T	F	F	T	T	T
F	T	T	F	F	F
F	F	T	T	F	F

3. (a) $(p \wedge \sim q) \vee q \vee (\sim p \wedge q)$

$\Rightarrow \{(p \vee q) \wedge (\sim q \vee q)\} \vee (\sim p \wedge q)$

$\Rightarrow \{(p \vee q) \wedge T\} \vee (\sim p \wedge q)$

$\Rightarrow (p \vee q) \vee (\sim p \wedge q)$

$\Rightarrow \{(p \vee q) \vee \sim p\} \wedge (p \vee q \vee q)$

$\Rightarrow T \wedge (p \vee q)$

$\Rightarrow p \vee q$

4. (b) $\sim[\sim s \vee (\sim r \wedge s)]$

$= s \wedge \sim(\sim r \wedge s)$

$= s \wedge (r \vee \sim s)$

$= (s \wedge r) \vee (s \wedge \sim s)$

$= (s \wedge r) \vee 0$

$= s \wedge r$

5. (c)

p	q	$\sim q$	$p \leftrightarrow \sim q$	$\sim (p \leftrightarrow \sim q)$
F	F	T	F	T
F	T	F	T	F
T	F	T	T	F
T	T	F	F	T

Clearly equivalent to $p \leftrightarrow q$

6. (b) Given statement is

$p \Rightarrow (q \vee r)$ which is equivalent to

$(p \Rightarrow q) \vee (p \Rightarrow r)$

7. (c) Given $\sim (p \vee \sim q) \vee \sim (p \vee q)$

$\equiv (\sim p \vee q) \vee (\sim p \vee \sim q)$

$\equiv \sim p \vee (q \vee \sim q)$

$\equiv \sim p$

8. (b) **Statement-2 :** $(p \rightarrow q) \leftrightarrow (\sim q \rightarrow \sim p)$

$\equiv (p \rightarrow q) \leftrightarrow (p \rightarrow q)$

which is always true.

So statement 2 is true

Statement-1: $(p \wedge \sim q) \wedge (\sim p \wedge q)$

$= p \wedge \sim q \wedge \sim p \wedge q$

$= p \wedge \sim p \wedge \sim q \wedge q$

$= f \wedge f = f$

So statement-1 is true

9. (c) $p \rightarrow (\sim p \vee q)$ has truth value F.

It means $p \rightarrow (\sim p \vee q)$ is false.

It means p is true and $\sim p \vee q$ is false.

$\Rightarrow$ p is true and both $\sim p$ and q are false.

$\Rightarrow$ p is true and q is false.

10. (a)

(2) $\frac{8}{4} = 2, \frac{64}{4} = 16$; but 4 is not prime.

Hence $P \wedge Q \rightarrow R$, false

(3) $\frac{(6)^2}{12} = \frac{36}{12} = 3$; but 12 is not prime

Hence $Q \rightarrow R$, false

(4) $\frac{(4)^2}{8} = \frac{16}{8} = 2$; $\frac{4}{8}$ is not an integer

Hence $Q \rightarrow P$, false

11. (b)

q	p	$q \rightarrow p$	$p \rightarrow (q \rightarrow p)$	$p \vee q$	$p \rightarrow (p \vee q)$
T	T	T	T	T	T
T	F	F	T	T	T
F	T	T	T	T	T
F	F	T	T	F	T

Since truth value of $p \rightarrow (q \rightarrow p)$ and $p \rightarrow (p \vee q)$ are same, hence $p \rightarrow (q \rightarrow p)$ is equivalent to $p \rightarrow (p \vee q)$.

12. (c)

A	B	~ A	A ∧ B	~ A ∨ B	(A ∧ B) → (~ A ∨ B)	~[(A ∧ B) → (~ A ∨ B)]
T	T	F	T	T	T	F
T	F	F	F	F	T	F
F	T	T	F	T	T	F
F	F	T	F	T	T	F

13. (b) Let p and q be two statements.
$p \to q$ is equivalent to $\sim p \vee q$.

14. (a) $(p \Rightarrow q) \wedge (q \Rightarrow p)$ means $p \Leftrightarrow q$

15. (c)

A	B	A ∨ B	A ∧ B	A ∧ (A ∨ B)	A ∨ (A ∧ B)	A → B	A ∧ (A → B)	[A ∧ (A → B) → B]	[B → [A ∧ (A → B)]
T	F	T	F	T	T	F	F	T	T
F	T	T	F	F	F	T	F	T	F
T	T	T	T	T	T	T	T	T	T
F	F	F	F	F	F	T	F	T	T

16. (b) The truth table for the logical statements, involved in statement 1, is as follows :

p	q	$\sim q$	$p \leftrightarrow \sim q$	$\sim(p \leftrightarrow \sim q)$	$p \leftrightarrow q$
T	T	F	F	T	T
T	F	T	T	F	F
F	T	F	T	F	F
F	F	T	F	T	T

We observe the columns for $\sim(p \leftrightarrow \sim q)$ and $p \leftrightarrow q$ are identical, therefore

$\sim(p \leftrightarrow \sim q)$ is equivalent to $p \leftrightarrow q$

But $\sim(p \leftrightarrow \sim q)$ is not a tautology as all entries in its column are not T.

∴ Statement-1 is true but statement-2 is false.

17. (b) Let us make the truth table for the given statements, as follows :

p	q	p∨q	q→p	p →(q→p)	p →(p∨q)
T	T	T	T	T	T
T	F	T	T	T	T
F	T	T	F	T	T
F	F	F	T	T	T

From table we observe

$p \to (q \to p)$ is equivalent to $p \to (p \vee q)$

18. (None)

p : x is an irrational number

q : y is a transcendental number

r : x is a rational number iff y is a transcendental number.

clearly $r : \sim p \leftrightarrow q$

Let us use truth table to check the equivalence of 'r' and 'q or p'; 'r' and $\sim(p \leftrightarrow \sim q)$

p	q	~p	~q	~p ↔q (1)	q or p (2)	p↔~q	~(p↔~q) (3)
T	T	F	F	F	T	F	T
T	F	F	T	T	T	T	F
F	T	T	F	T	T	T	F
F	F	T	T	F	F	F	T

From columns (1), (2) and (3), we observe, none of the these statements are equivalent to each other.

∴ Statement 1as well as statement 2 both are false.

∴ None of the options is correct.

19. (a) $p \to q$

then $\sim q \to \sim p$

∴ If the square of two numbers are equal, then the numbers are equal.

20. (c) Contrapositive of $p \to q$ is given by $\sim q \to \sim p$

So (c) is the right option.

21. (a) Contrapositive of P :

T is not divisible by 2 ⇒ T is not odd number

$T \Rightarrow F : F(V_1)$

Contra positive Q :

T is not odd number ⇒ T is not a prime number

$F \Rightarrow F : T(V_2)$

22. (d) Suman is brilliant and dishonest can be expressed as

$P \wedge \sim R$

therefore given statement is equal to $(P \wedge \sim R) \leftrightarrow Q$

Negation of the above statement is $\sim Q \leftrightarrow P \wedge \sim R$

23. (d) The centre positive of the statement is "If i will come, then it is not raining".

24. (c) Given statement can be written in implication form as

I am not feeling well ⇒ I will go to the doctor.

Contrapositive form :

I will not go to the doctor ⇒ I am feeling well.

i.e. - If I will not go to the doctor, then I am feeling well.

25. (b) let p = If it does not rain

q = I go to school

According to law of contrapositive

$p \Rightarrow q \equiv \sim q \Rightarrow \sim p$

i.e. $\sim q$ = I do not go to school

$\sim p$ = It rains

$\sim q \Rightarrow \sim p$ is If I do not go to school, it rains.

26. (a) Let p : I become a teacher.

q : I will open a school

Negation of $p \to q$ is $\sim(p \to q) = p \wedge \sim q$

i.e. I will become a teacher and I will not open a school.

27. **(c)** Let p : The sun is shining.
q : I shall play tennis in the afternoon.
Negation of $p \rightarrow q$ is $\sim(p \rightarrow q) = p \wedge \sim q$

28. **(a)** Only statement given in option
(a) is true.
(b) The converse of $\tan x = 0 \Rightarrow x = 0$ is $x = 0 \Rightarrow \tan x = 0$
$\therefore$ Statement (b) is false
(c) $\sim(p \Rightarrow q)$ is equivalent to $p \wedge \sim q$
$\therefore$ Statement given in option (c) is false.
(d) No, $p \vee q$ and $p \wedge q$ does not have the same truth value.

29. **(b)** P : there is a rational number $x \in S$ such that $x > 0$
$\sim$P : Every rational number $x \in S$ satisfies $x \leq 0$

Statistics

TOPIC-1 : Arithmetic Mean, Geometric Mean, Harmonic Mean, Median & Mode

1. The mean age of 25 teachers in a school is 40 years. A teacher retires at the age of 60 years and a new teacher is appointed in his place. If now the mean age of the teachers in this school is 39 years, then the age (in years) of the newly appointed teacher is : **[Online April 8, 2017]**
(a) 25 (b) 30
(c) 35 (d) 40

2. The mean of the data set comprising of 16 observations is 16. If one of the observation valued 16 is deleted and three new observations valued 3, 4 and 5 are added to the data, then the mean of the resultant data, is: **[2015]**
(a) 15.8 (b) 14.0
(c) 16.8 (d) 16.0

3. Let the sum of the first three terms of an A. P, be 39 and the sum of its last four terms be 178. If the first term of this A.P. is 10, then the median of the A.P. is : **[Online April 10, 2015]**
(a) 28 (b) 26.5
(c) 29.5 (d) 31

4. A factory is operating in two shifts, day and night, with 70 and 30 workers respectively. If per day mean wage of the day shift workers is ₹ 54 and per day mean wage of all the workers is ₹ 60, then per day mean wage of the night shift workers (in ₹) is : **[Online April 10, 2015]**
(a) 69 (b) 66
(c) 74 (d) 75

5. In a set of 2n distinct observations, each of the observations below the median of all the observations is increased by 5 and each of the remaining observations is decreased by 3. Then the mean of the new set of observations: **[Online April 9, 2014]**
(a) increases by 1 (b) decreases by 1
(c) decreases by 2 (d) increases by 2

6. If the median and the range of four numbers $\{x, y, 2x + y, x - y\}$, where $0 < y < x < 2y$, are 10 and 28 respectively, then the mean of the numbers is : **[Online April 23, 2013]**
(a) 18 (b) 10
(c) 5 (d) 14

7. The mean of a data set consisting of 20 observations is 40. If one observation 53 was wrongly recorded as 33, then the correct mean will be : **[Online April 9, 2013]**
(a) 41 (b) 49
(c) 40.5 (d) 42.5

8. The median of 100 observations grouped in classes of equal width is 25. If the median class interval is 20 - 30 and the number of observations less than 20 is 45, then the frequency of median class is **[Online May 19, 2012]**
(a) 10 (b) 20
(c) 15 (d) 12

9. The frequency distribution of daily working expenditure of families in a locality is as follows:

Expenditure in ₹. (x):	0-50	50-100	100-150	150-200	200-250
No. of families (f):	24	33	37	b	25

If the mode of the distribution is ₹ 140, then the value of b is **[Online May 7, 2012]**
(a) 34 (b) 31
(c) 26 (d) 36

10. The average marks of boys in class is 52 and that of girls is 42. The average marks of boys and girls combined is 50. The percentage of boys in the class is **[2007]**
(a) 80 (b) 60
(c) 40 (d) 20.

11. Let x_1, x_2, ... x_n be n observations such that $\sum x_i^2 = 400$ and $\sum x_i = 80$. Then the possible value of n among the following is **[2005]**
(a) 15 (b) 18
(c) 9 (d) 12

12. If in a frequency distribution, the mean and median are 21 and 22 respectively, then its mode is approximately **[2005]**
(a) 22.0 (b) 20.5
(c) 25.5 (d) 24.0

13. The median of a set of 9 distinct observations is 20.5. If each of the largest 4 observations of the set is increased by 2, then the median of the new set **[2003]**
(a) remains the same as that of the original set
(b) is increased by 2
(c) is decreased by 2
(d) is two times the original median.

14. In a class of 100 students there are 70 boys whose average marks in a subject are 75. If the average marks of the complete class is 72, then what is the average of the girls?
(a) 73 (b) 65 **[2002]**
(c) 68 (d) 74

TOPIC-2 : Quartile, Measures of Dispersion, Quartile Deviation, Mean Deviation, Variance & Standard Deviation, Coefficient of Variation

15. The sum of 100 observations and the sum of their squares are 400 and 2475, respectively. Later on, three observations, 3, 4 and 5, were found to be incorrect. If the incorrect observations are omitted, then the variance of the remaining observations is : **[Online April 9, 2017]**

(a) 8.25 (b) 8.50
(c) 8.00 (d) 9.00

16. If the standard deviation of the numbers 2, 3, a and 11 is 3.5, then which of the following is true? **[2016]**

(a) $3a^2 - 34a + 91 = 0$
(b) $3a^2 - 23a + 44 = 0$
(c) $3a^2 - 26a + 55 = 0$
(d) $3a^2 - 32a + 84 = 0$

17. The mean of 5 observations is 5 and their variance is 124. If three of the observations are 1, 2 and 6; then the mean deviation from the mean of the data is : **[Online April 10, 2016]**

(a) 2.5 (b) 2.6
(c) 2.8 (d) 2.4

18. If the mean deviation of the numbers 1, 1 + d, ..., 1 + 100d from their mean is 255, then a value of d is : **[Online April 9, 2016]**

(a) 10.1 (b) 5.05
(c) 20.2 (d) 10

19. The variance of first 50 even natural numbers is **[2014]**

(a) 437 (b) $\frac{437}{4}$
(c) $\frac{833}{4}$ (d) 833

20. Let $\bar{x}$, M and σ^2 be respectively the mean, mode and variance of n observations $x_1, x_2, ..., x_n$ and $d_i = -x_i - a$, $i = 1, 2, ..., n$, where a is any number.
Statement I: Variance of $d_1, d_2, ... d_n$ is σ^2.
Statement II: Mean and mode of $d_1, d_2, ... d_n$ are $-\bar{x} - a$ and $-M - a$, respectively. **[Online April 19, 2014]**

(a) Statement I and Statement II are both false
(b) Statement I and Statement II are both true
(c) Statement I is true and Statement II is false
(d) Statement I is false and Statement II is true

21. Let $\overline{X}$ and M.D. be the mean and the mean deviation about $\overline{X}$ of n observations x_i, i = 1, 2, ..., n. If each of the observations is increased by 5, then the new mean and the mean deviation about the new mean, respectively, are : **[Online April 12, 2014]**

(a) $\overline{X}$, M.D. (b) $\overline{X} + 5$, M.D.
(c) $\overline{X}$, M.D. + 5 (d) $\overline{X} + 5$, M.D. + 5

22. All the students of a class performed poorly in Mathematics. The teacher decided to give grace marks of 10 to each of the students. Which of the following statistical measures will not change even after the grace marks were given ? **[2013]**

(a) mean (b) median
(c) mode (d) variance

23. In a set of 2n observations, half of them are equal to 'a' and the remaining half are equal to '–a'. If the standard deviation of all the observations is 2 ; then the value of $|a|$ is : **[Online April 25, 2013]**

(a) 2 (b) $\sqrt{2}$
(c) 4 (d) $2\sqrt{2}$

24. Mean of 5 observations is 7. If four of these observations are 6, 7, 8, 10 and one is missing then the variance of all the five observations is : **[Online April 22, 2013]**

(a) 4 (b) 6
(c) 8 (d) 2

25. Let $x_1, x_2, ..., x_n$ be n observations, and let $\bar{x}$ be their arithmetic mean and σ^2 be the variance.
Statement-1 : Variance of $2x_1, 2x_2, ..., 2x_n$ is $4\sigma^2$.
Statement-2 : Arithmetic mean $2x_1, 2x_2, ..., 2x_n$ is $4\bar{x}$. **[2012]**

(a) Statement-1 is false, Statement-2 is true.
(b) Statement-1 is true, statement-2 is true; statement-2 is a correct explanation for Statement-1.
(c) Statement-1 is true, statement-2 is true; statement-2 is *not* a correct explanation for Statement-1.
(d) Statement-1 is true, statement-2 is false.

26. **Statement 1:** The variance of first *n* odd natural numbers is $\frac{n^2 - 1}{3}$

Statement 2: The sum of first n odd natural number is n^2 and the sum of square of first *n* odd natural numbers is $\frac{n(4n^2 + 1)}{3}$. **[Online May 26, 2012]**

(a) Statement 1 is true, Statement 2 is false.
(b) Statement 1 is true, Statement 2 is true; Statement 2 is not a correct explanation for Statement 1.
(c) Statement 1 is false, Statement 2 is true.
(d) Statement 1 is true, Statement 2 is true, Statement 2 is a correct explanation for Statement 1.

27. If the mean of 4, 7, 2, 8, 6 and a is 7, then the mean deviation from the median of these observations is **[Online May 12, 2012]**

(a) 8 (b) 5
(c) 1 (d) 3

28. A scientist is weighing each of 30 fishes. Their mean weight worked out is 30 gm and a standarion deviation of 2 gm. Later, it was found that the measuring scale was misaligned and always under reported every fish weight by 2 gm. The correct mean and standard deviation (in gm) of fishes are respectively : **[2011RS]**

(a) 32, 2 (b) 32, 4
(c) 28, 2 (d) 28, 4

29. If the mean deviation about the median of the numbers a, $2a$,.......,$50a$ is 50, then $|a|$ equals **[2011]**

(a) 3 (b) 4
(c) 5 (d) 2

30. For two data sets, each of size 5, the variances are given to be 4 and 5 and the corresponding means are given to be 2 and 4, respectively. The variance of the combined data set is **[2010]**

(a) $\frac{11}{2}$ (b) 6
(c) $\frac{13}{2}$ (d) $\frac{5}{2}$

31. If the mean deviation of the numbers 1, 1 + d, 1 + 2d, ... 1 + 100d from their mean is 255, then d is equal to : **[2009]**

(a) 20.0 (b) 10.1
(c) 20.2 (d) 10.0

32. **Statement-1 :** The variance of first n even natural numbers is $\frac{n^2-1}{4}$.

Statement-2 : The sum of first n natural numbers is $\frac{n(n+1)}{2}$ and the sum of squares of first n natural numbers is $\frac{n(n+1)(2n+1)}{6}$. **[2009]**

(a) Statement-1 is true, Statement-2 is true. Statement-2 is not a correct explanation for Statement-1.
(b) Statement-1 is true, Statement-2 is false.
(c) Statement-1 is false, Statement-2 is true.
(d) Statement-1 is true, Statement-2 is true. Statement-2 is a correct explanation for Statement-1.

33. The mean of the numbers a, b, 8, 5, 10 is 6 and the variance is 6.80. Then which one of the following gives possible values of a and b? **[2008]**

(a) $a=0, b=7$ (b) $a=5, b=2$
(c) $a=1, b=6$ (d) $a=3, b=4$

34. Suppose a population A has 100 observations 101, 102, ..., 200 and another population B has 100 obsevrations 151, 152, ... 250. If V_A and V_B represent the variances of the two populations, respectively then $\frac{V_A}{V_B}$ is **[2006]**

(a) 1 (b) $\frac{9}{4}$
(c) $\frac{4}{9}$ (d) $\frac{2}{3}$

35. In a series of 2 n observations, half of them equal a and remaining half equal $-a$. If the standard deviation of the observations is 2, then $|a|$ equals. **[2004]**

(a) $\frac{\sqrt{2}}{n}$ (b) $\sqrt{2}$
(c) 2 (d) $\frac{1}{n}$

36. Consider the following statements :

(A) Mode can be computed from histogram
(B) Median is not independent of change of scale
(C) Variance is independent of change of origin and scale.

Which of these is / are correct ? **[2004]**

(a) (A), (B) and (C) (b) only (B)
(c) only (A) and (B) (d) only (A)

37. In an experiment with 15 observations on x, the following results were available: **[2003]**

$\Sigma x^2 = 2830, \Sigma x = 170$

One observation that was 20 was found to be wrong and was replaced by the correct value 30. The corrected variance is **[2003]**

(a) 8.33 (b) 78.00
(c) 188.66 (d) 177.33

Hints & Solutions

1. (c) Let; $\frac{x_1+x_2+.......+x_{25}}{25}=\bar{x}=40$

$\Rightarrow x_1+x_2+.........+x_{25}=1000$

$\therefore x_2+x_2+.........+x_{25}-60+A=39\times 25$

Let A be the age of new teacher.

$\Rightarrow 1000-60+A=975$

$\Rightarrow A=975-940=35$

2. (b) Sum of 16 observations $=16\times 16=256$

Sum of resultant 18 observations $=256-16+(3+4+5)$

$=252$

Mean of observations $=\frac{252}{18}=14$

3. (c) $a_1+a_2+a_3=39$

$\Rightarrow a_1+(a_1+d)+(a_1+2d)=39$

$\Rightarrow 3a_1+3d=39\,[\because a_1=10]$

$\Rightarrow d=3$

Sum of last four term = 178

Their mean $=\frac{178}{4}=44.5$

$a_n=44.5+1.5+3=49$

Median $=\frac{10+49}{2}=\frac{59}{2}=29.5$

4. (c) Let average wage of Night shift worker is x

$70\times 54+30\times x=60\times 100$

$x=74$

5. (a) There are $2n$ observations $x_1, x_2, ..., x_{2n}$

So, mean $=\sum_{i=1}^{2n}\frac{x_i}{2n}$

Let these observations be divided into two parts $x_1, x_2, ..., x_n$ and $x_{n+1}, ..., x_{2n}$

Each in 1st part 5 is added, so total of first part is

$\sum_{i=1}^{n}x_i+5n$

In second part 3 is subtracted from each

So, total of second part is $\sum_{i=n+1}^{2n}x_i-3n$

Total of $2n$ terms are

$\sum_{i=1}^{n}x_i+5n+\sum_{i=n+1}^{2n}x_i-3n=\sum_{i=1}^{2n}x_i+2n$

Mean $=\sum_{i=1}^{2n}\frac{x_i+2n}{2n}=\sum_{i=1}^{2n}\frac{x_i}{2n}+1$

So, it increase by 1.

6. (d) Since $0<y<x<2y$

$\therefore\ y>\frac{x}{2}\Rightarrow x-y<\frac{x}{2}$

$\therefore\ x-y<y<x<2x+y$

Hence median $=\frac{y+x}{2}=10$

$\Rightarrow x+y=20$ ...(i)

And range $=(2x+y)-(x-y)=x+2y$

But range = 28

$\therefore x+2y=28$ ...(ii)

From equations (i) and (ii),

$x=12, y=8$

$\therefore$ Mean $=\frac{(x-y)+y+x+(2x+y)}{4}=\frac{4x+y}{4}$

$=x+\frac{y}{4}=12+\frac{8}{4}=14$

7. (a) Correct mean $=\frac{20\times 40-33+55}{20}=41.1$

Nearest option : (a) 41

8. (a) Median is given as

$$M=l+\frac{\frac{N}{2}-F}{f}\times C$$

where

$l=$ lower limit of the median - class

$f=$ frequency of the median class

$N=$ total frequency

$F=$ cumulative frequency of the class just before the median class

$C=$ length of median class

Now, given, $M=25, N=100, F=45,$

$C=20-30=10,\ l=20.$

$\therefore$ By using formula, we have

$$25=20+\frac{50-45}{f}\times 10$$

$$25-20=\frac{50}{f}\Rightarrow 5=\frac{50}{f}\Rightarrow f=10$$

9. **(d)** Frequency distribution is given as

Expenditure	No. of families (f)
0-50	24
50-100	33
100-150	37
150-200	b
200-250	25

Clearly, modal class is 100-150, as the maximum frequency occurs in this class.
Given, Mode = 140
We have

$$\text{Mode} = \ell + \frac{f_0 - f_{-1}}{2f_0 - f_{-1} - f_1} \times i$$

where
$\ell = 100, f_0 = 37, f_{-1} = 33, f_1 = b$
$i = 50$
Thus, we get

$$140 = 100 + \left[\frac{37-33}{2(37)-33-b}\right] \times 50$$

$$= 100 + \left[\frac{4}{74-33-b}\right] \times 50$$

$$= 100 + \frac{200}{41-b}$$

$\Rightarrow \quad 5740 = 4300 + 40b \Rightarrow b = 36$

10. **(a)** Let the number of boys be x and that of girls be y.
$\Rightarrow 52x + 42y = 50(x+y)$
$\Rightarrow 52x - 50x = 50y - 42y$

$$\Rightarrow \quad 2x = 8y \Rightarrow \frac{x}{y} = \frac{4}{1} \text{ and } \frac{x}{x+y} = \frac{4}{5}$$

$$\text{Required \% of boys} = \frac{x}{x+y} \times 100 = \frac{4}{5} \times 100 = 80\ \%$$

11. **(b)** We know that for positive real numbers $x_1, x_2, ..., x_n$, A.M. of kth powers of $x'_i s \geq k^{th}$ the power of A.M. of $x'_i s$

$$\Rightarrow \frac{\sum x_1^2}{n} \geq \left(\frac{\sum x_1}{n}\right)^2 \Rightarrow \frac{400}{n} \geq \left(\frac{80}{n}\right)^2$$

$\Rightarrow n \geq 16$. So only possible value for $n = 18$
$\Rightarrow \text{Mode} = 3 \times 22 - 2 \times 21 = 66 - 42 = 24.$

12. **(d)** Mode + 2Mean = 3 Median

13. **(a)** $n = 9$ then median term $= \left(\frac{9+1}{2}\right)^{th} = 5^{th}$ term. Last four observations are increased by 2. The median is 5th observation which is remaining unchanged.
$\therefore$ there will be no change in median.

14. **(b)** Total student = 100;
for 70 students total marks = 75 × 70 = 5250
$\Rightarrow$ Total marks of girls = 7200 – 5250 = 1950

$$\text{Average of girls} = \frac{1950}{30} = 65$$

15. **(d)** $\sum_{i=1}^{100} x_i = 400 \qquad \sum_{i=1}^{100} x_i^2 = 2475$

$$\text{Variance} = \sigma^2 = \frac{\sum x_i^2}{N} - \left(\frac{\sum x_i}{N}\right)^2$$

$$= \frac{2475}{97} - \left(\frac{388}{97}\right)^2$$

$$= \frac{2425-1552}{97} = \frac{873}{97} = 9$$

16. **(d)** $\bar{x} = \frac{2+3+a+11}{4} = \frac{a}{4} + 4$

$$\sigma = \sqrt{\sum \frac{x_i^2}{n} - (\bar{x})^2}$$

$$\Rightarrow 3.5 = \sqrt{\frac{4+9+a^2+121}{4} - \left(\frac{a}{4}+4\right)^2}$$

$$\Rightarrow \frac{49}{4} = \frac{4(134+a^2)-(a^2+256+32a)}{16}$$

$$\Rightarrow 3a^2 - 32a + 84 = 0$$

17. **(c)** $n = 5$
$\bar{x} = 5$
variance = 124
$x_1 = 1,\ x_2 = 2,\ x_3 = 6$
$\bar{x} = 5$

$$\frac{x_1 + x_2 + x_3 + x_4 + x_5}{5} = 5$$

$\Rightarrow x_4 + x_5 + 9 = 25$
$\Rightarrow x_4 + x_5 = 16$

$\Rightarrow x_4 + x_5 + 10 - 10 = 16$
$\Rightarrow (x_4 - 5) + (x_5 - 5) = 16 - 10$
$\Rightarrow (x_4 - 5) + (x_5 - 5) = 6$

Mean deviation $= \frac{\Sigma |x_i - \bar{x}|}{N}$

$= \frac{|x_1 - 5| + |x_2 - 5| + |x_3 - 5| + |x_4 - 5| + |x_5 - 5|}{5}$

$= \frac{4+3+1+6}{5} = \frac{14}{5} = 2.8$

18. (a) $\bar{x} = \frac{1}{101}[1 + (1+d) + (1+2d)] \ldots.. (1+100d)]$

$= \frac{1}{101} \times \frac{101}{2}[1 + (1+100d)] = 1 + 50d$

mean deviation from mean

$= \frac{1}{101}[|1 - (1+50d)| + |(1+d) - (1+50d)| \ldots..| [1+100d] - (1+50d)|]$

$= \frac{2|d|}{101}(1 + 2 + 3 \ldots.. + 50)$

$= \frac{2|d|}{101} \times \frac{50 \times 51}{2} = \frac{2550}{101}|d|$

$= \frac{2550}{101}|d| = 225 \Rightarrow |d| = 10.1$

19. (d) First 50 even natural numbers are 2, 4, 6 ....., 100

Variance $= \frac{\sum x_i^2}{N} - (\bar{x})^2$

$\Rightarrow \sigma^2 = \frac{2^2 + 4^2 + \ldots + 100^2}{50} - \left(\frac{2 + 4 + \ldots + 100}{50}\right)^2$

$= \frac{4(1^2 + 2^2 + 3^2 + \ldots. + 50^2)}{50} - (51)^2$

$= 4\left(\frac{50 \times 51 \times 101}{50 \times 6}\right) - (51)^2 = 3434 - 2601 \Rightarrow \sigma^2 = 833$

20. (b) $\bar{x} = \frac{x_1 + x_2 + x_3 + \ldots + x_n}{n}$

$\sigma^2 = \frac{1}{n}\sum_{i=1}^{n}(x_i - \bar{x})^2$

Mean of $d_1, d_2, d_3, \ldots., d_n$

$= \frac{d_1 + d_2 + d_3 + \ldots. + d_n}{n}$

$= \frac{(-x_1 - a) + (-x_2 - a) + (-x_3 - a) + \ldots. + (-x_n - a)}{n}$

$= -\left[\frac{x_1 + x_2 + x_3 + \ldots. + x_n}{n}\right] - \frac{na}{n}$

$= -\bar{x} - a$

Since, $d_i = -x_i - a$ and we multiply or subtract each observation by any number the mode remains the same. Hence mode of $-x_i - a$ i.e. d_i and x_i are same. Now variance of $d_1, d_2, \ldots., d_n$

$= \frac{1}{n}\sum_{i=1}^{n}[d_i - (-\bar{x} - a)]^2$

$= \frac{1}{n}\sum_{i=1}^{n}[-x_i - a + \bar{x} + a]^2$

$= \frac{1}{n}\sum_{i=1}^{n}(-x_i + \bar{x})^2$

$= \frac{1}{n}\sum_{i=1}^{n}(\bar{x} - x_i)^2 = \sigma^2$

21. (b) Let x_i be n observations, $i = 1, 2, \ldots n$

Let $\bar{X}$ be the mean and M.D be the mean deviation about $\bar{X}$.

If each observation is increased by 5 then new mean will be $\bar{X} + 5$ and new M.D. about new mean will be M.D.

$\left(\because \text{Mean} = \sum_{i=1}^{n}\frac{x_i}{n}\right)$

22. (d) If initially all marks were x_i then

$\sigma_1^2 = \frac{\sum_i (x_i - \bar{x})^2}{N}$

Now each is increased by 10

$\sigma_1^2 = \frac{\sum_i [(x_i + 10) - (\bar{x} + 10)]^2}{N} = \frac{\sum_i (x_i - \bar{x})^2}{N}$

$= \sigma_1^2$

Hence, variance will not change even after the grace marks were given.

23. (a) Clearly mean A = 0

Now, standard deviation $\sigma = \sqrt{\frac{\Sigma(x - A)^2}{2n}}$

$2 = \sqrt{\frac{(a-0)^2 + (a-0)^2 + \ldots\ldots + (0-a)^2 + \ldots\ldots}{2n}}$

$= \sqrt{\frac{a^2.2n}{2n}} = |a|$

Hence, $|a| = 2$

24. **(d)** Let 5th observation be x.
Given mean = 7

$$\therefore\ 7=\frac{6+7+8+10+x}{5}$$

$\Rightarrow\ x=4$
Now, Variance

$$=\sqrt{\frac{(6-7)^2+(7-7)^2+(8-7)^2+(10-7)^2+(4-7)^2}{5}}$$

$$=\sqrt{\frac{1^2+0^2+1^2+3^2+3^2}{5}}=\sqrt{\frac{20}{5}}=\sqrt{4}=2$$

25. **(d)** A.M. of $2x_1, 2x_2, ..., 2x_n$ is

$$\frac{2x_1+2x_2+...+2x_n}{n}$$

$$=2\left(\frac{x_1+x_2+....+x_n}{n}\right)=2\bar{x}$$

$$\left(\because\ \text{Mean}=\frac{\text{sum of observations}}{\text{Number of observations}}\right)$$

So statement-2 is false.
variance $(2x_i)=2^2$ variance $(x_i)=4\sigma^2$ where $i=1, 2,......n$
So statement-1 is true.

26. **(a)** Statement 2 : Sum of first n odd natural numbers is not equal to n^2.
So, statement - 2 is false.

27. **(d)** Given observations are 4, 7, 2, 8, 6, a and mean is 7.
We know

$$\text{Mean}=\frac{4+7+2+8+6+a}{6}$$

$$\Rightarrow\quad 7=\frac{4+7+2+8+6+a}{6}\Rightarrow a=15$$

Now, given observations can be written in ascending order which is 2, 4, 6, 7, 8, 15
Since, No. of observation is even
$\therefore$ Median

$$=\frac{\left(\frac{6}{2}\right)\text{th observation}+\left(\frac{6}{2}+1\right)\text{th observation}}{2}$$

$$=\frac{\text{3rd observation}+\text{4th observation}}{2}$$

$$=\frac{6+7}{2}=\frac{13}{2}$$

$$\text{Now, Mean deviation}=\frac{\sum_{i=1}^{6}\left|x_i-\frac{13}{2}\right|}{6}$$

$$=\frac{\left|4-\frac{13}{2}\right|+\left|7-\frac{13}{2}\right|+\left|2-\frac{13}{2}\right|+\left|8-\frac{13}{2}\right|+\left|6-\frac{13}{2}\right|+\left|15-\frac{13}{2}\right|}{6}$$

$$=\frac{\frac{5}{2}+\frac{1}{2}+\frac{9}{2}+\frac{3}{2}+\frac{1}{2}+\frac{17}{2}}{6}=\frac{18}{6}=3$$

28. **(a)** Correct mean = observed mean + 2 = 30 + 2 = 32
Correct S. D. = observed S.D. = 2

29. **(b)** Median is the mean of 25th and 26th observation

$$\therefore\ M=\frac{25a+26a}{2}=25.5a$$

$$M.D\,(M)=\frac{\Sigma|x_i-M|}{N}$$

$$\Rightarrow\ 50=\frac{1}{50}[2\times|a|\times(0.5+1.5+2.5+....24.5)]$$

$$\Rightarrow\ 2500=2|a|\times\frac{25}{2}(25)$$

$$\Rightarrow\ |a|=4$$

30. **(a)** $\sigma_x^2=4, \sigma_y^2=5,\ x=2,\ y=4$

$$\frac{1}{5}\sum x_i^2-(2)^2=4;\ \frac{1}{5}\sum y_i^2-(4)^2=5$$

$$\sum x_i^2=40; \sum y_i^2=105$$

$$\Rightarrow\ \sum\left(x_i^2+y_i^2\right)=145$$

$$\Rightarrow\ \sum(x_i+y_i)=5(2)+5(4)=30$$

Variance of combined data

$$=\frac{1}{10}\sum\left(x_i^2+y_i^2\right)-\left(\frac{1}{10}\sum(x_i+y_i)\right)^2$$

$$=\frac{145}{10}-9=\frac{11}{2}$$

31. **(b)** $\text{Mean}=\dfrac{101+d(1+2+3+......+100)}{101}$

$$=1+\frac{d\times100\times101}{101\times2}=1+50d$$

$\because$ Mean deviation from the mean = 255

$$\Rightarrow\ \frac{1}{101}[|1-(1+50d)|+|(1+d)-(1+50d)|$$

$$+|(1+2d)-(1+50d)|+....+|(1+100d)-(1+50d)|]=255$$

$$\Rightarrow\ 2d[1+2+3+...+50]=101\times255$$

$$\Rightarrow\ 2d\times\frac{50\times51}{2}=101\times255$$

$$\Rightarrow\ d=\frac{101\times255}{50\times51}=10.1$$

32. **(c)** For the numbers 2, 4, 6, 8, ..., $2n$

$$\bar{x} = \frac{2[n(n+1)]}{2n} = (n+1)$$

And $Var = \frac{\Sigma(x-\bar{x})^2}{2n} = \frac{\Sigma x^2}{n} - (\bar{x})^2$

$$= \frac{4\Sigma n^2}{n} - (n+1)^2$$

$$= \frac{4n(n+1)(2n+1)}{6n} - (n+1)^2$$

$$= \frac{2(2n+1)(n+1)}{3} - (n+1)^2$$

$$= (n+1)\left[\frac{4n+2-3n-3}{3}\right]$$

$$= \frac{(n+1)(n-1)}{3} = \frac{n^2-1}{3}$$

$\therefore$ Statement-1 is false. Clearly, statement - 2 is true.

33. **(d)** Mean of $a, b, 8, 5, 10$ is 6

$$\Rightarrow \frac{a+b+8+5+10}{5} = 10$$

$\Rightarrow a+b=7$ ...(i)

Variance of $a, b, 8, 5, 10$ is 6.80

$$\Rightarrow \frac{(a-6)^2+(b-6)^2+(8-6)^2+(5-6)^2+(10-6)^2}{5} = 6.80$$

$\Rightarrow a^2-12a+36+(1-a)^2+21=34$

[using eq. (i)]

$\Rightarrow 2a^2-14a+24=0 \Rightarrow a^2-7a+12=0$

$\Rightarrow a=3$ or $4 \Rightarrow b=4$ or 3

$\therefore$ The possible values of a and b are $a=3$ and $b=4$

or, $a=4$ and $b=3$

34. **(a)** $\sigma_x^2 = \frac{\sum d_i^2}{n}$ (Here deviations are taken from the mean).

Since A and B both have 100 consecutive integers, therefore both have same standard deviation and hence the variance. $\therefore \frac{V_A}{V_B} = 1$

(As $\sum d_i^2$ is same in both the cases)

35. **(c)** Clearly mean $A=0$

Standard deviation $\sigma = \sqrt{\frac{\sum(x-A)^2}{2n}}$

$$2 = \sqrt{\frac{(a-0)^2+(a-0)^2+...(0-a)^2+...}{2n}}$$

$$= \sqrt{\frac{a^2.2n}{2n}} = |a|$$

Hence $|a|=2$

36. **(c)** Only first (A) and second (B) statements are correct.

37. **(b)** $\Sigma x=170, \Sigma x^2=2830$ increase in $\Sigma x=10$, then

$\Sigma x' = 170+10=180$

Increase in $\Sigma x^2 = 900-400 = 500$ then

$\Sigma x'^2 = 2830+500=3330$

$$\text{Variance} = \frac{1}{n}\Sigma x'^2 - \left(\frac{1}{n}\Sigma x'\right)^2$$

$$= \frac{1}{15}\times 3330 - \left(\frac{1}{15}\times 180\right)^2 = 222-144=78.$$

Probability

TOPIC-1 : Random Experiment, Sample Space, Events, Probability of an Event, Mutually Exclusive & Exhaustive Events, Equally Likely Events

1. If the lengths of the sides of a triangle are decided by the three throws of a single fair die, then the probability that the triangle is of maximum area given that it is an isosceles triangle, is : **[Online April 11, 2015]**

   (a) $\frac{1}{21}$ (b) $\frac{1}{27}$

   (c) $\frac{1}{15}$ (d) $\frac{1}{26}$

2. A number x is chosen at random from the set $\{1, 2, 3, 4, ..., 100\}$. Define the event: A = the chosen number x satisfies

   $\frac{(x-10)(x-50)}{(x-30)} \geq 0$

   Then P (A) is: **[Online April 12, 2014]**

   (a) 0.71 (b) 0.70

   (c) 0.51 (d) 0.20

3. A set S contains 7 elements. A non-empty subset A of S and an element x of S are chosen at random. Then the probability that $x \in A$ is: **[Online April 11, 2014]**

   (a) $\frac{1}{2}$ (b) $\frac{64}{127}$

   (c) $\frac{63}{128}$ (d) $\frac{31}{128}$

4. There are two balls in an urn. Each ball can be either white or black. If a white ball is put into the urn and there after a ball is drawn at random from the urn, then the probability that it is white is **[Online May 26, 2012]**

   (a) $\frac{1}{4}$ (b) $\frac{2}{3}$

   (c) $\frac{1}{5}$ (d) $\frac{1}{3}$

5. If six students, including two particular students *A* and *B*, stand in a row, then the probability that *A* and *B* are separated with one student in between them is **[Online May 19, 2012]**

   (a) $\frac{8}{15}$ (b) $\frac{4}{15}$

   (c) $\frac{2}{15}$ (d) $\frac{1}{15}$

6. A number n is randomly selected from the set $\{1, 2, 3, ..., 1000\}$. The probability that $\frac{\sum_{i=1}^{n} i^2}{\sum_{i=1}^{n} i}$ is an integer is **[Online May 12, 2012]**

   (a) 0.331 (b) 0.333

   (c) 0.334 (d) 0.332

7. Four numbers are chosen at random (without replacement) from the set $\{1, 2, 3, ...20\}$. **[2010]**

   Statement -1: The probability that the chosen numbers when arranged in some order will form an AP is $\frac{1}{85}$.

   Statement -2 : If the four chosen numbers form an AP, then the set of all possible values of common difference is $(\pm 1, \pm 2, \pm 3, \pm 4, \pm 5)$.

   (a) Statement -1 is true, Statement -2 is true; Statement -2 is **not** a correct explanation for Statement - 1

   (b) Statement - 1 is true, Statment -2 is false

   (c) Statement - 1 is false, Statment -2 is true.

   (d) Statement - 1 is true, Statement -2 is true ; Statement -2 is a correct explanation for Statement -1.

8. An urn contains nine balls of which three are red, four are blue and two are green. Three balls are drawn at random without replacement from the urn. The probability that the three balls have different colours is **[2010]**

   (a) $\frac{2}{7}$ (b) $\frac{1}{21}$

   (c) $\frac{2}{23}$ (d) $\frac{1}{3}$

9. Five horses are in a race. Mr. A selects two of the horses at random and bets on them. The probability that Mr. A selected the winning horse is **[2003]**

(a) $\frac{2}{5}$ (b) $\frac{4}{5}$

(c) $\frac{3}{5}$ (d) $\frac{1}{5}$

TOPIC-2 : Odds Against & Odds in Favour of an Event, Addition Theorem, Boole's Inequality, Demorgan's Law

10. For three events A, B and C,
P(Exactly one of A or B occurs)
= P(Exactly one of B or C occurs)
= P(Exactly one of C or A occurs) = $\frac{1}{4}$ and
P(All the three events occur simultaneously) = $\frac{1}{16}$.
Then the probability that at least one of the events occurs, is : **[2017]**

(a) $\frac{3}{16}$ (b) $\frac{7}{32}$

(c) $\frac{7}{16}$ (d) $\frac{7}{64}$

11. From a group of 10 men and 5 women, four member committees are to be formed each of which must contain at least one woman. Then the probability for these committees to have more women than men, is : **[Online April 9, 2017]**

(a) $\frac{21}{220}$ (b) $\frac{3}{11}$

(c) $\frac{1}{11}$ (d) $\frac{2}{23}$

12. If 12 identical balls are to be placed in 3 identical boxes, then the probability that one of the boxes contains exactly 3 balls is : **(2015)**

(a) $220\left(\frac{1}{3}\right)^{12}$ (b) $22\left(\frac{1}{3}\right)^{11}$

(c) $\frac{55}{3}\left(\frac{2}{3}\right)^{11}$ (d) $55\left(\frac{2}{3}\right)^{10}$

13. If A and B are two events such that $P(A \cup B) = P(A \cap B)$, then the incorrect statement amongst the following statements is: **[Online April 9, 2014]**

(a) A and B are equally likely

(b) $P(A \cap B') = 0$

(c) $P(A' \cap B) = 0$

(d) $P(A) + P(B) = 1$

14. If the events A and B are mutually exclusive events such that $P(A) = \frac{3x+1}{3}$ and $P(B) = \frac{1-x}{4}$, then the set of possible values of x lies in the interval : **[Online April 25, 2013]**

(a) $[0, 1]$ (b) $\left[\frac{1}{3}, \frac{2}{3}\right]$

(c) $\left[-\frac{1}{3}, \frac{5}{9}\right]$ (d) $\left[-\frac{7}{9}, \frac{4}{9}\right]$

15. Let X and Y are two events such that $P(X \cup Y) = P(X \cap Y)$.

Statement 1: $P(X \cap Y') = P(X' \cap Y) = 0$

Statement 2: $P(X) + P(Y) = 2P(X \cap Y)$

[Online May 7, 2012]

(a) Statement 1 is false, Statement 2 is true.

(b) Statement 1 is true, Statement 2 is true, Statement 2 is not a correct explanation of Statement 1.

(c) Statement 1 is true, Statement 2 is false.

(d) Statement 1 is true, Statement 2 is true; Statement 2 is a correct explanation of Statement 1.

16. A die is thrown. Let A be the event that the number obtained is greater than 3. Let B be the event that the number obtained is less than 5. Then $P(A \cup B)$ is **[2008]**

(a) $\frac{3}{5}$ (b) 0

(c) 1 (d) $\frac{2}{5}$

17. Events A, B, C are mutually exclusive events such that $P(A) = \frac{3x+1}{3}$; $P(B) = \frac{1-x}{4}$ and $P(C) = \frac{1-2x}{2}$ The set of possible values of x are in the interval. **[2003]**

(a) $[0, 1]$ (b) $\left[\frac{1}{3}, \frac{1}{2}\right]$

(c) $\left[\frac{1}{3}, \frac{2}{3}\right]$ (d) $\left[\frac{1}{3}, \frac{13}{3}\right]$

18. A and B are events such that $P(A \cup B) = 3/4$, $P(A \cap B) = 1/4$, $P(\overline{A}) = 2/3$ then $P(\overline{A} \cap B)$ is **[2002]**

(a) 5/12 (b) 3/8

(c) 5/8 (d) 1/4

Hints & Solutions

1. **(b)** Favourable case = (6, 6, 6)
Total case = {(1, 1, 1) (2, 2, 1), (2, 2, 2), (2, 2, 3), (3, 3, 1) ..... (3, 3, 5) (4, 4, 1).... (4, 4, 6) (5, 5, 1).... (5, 5, 6) (6, 6, 1).... (6, 6, 6)}
which satisfies condition a + b > c
Number of total case = 27

Probability = $\frac{1}{27}$

2. **(a)** Given $\frac{(x-10)(x-50)}{(x-30)} \geq 0$

Let $x \geq 10$, $x \geq 50$ equation will be true $\forall x \geq 50$

as $\left(\frac{x-50}{x-30}\right) \geq 0, \ \forall x \in [10, 30)$

$\frac{(x-10)(x-50)}{x-30} \geq 0 \ \forall x \in [10, 30)$

Total value of x between 10 to 30 is 20.
Total values of x between 50 to 100 including 50 and 100 is 51.
Total values of x = 51 + 20 = 71

$P(A) = \frac{71}{100} = 0.71$

3. **(b)** Let S = $\{x_1, x_2, x_3, x_4, x_5, x_6, x_7\}$
Let the chosen element be x_i.
Total number of subsets of S = 2^7 = 128
No. of non-empty subsets of S = 128 – 1 = 127
We need to find number of those subsets that contains x_i.

2	2	2	2	1	2	2

$x_1 \ x_2$ ------- x_i ---- x_7

For those subsets containing x_i, each element has 2 choices.
i.e., (included or not included) in subset,
However as the subset must contain x_i, x_i has only one choice. (included one)
So, total no. of subsets containing $x_i = 2 \times 2 \times 2 \times 2 \times 1 \times 2 \times 2 = 64$

Required prob $= \frac{\text{No. of subsets containing } x_i}{\text{Total no. of non-empty subsets}}$

$= \frac{64}{127}$

4. **(b)** Total possible event when one ball is taken out $= {}^3C_1$

Let E : The event of 1 white ball coming out
No. of ways to 1 white ball coming out $= {}^2C_1$

$\therefore P(E) = \frac{{}^2C_1}{{}^3C_1} = \frac{2}{3}$

5. **(b)** Consider a group of three students A, B and an other student in between A and B. Choice for a student between A and B is 4. A and B can interchange their places in the group in 2 ways.
Now the group of three students (student A, student B and a student in between A and B) and the remaining 3 students can be stand in a row in 4! ways.
Hence total number of ways to stand in a row such that A and B are separated with one student in between them
= 4 × 2 × 4!
Now total number of ways to stand 6 student stand in a row without any restriction = 6!
Hence required probability

$= \frac{4 \times 2 \times 4!}{6!} = \frac{4 \times 2}{6 \times 5} = \frac{4}{15}$

6. **(c)** $\frac{\sum_{i=1}^{n} i^2}{\sum_{i=1}^{n} i} = \frac{\frac{n(n+1)(2n+1)}{6}}{\frac{n(n+1)}{2}} = \frac{2n+1}{3}$

For n = 1, 2, 3, ..., 1000

Value of $\frac{2n+1}{3} = \frac{3}{3}, \frac{5}{3}, \frac{7}{3}, \ldots\ldots\ldots, \frac{2001}{3}$ respectively.

Out of $\frac{3}{3}, \frac{5}{3}, \frac{7}{3}, \ldots\ldots\ldots, \frac{2001}{3}$ only first term $\left(\frac{3}{3} = 1\right)$, fourth term $\left(\frac{9}{3} = 3\right)$, 667th term $\left(\frac{2001}{3} = 667\right)$ are integers.

Hence, out of 1000 values of $\frac{2n+1}{3}$,

total number of integral values of $\frac{2n+1}{3}$

= 333 + 1 = 334

$\therefore$ Required probability $= \frac{334}{1000} = 0.334$

7. (b) $n(S) = {}^{20}C_4$

Statement-1:

common difference is 1; total number of cases = 17

common difference is 2; total number of cases = 14

common difference is 3; total number of cases = 11

common difference is 4; total number of cases = 8

common difference is 5; total number of cases = 5

common difference is 6; total number of cases = 2

$$\text{Prob.} = \frac{17+14+11+8+5+2}{{}^{20}C_4} = \frac{1}{85}$$

Statement -2 is false, because common difference can be 6 also.

8. (a) $n(S) = {}^9C_3$

$n(E) = {}^3C_1 \times {}^4C_1 \times {}^2C_1$

$$\text{Probability} = \frac{3\times4\times2}{{}^9C_3} = \frac{24\times3!}{9!}\times6! = \frac{24\times6}{9\times8\times7} = \frac{2}{7}$$

9. (a) Let 5 horses are H_1, H_2, H_3, H_4 and H_5. Selected pair of horses will be one of the 10 pairs (i.e.; ${}^5C_2$): H_1H_2, H_1H_3, H_1H_4, H_1H_5, H_2H_3, H_2H_4, H_2H_5, H_3H_4, H_3H_5 and H_4H_5.

Any horse can win the race in 4 ways.

For example : Horses H_2 win the race in 4 ways H_1H_2, H_2H_3, H_2H_4 and H_2H_5.

$$\text{Hence required probability} = \frac{4}{10} = \frac{2}{5}$$

10. (c) P (exactly one of A or B occurs)

$$= P(A) + P(B) - 2P(A \cap B) = \frac{1}{4} \quad ...(1)$$

P (Exactly one of B or C occurs)

$$= P(B) + P(C) - 2P(B \cap C) = \frac{1}{4} \quad ...(2)$$

P (Exactly one of C or A occurs)

$$= P(C) + P(A) - 2P(C \cap A) = \frac{1}{4} \quad ...(3)$$

Adding (1), (2) and (3), we get

$$2\Sigma P(A) - 2\Sigma P(A \cap B) = \frac{3}{4}$$

$$\therefore \Sigma P(A) - \Sigma P(A \cap B) = \frac{3}{8}$$

$$\text{Now, } P(A \cap B \cap C) = \frac{1}{16}$$

$\therefore P(A \cup B \cup C)$

$= \Sigma P(A) - \Sigma P(A \cap B) + P(A \cap B \cap C)$

$$= \frac{3}{8} + \frac{1}{16} = \frac{7}{16}$$

11. (c) Probability of 4 member committee which contain atleast one woman.

$\Rightarrow P(3M, 1W) + P(2M, 2W) + P(1M, 3W) + P(0M, 4W)$

$$\Rightarrow \frac{{}^{10}C_3\,{}^5C_1}{{}^{15}C_4} + \frac{{}^{10}C_2\,{}^5C_2}{{}^{15}C_4} + \frac{{}^{10}C_1\,{}^5C_3}{{}^{15}C_4} + \frac{{}^{10}C_0\,{}^5C_4}{{}^{15}C_4}$$

$$\Rightarrow \frac{600}{1365} + \frac{450}{1365} + \frac{100}{1365} + \frac{5}{1365}$$

$$\Rightarrow \frac{1155}{1365}$$

$\therefore$ Probability of committees to have more women than men.

$$= \frac{P(1M,3W) + P(0M,4W)}{P(3M,1W) + P(2M,2W) + P(1M,3W) + P(0M,4W)}$$

$$= \frac{\frac{105}{1365}}{\frac{1155}{1365}} = \frac{1}{11}$$

12. (c) **Note:-** The question should state '3 different' boxes instead of '3 identical boxes' and one particular box has 3 balls. Then the solution would be:

$$\text{Required probability} = \frac{{}^{12}C_3 \times 2^9}{3^{12}}$$

$$= \frac{55}{3}\left(\frac{2}{3}\right)^{11}$$

13. (d) Let A and B be two events such that

$P(A \cup B) = P(A \cap B)$

and $P(A \cup B) = P(A) + P(B) - P(A \cap B)$

option (a) : since $P(A \cup B) = P(A \cap B)$ (given)

therefore A and B are equally likely

Suppose option (b) and option (c) are correct.

$\therefore P(A \cap B') = 0$ and $P(A' \cap B) = 0$

$\Rightarrow P(A) - P(A \cap B) = 0$ and $P(B) - P(A \cap B) = 0$

$\Rightarrow P(A) = P(A \cap B)$ and $P(B) = P(A \cap B)$

Thus $P(A) = P(B) = P(A \cap B) = P(A \cup B)$

[$\because$ Given $P(A \cap B) = P(A \cup B)$]

Also, we know

$P(A \cup B) = P(A) + P(B) - P(A \cap B)$

$= P(A \cap B) + P(A \cap B) - P(A \cap B)$

$= P(A \cap B)$

which is true from given condition

Hence, option (a), (b) and (c) are correct.

14. (c) Since events A and B are mutually exclusive

$\therefore$ P(A) + P(B) = 1

$\Rightarrow \frac{3x+1}{3}+\frac{1-x}{4}=1$

$\Rightarrow 12x+4+3-3x=12$

$\Rightarrow 9x=5 \Rightarrow x=\frac{5}{9}$

$\therefore x\in\left[-\frac{1}{3},\frac{5}{9}\right]$

15. (b) Let X and Y be two events such that

$P(X\cup Y)=P(X\cap Y)$ ...(1)

We know

$P(X\cup Y)=P(X)+P(Y)-P(X\cap Y)$

$P(X\cap Y)=P(X)+P(Y)-P(X\cap Y)$ (from (1))

$\Rightarrow P(X)+P(Y)=2P(X\cap Y)$

Hence, Statement - 2 is true.

Now, $P(X\cap Y')=P(X)-P(X\cap Y)$

and $P(X'\cap Y)=P(Y)-P(X\cap Y)$

This implies statement-1 is also true.

16. (c) $A\equiv$ number is greater than 3

$\Rightarrow P(A)=\frac{3}{6}=\frac{1}{2}$

$B\equiv$ number is less than 5 $\Rightarrow P(B)=\frac{4}{6}=\frac{2}{3}$

$A\cap B\equiv$ number is greater than 3 but less than 5.

$\Rightarrow P(A\cap B)=\frac{1}{6}$

$\therefore P(A\cup B)=P(A)+P(B)-P(A\cap B)$

$=\frac{1}{2}+\frac{2}{3}-\frac{1}{6}=\frac{3+4-1}{6}=1$

17. (b) $P(A)=\frac{3x+1}{3},\ P(B)=\frac{1-x}{4},$

$P(C)=\frac{1-2x}{2}$

$\because$ For any event $E, 0\le P(E)\le 1$

$\Rightarrow 0\le\frac{3x+1}{3}\le 1,\ 0\le\frac{1-x}{4}\le 1$ and $0\le\frac{1-2x}{2}\le 1$

$\Rightarrow -1\le 3x\le 2, -3\le x\le 1$ and $-1\le 2x\le 1$

$\Rightarrow -\frac{1}{3}\le x\le\frac{2}{3}\le -3\le x\le 1,$ and $-\frac{1}{2}\le x\le\frac{1}{2}$

Also for mutually exclusive events $A, B, C,$

$P(A\cup B\cup C)=P(A)+P(B)+P(C)$

$\Rightarrow P(A\cup B\cup C)=\frac{3x+1}{3}+\frac{1-x}{4}+\frac{1-2x}{2}$

$\therefore 0\le\frac{1+3x}{3}+\frac{1-x}{4}+\frac{1-2x}{2}\le 1$

$0\le 13-3x\le 12 \Rightarrow 1\le 3x\le 13$

$\Rightarrow \frac{1}{3}\le x\le\frac{13}{3}$

Considering all inequations, we get

$\max\left\{-\frac{1}{3},-3,-\frac{1}{2},\frac{1}{3}\right\}\le x\le\min\left\{\frac{2}{3},1,\frac{1}{2},\frac{13}{3}\right\}$

$\frac{1}{3}\le x\le\frac{1}{2}\Rightarrow x\in\left[\frac{1}{3},\frac{1}{2}\right]$

18. (a) $P(A\cup B)=P(A)+P(B)-P(A\cap B);$

$\Rightarrow \frac{3}{4}=1-P(\overline{A})+P(B)-\frac{1}{4}$

$\Rightarrow 1=1-\frac{2}{3}+P(B)\Rightarrow P(B)=\frac{2}{3};$

Now, $P(\overline{A}\cap B)=P(B)-P(A\cap B)$

$=\frac{2}{3}-\frac{1}{4}=\frac{5}{12}.$

Chapter 16 Relations and Functions

TOPIC-1 : Types of Relations, Inverse of a Relation, Mappings, Mapping of Functions, Kinds of Mapping of Functions

1. The function $f: R \to \left[-\frac{1}{2}, \frac{1}{2}\right]$ defined as $f(x) = \frac{x}{1+x^2}$, is: **[2017]**

(a) neither injective nor surjective
(b) invertible
(c) injective but not surjective
(d) surjective but not injective

2. The function $f: N \to N$ defined by $f(x) = x - 5\left[\frac{x}{5}\right]$, where N is set of natural numbers and $[x]$ denotes the greatest integer less than or equal to x, is : **[Online April 9, 2017]**

(a) one-one and onto.
(b) one-one but not onto.
(c) onto but not one-one.
(d) neither one-one nor onto.

3. Let $A = \{x_1, x_2, ..., x_7\}$ and $B = \{y_1, y_2, y_3\}$ be two sets containing seven and three distinct elements respectively. Then the total number of functions $f : A \to B$ that are onto, if there exist exactly three elements x in A such that $f(x) = y_2$, is equal to : **(Online April 11, 2015)**

(a) $14.{}^7C_3$ (b) $16.{}^7C_3$
(c) $14.{}^7C_2$ (d) $12.{}^7C_2$

4. Let $f: R \to R$ be defined by $f(x) = \frac{|x|-1}{|x|+1}$ then f is: **[Online April 19, 2014]**

(a) both one-one and onto
(b) one-one but not onto
(c) onto but not one-one
(d) neither one-one nor onto.

5. Let P be the relation defined on the set of all real numbers such that
$P = \{(a, b) : \sec^2 a - \tan^2 b = 1\}$. Then P is: **[Online April 9, 2014]**

(a) reflexive and symmetric but not transitive.
(b) reflexive and transitive but not symmetric.
(c) symmetric and transitive but not reflexive.
(d) an equivalence relation.

6. Let $R = \{(x, y) : x, y \in N \text{ and } x^2 - 4xy + 3y^2 = 0\}$, where N is the set of all natural numbers. Then the relation R is : **[Online April 23, 2013]**

(a) reflexive but neither symmetric nor transitive.
(b) symmetric and transitive.
(c) reflexive and symmetric,
(d) reflexive and transitive.

7. Let $R = \{(3, 3) (5, 5), (9, 9), (12, 12), (5, 12), (3, 9), (3, 12), (3, 5)\}$ be a relation on the set $A = \{3, 5, 9, 12\}$. Then, R is : **[Online April 22, 2013]**

(a) reflexive, symmetric but not transitive.
(b) symmetric, transitive but not reflexive.
(c) an equivalence relation.
(d) reflexive, transitive but not symmetric.

8. Let $A = \{1, 2, 3, 4\}$ and $R : A \to A$ be the relation defined by $R = \{(1, 1), (2, 3), (3, 4), (4, 2)\}$. The correct statement is : **[Online April 9, 2013]**

(a) R does not have an inverse.
(b) R is not a one to one function.
(c) R is an onto function.
(d) R is not a function.

9. If $P(S)$ denotes the set of all subsets of a given set S, then the number of one-to-one functions from the set $S = \{1, 2, 3\}$ to the set $P(S)$ is **[Online May 19, 2012]**

(a) 24 (b) 8
(c) 336 (d) 320

10. If $A = \{x \in z^+ : x < 10$ and x is a multiple of 3 or 4$\}$, where z^+ is the set of positive integers, then the total number of symmetric relations on A is **[Online May 12, 2012]**

(a) 2^5 (b) 2^{15}
(c) 2^{10} (d) 2^{20}

11. Let R be the set of real numbers. **[2011]**
Statement-1: $A = \{(x, y) \in R \times R : y - x \text{ is an integer}\}$ is an equivalence relation on R.
Statement-2: $B = \{(x, y) \in R \times R : x = \alpha y$ for some rational number $\alpha\}$ is an equivalence relation on R.
(a) Statement-1 is true, Statement-2 is true; Statement-2 is not a correct explanation for Statement-1.
(b) Statement-1 is true, Statement-2 is false.
(c) Statement-1 is false, Statement-2 is true.
(d) Statement-1 is true, Statement-2 is true; Statement-2 is a correct explanation for Statement-1.

12. Consider the following relations:
R = $\{(x, y) \mid x, y$ are real numbers and $x = wy$ for some rational number $w\}$;
$S = \{\left(\frac{m}{n}, \frac{p}{q}\right) \mid m, n, p$ and q are integers such that $n, q \neq 0$ and $qm = pn\}$.
Then **[2010]**
(a) Neither R nor S is an equivalence relation
(b) S is an equivalence relation but R is not an equivalence relation
(c) R and S both are equivalence relations
(d) R is an equivalence relation but S is not an equivalence relation

13. Let R be the real line. Consider the following subsets of the plane $R \times R$:
$S = \{(x, y): y = x + 1 \text{ and } 0 < x < 2\}$
$T = \{(x, y): x - y \text{ is an integer}\}$,
Which one of the following is true? **[2008]**
(a) Neither S nor T is an equivalence relation on R
(b) Both S and T are equivalence relation on R
(c) S is an equivalence relation on R but T is not
(d) T is an equivalence relation on R but S is not

14. Let W denote the words in the English dictionary. Define the relation R by $R = \{(x, y) \in W \times W |$ the words x and y have at least one letter in common.$\}$ Then R is **[2006]**
(a) not reflexive, symmetric and transitive
(b) relexive, symmetric and not transitive
(c) reflexive, symmetric and transitive
(d) reflexive, not symmetric and transitive

15. Let R = {(3, 3), (6, 6), (9, 9), (12, 12), (6, 12), (3, 9), (3, 12), (3, 6)} be a relation on the set $A = \{3, 6, 9, 12\}$. The relation is **[2005]**
(a) reflexive and transitive only
(b) reflexive only
(c) an equivalence relation
(d) reflexive and symmetric only

16. Let $f : (-1, 1) \to B$, be a function defined by $f(x) = \tan^{-1}\frac{2x}{1-x^2}$, then f is both one - one and onto when B is the interval **[2005]**
(a) $\left(0, \frac{\pi}{2}\right)$ (b) $\left[0, \frac{\pi}{2}\right)$
(c) $\left[-\frac{\pi}{2}, \frac{\pi}{2}\right]$ (d) $\left(-\frac{\pi}{2}, \frac{\pi}{2}\right)$

17. Let R = $\{(1,3), (4,2), (2,4), (2,3), (3,1)\}$ be a relation on the set $A = \{1, 2, 3, 4\}$.. The relation R is **[2004]**
(a) reflexive (b) transitive
(c) not symmetric (d) a function

18. If $f : R \to S$, defined by $f(x) = \sin x - \sqrt{3}\cos x + 1$, is onto, then the interval of S is **[2004]**
(a) $[-1, 3]$ (b) $[-1, 1]$
(c) $[0, 1]$ (d) $[0, 3]$

19. A function f from the set of natural numbers to integers defined by **[2003]**
$$f(n) = \begin{cases} \frac{n-1}{2}, & \text{when n is odd} \\ -\frac{n}{2}, & \text{when n is even} \end{cases} \text{ is}$$
(a) neither one -one nor onto
(b) one-one but not onto
(c) onto but not one-one
(d) one-one and onto both.

TOPIC-2 : Composite Functions & Relations, Inverse of a Function, Binary Operations

20. Let $f(x) = 2^{10} \cdot x + 1$ and $g(x) = 3^{10} \cdot x - 1$. If $(fog)(x) = x$, then x is equal to : **[Online April 8, 2017]**
(a) $\frac{3^{10}-1}{3^{10}-2^{-10}}$ (b) $\frac{2^{10}-1}{2^{10}-3^{-10}}$
(c) $\frac{1-3^{-10}}{2^{10}-3^{-10}}$ (d) $\frac{1-2^{-10}}{3^{10}-2^{-10}}$

21. For $x \in R, x \neq 0$, let $f_0(x) = \frac{1}{1-x}$ and $f_{n+1}(x) = f_0(f_n(x))$, $n = 0, 1, 2, ...$ Then the value of $f_{100}(3) + f_1\left(\frac{2}{3}\right) + f_2\left(\frac{3}{2}\right)$ is equal to : **[Online April 9, 2016]**
(a) $\frac{8}{3}$ (b) $\frac{4}{3}$
(c) $\frac{5}{3}$ (d) $\frac{1}{3}$

22. If g is the inverse of a function f and $f'(x)=\dfrac{1}{1+x^5}$, then $g'(x)$ is equal to: **[2014]**

(a) $\dfrac{1}{1+\{g(x)\}^5}$ (b) $1+\{g(x)\}^5$

(c) $1+x^5$ (d) $5x^4$

23. Let A and B be non empty sets in R and $f: A \to B$ is a bijective function. **[Online May 26, 2012]**

Statement 1: f is an onto function.

Statement 2: There exists a function $g: B \to A$ such that fog $= I_B$.

(a) Statement 1 is true, Statement 2 is false.

(b) Statement 1 is true, Statement 2 is true; Statement 2 is a correct explanation for Statement 1.

(c) Statement 1 is false, Statement 2 is true.

(d) Statement 1 is true, Statement 2 is true, Statement 2 is not the correct explanation for Statement 1.

24. Let f be a function defined by

$f(x)=(x-1)^2+1, (x\geq 1)$. **[2011RS]**

Statement - 1 :

The set $\{x: f(x)=f^{-1}(x)\}=\{1,2\}$.

Statement - 2:

f is a bijection and $f^{-1}(x)=1+\sqrt{x-1}, x\geq 1$.

(a) Statement-1 is true, Statement-2 is true; Statement-2 is a correct explanation for Statement-1.

(b) Statement-1 is true, Statement-2 is true; Statement-2 is NOT a correct explanation for Statement-1.

(c) Statement-1 is true, Statement-2 is false.

(d) Statement-1 is false, Statement-2 is true.

25. Let $f(x) = (x+1)^2 - 1, x \geq -1$

Statement -1 : The set $\{x : f(x) = f^{-1}(x) = \{0, -1\}$

Statement-2 : f is a bijection. **[2009]**

(a) Statement-1 is true, Statement-2 is true. Statement-2 is not a correct explanation for Statement-1.

(b) Statement-1 is true, Statement-2 is false.

(c) Statement-1 is false, Statement-2 is true.

(d) Statement-1 is true, Statement-2 is true. Statement-2 is not a correct explanation for Statement-1.

26. Let $f: N \to Y$ be a function defined as $f(x) = 4x + 3$ where $Y = \{y \in N : y = 4x + 3$ for some $x \in N\}$.
Show that f is invertible and its inverse is **[2008]**

(a) $g(y)=\dfrac{3y+4}{3}$ (b) $g(y)=4+\dfrac{y+3}{4}$

(c) $g(y)=\dfrac{y+3}{4}$ (d) $g(y)=\dfrac{y-3}{4}$

Hints & Solutions

1. (d) we have $f: R \rightarrow \left[-\frac{1}{2}, \frac{1}{2}\right]$,

$$f(x) = \frac{x}{1+x^2} \forall x \in R$$

$$\Rightarrow f'(x) = \frac{(1+x^2).1 - x.2x}{(1+x^2)^2} = \frac{-(x+1)(x-1)}{(1+x^2)^2}$$

– + – sign of f′ (x)

x = –1 x = 1

$\Rightarrow$ f′ (x) changes sign in different intervals.

$\therefore$ Not injective

Now $y = \frac{x}{1+x^2}$

$\Rightarrow y + yx^2 = x$

$\Rightarrow yx^2 - x + y = 0$

For $y \neq 0$, $D = 1 - 4y^2 \geq 0$

$\Rightarrow y \in \left[\frac{-1}{2}, \frac{1}{2}\right] - \{0\}$

For $y = 0 \Rightarrow x = 0$

$\therefore$ Range is $\left[\frac{-1}{2}, \frac{1}{2}\right]$

$\Rightarrow$ Surjective but not injective

2. (d) $\left.\begin{array}{l} f(1) = 1 - 5[1/5] = 1 \\ f(6) = 6 - 5[6/5] = 1 \end{array}\right\} \rightarrow$ Many one

$f(10) = 10 - 5(2) = 0$ which is not in co–domain.

Neither one–one nor onto.

3. (a) Number of onto function such that exactly three elements in $x \in A$ such that $f(x) = \frac{1}{2}$ is equal to $= {}^7C_3$,

$\{2^4 - 2\} = 14. {}^7C_3$

4. (d) $P = \{(a, b): \sec^2 a - \tan^2 b = 1\}$

For reflexive :

$\sec^2 a - \tan^2 a = 1$ (true $\forall a$)

For symmetric :

$\sec^2 b - \tan^2 a = 1$

L.H.S

$1 + \tan^2 b - (\sec^2 a - 1) = 1 + \tan^2 b - \sec^2 a + 1$

$= -(\sec^2 a - \tan^2 b) + 2$

$= -1 + 2 = 1$

So, Relation is symmetric

For transitive :

if $\sec^2 a - \tan^2 b = 1$ and $\sec^2 b - \tan^2 c = 1$

$\sec^2 a - \tan^2 c = (1 + \tan^2 b) - (\sec^2 b - 1)$

$= -\sec^2 b + \tan^2 b + 2$

$= -1 + 2 = 1$

So, Relation is transitive.

Hence, Relation P is an equivalence relation

5. (c) $f(x) = \frac{|x|-1}{|x|+1}$

for one-one function if $f(x_1) = f(x_2)$ then x_1 must be equal to x_2

Let $f(x_1) = f(x_2)$

$$\frac{|x_1|-1}{|x_1|+1} = \frac{|x_2|-1}{|x_2|+1}$$

$$|x_1||x_2| + |x_1| - |x_2| - 1 = |x_1||x_2| - |x_1| + |x_2| - 1$$

$$\Rightarrow |x_1| - |x_2| = |x_2| - |x_1|$$

$$2|x_1| = 2|x_2|$$

$$|x_1| = |x_2|$$

$x_1 = x_2$, $x_1 = -x_2$

here x_1 has two values therefore function is many one function.

For onto : $f(x) = \frac{|x|-1}{|x|+1}$

for every value of $f(x)$ there is a value of x in domain set.

If $f(x)$ is negative then $x = 0$

for all positive value of $f(x)$, domain contain atleast one element. Hence $f(x)$ is onto function.

6. (c) Domain = {1, 2, 3, 4}

Range = {1, 2, 3, 4}

$\therefore$ Domain = Range

Hence the relation R is onto function.

7. (d) Let R = {(3, 3), (5, 5), (9, 9), (12, 12), (5, 12), (3, 9), (3, 12), (3, 5)} be a relation on set

A = {3, 5, 9, 12}

Clearly, every element of A is related to itself.

Therefore, it is a reflexive.

Now, R is not symmetry because 3 is related to 5 but 5 is not related to 3.

Also R is transitive relation because it satisfies the property that if a R b and b R c then a R c.

8. **(d)** $R = \{(x, y) : x, y \in N \text{ and } x^2 - 4xy + 3y^2 = 0\}$

Now, $x^2 - 4xy + 3y^2 = 0$

$\Rightarrow (x - y)(x - 3y) = 0$

$\therefore x = y$ or $x = 3y$

$\therefore$ R = {(1, 1), (3, 1), (2, 2), (6, 2), (3, 3), (9, 3),......}

Since (1, 1), (2, 2), (3, 3),...... are present in the relation, therefore R is reflexive.

Since (3, 1) is an element of R but (1, 3) is not the element of R, therefore R is not symmetric

Here $(3, 1) \in R$ and $(1, 1) \in R \Rightarrow (3, 1) \in R$

$(6, 2) \in R$ and $(2, 2) \in R \Rightarrow (6, 2) \in R$

For all such $(a, b) \in R$ and $(b, c) \in R \Rightarrow (a, c) \in R$

Hence R is transitive.

9. **(b)** A relation on a set A is said to be symmetric iff

$(a, b) \in A \Rightarrow (b, a) \in A, \ \forall \ a, b \in A$

Here $A = \{3, 4, 6, 8, 9\}$

Number of order pairs of $A \times A = 5 \times 5 = 25$

Divide 25 order pairs of $A \times A$ in 3 parts as follows :

Part – A : (3, 3), (4, 4), (6, 6), (8, 8), (9, 9)

Part – B : (3, 4), (3, 6), (3, 8), (3, 9), (4, 6), (4, 8), (4, 9), (6, 8), (6, 9), (8, 9)

Part – C : (4, 3), (6, 3), (8, 3), (9, 3), (6, 4), (8, 4), (9, 4), (8, 6), (9, 6), (9, 8)

In part – A, both components of each order pair are same.

In part – B, both components are different but not two such order pairs are present in which first component of one order pair is the second component of another order pair and vice-versa.

In part–C, only reverse of the order pairs of part –B are present i.e., if (a, b) is present in part – B, then (b, a) will be present in part –C

For example (3, 4) is present in part – B and (4, 3) present in part –C.

Number of order pair in A, B and C are 5, 10 and 10 respectively.

In any symmetric relation on set A, if any order pair of part –B is present then its reverse order pair of part –C will must be also present.

Hence number of symmetric relation on set A is equal to the number of all relations on a set D, which contains all the order pairs of part –A and part– B.

Now $n(D) = n(A) + n(B) = 5 + 10 = 15$

Hence number of all relations on set $D = (2)^{15}$

$\Rightarrow$ Number of symmetric relations on set $D = (2)^{15}$

10. **(c)** Let $S = \{1, 2, 3\} \Rightarrow n(S) = 3$

Now, $P(S)$ = set of all subsets of S

total no. of subsets $= 2^3 = 8$

$\therefore n[P(S)] = 8$

Now, number of one-to-one functions from $S \to P(S)$ is

$${}^8P_3 = \frac{8!}{5!} = 8 \times 7 \times 6 = 336.$$

11. **(a)** Let for statement 1: $xRy = x - y \in I$. As xRx is an integer and yRx as well as xRz (for xRy and yRz) is also an integer.

Hence equivalence.

Similarly as $x = \alpha y$ hence $\alpha = 1$ for reflexive and $\frac{1}{\alpha}$ being a rational for symmetric for some non zero α and product of rationals also being rational $\Rightarrow$ equivalence

But not symmetric because of $\alpha = 0$ case

Both relations are equivalence but not the correct explanation.

12. **(b)** x Ry need not implies yRx

$S : \frac{m}{n} s \frac{p}{q}$

Given $qm = pn \Rightarrow \frac{p}{q} = \frac{m}{n}$

$\therefore \frac{m}{n} s \frac{m}{n}$ reflexive $\frac{m}{n} s \frac{p}{q} \Rightarrow \frac{p}{q} s \frac{m}{n}$ symmetric

$\frac{m}{n} s \frac{p}{q}, \frac{p}{q} s \frac{r}{s} \Rightarrow qm = pn, ps = rq$

$\Rightarrow \frac{p}{q} = \frac{m}{n} = \frac{r}{s} \Rightarrow$ ms = rn transitive.

S is an equivalence relation.

13. **(d)** Given $S = \{(x, y) : y = x + 1 \text{ and } 0 < x < 2\}$

$\because x \neq x + 1$ for any $x \in (0, 2)$

$\Rightarrow (x, x) \notin S$

$\therefore S$ is not reflexive.

Hence S in not an equivalence relation.

Also $T = \{x, y) : x - y$ is an integer}

$\because x - x = 0$ is an integer $\forall x \in R$

$\therefore T$ is reflexive.

If $x - y$ is an integer then $y - x$ is also an integer

$\therefore T$ is symmetric

If $x - y$ is an integer and $y - z$ is an integer then $(x - y) + (y - z) = x - z$ is also an integer.

$\therefore T$ is transitive

14. **(b)** Clearly $(x, x) \in R \forall x \in W$. So R is reflexive.

Let $(x, y) \in R$, then $(y, x) \in R$ as x and y have at least one letter in common. So, R is symmetric.

But R is not transitive for example

Let x = INDIA, y = BOMBAY and z = JOKER

then $(x, y) \in R$ (A is common) and $(y, z) \in R$ (O is common) but $(x, z) \notin R$. (as no letter is common)

15. (a) Reflexive and transitive only.

e.g. (3, 3), (6, 6), (9, 9), (12, 12) [Reflexive]

(3, 6), (6, 12), (3, 12) [Transitive].

(3, 6) $\in R$ but (6, 3) $\notin R$ [non symmetric]

16. (d) Given $f(x)=\tan^{-1}\left(\frac{2x}{1-x^2}\right)=2\tan^{-1}x$

for $x\in(-1,1)$

If $x\in(-1,1)\Rightarrow\tan^{-1}x\in\left(\frac{-\pi}{4},\frac{\pi}{4}\right)$

$\Rightarrow 2\tan^{-1}x\in\left(\frac{-\pi}{2},\frac{\pi}{2}\right)$

Clearly, range of $f(x)=\left(-\frac{\pi}{2},\frac{\pi}{2}\right)$

For f to be onto, codomain = range

$\therefore$ Co-domain of function $=B=\left(-\frac{\pi}{2},\frac{\pi}{2}\right)$.

17. (c) $\because (1,1)\notin R\Rightarrow R$ is not reflexive $(2,3)\in R$ but $(3,2)\notin R$

$\therefore$ R is not symmetric

18. (a) $f(x)$ is onto $\therefore S=$ range of $f(x)$

Now $f(x)=\sin x-\sqrt{3}\cos x+1$

$=2\sin\left(x-\frac{\pi}{3}\right)+1$

$\because -1\le\sin\left(x-\frac{\pi}{3}\right)\le 1$

$-1\le 2\sin\left(x-\frac{\pi}{3}\right)+1\le 3$

$\therefore f(x)\in[-1,3]=S$

ALTERNATE SOLUTION

We know that

$-\sqrt{a^2+b^2}\le a\sin\theta+b\cos\theta\le\sqrt{a^2+b^2}$

$\therefore\ -2\le\sin x-\sqrt{3}\cos x\le 2$

$\Rightarrow -1\le\sin x-\sqrt{3}\cos x+1\le 3$

$\therefore f(x)\in[-1,3]$

19. (d) We have $f:N\to I$

If x and y are two even natural numbers,

then $f(x)=f(y)\Rightarrow\frac{-x}{2}=\frac{-y}{2}\Rightarrow x=y$

Again if x and y are two odd natural numbers then

$f(x)=f(y)\Rightarrow\frac{x-1}{2}=\frac{y-1}{2}\Rightarrow x=y$

$\therefore f$ is onto.

Also each negative integer is an image of even natural number and each positive integer is an image of odd natural number.

$\therefore f$ is onto.

Hence f is one one and onto both.

20. (d) $f(g(x))=x$

$\Rightarrow\ f(3^{10}x-1)=2^{10}(3^{10}.x-1)+1=x$

$\Rightarrow\ 2^{10}(3^{10}x-1)+1=x$

$\Rightarrow\ x(6^{10}-1)=2^{10}-1$

$\Rightarrow\ x=\frac{2^{10}-1}{6^{10}-1}=\frac{1-2^{-10}}{3^{10}-2^{-10}}$

21. (c) $f_1(x)=f_{0+1}(x)=f_0(f_0(x))=\frac{1}{1-\frac{1}{1-x}}=\frac{x-1}{x}$

$f_2(x)=f_{1+1}(x)=f_0(f_1(x))=\frac{1}{1-\frac{x-1}{x}}=x$

$f_3(x)=f_{2+1}(x)=f_0(f_2(x))=f_0(x)=\frac{1}{1-x}$

$f_4(x)=f_{3+1}(x)=f_0(f_3(x))=\frac{x-1}{x}$

$\therefore\ f_0=f_3=f_6=\ldots\ldots\ldots=\frac{1}{1-x}$

$f_1=f_4=f_7=\ldots\ldots\ldots=\frac{x-1}{x}$

$f_2=f_5=f_8=\ldots\ldots\ldots=x$

$f_{100}(3)=\frac{3-1}{3}=\frac{2}{3}f_1\left(\frac{2}{3}\right)=\frac{\frac{2}{3}-1}{\frac{2}{3}}=-\frac{1}{2}$

$f_2\left(\frac{3}{2}\right)=\frac{3}{2}$

$\therefore\ f_{100}(3)+f_1\left(\frac{2}{3}\right)+f_2\left(\frac{3}{2}\right)=\frac{5}{3}$

22. (b) Since $f(x)$ and $g(x)$ are inverse of each other

$\therefore\ g'(f(x))=\frac{1}{f'(x)}$

$\Rightarrow\ g'(f(x))=1+x^5\qquad\left(\because\ f'(x)=\frac{1}{1+x^5}\right)$

Here $x = g(y)$

$\therefore \quad g'(y) = 1 + [g(y)]^5$

$\Rightarrow g'(x) = 1 + (g(x))^5$

23. (d) Let A and B be non-empty sets in R.

Let $f : A \to B$ is bijective function.

Clearly statement - 1 is true which says that f is an onto function.

Statement - 2 is also true statement but it is not the correct explanation for statement-1

24. (a) $f(x) = (x-1)^2 + 1, x \geq 1$

Since f is a bijective function

$\therefore \quad f : [1, \infty) \to [1, \infty)$

$\Rightarrow \quad y = (x-1)^2 + 1 \Rightarrow (x-1)^2 = y - 1$

$\Rightarrow x = 1 \pm \sqrt{y-1} \Rightarrow f^{-1}(y) = 1 \pm \sqrt{y-1}$

$\Rightarrow \quad f^{-1}(x) = 1 + \sqrt{x-1} \ \{\because x \geq 1\}$

Hence statement-2 is correct

Now $f(x) = f^{-1}(x)$

$\Rightarrow f(x) = x \Rightarrow (x-1)^2 + 1 = x$

$\Rightarrow \quad x^2 - 3x + 2 = 0 \Rightarrow x = 1, 2$

Hence statement-1 is correct,

25. (b) Given that $f(x) = (x+1)^2 - 1, \ x \geq -1$

Clearly $D_f = [-1, \infty)$ but co-domain is not given. Therefore $f(x)$ need not be necessarily onto.

But if $f(x)$ is onto then as $f(x)$ is one one also, $(x+1)$ being something +ve,

$f^{-1}(x)$ will exist where

$(x+1)^2 - 1 = y$

$\Rightarrow x + 1 = \sqrt{y+1}$

(+ve square root as $x + 1 \geq 0$)

$\Rightarrow x = -1 + \sqrt{y+1}$

$\Rightarrow f^{-1}(x) = \sqrt{x+1} - 1$

Then $\quad f(x) = f^{-1}(x)$

$\Rightarrow (x+1)^2 - 1 = \sqrt{x+1} - 1$

$\Rightarrow (x+1)^2 = \sqrt{x+1} \Rightarrow (x+1)^4 = (x+1)$

$\Rightarrow (x+1)[(x+1)^3 - 1] = 0 \Rightarrow x = -1, 0$

$\therefore$ The statement-1 is correct but statement-2 is false.

26. (d) Clearly f is one one and onto, so invertible

Also $f(x) = 4x + 3 = y$

$\Rightarrow x = \dfrac{y-3}{4} \quad \therefore \ g(y) = \dfrac{y-3}{4}$

Inverse Trigonometric Functions

TOPIC-1 : Trigometric Functions & Their Inverses, Domain & Range of Inverse Trigonometric Functions, Principal Value of Inverse Trigonometric Functions, Intervals for Inverse Trigonometric Functions

1. A value of x satisfying the equation $\sin[\cot^{-1}(1+x)] = \cos[\tan^{-1}x]$, is : **[Online April 9, 2017]**

(a) $-\frac{1}{2}$ (b) -1

(c) 0 (d) $\frac{1}{2}$

2. The principal value of $\tan^{-1}\left(\cot\frac{43\pi}{4}\right)$ is: **[Online April 19, 2014]**

(a) $-\frac{3\pi}{4}$ (b) $\frac{3\pi}{4}$

(c) $-\frac{\pi}{4}$ (d) $\frac{\pi}{4}$

3. The number of solutions of the equation, $\sin^{-1}x = 2\tan^{-1}x$ (in principal values) is : **[Online April 22, 2013]**

(a) 1 (b) 4
(c) 2 (d) 3

4. A value of $\tan^{-1}\left(\sin\left(\cos^{-1}\left(\sqrt{\frac{2}{3}}\right)\right)\right)$ is **[Online May 19, 2012]**

(a) $\frac{\pi}{4}$ (b) $\frac{\pi}{2}$

(c) $\frac{\pi}{3}$ (d) $\frac{\pi}{6}$

5. The largest interval lying in $\left(\frac{-\pi}{2}, \frac{\pi}{2}\right)$ for which the function,

$f(x) = 4^{-x^2} + \cos^{-1}\left(\frac{x}{2}-1\right) + \log(\cos x)$, is defined, is

(a) $\left[-\frac{\pi}{4}, \frac{\pi}{2}\right)$ (b) $\left[0, \frac{\pi}{2}\right)$ **[2007]**

(c) $[0, \pi]$ (d) $\left(-\frac{\pi}{2}, \frac{\pi}{2}\right)$

6. The domain of the function $f(x) = \frac{\sin^{-1}(x-3)}{\sqrt{9-x^2}}$ is

(a) $[1, 2]$ (b) $[2, 3)$ **[2004]**
(c) $[1, 2]$ (d) $[2, 3]$

7. The trigonometric equation $\sin^{-1}x = 2\sin^{-1}a$ has a solution for **[2003]**

(a) $|a| \le \frac{1}{\sqrt{2}}$ (b) $\frac{1}{2} < |a| < \frac{1}{\sqrt{2}}$

(c) all real values of a (d) $|a| < \frac{1}{2}$

8. $\cot^{-1}(\sqrt{\cos\alpha}) - \tan^{-1}(\sqrt{\cos\alpha}) = x$, then $\sin x =$

(a) $\tan^2\left(\frac{\alpha}{2}\right)$ (b) $\cot^2\left(\frac{\alpha}{2}\right)$ **[2002]**

(c) $\tan\alpha$ (d) $\cot\left(\frac{\alpha}{2}\right)$

9. The domain of $\sin^{-1}[\log_3(x/3)]$ is **[2002]**
(a) $[1, 9]$ (b) $[-1, 9]$
(c) $[-9, 1]$ (d) $[-9, -1]$

TOPIC-2 : Properties of Inverse Trigonometric Functions, Infinite Series of Inverse Trigonometric Functions

10. The value of $\tan^{-1}\left[\frac{\sqrt{1+x^2}+\sqrt{1-x^2}}{\sqrt{1+x^2}-\sqrt{1-x^2}}\right]$, $|x| < \frac{1}{2}, x \neq 0$, is equal to **[Online April 8, 2017]**

(a) $\frac{\pi}{4}+\frac{1}{2}\cos^{-1}x^2$ (b) $\frac{\pi}{4}+\cos^{-1}x^2$

(c) $\frac{\pi}{4}-\frac{1}{2}\cos^{-1}x^2$ (d) $\frac{\pi}{4}-\cos^{-1}x^2$

11. Let

$\tan^{-1} y = \tan^{-1} x + \tan^{-1}\left(\frac{2x}{1-x^2}\right),$

where or $|x| < \frac{1}{\sqrt{3}}$. Then a value of y is : **[2015]**

(a) $\frac{3x - x^3}{1+3x^2}$ (b) $\frac{3x + x^3}{1+3x^2}$

(c) $\frac{3x - x^3}{1-3x^2}$ (d) $\frac{3x + x^3}{1-3x^2}$

12. If $f(x) = 2\tan^{-1} x + \sin^{-1}\left(\frac{2x}{1+x^2}\right), x > 1$ then $f(5)$ is equal to : **[Online April 10, 2015]**

(a) $\tan^{-1}\left(\frac{65}{156}\right)$ (b) $\frac{\pi}{2}$

(c) π (d) $4\tan^{-1}(5)$

13. **Statement I:** The equation $(\sin^{-1}x)^3 + (\cos^{-1}x)^3 - a\pi^3 = 0$ has a solution for all $a \geq \frac{1}{32}$.

Statement II: For any $x \in R$, $\sin^{-1}x + \cos^{-1}x = \frac{\pi}{2}$ and

$0 \leq \left(\sin^{-1}x - \frac{\pi}{4}\right)^2 \leq \frac{9\pi^2}{16}$ **[Online April 12, 2014]**

(a) Both statements I and II are true.
(b) Both statements I and II are false.
(c) Statement I is true and statement II is false.
(d) Statement I is false and statement II is true.

14. If x, y, z are in A.P. and $\tan^{-1}x$, $\tan^{-1}y$ and $\tan^{-1}z$ are also in A.P., then **[2013]**

(a) $x = y = z$ (b) $2x = 3y = 6z$

(c) $6x = 3y = 2z$ (d) $6x = 4y = 3z$

15. Let $x \in (0, 1)$. The set of all x such that $\sin^{-1}x > \cos^{-1}x$, is the interval: **[Online April 25, 2013]**

(a) $\left(\frac{1}{2}, \frac{1}{\sqrt{2}}\right)$ (b) $\left(\frac{1}{\sqrt{2}}, 1\right)$

(c) $(0, 1)$ (d) $\left(0, \frac{\sqrt{3}}{2}\right)$

16. $S = \tan^{-1}\left(\frac{1}{n^2+n+1}\right) + \tan^{-1}\left(\frac{1}{n^2+3n+3}\right) + \ldots$

$+ \tan^{-1}\left(\frac{1}{1+(n+19)(n+20)}\right)$, then $\tan S$ is equal to : **[Online April 23, 2013]**

(a) $\frac{20}{401+20n}$ (b) $\frac{n}{n^2+20n+1}$

(c) $\frac{20}{n^2+20n+1}$ (d) $\frac{n}{401+20n}$

17. A value of x for which $\sin(\cot^{-1}(1+x)) = \cos(\tan^{-1}x)$, is : **[Online April 9, 2013]**

(a) $-\frac{1}{2}$ (b) 1

(c) 0 (d) $\frac{1}{2}$

18. If $\sin^{-1}\left(\frac{x}{5}\right) + \text{cosec}^{-1}\left(\frac{5}{4}\right) = \frac{\pi}{2}$, then the values of x is **[2007]**

(a) 4 (b) 5

(c) 1 (d) 3

19. If $\cos^{-1}x - \cos^{-1}\frac{y}{2} = \alpha$, then $4x^2 - 4xy\cos\alpha + y^2$ is equal to **[2005]**

(a) $2\sin 2\alpha$ (b) 4

(c) $4\sin^2\alpha$ (d) $-4\sin^2\alpha$

Hints & Solutions

1. (a) $\sin\left[\cot^{-1}(1+x)\right]=\cos\left(\tan^{-1}x\right)$

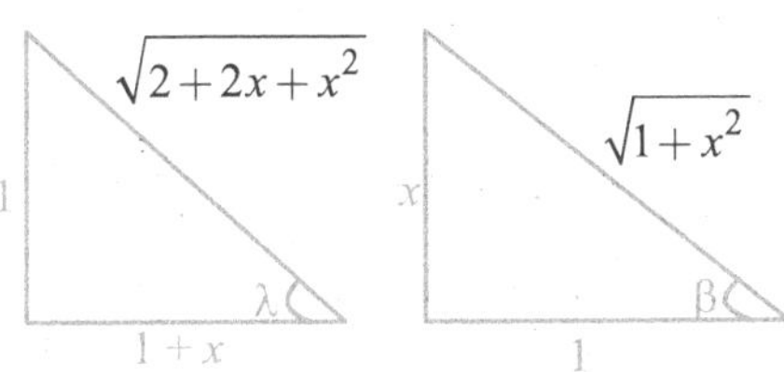

Let; $\cot\lambda = 1+x$
$\tan\beta = x$

$\Rightarrow \sin\lambda=\cos\beta$

$$\Rightarrow \frac{1}{\sqrt{x^2+2x+2}}=\frac{1}{1\sqrt{1+x^2}}$$

$$\Rightarrow x^2+2x+2=x^2+1$$

$$\Rightarrow \boxed{x=-1/2}$$

2. (c) Consider

$$\tan^{-1}\left[\cot\frac{43\pi}{4}\right]=\tan^{-1}\left[\cot\left(10\pi+\frac{3\pi}{4}\right)\right]$$

$$=\tan^{-1}\left[\cot\frac{3\pi}{4}\right] \quad [\because \cot(2n\pi+\theta)=\cot\theta]$$

$$=\tan^{-1}\left[\tan\left(\frac{\pi}{2}-\frac{3\pi}{4}\right)\right]$$

$$=\frac{\pi}{2}-\frac{3\pi}{4}=\frac{2\pi-3\pi}{4}=\frac{-\pi}{4}$$

3. (a) Given equation is
$\sin^{-1}x=2\tan^{-1}x$
Now, this equation has only one solution.

$\therefore$ LHS $=\sin^{-1}1=\frac{\pi}{2}$

and RHS $=2\tan^{-1}1=2\times\frac{\pi}{4}=\frac{\pi}{2}$

Also, $x=1$ gives angle value as $\frac{\pi}{4}$ and $\frac{5\pi}{4}$

$\frac{5\pi}{4}$ is outside the principal value.

4. (d) Consider $\tan^{-1}\left[\sin\left(\cos^{-1}\sqrt{\frac{2}{3}}\right)\right]$

Let $\cos^{-1}\sqrt{\frac{2}{3}}=\theta \Rightarrow \cos\theta=\sqrt{\frac{2}{3}}$

$$\Rightarrow \sin\theta=\sqrt{1-\cos^2\theta}=\sqrt{1-\frac{2}{3}}=\sqrt{\frac{1}{3}}$$

$$\therefore \tan^{-1}\left[\sin\left(\cos^{-1}\sqrt{\frac{2}{3}}\right)\right]=\tan^{-1}[\sin\theta]$$

$$=\tan^{-1}\left[\sqrt{\frac{1}{3}}\right]=\tan^{-1}\left(\frac{1}{\sqrt{3}}\right)$$

$$=\frac{\pi}{6}$$

5. (b) $f(x)=4^{-x^2}+\cos^{-1}\left(\frac{x}{2}-1\right)+\log(\cos x)$

$f(x)$ is defined if $-1\le\left(\frac{x}{2}-1\right)\le 1$ and $\cos x>0$

or $\quad 0\le\frac{x}{2}\le 2$ and $-\frac{\pi}{2}<x<\frac{\pi}{2}$

or $\quad 0\le x\le 4$ and $-\frac{\pi}{2}<x<\frac{\pi}{2}$

$\therefore \quad x\in\left[0,\frac{\pi}{2}\right)$

6. (b) $f(x)=\frac{\sin^{-1}(x-3)}{\sqrt{9-x^2}}$ is defined

if (i) $-1\le x-3\le 1\Rightarrow 2\le x\le 4$

and (ii) $9-x^2>0\Rightarrow -3<x<3$
Taking common solution of (i) and (ii),
we get $2\le x<3$ $\therefore$ Domain $=[2,3)$

7. (a) $\sin^{-1}x=2\sin^{-1}a$

$-\frac{\pi}{2}\le\sin^{-1}x\le\frac{\pi}{2}$; $\therefore -\frac{\pi}{2}\le 2\sin^{-1}a\le\frac{\pi}{2}$

$-\frac{\pi}{4}\le\sin^{-1}a\le\frac{\pi}{4}$ or $\frac{-1}{\sqrt{2}}\le a\le\frac{1}{\sqrt{2}}$

$\therefore |a|\le\frac{1}{\sqrt{2}}$

8. **(a)** $\cot^{-1}(\sqrt{\cos\alpha}) - \tan^{-1}(\sqrt{\cos\alpha}) = x$

$\tan^{-1}\left(\frac{1}{\sqrt{\cos\alpha}}\right) - \tan^{-1}(\sqrt{\cos\alpha}) = x$

$\Rightarrow \tan^{-1}\dfrac{\frac{1}{\sqrt{\cos\alpha}} - \sqrt{\cos\alpha}}{1 + \frac{1}{\sqrt{\cos\alpha}}.\sqrt{\cos\alpha}} = x$

$\Rightarrow \tan^{-1}\dfrac{1-\cos\alpha}{2\sqrt{\cos\alpha}} = x$

$\Rightarrow \tan x = \dfrac{1-\cos\alpha}{2\sqrt{\cos\alpha}}$ OR $\cot x = \dfrac{2\sqrt{\cos\alpha}}{1-\cos\alpha}$

[Considering a Δ with perpendicular $= (1-\cos\alpha)$ and base $= 2\sqrt{\cos\alpha}$]

$\Rightarrow \sin x = \dfrac{1-\cos\alpha}{1+\cos\alpha} = \dfrac{1-(1-2\sin^2\alpha/2)}{1+2\cos^2\alpha/2-1}$

or $\sin x = \tan^2\dfrac{\alpha}{2}$

9. **(a)** $f(x) = \sin^{-1}\left(\log_3\left(\frac{x}{3}\right)\right)$ exists

if $-1 \le \log_3\left(\frac{x}{3}\right) \le 1 \Leftrightarrow 3^{-1} \le \frac{x}{3} \le 3^1$

$\Leftrightarrow 1 \le x \le 9$ or $x \in [1, 9]$

10. **(a)** Let $x^2 = \cos 2\theta$; $\Rightarrow \theta = \frac{1}{2}\cos^{-1}x^2$

$\Rightarrow \tan^{-1}\left[\dfrac{\sqrt{1+x^2}}{\sqrt{1+x^2}} - \dfrac{\sqrt{1-x^2}}{\sqrt{1-x^2}}\right] = \left[\dfrac{\sqrt{1+\cos 2\theta}+\sqrt{1-\cos 2\theta}}{\sqrt{1+\cos 2\theta}-\sqrt{1-\cos 2\theta}}\right]$

$\Rightarrow \tan^{-1}\left[\dfrac{1+\tan\theta}{1-\tan\theta}\right] = \tan^{-1}\left[\tan\left(\frac{\pi}{4}+\theta\right)\right]$

$= \frac{\pi}{4} + \frac{1}{2}\cos^{-1}x^2$

11. **(c)** $\tan^{-1}y = \tan^{-1}x + \tan^{-1}\left[\dfrac{2x}{1-x^2}\right]$

$= \tan^{-1}x + 2\tan^{-1}x$

$= 3\tan^{-1}x$

$\tan^{-1}y = \tan^{-1}\left[\dfrac{3x-x^3}{1-3x^2}\right]$

$y = \dfrac{3x-x^3}{1-3x^2}$

12. **(c)** $f(x) = 2\tan^{-1}x + \sin^{-1}\left(\dfrac{2x}{1+x^2}\right)$

$\Rightarrow f(x) = 2\tan^{-1}x + \pi - 2\tan^{-1}x$

$\Rightarrow f(x) = \pi$

$\Rightarrow f(5) = \pi$

13. **(a)** $\sin^{-1}x \in \left[-\frac{\pi}{2}, \frac{\pi}{2}\right]$

$\Rightarrow -\frac{3\pi}{4} \le \left(\sin^{-1}x - \frac{\pi}{4}\right) \le \frac{\pi}{4}$

$0 \le \left(\sin^{-1}x - \frac{\pi}{4}\right)^2 \le \frac{9}{16}\pi^2$ ..(1)

Statement II is true

$(\sin^{-1}x)^3 + (\cos^{-1}x)^3 = a\pi^3$

$\Rightarrow (\sin^{-1}x + \cos^{-1}x)\left[(\sin^{-1}x+\cos^{-1}x)^2 - 3\sin^{-1}x\cos^{-1}x\right] = a\pi^3$

$\Rightarrow \frac{\pi^2}{4} - 3\sin^{-1}x\cos^{-1}x = 2a\pi^2$

$\Rightarrow \sin^{-1}x\left(\frac{\pi}{2} - \sin^{-1}x\right) = \frac{\pi^2}{12}(1-8a)$

$\Rightarrow \left(\sin^{-1}x - \frac{\pi}{4}\right)^2 = \frac{\pi^2}{12}(8a-1) + \frac{\pi^2}{16}$

$\Rightarrow \left(\sin^{-1}x - \frac{\pi}{4}\right)^2 = \frac{\pi^2}{48}(32a-1)$

Putting this value in equation (1)

$0 \le \frac{\pi^2}{48}(32a-1) \le \frac{9}{16}\pi^2$

$\Rightarrow 0 \le 32a - 1 \le 27$

$\frac{1}{32} \le a \le \frac{7}{8}$

Statement-I is also true

14. **(a)** Since, x, y, z are in A.P.

$\therefore\ 2y = x + z$

Also, we have

$2\tan^{-1}y = \tan^{-1}x + \tan^{-1}(z)$

$\Rightarrow \tan^{-1}\left(\dfrac{2y}{1-y^2}\right) = \tan^{-1}\left(\dfrac{x+z}{1-xz}\right)$

$\Rightarrow \dfrac{x+z}{1-y^2} = \dfrac{x+z}{1-xz}$ $(\because\ 2y = x+z)$

$\Rightarrow y^2 = xz$ or $x + z = 0 \Rightarrow x = y = z$

15. **(b)** Given $\sin^{-1}x > \cos^{-1}x$ where $x \in (0, 1)$

$\Rightarrow \sin^{-1}x > \frac{\pi}{2} - \sin^{-1}x$

$\Rightarrow 2\sin^{-1}x > \frac{\pi}{2} \Rightarrow \sin^{-1}x > \frac{\pi}{4}$

$\Rightarrow\ x > \sin\frac{\pi}{4} \Rightarrow x > \frac{1}{\sqrt{2}}$

Maximum value of $\sin^{-1} x$ is $\frac{\pi}{2}$

So, maximum value of x is 1. So, $x \in \left(\frac{1}{\sqrt{2}}, 1\right)$.

16. (c) We know that,

$$\tan^{-1}\frac{1}{1+2} + \tan^{-1}\frac{1}{1+2\times 3} + \tan^{-1}\frac{1}{1+3\times 4} + ...+$$

$$\tan^{-1}\frac{1}{1+(n-1)n} + \tan^{-1}\frac{1}{1+n(n+1)} + ...+$$

$$\tan^{-1}\frac{1}{1+(n+19)(n+20)} = \tan^{-1}\frac{n+19}{n+21}$$

$$\Rightarrow \tan^{-1}\frac{n-1}{n+1} + \tan^{-1}\frac{1}{1+n(n+1)} + \tan^{-1}\frac{1}{1+(n+1)(n+2)}$$

$$+......+\frac{1}{1+(n+19)(n+20)} = \tan^{-1}\frac{n+19}{n+21}$$

$$\Rightarrow \tan^{-1}\frac{1}{1+n(n+1)} + \tan^{-1}\frac{1}{1+(n+1)(n+2)} + ...+$$

$$\frac{1}{1+(n+19)(n+20)} = \tan^{-1}\frac{n+19}{n+21} - \tan^{-1}\frac{n-1}{n+1}$$

$$\Rightarrow \tan^{-1}\left(\frac{1}{n^2+n+1}\right) + \tan^{-1}\left(\frac{1}{n^2+3n+3}\right) + ...+$$

$$\tan^{-1}\frac{1}{1+(n+19)(n+20)}$$

$$= \tan^{-1}\left(\frac{\frac{n+19}{n+21} - \frac{n-1}{n+1}}{1+\frac{n+19}{n+21}\times\frac{n-1}{n+1}}\right)$$

$$= \tan^{-1}\frac{20}{n^2+20n+1} = S$$

$$\therefore\ \tan^{-1} S = \frac{20}{n^2+20n+1}$$

17. (a) $\sin(\cot^{-1}(1+x)) = \cos(\tan^{-1} x)$

$\Rightarrow \operatorname{cosec}^2(\cot^{-1}(1+x)) = \sec^2(\tan^{-1} x)$

$\Rightarrow 1 + [\cot(\cot^{-1}(1+x))]^2 = 1 + [\tan(\tan^{-1} x)]^2$

$\Rightarrow (1+x)^2 = x^2 \Rightarrow x = -\frac{1}{2}$

18. (d) $\sin^{-1}\left(\frac{x}{5}\right) + \operatorname{cosec}^{-1}\left(\frac{5}{4}\right) = \frac{\pi}{2}$

$\Rightarrow\ \sin^{-1}\left(\frac{x}{5}\right) = \frac{\pi}{2} - \operatorname{cosec}^{-1}\left(\frac{5}{4}\right)$

$\Rightarrow\ \sin^{-1}\left(\frac{x}{5}\right) = \frac{\pi}{2} - \sin^{-1}\left(\frac{4}{5}\right)$

$[\because \sin^{-1} x + \cos^{-1} x = \pi/2]$

$\Rightarrow\ \sin^{-1}\left(\frac{x}{5}\right) = \cos^{-1}\left(\frac{4}{5}\right)$ ....(i)

Let $\cos^{-1}\frac{4}{5} = A \Rightarrow \cos A = \frac{4}{5}$

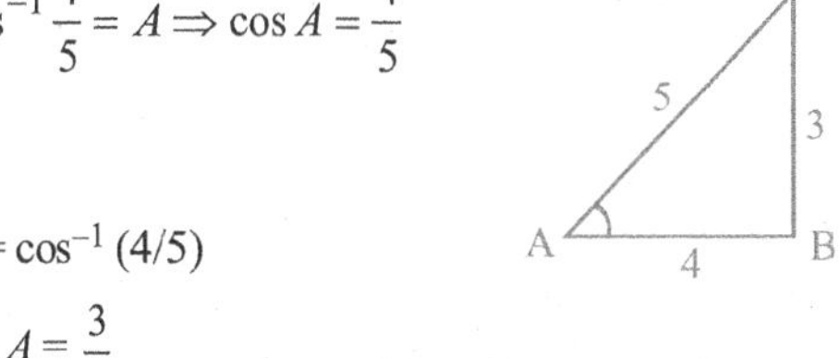

$\Rightarrow A = \cos^{-1}(4/5)$

$\Rightarrow \sin A = \frac{3}{5}$

$\Rightarrow A = \sin^{-1}\frac{3}{5}$

$\therefore\ \cos^{-1}(4/5) = \sin^{-1}(3/5)$

$\therefore$ equation (i) become,

$\sin^{-1}\frac{x}{5} = \sin^{-1}\frac{3}{5} \Rightarrow \frac{x}{5} = \frac{3}{5} \Rightarrow x = 3$

19. (c) $\cos^{-1} x - \cos^{-1}\frac{y}{2} = \alpha$

$$\cos^{-1}\left(\frac{xy}{2} + \sqrt{(1-x^2)\left(1-\frac{y^2}{4}\right)}\right) = \alpha$$

$$\cos^{-1}\left(\frac{xy + \sqrt{4-y^2-4x^2+x^2y^2}}{2}\right) = \alpha$$

$\Rightarrow 4 - y^2 - 4x^2 + x^2y^2$

$= 4\cos^2\alpha + x^2y^2 - 4xy\cos\alpha$

$\Rightarrow\ 4x^2 + y^2 - 4xy\cos\alpha = 4\sin^2\alpha\cdot$

Matrices

TOPIC-1 : Order of Matrices, Types of Matrices, Addition & Subtraction of Matrices, Scalar Multiplication of Matrices, Multiplication of Matrices

1. If $A=\begin{bmatrix}0 & -1\\ 1 & 0\end{bmatrix}$, then which one of the following statements is not correct? **[Online April 10, 2015]**
(a) $A^2+I=A(A^2-I)$
(b) $A^4-I=A^2+I$
(c) $A^3+I=A(A^3-I)$
(d) $A^3-I=A(A-I)$

2. If $A=\begin{bmatrix}1 & 2 & x\\ 3 & -1 & 2\end{bmatrix}$ and $B=\begin{bmatrix}y\\ x\\ 1\end{bmatrix}$ be such that $AB=\begin{bmatrix}6\\ 8\end{bmatrix}$, then: **[Online April 12, 2014]**
(a) $y=2x$
(b) $y=-2x$
(c) $y=x$
(d) $y=-x$

3. If p, q, r are 3 real numbers satisfying the matrix equation,
$$[pqr]\begin{bmatrix}3 & 4 & 1\\ 3 & 2 & 3\\ 2 & 0 & 2\end{bmatrix}=[3\ \ 0\ \ 1] \text{ then}$$
$2p+q-r$ equals : **[Online April 22, 2013]**
(a) -3
(b) -1
(c) 4
(d) 2

4. The matrix $A^2+4A-5I$, where I is identity matrix and $A=\begin{bmatrix}1 & 2\\ 4 & -3\end{bmatrix}$, equals **[Online April 9, 2013]**
(a) $4\begin{bmatrix}2 & 1\\ 2 & 0\end{bmatrix}$
(b) $4\begin{bmatrix}0 & -1\\ 2 & 2\end{bmatrix}$
(c) $32\begin{bmatrix}2 & 1\\ 2 & 0\end{bmatrix}$
(d) $32\begin{bmatrix}1 & 1\\ 1 & 0\end{bmatrix}$

5. If $A=\begin{bmatrix}1 & 0 & 0\\ 2 & 1 & 0\\ -3 & 2 & 1\end{bmatrix}$ and $B=\begin{bmatrix}1 & 0 & 0\\ -2 & 1 & 0\\ 7 & -2 & 1\end{bmatrix}$ then AB equals **[Online May 26, 2012]**
(a) I
(b) A
(c) B
(d) 0

6. If $\omega \neq 1$ is the complex cube root of unity and matrix $H=\begin{bmatrix}\omega & 0\\ 0 & \omega\end{bmatrix}$, then H^{70} is equal to **[2011RS]**
(a) 0
(b) $-H$
(c) H^2
(d) H

7. The number of 3×3 non-singular matrices, with four entries as 1 and all other entries as 0, is **[2010]**
(a) 5
(b) 6
(c) at least 7
(d) less than 4

8. Let $A=\begin{pmatrix}1 & 2\\ 3 & 4\end{pmatrix}$ and $B=\begin{pmatrix}a & 0\\ 0 & b\end{pmatrix}$, $a,b\in N$. Then **[2006]**
(a) there cannot exist any B such that AB = BA
(b) there exist more than one but finite number of B′s such that AB = BA
(c) there exists exactly one B such that AB = BA
(d) there exist infinitely many B′s such that AB = BA

9. If A and B are square matrices of size $n \times n$ such that $A^2-B^2=(A-B)(A+B)$, then which of the following will be always true? **[2006]**
(a) $A=B$
(b) $AB=BA$
(c) either of A or B is a zero matrix
(d) either of A or B is identity matrix

10. If $A=\begin{bmatrix}1 & 0\\ 1 & 1\end{bmatrix}$ and $I=\begin{bmatrix}1 & 0\\ 0 & 1\end{bmatrix}$, then which one of the following holds for all $n\geq 1$, by the principle of mathematical induction **[2005]**
(a) $A^n=nA-(n-1)I$
(b) $A^n=2^{n-1}A-(n-1)I$
(c) $A^n=nA+(n-1)I$
(d) $A^n=2^{n-1}A+(n-1)I$

11. If $A=\begin{bmatrix}a & b\\ b & a\end{bmatrix}$ and $A^2=\begin{bmatrix}\alpha & \beta\\ \beta & \alpha\end{bmatrix}$, then **[2003]**
(a) $\alpha=2ab, \beta=a^2+b^2$
(b) $\alpha=a^2+b^2,\ \beta=ab$
(c) $\alpha=a^2+b^2,\ \beta=2ab$
(d) $\alpha=a^2+b^2,\ \beta=a^2-b^2$.

TOPIC-2 : Transpose of Matrices, Symmetric & Skew Symmetric Matrices, Inverse of a Matrix by Elementary Row Operations

12. For two 3×3 matrices A and B, let $A + B = 2B^T$ and $3A + 2B = I_3$, where B^T is the transpose of B and I_3 is 3×3 identity matrix. Then : **[Online April 9, 2017]**

(a) $5A + 10B = 2I_3$ (b) $10A + 5B = 3I_3$
(c) $B + 2A = I_3$ (d) $3A + 6B = 2I_3$

13. If $P = \begin{bmatrix} \frac{\sqrt{3}}{2} & \frac{1}{2} \\ -\frac{1}{2} & \frac{\sqrt{3}}{2} \end{bmatrix}$, $A = \begin{bmatrix} 1 & 1 \\ 0 & 1 \end{bmatrix}$ and $Q = PAP^T$, then $P^T Q^{2015} P$ is ; **[Online April 9, 2016]**

(a) $\begin{bmatrix} 0 & 2015 \\ 0 & 0 \end{bmatrix}$ (b) $\begin{bmatrix} 2015 & 0 \\ 1 & 2015 \end{bmatrix}$

(c) $\begin{bmatrix} 1 & 2015 \\ 0 & 1 \end{bmatrix}$ (d) $\begin{bmatrix} 2015 & 1 \\ 0 & 2015 \end{bmatrix}$

14. If $A = \begin{bmatrix} 1 & 2 & 2 \\ 2 & 1 & -2 \\ a & 2 & b \end{bmatrix}$ is a matrix satisfying the equation $AA^T = 9I$, where I is 3×3 identity matrix, then the ordered pair (a, b) is equal to: **[2015]**

(a) (2, 1) (b) (–2, – 1)
(c) (2, – 1) (d) (–2, 1)

15. Let A and B be any two 3×3 matrices. If A is symmetric and B is skewsymmetric, then the matrix AB – BA is: **[Online April 19, 2014]**

(a) skewsymmetric
(b) symmetric
(c) neither symmetric nor skewsymmetric
(d) I or – I, where I is an identity matrix.

16. If $A = \begin{pmatrix} \alpha - 1 \\ 0 \\ 0 \end{pmatrix}$, $B = \begin{pmatrix} \alpha + 1 \\ 0 \\ 0 \end{pmatrix}$ be two matrices, then AB^T is a non-zero matrix for $|\alpha|$ not equal to **[Online May 7, 2012]**

(a) 2 (b) 0
(c) 1 (d) 3

17. Let A and B be two symmetric matrices of order 3. **[2011]**
Statement-1: $A(BA)$ and $(AB)A$ are symmetric matrices.
Statement-2: AB is symmetric matrix if matrix multiplication of A with B is commutative.

(a) Statement-1 is true, Statement-2 is true; Statement-2 is **not a** correct explanation for Statement-1.
(b) Statement-1 is true, Statement-2 is false.
(c) Statement-1 is false, Statement-2 is true.
(d) Statement-1 is true, Statement-2 is true; Statement-2 is a correct explanation for Statement-1.

Hints & Solutions

1. (a) Given that

$$A = \begin{bmatrix} 0 & -1 \\ 1 & 0 \end{bmatrix}$$

$$A^2 = \begin{bmatrix} -1 & 0 \\ 0 & -1 \end{bmatrix} \Rightarrow A^2 = -I$$

$$A^3 = \begin{bmatrix} 0 & 1 \\ -1 & 0 \end{bmatrix}$$

$$A^4 = \begin{bmatrix} 1 & 0 \\ 0 & 1 \end{bmatrix} = I$$

$A^2 + I = A^3 - A$

$-I + I = A^3 - A$

$A^3 \neq A$

2. (a) Let $A = \begin{bmatrix} 1 & 2 & x \\ 3 & -1 & 2 \end{bmatrix}$ and $B = \begin{bmatrix} y \\ x \\ 1 \end{bmatrix}$

$$AB = \begin{bmatrix} 1 & 2 & x \\ 3 & -1 & 2 \end{bmatrix} \begin{bmatrix} y \\ x \\ 1 \end{bmatrix}$$

$$\Rightarrow \begin{bmatrix} 6 \\ 8 \end{bmatrix} = \begin{bmatrix} y+2x+x \\ 3y-x+2 \end{bmatrix}$$

$$\Rightarrow \begin{bmatrix} 6 \\ 8 \end{bmatrix} = \begin{bmatrix} y+3x \\ 3y-x+2 \end{bmatrix}$$

$\Rightarrow y + 3x = 6$ and $3y - x = 6$

On solving, we get

$x = \dfrac{6}{5}$ and $y = \dfrac{12}{5}$

$\Rightarrow y = 2x$

3. (a) Given

$$[p \quad q \quad r] \begin{bmatrix} 3 & 4 & 1 \\ 3 & 2 & 3 \\ 2 & 0 & 2 \end{bmatrix} = [3 \quad 0 \quad 1]$$

$\Rightarrow [3p+3q+2r \quad 4p+2q \quad p+3q+2r] = [3 \quad 0 \quad 1]$

$\Rightarrow 3p+3q+2r = 3$ ...(i)

$4p+2q = 0 \Rightarrow q = -2p$ ...(ii)

$p+3q+2r = 1$ ...(iii)

On solving (i), (ii) and (iii), we get

$p = 1, q = -2, r = 3$

$\therefore\ 2p+q-r = 2(1)+(-2)-(3) = -3.$

4. (a) $A^2 + 4A - 5I = A \times A + 4A - 5I$

$$= \begin{bmatrix} 1 & 2 \\ 4 & -3 \end{bmatrix} \times \begin{bmatrix} 1 & 2 \\ 4 & -3 \end{bmatrix} + 4\begin{bmatrix} 1 & 2 \\ 4 & -3 \end{bmatrix} - 5\begin{bmatrix} 1 & 0 \\ 0 & 1 \end{bmatrix}$$

$$= \begin{bmatrix} 9 & -4 \\ -8 & 17 \end{bmatrix} + \begin{bmatrix} 4 & 8 \\ 16 & -12 \end{bmatrix} - \begin{bmatrix} 5 & 0 \\ 0 & 5 \end{bmatrix}$$

$$= \begin{bmatrix} 9+4-5 & -4+8-0 \\ -8+16-0 & 17-12-5 \end{bmatrix} = \begin{bmatrix} 8 & 4 \\ 8 & 0 \end{bmatrix}$$

$$= 4\begin{bmatrix} 2 & 1 \\ 2 & 0 \end{bmatrix}$$

5. (a) $A = \begin{bmatrix} 1 & 0 & 0 \\ 2 & 1 & 0 \\ -3 & 2 & 1 \end{bmatrix}$, $B = \begin{bmatrix} 1 & 0 & 0 \\ -2 & 1 & 0 \\ 7 & -2 & 1 \end{bmatrix}$

$$AB = \begin{bmatrix} 1 & 0 & 0 \\ 0 & 1 & 0 \\ 0 & 0 & 1 \end{bmatrix} = I$$

6. (d) $H^2 = \begin{bmatrix} \omega & 0 \\ 0 & \omega \end{bmatrix} \begin{bmatrix} \omega & 0 \\ 0 & \omega \end{bmatrix} = \begin{bmatrix} \omega^2 & 0 \\ 0 & \omega^2 \end{bmatrix}$

If $H^k = \begin{bmatrix} \omega^k & 0 \\ 0 & \omega \end{bmatrix}$ then $H^{k+1} = \begin{bmatrix} \omega^{k+1} & 0 \\ 0 & \omega^{k+1} \end{bmatrix}$

So by principle of mathematical induction,

$$H^{70} = \begin{bmatrix} \omega^{70} & 0 \\ 0 & \omega^{70} \end{bmatrix} = \begin{bmatrix} \omega^{69}\omega & 0 \\ 0 & \omega^{69}\omega \end{bmatrix} = \begin{bmatrix} \omega & 0 \\ 0 & \omega \end{bmatrix} = H$$

7. (c) $\begin{bmatrix} 1 & \ldots & \ldots \\ \ldots & 1 & \ldots \\ \ldots & \ldots & 1 \end{bmatrix}$ are 6 non-singular matrices because 6 blanks will be filled by 5 zeros and 1 one.

Similarly, $\begin{bmatrix} \ldots & \ldots & 1 \\ \ldots & 1 & \ldots \\ 1 & \ldots & \ldots \end{bmatrix}$ are 6 non-singular matrices.

So, required cases are more than 7, non-singular 3×3 matrices.

8. (d) $A=\begin{bmatrix}1&2\\3&4\end{bmatrix}$ $B=\begin{bmatrix}a&0\\0&b\end{bmatrix}$

$AB=\begin{bmatrix}a&2b\\3a&4b\end{bmatrix}$

$BA=\begin{bmatrix}a&0\\0&b\end{bmatrix}\begin{bmatrix}1&2\\3&4\end{bmatrix}=\begin{bmatrix}a&2a\\3b&4b\end{bmatrix}$

Hence, $AB=BA$ only when $a=b$

$\therefore$ There can be infinitely many B's for which $AB=BA$

9. (b) $A^2-B^2=(A-B)(A+B)$

$A^2-B^2=A^2+AB-BA-B^2$

$\Rightarrow AB=BA$

10. (a) We observe that

$A^2=\begin{bmatrix}1&0\\2&1\end{bmatrix}, A^3=\begin{bmatrix}1&0\\3&1\end{bmatrix}$ and we can prove by induction that $A^n=\begin{bmatrix}1&0\\n&1\end{bmatrix}$

Now $nA-(n-1)I=\begin{bmatrix}n&0\\n&n\end{bmatrix}-\begin{bmatrix}n-1&0\\0&n-1\end{bmatrix}$

$=\begin{bmatrix}1&0\\n&1\end{bmatrix}=A^n$

$\therefore nA-(n-1)I=A^n$

11. (c) $A^2=\begin{bmatrix}\alpha&\beta\\\beta&\alpha\end{bmatrix}=\begin{bmatrix}a&b\\b&a\end{bmatrix}\begin{bmatrix}a&b\\b&a\end{bmatrix}$

$=\begin{bmatrix}a^2+b^2&2ab\\2ab&a^2+b^2\end{bmatrix}$

$\alpha=a^2+b^2;\ \beta=2ab$

12. (b) $A^T+B^T=2B$

$\because\ [(A+B)^T=(2B^T)^T]$

$\Rightarrow\ B=\dfrac{A^T+B^T}{2}=A+\left(\dfrac{B^T+A^T}{2}\right)=2B^T$

$\Rightarrow\ 2A+A^T=3B^T$

$\Rightarrow\ A=\dfrac{3B^T-A^T}{2}$

Also, $3A+2B=I_3$ ...(i)

$\Rightarrow\ 3\left(\dfrac{3B^T-A^T}{2}\right)+2\left(\dfrac{A^T+B^T}{2}\right)=I_3$

$\Rightarrow\ 11B^T-A^T=2I_3$ ...(ii)

Add (i) and (ii)

$35B=7I_3$

$\Rightarrow\ B=\dfrac{I_3}{5}$

$\Rightarrow\ 11\dfrac{I_3}{5}-A=2I_3$

$\Rightarrow\ 11\dfrac{I_3}{5}-2I_3=A$

$\Rightarrow\ A=\dfrac{I_3}{5}$

$\because\ 5A=5B=I_3$

$\Rightarrow\ 10A+5B=3I_3$

13. (c) $P=\begin{bmatrix}\frac{\sqrt{3}}{2}&\frac{1}{2}\\-\frac{1}{2}&\frac{\sqrt{3}}{2}\end{bmatrix}$ $P^T=\begin{bmatrix}\frac{\sqrt{3}}{2}&\frac{-1}{2}\\\frac{1}{2}&\frac{\sqrt{3}}{2}\end{bmatrix}$

$PP^T=P^TP=I$

$Q^{2015}=(PAP^T)(PAP^T)$ ——— (2015 terms)

$=PA^{2015}P^T$

$P^TQ^{2015}P=A^{2015}$

$A^2=\begin{bmatrix}1&1\\0&1\end{bmatrix}\begin{bmatrix}1&1\\0&1\end{bmatrix}=\begin{bmatrix}1&2\\0&1\end{bmatrix}$

$A^3=\begin{bmatrix}1&2\\0&1\end{bmatrix}\begin{bmatrix}1&1\\0&1\end{bmatrix}=\begin{bmatrix}1&3\\0&1\end{bmatrix}$

$\therefore\ A^{2015}=\begin{bmatrix}1&2015\\0&1\end{bmatrix}$

14. (b) $\begin{bmatrix}1&2&2\\2&1&-2\\a&2&b\end{bmatrix}\begin{bmatrix}1&2&a\\2&1&2\\2&-2&b\end{bmatrix}=\begin{bmatrix}9&0&0\\0&9&0\\0&0&9\end{bmatrix}$

$\Rightarrow\begin{bmatrix}1+4+4&2+2-4&a+4+2b\\2+2-4&4+1+4&2a+2-2b\\a+4+2b&2a+2-2b&a^2+4+b^2\end{bmatrix}=\begin{bmatrix}9&0&0\\0&9&0\\0&0&9\end{bmatrix}$

$\Rightarrow a+4+2b=0\Rightarrow a+2b=-4$ ...(i)

$2a+2-2b=0\Rightarrow 2a-2b=-2$

$\Rightarrow a-b=-1$ ...(ii)

On solving (i) and (ii) we get

$-1+b+2b=-4$ ...(i)

$$-1+3b = -4$$
$$3b = -3$$
$$b = -1$$

and $a = -2$

$(a, b) = (-2, -1)$

15. **(b)** Let A be symmetric matrix and B be skew symmetric matrix.

$\therefore A^T = A$ and $B^T = -B$

Consider

$(AB - BA)^T = (AB)^T - (BA)^T$

$= B^T A^T - A^T B^T$

$= (-B)(A) - (A)(-B)$

$= -BA + AB = AB - BA$

This shows AB – BA is symmetric matrix.

16. **(c)** Let $A = \begin{pmatrix} \alpha-1 \\ 0 \\ 0 \end{pmatrix}$, $B = \begin{pmatrix} \alpha+1 \\ 0 \\ 0 \end{pmatrix}$ be two matrices.

$$AB^T = \begin{pmatrix} \alpha-1 \\ 0 \\ 0 \end{pmatrix} \begin{pmatrix} \alpha+1 & 0 & 0 \end{pmatrix}$$

$$= \begin{pmatrix} \alpha^2-1 & 0 & 0 \\ 0 & 0 & 0 \\ 0 & 0 & 0 \end{pmatrix}$$

Thus, AB^T is non-zero matrix for $|\alpha| \neq 1$

17. **(a)** $\therefore A' = A$

$B' = B$

Now $(A(BA))' = (BA)'A'$

$= (A'B')A' = (AB)A = A(BA)$

Similarly $((AB)A)' = (AB)A$

So, A(BA) and (AB)A are symmetric matrices.

Again $(AB)' = B'A' = BA$

Now if BA = AB, then AB is symmetric matrix.

Determinants

TOPIC-1 : Minor & Co-factor of an Element of a Determinant, Value of a Determinant, Property of Determinant of Matrices, Singular & Non-Singular Matrices, Multiplication of two Determinants

1. If S = $\left\{x \in [0, 2\pi] : \begin{vmatrix} 0 & \cos x & -\sin x \\ \sin x & 0 & \cos x \\ \cos x & \sin x & 0 \end{vmatrix} = 0\right\}$, then $\sum_{x \in S} \tan\left(\frac{\pi}{3} + x\right)$ is equal to **[Online April 8, 2017]**

(a) $4 + 2\sqrt{3}$ (b) $-2 + \sqrt{3}$
(c) $-2 - \sqrt{3}$ (d) $-4 - 2\sqrt{3}$

2. If A = $\begin{bmatrix} -4 & -1 \\ 3 & 1 \end{bmatrix}$, then the determinant of the matrix $(A^{2016} - 2A^{2015} - A^{2014})$ is : **[Online April 10, 2016]**

(a) –175 (b) 2014
(c) 2016 (d) –25

3. if $\begin{vmatrix} x^2 + x & x+1 & x-2 \\ 2x^2 + 3x - 1 & 3x & 3x-3 \\ x^2 + 2x + 3 & 2x-1 & 2x-1 \end{vmatrix} = ax - 12$, then '$a$' is equal to : **[Online April 11, 2015]**

(a) 24 (b) –12
(c) –24 (d) 12

4. The least value of the product xyz for which the determinant $\begin{vmatrix} x & 1 & 1 \\ 1 & y & 1 \\ 1 & 1 & z \end{vmatrix}$ is non-negative, is : **[Online April 10, 2015]**

(a) $-2\sqrt{2}$ (b) –1
(c) $-16\sqrt{2}$ (d) –8

5. If $f(\theta) = \begin{vmatrix} 1 & \cos\theta & 1 \\ -\sin\theta & 1 & -\cos\theta \\ -1 & \sin\theta & 1 \end{vmatrix}$ and A and B are respectively the maximum and the minimum values of $f(\theta)$, then (A, B) is equal to: **[Online April 12, 2014]**

(a) $(3, -1)$ (b) $\left(4, 2 - \sqrt{2}\right)$
(c) $\left(2 + \sqrt{2}, 2 - \sqrt{2}\right)$ (d) $\left(2 + \sqrt{2}, -1\right)$

6. If B is a 3 × 3 matrix such that $B^2 = 0$, then det. $[(I + B)^{50} - 50B]$ is equal to: **[Online April 9, 2014]**

(a) 1 (b) 2
(c) 3 (d) 50

7. Let $S = \left\{\begin{pmatrix} a_{11} & a_{12} \\ a_{21} & a_{22} \end{pmatrix} : a_{ij} \in \{0, 1, 2\}, a_{11} = a_{22}\right\}$

Then the number of non-singular matrices in the set S is : **[Online April 25, 2013]**

(a) 27 (b) 24
(c) 10 (d) 20

8. Let A, other than I or – I, be a 2 × 2 real matrix such that $A^2 = I$, I being the unit matrix. Let Tr (A) be the sum of diagonal elements of A. **[Online April 23, 2013]**

Statement-1: Tr (A) = 0

Statement-2: det (A) = – 1

(a) Statement-1 is true; Statement-2 is false.
(b) Statement-1 is true; Statement-2 is true; Statement-2 is **not** a correct explanation for Statement-1.
(c) Statement-1 is true; Statement-2 is true; Statement-2 is a correct explanation for Statement-1.
(d) Statement-1 is false; Statement-2 is true.

9. **Statement - 1:** **[2011RS]**

Determinant of a skew-symmetric matrix of order 3 is zero.

Statement - 2 :

For any matrix A, $\det(A)^T = \det(A)$ and $\det(-A) = -\det(A)$. Where det (B) denotes the determinant of matrix B. Then :

(a) Both statements are true
(b) Both statements are false
(c) Statement-1 is false and statement-2 is true
(d) Statement-1 is true and statement-2 is false

10. Let A be a 2 × 2 matrix with non-zero entries and let $A^2 = I$, where I is 2 × 2 identity matrix. Define

$\text{Tr}(A)$ = sum of diagonal elements of A and

$|A|$ = determinant of matrix A.

Statement - 1 : $\text{Tr}(A) = 0$.

Statement -2 : $|A|=1$. **[2010]**

(a) Statement -1 is true, Statement -2 is true ; Statement -2 is **not** a correct explanation for Statement -1.
(b) Statement -1 is true, Statement -2 is false.
(c) Statement -1 is false, Statement -2 is true .
(d) Statement - 1 is true, Statement 2 is true ; Statement -2 is a correct explanation for Statement -1.

11. Let A be a 2×2 matrix with real entries. Let I be the 2×2 identity matrix. Denote by tr(A), the sum of diagonal entries of a. Assume that $A^2 = I$. **[2008]**

Statement-1 : If $A \neq I$ and $A \neq -I$, then det $(A) = -1$

Statement-2 : If $A \neq I$ and $A \neq -I$, then tr $(A) \neq 0$.

(a) Statement -1 is false, Statement-2 is true
(b) Statement -1 is true, Statement-2 is true; Statement -2 is a correct explanation for Statement-1
(c) Statement -1 is true, Statement-2 is true; Statement -2 is not a correct explanation for Statement-1
(d) Statement -1 is true, Statement-2 is false

12. Let $A = \begin{vmatrix} 5 & 5\alpha & \alpha \\ 0 & \alpha & 5\alpha \\ 0 & 0 & 5 \end{vmatrix}$. If $\left|A^2\right| = 25$, then $|\alpha|$ equals **[2007]**

(a) 1/5 (b) 5
(c) 5^2 (d) 1

13. If $1, \omega, \omega^2$ are the cube roots of unity, then

$$\Delta = \begin{vmatrix} 1 & \omega^n & \omega^{2n} \\ \omega^n & \omega^{2n} & 1 \\ \omega^{2n} & 1 & \omega^n \end{vmatrix}$$ is equal to **[2003]**

(a) ω^2 (b) 0
(c) 1 (d) ω

TOPIC-2 : Properties of Determinants, Area of a Triangle

14. Let k be an integer such that triangle with vertices (k, –3k), (5, k) and (–k, 2) has area 28 sq. units. Then the orthocentre of this triangle is at the point : **[2017]**

(a) $\left(2, \frac{1}{2}\right)$ (b) $\left(2, -\frac{1}{2}\right)$
(c) $\left(1, \frac{3}{4}\right)$ (d) $\left(1, -\frac{3}{4}\right)$

15. Let ω be a complex number such that $2\omega + 1 = z$ where $z = \sqrt{-3}$. If $\begin{vmatrix} 1 & 1 & 1 \\ 1 & -\omega^2 - 1 & \omega^2 \\ 1 & \omega^2 & \omega^7 \end{vmatrix} = 3k$, then k is equal to : **[2017]**

(a) 1 (b) –z
(c) z (d) –1

16. The number of distinct real roots of the equaiton,

$$\begin{vmatrix} \cos x & \sin x & \sin x \\ \sin x & \cos x & \sin x \\ \sin x & \sin x & \cos x \end{vmatrix} = 0 \text{ in the interval } \left[-\frac{\pi}{4}, \frac{\pi}{4}\right] \text{ is :}$$

[Online April 9, 2016]

(a) 1 (b) 4
(c) 2 (d) 3

17. If $\alpha, \beta \neq 0$, and $f(n) = \alpha^n + \beta^n$ and

$$\begin{vmatrix} 3 & 1+f(1) & 1+f(2) \\ 1+f(1) & 1+f(2) & 1+f(3) \\ 1+f(2) & 1+f(3) & 1+f(4) \end{vmatrix} = K(1-\alpha)^2(1-\beta)^2(\alpha-\beta)^2,$$

then K is equal to: **[2014]**

(a) 1 (b) –1
(c) $\alpha\beta$ (d) $\frac{1}{\alpha\beta}$

18. If $\Delta_r = \begin{vmatrix} r & 2r-1 & 3r-2 \\ \frac{n}{2} & n-1 & a \\ \frac{1}{2}n(n-1) & (n-1)^2 & \frac{1}{2}(n-1)(3n-4) \end{vmatrix}$

then the value of $\sum_{r=1}^{n-1} \Delta_r$

[Online April 19, 2014]

(a) depends only on a
(b) depends only on n
(c) depends both on a and n
(d) is independent of both a and n

19. If

$$\begin{vmatrix} a^2 & b^2 & c^2 \\ (a+\lambda)^2 & (b+\lambda)^2 & (c+\lambda)^2 \\ (a-\lambda)^2 & (b-\lambda)^2 & (c-\lambda)^2 \end{vmatrix} = k\lambda \begin{vmatrix} a^2 & b^2 & c^2 \\ a & b & c \\ 1 & 1 & 1 \end{vmatrix}, \lambda \neq 0$$

then k is equal to: **[Online April 12, 2014]**

(a) $4\lambda abc$ (b) $-4\lambda abc$
(c) $4\lambda^2$ (d) $-4\lambda^2$

20. If a, b, c are sides of a scalene triangle, then the value of

$$\begin{vmatrix} a & b & c \\ b & c & a \\ c & a & b \end{vmatrix} \text{ is :}$$ **[Online April 9, 2013]**

(a) non - negative (b) negative
(c) positive (d) non-positive

21. If a, b, c, are non zero complex numbers satisfying $a^2 + b^2 + c^2 = 0$ and

$$\begin{vmatrix} b^2+c^2 & ab & ac \\ ab & c^2+a^2 & bc \\ ac & bc & a^2+b^2 \end{vmatrix} = ka^2b^2c^2, \text{ then } k \text{ is equal to}$$

[Online May 19, 2012]

(a) 1 (b) 3
(c) 4 (d) 2

22. If $\begin{vmatrix} -2a & a+b & a+c \\ b+a & -2b & b+c \\ c+a & b+c & -2c \end{vmatrix} = \alpha(a+b)(b+c)(c+a) \neq 0$

then α is equal to **[Online May 12, 2012]**

(a) $a+b+c$ (b) abc
(c) 4 (d) 1

23. The area of the triangle whose vertices are complex numbers $z, iz, z + iz$ in the Argand diagram is **[Online May 12, 2012]**

(a) $2|z|^2$ (b) $1/2|z|^2$
(c) $4|z|^2$ (d) $|z|^2$

24. The area of triangle formed by the lines joining the vertex of the parabola, $x^2 = 8y$, to the extremities of its latus rectum is **[Online May 12, 2012]**

(a) 2 (b) 8
(c) 1 (d) 4

25. Let a, b, c be such that $b(a + c) \neq 0$ if **[2009]**

$$\begin{vmatrix} a & a+1 & a-1 \\ -b & b+1 & b-1 \\ c & c-1 & c+1 \end{vmatrix} + \begin{vmatrix} a+1 & b+1 & c-1 \\ a-1 & b-1 & c+1 \\ (-1)^{n+2}a & (-1)^{n+1}b & (-1)^n c \end{vmatrix} = 0,$$

then the value of n is :

(a) any even integer (b) any odd integer
(c) any integer (d) zero

26. If $D = \begin{vmatrix} 1 & 1 & 1 \\ 1 & 1+x & 1 \\ 1 & 1 & 1+y \end{vmatrix}$ for $x \neq 0, y \neq 0$, then D is

(a) divisible by x but not y **[2007]**
(b) divisible by y but not x
(c) divisible by neither x nor y
(d) divisible by both x and y

27. If $a_1, a_2, a_3, \ldots\ldots\ldots\ldots, a_n, \ldots\ldots$ are in G.P., then the determinant

$$\Delta = \begin{vmatrix} \log a_n & \log a_{n+1} & \log a_{n+2} \\ \log a_{n+3} & \log a_{n+4} & \log a_{n+5} \\ \log a_{n+6} & \log a_{n+7} & \log a_{n+8} \end{vmatrix}$$

is equal to **[2005]**

(a) 1 (b) 0
(c) 4 (d) 2

28. If $a^2 + b^2 + c^2 = -2$ and **[2005]**

$$f(x) = \begin{vmatrix} 1+a^2x & (1+b^2)x & (1+c^2)x \\ (1+a^2)x & 1+b^2x & (1+c^2)x \\ (1+a^2)x & (1+b^2)x & 1+c^2x \end{vmatrix},$$

then f(x) is a polynomial of degree

(a) 1 (b) 0
(c) 3 (d) 2

29. If $a_1, a_2, a_3, \ldots\ldots, a_n, \ldots.$ are in G.P., then the value of the determinant **[2004]**

$$\begin{vmatrix} \log a_n & \log a_{n+1} & \log a_{n+2} \\ \log a_{n+3} & \log a_{n+4} & \log a_{n+5} \\ \log a_{n+6} & \log a_{n+7} & \log a_{n+8} \end{vmatrix}, \text{ is}$$

(a) –2 (b) 1
(c) 2 (d) 0

30. If $a > 0$ and discriminant of $ax^2+2bx+c$ is –ve, then

$$\begin{vmatrix} a & b & ax+b \\ b & c & bx+c \\ ax+b & bx+c & 0 \end{vmatrix} \text{ is equal to}$$ **[2002]**

(a) +ve (b) $(ac-b^2)(ax^2+2bx+c)$
(c) –ve (d) 0

31. l, m, n are the pth, q^{th} and r^{th} term of a G. P. all positive,

then $\begin{vmatrix} \log l & p & 1 \\ \log m & q & 1 \\ \log n & r & 1 \end{vmatrix}$ equals **[2002]**

(a) –1 (b) 2
(c) 1 (d) 0

TOPIC-3 : Adjoint of a Matrix, Inverse of a Matrix, Some Special Cases of Matrix, Rank of a Matrix

32. If $A = \begin{bmatrix} 2 & -3 \\ -4 & 1 \end{bmatrix}$, then adj $(3A^2 + 12A)$ is equal to : **[2017]**

(a) $\begin{bmatrix} 72 & -63 \\ -84 & 51 \end{bmatrix}$ (b) $\begin{bmatrix} 72 & -84 \\ -63 & 51 \end{bmatrix}$

(c) $\begin{bmatrix} 51 & 63 \\ 84 & 72 \end{bmatrix}$ (d) $\begin{bmatrix} 51 & 84 \\ 63 & 72 \end{bmatrix}$

33. Let A be any 3 × 3 invertible matrix. Then which one of the following is not always true ? **[Online April 8, 2017]**

(a) adj (A) $= |A| \cdot A^{-1}$
(b) adj (adj(A)) $= |A| . A$
(c) adj (adj(A)) $= |A|^2 . (\text{adj}(A))^{-1}$
(d) adj (adj(A)) $= |A| . (\text{adj}(A))^{-1}$

34. If $A = \begin{bmatrix} 5a & -b \\ 3 & 2 \end{bmatrix}$ and A adj $A = A A^T$, then 5a + b is equal to : **[2016]**

(a) 4 (b) 13
(c) –1 (d) 5

35. Let A be a 3 × 3 matrix such that $A^2 - 5A + 7I = 0$.

Statement–I : $A^{-1} = \frac{1}{7}(5I - A)$.

Statement II : the polynomial $A^3 - 2A^2 - 3A + I$ can be reduced to 5 (A – 4I). **[Online April 10, 2016]**

Then :

(a) Both the statements are true.
(b) Both the statements are false.
(c) Statement–I is true, but Statement-II is false.
(d) Statement I is false, but Statement-II is true.

36. If A is a 3 × 3 matrix such that |5.adjA| = 5, then |A| is equal to : **[Online April 11, 2015]**

(a) $\pm\frac{1}{5}$ (b) $\pm\frac{1}{25}$
(c) ±1 (d) ±5

37. If A is an 3 × 3 non-singular matrix such that $AA' = A'A$ and $B = A^{-1}A'$, then BB' equals: **[2014]**

(a) B^{-1} (b) $(B^{-1})'$
(c) $I + B$ (d) I

38. Let A be a 3 × 3 matrix such that

$$A\begin{bmatrix} 1 & 2 & 3 \\ 0 & 2 & 3 \\ 0 & 1 & 1 \end{bmatrix} = \begin{bmatrix} 0 & 0 & 1 \\ 1 & 0 & 0 \\ 0 & 1 & 0 \end{bmatrix}$$

Then A^{-1} is: **[Online April 11, 2014]**

(a) $\begin{bmatrix} 3 & 1 & 2 \\ 3 & 0 & 2 \\ 1 & 0 & 1 \end{bmatrix}$ (b) $\begin{bmatrix} 3 & 2 & 1 \\ 3 & 2 & 0 \\ 1 & 1 & 0 \end{bmatrix}$

(c) $\begin{bmatrix} 0 & 1 & 3 \\ 0 & 2 & 3 \\ 1 & 1 & 1 \end{bmatrix}$ (d) $\begin{bmatrix} 1 & 2 & 3 \\ 0 & 1 & 1 \\ 0 & 2 & 3 \end{bmatrix}$

39. If $P = \begin{bmatrix} 1 & \alpha & 3 \\ 1 & 3 & 3 \\ 2 & 4 & 4 \end{bmatrix}$ is the adjoint of a 3 × 3 matrix A and |A| = 4, then α is equal to : **[2013]**

(a) 4 (b) 11
(c) 5 (d) 0

40. Let P and Q be 3 × 3 matrices $P \neq Q$. If $P^3 = Q^3$ and $P^2Q = Q^2P$ then determinant of $(P^2 + Q^2)$ is equal to : **[2012]**

(a) –2 (b) 1
(c) 0 (d) –1

41. Let $A = \begin{pmatrix} 1 & 0 & 0 \\ 2 & 1 & 0 \\ 3 & 2 & 1 \end{pmatrix}$. If u_1 and u_2 are column matrices such that $Au_1 = \begin{pmatrix} 1 \\ 0 \\ 0 \end{pmatrix}$ and $Au_2 = \begin{pmatrix} 0 \\ 1 \\ 0 \end{pmatrix}$, then $u_1 + u_2$ is equal to : **[2012]**

(a) $\begin{pmatrix} -1 \\ 1 \\ 0 \end{pmatrix}$ (b) $\begin{pmatrix} -1 \\ 1 \\ -1 \end{pmatrix}$

(c) $\begin{pmatrix} -1 \\ -1 \\ 0 \end{pmatrix}$ (d) $\begin{pmatrix} 1 \\ -1 \\ -1 \end{pmatrix}$

42. If A^T denotes the transpose of the matrix $A = \begin{bmatrix} 0 & 0 & a \\ 0 & b & c \\ d & e & f \end{bmatrix}$, where a, b, c, d, e and f are integers such that $abd \neq 0$, then the number of such matrices for which $A^{-1} = A^T$ is **[Online May 19, 2012]**

(a) 2(3!) (b) 3(2!)
(c) 2^3 (d) 3^2

43. Let A and B be real matrices of the form $\begin{bmatrix} \alpha & 0 \\ 0 & \beta \end{bmatrix}$ and $\begin{bmatrix} 0 & \gamma \\ \delta & 0 \end{bmatrix}$, respectively. **[Online May 12, 2012]**

Statement 1: $AB - BA$ is always an invertible matrix.

Statement 2: $AB - BA$ is never an identity matrix.

(a) Statement 1 is true, Statement 2 is false.
(b) Statement 1 is false, Statement 2 is true.
(c) Statement 1 is true, Statement 2 is true; Statement 2 is a correct explanation of Statement 1.
(d) Statement 1 is true, Statement 2 is true, Statement 2 is not a correct explanation of Statement 1.

44. Consider the following relation R on the set of real square matrices of order 3. **[2011RS]**

$R = \{(A, B) | A = P^{-1}BP$ for some invertible matrix $P\}$

Statement-1 : R is equivalence relation.

Statement-2 : For any two invertible 3 × 3 matrices M and N, $(MN)^{-1} = N^{-1}M^{-1}$.

(a) Statement-1 is true, statement-2 is true and statement-2 is a correct explanation for statement-1.
(b) Statement-1 is true, statement-2 is true; statement-2 is not a correct explanation for statement-1.
(c) Statement-1 is true, stement-2 is false.
(d) Statement-1 is false, statement-2 is true.

45. Let A be a 2×2 matrix

Statement-1 : adj (adj A) = A

Statement-2 : |adj A| = |A| **[2009]**

(a) Statement-1 is true, Statement-2 is true. Statement-2 is not a correct explanation for Statement-1.
(b) Statement-1 is true, Statement-2 is false.
(c) Statement-1 is false, Statement-2 is true.
(d) Statement-1 is true, Statement-2 is true. Statement-2 is a correct explanation for Statement-1.

46. Let A be a square matrix all of whose entries are integers. Then which one of the following is true? **[2008]**

(a) If det $A = \pm 1$, then A^{-1} exists but all its entries are not necessarily integers
(b) If det $A \neq \pm 1$, then A^{-1} exists and all its entries are non integers
(c) If det $A = \pm 1$, then A^{-1} exists but all its entries are integers
(d) If det $A = \pm 1$, then A^{-1} need not exists

47. If $A^2 - A + I = 0$, then the inverse of A is **[2005]**

(a) $A+I$ (b) A
(c) $A-I$ (d) $I-A$

48. Let $A = \begin{pmatrix} 1 & -1 & 1 \\ 2 & 1 & -3 \\ 1 & 1 & 1 \end{pmatrix}$. and $B = \begin{pmatrix} 4 & 2 & 2 \\ -5 & 0 & \alpha \\ 1 & -2 & 3 \end{pmatrix}$. If B is the inverse of matrix A, then α is **[2004]**

(a) 5 (b) –1
(c) 2 (d) –2

49. Let $A = \begin{pmatrix} 0 & 0 & -1 \\ 0 & -1 & 0 \\ -1 & 0 & 0 \end{pmatrix}$. The only correct statement about the matrix A is **[2004]**

(a) $A^2 = I$
(b) $A = (-1)I$, where I is a unit matrix
(c) A^{-1} does not exist
(d) A is a zero matrix

TOPIC-4 : Solution of System of Linear Equations

50. If S is the set of distinct values of 'b' for which the following system of linear equations **[2017]**

$x + y + z = 1$
$x + ay + z = 1$
$ax + by + z = 0$

has no solution, then S is :

(a) a singleton
(b) an empty set
(c) an infinite set
(d) a finite set containing two or more elements

51. The number of real values of λ for which the system of linear equations

$2x + 4y - \lambda z = 0$
$4x + \lambda y + 2z = 0$
$\lambda x + 2y + 2z = 0$

has infinitely many solutions, is : **[Online April 8, 2017]**

(a) 0 (b) 1
(c) 2 (d) 3

52. The system of linear equations

$x + \lambda y - z = 0$
$\lambda x - y - z = 0$
$x + y - \lambda z = 0$

has a non-trivial solution for: **[2016]**

(a) exactly two values of λ.
(b) exactly three values of λ.
(c) infinitely many values of λ.
(d) exactly one value of λ.

53. The set of all values of λ for which the system of linear equations : **[2015]**

$2x_1 - 2x_2 + x_3 = \lambda x_1$
$2x_1 - 3x_2 + 2x_3 = \lambda x_2$
$-x_1 + 2x_2 = \lambda x_3$

has a non-trivial solution,

(a) contains two elements.
(b) contains more than two elements
(c) is an empty set.
(d) is a singleton

54. If a, b, c are non-zero real numbers and if the system of equations **[Online April 9, 2014]**

$(a-1)x = y + z,$
$(b-1)y = z + x,$
$(c-1)z = x + y,$

has a non-trivial solution, then ab + bc + ca equals:

(a) a + b + c (b) abc
(c) 1 (d) – 1

55. The number of values of k, for which the system of equations :

$(k+1)x + 8y = 4k$
$kx + (k+3)y = 3k - 1$

has no solution, is **[2013]**

(a) infinite (b) 1
(c) 2 (d) 3

56. Consider the system of equations :

$x + ay = 0$, $y + az = 0$ and $z + ax = 0$. Then the set of all real values of 'a' for which the system has a unique solution is: **[Online April 25, 2013]**

(a) $R - \{1\}$ (b) $R - \{-1\}$
(c) $\{1, -1\}$ (d) $\{1, 0, -1\}$

57. Statement-1: The system of linear equations

$x + (\sin\alpha)y + (\cos\alpha)z = 0$
$x + (\cos\alpha)y + (\sin\alpha)z = 0$
$x - (\sin\alpha)y - (\cos\alpha)z = 0$

has a non-trivial solution for only one value of α lying in the interval $\left(0, \frac{\pi}{2}\right)$.

Statement-2: The equation in α

$$\begin{vmatrix} \cos\alpha & \sin\alpha & \cos\alpha \\ \sin\alpha & \cos\alpha & \sin\alpha \\ \cos\alpha & -\sin\alpha & -\cos\alpha \end{vmatrix} = 0$$

has only one solution lying in the interval $\left(0, \frac{\pi}{2}\right)$.

[Online April 23, 2013]

(a) Statement-1 is true, Statement-2 is true, Statement-2 is **not** correct explantion for Statement-1.
(b) Statement-1 is true, Statement-2 is true, Statement-2 is a correct explantion for Statement-1.
(c) Statement-1 is true, Statement-2 is false.
(d) Statememt-1 is false, Statement-2 is true.

58. If the system of linear equations :

$$x_1 + 2x_2 + 3x_3 = 6$$
$$x_1 + 3x_2 + 5x_3 = 9$$
$$2x_1 + 5x_2 + ax_3 = b$$

is consistent and has infinite number of solutions, then : **[Online April 22, 2013]**

(a) $a = 8$, b can be any real number
(b) $b = 15$, a can be any real number
(c) $a \in R - \{8\}$ and $b \in R - \{15\}$
(d) $a = 8, b = 15$

59. Statement 1: If the system of equations $x + ky + 3z = 0$, $3x + ky - 2z = 0$, $2x + 3y - 4z = 0$ has a non-trivial solution, then the value of k is $\frac{31}{2}$.

Statement 2: A system of three homogeneous equations in three variables has a non trivial solution if the determinant of the coefficient matrix is zero. **[Online May 26, 2012]**

(a) Statement 1 is false, Statement 2 is true.
(b) Statement 1 is true, Statement 2 is true, Statement 2 is a correct explanation for Statement 1.
(c) Statement 1 is true, Statement 2 is true, , Statement 2 is not a correct explanation for Statement 1.
(d) Statement 1 is true, Statement 2 is false.

60. If the system of equations **[Online May 7, 2012]**

$$x + y + z = 6$$
$$x + 2y + 3z = 10$$
$$x + 2y + \lambda z = 0$$

has a unique solution, then λ is not equal to

(a) 1 (b) 0
(c) 2 (d) 3

61. If the trivial solution is the only solution of the system of equations **[2011RS]**

$$x - ky + z = 0$$
$$kx + 3y - kz = 0$$
$$3x + y - z = 0$$

then the set of all values of k is :

(a) $R - \{2, -3\}$ (b) $R - \{2\}$
(c) $R - \{-3\}$ (d) $\{2, -3\}$

62. The number of values of k for which the linear equations $4x + ky + 2z = 0$, $kx + 4y + z = 0$ and $2x + 2y + z = 0$ possess a non-zero solution is **[2011]**

(a) 2 (b) 1
(c) zero (d) 3

63. Consider the system of linear equations; **[2010]**

$$x_1 + 2x_2 + x_3 = 3$$
$$2x_1 + 3x_2 + x_3 = 3$$
$$3x_1 + 5x_2 + 2x_3 = 1$$

The system has

(a) exactly 3 solutions
(b) a unique solution
(c) no solution
(d) infinite number of solutions

64. Let a, b, c be any real numbers. Suppose that there are real numbers x, y, z not all zero such that $x = cy + bz$, $y = az + cx$, and $z = bx + ay$. Then $a^2 + b^2 + c^2 + 2abc$ is equal to **[2008]**

(a) 2 (b) –1
(c) 0 (d) 1

65. The system of equations

$$\alpha x + y + z = \alpha - 1$$
$$x + \alpha y + z = \alpha - 1$$
$$x + y + \alpha z = \alpha - 1$$

has infinite solutions, if α is **[2005]**

(a) – 2 (b) either – 2 or 1
(c) not – 2 (d) 1

66. If the system of linear equations **[2003]**

$x + 2ay + az = 0$; $x + 3by + bz = 0$;

$x + 4cy + cz = 0$ has a non - zero solution, then a, b, c.

(a) satisfy $a + 2b + 3c = 0$ (b) are in A.P
(c) are in G.P (d) are in H.P.

Hints & Solutions

1. (c) Since the given determinant is equal to zero.
$\Rightarrow$ $0\,(0-\cos x \sin x)-\cos x(0-\cos^2 x)-\sin x\,(\sin^2 x-0)=0$
$\Rightarrow$ $\cos^3 x-\sin^3 x=0$
$\Rightarrow$ $\tan^3=1 \Rightarrow \tan x=1$

$$\therefore \sum_{x\in s}\tan\left(\frac{\pi}{3}+x\right)=\sum_{x\in s}\frac{\tan\pi/3+\tan x}{1-\tan\pi/3.\tan x}$$

$$\sum_{x\in s}\frac{\sqrt{3}+1}{1-\sqrt{3}}$$

$$\sum_{x\in s}\frac{\sqrt{3}+1}{1-\sqrt{3}}\times\frac{1+\sqrt{3}}{1+\sqrt{3}}\Rightarrow\sum_{x\in s}\frac{1+3+2\sqrt{3}}{-2}$$

$$=-2-\sqrt{3}$$

2. (d) $A=\begin{bmatrix}-4 & -1\\ 3 & 1\end{bmatrix}\Rightarrow A^2=\begin{bmatrix}-4 & -1\\ 3 & 1\end{bmatrix}\begin{bmatrix}-4 & -1\\ 3 & 1\end{bmatrix}$

$=\begin{bmatrix}13 & 3\\ -9 & -2\end{bmatrix}$ and $|A|=1$.

Now, $A^{2016}-2A^{2015}-A^{2014}=A^{2014}(A^2-2A-I)$

$\Rightarrow$ $|A^{2016}-2A^{2015}-A^{2014}|=|A^{2014}||A^2-2A-I|$

$=|A|^{2014}\begin{vmatrix}20 & 5\\ -15 & -5\end{vmatrix}=-25$

3. (a) Let $\begin{vmatrix}x^2+x & x+1 & x-2\\ 2x^2+3x-1 & 3x & 3x-3\\ x^2+2x+3 & 2x-1 & 2x-1\end{vmatrix}=ax-12$

Put $x=-1$, we get

$\begin{vmatrix}0 & 0 & -3\\ -2 & -3 & 0\\ 2 & -3 & -3\end{vmatrix}=-a-12$

$\Rightarrow -3\,(6+6)=-a-12\Rightarrow -36+12=a$
$\Rightarrow a=24$

4. (d) $\begin{vmatrix}x & 1 & 1\\ 1 & y & 1\\ 1 & 1 & z\end{vmatrix}\geq 0$

$xyz-x-y-z+2\geq 0$

$xyz+2\geq x+y+z\geq 3\,(xyz)^{1/3}$
$xyz+2-3(xyz)^{1/3}\geq 0$
$ut(xyz)=t^3$
$t^3-3t+2\geq 0$
$(t+2)\,(t-1)^2\geq 0$
$[t=-2]\;t^3=-8$

5. (c) Let $f(\theta)=\begin{vmatrix}1 & \cos\theta & 1\\ -\sin\theta & 1 & -\cos\theta\\ -1 & \sin\theta & 1\end{vmatrix}$

$=(1+\sin\theta\cos\theta)-\cos\theta(-\sin\theta-\cos\theta)+1(-\sin^2\theta+1)$

$=1+\sin\theta\cos\theta+\sin\theta\cos\theta+\cos^2\theta-\sin^2\theta+1$

$=2+2\sin\theta\cos\theta+\cos 2\theta$

$=2+\sin 2\theta+\cos 2\theta$ ...(1)

Now, maximum value of (1)

is $2+\sqrt{1^2+1^2}=2+\sqrt{2}$

and minimum value of (1) is

$2-\sqrt{1^2+1^2}=2-\sqrt{2}$.

6. (a) $\det[(I+B)^{50}-50B]$
$=\det[{}^{50}C_0\,I+{}^{50}C_1\,B+{}^{50}C_2\,B^2+{}^{50}C_3\,B^3+\ldots+{}^{50}C_{50}\,B^{50}\,B^{50}-50B]$
{All terms having B^n, $2\leq n\leq 50$ will be zero because given that $B^2=0$}
$=\det[I+50B-50B]=\det[I]=1$

7. (d) The matrices in the form

$\begin{bmatrix}a_{11} & a_{12}\\ a_{21} & a_{22}\end{bmatrix}$, $a_{ij}\in\{0,1,2\}$, $a_{11}=a_{12}$ are

$\begin{bmatrix}0 & 0/1/2\\ 0/1/2 & 0\end{bmatrix},\begin{bmatrix}1 & 0/1/2\\ 0/1/2 & 1\end{bmatrix},\begin{bmatrix}2 & 0/1/2\\ 0/1/2 & 2\end{bmatrix}$

At any place, 0/1/2 means 0, 1 or 2 will be the element at that place.
Hence there are total $27=3\times3+3\times3+3\times3$) matrices of the above form. Out of which the matrices which are singular are

$\begin{bmatrix}0 & 0/1/2\\ 0 & 0\end{bmatrix},\begin{bmatrix}0 & 0\\ 1/2 & 0\end{bmatrix},\begin{bmatrix}1 & 1\\ 1 & 1\end{bmatrix},\begin{bmatrix}2 & 2\\ 2 & 2\end{bmatrix}$

Hence there are total $7(=3+2+1+1)$ singular matrices. Therefore number of all non-singular matrices in the given form $=27-7=20$

8. (b) $\begin{bmatrix} a & b \\ c & d \end{bmatrix}\begin{bmatrix} a & b \\ c & d \end{bmatrix}=\begin{bmatrix} 1 & 0 \\ 0 & 1 \end{bmatrix}$

$\begin{bmatrix} a^2+bc & ab+bd \\ ac+cd & bc+d^2 \end{bmatrix}=\begin{bmatrix} 1 & 0 \\ 0 & 1 \end{bmatrix}$

$b(a+d)=0, b=0$ or $a=-d$ ...(1)

$c(a+d)=0, c=0$ or $a=-d$ ...(2)

$a^2+bc=1, bc+d^2=1$ ...(3)

'a' and 'd' are diagonal elements $a+d=0$ statement-1 is correct.

Now, $\det(A)=ad-bc$

Now, from (3) $a^2+bc=1$ and $d^2+bc=1$

So, $a^2-d^2=0$

Adding $a^2+d^2+2bc=2$

$\Rightarrow (a+d)^2-2ad+2bc=2$

or $0-2(ad-bc)=2$

So, $ad-bc=1 \Rightarrow \det(A)=-1$

So, statement – 2 is also true.

But statement – 2 is not the correct explanation of statement-1.

9. (d) **Statement-1 :** Determinant of skew symmetric matrix of odd order is zero.

Statement-2 : $\det\left(A^T\right)=\det(A)$.

$\det(-A)=-(-1)^n\det(A)$.

where A is a $n\times n$ order matrix.

10. (b) Let $A=\begin{pmatrix} a & b \\ c & d \end{pmatrix}$ where a, b, c, d $\neq 0$

$A^2=\begin{pmatrix} a & b \\ c & d \end{pmatrix}\begin{pmatrix} a & b \\ c & d \end{pmatrix}$

$\Rightarrow A^2=\begin{pmatrix} a^2+bc & ab+bd \\ ac+cd & bc+d^2 \end{pmatrix}$

$\Rightarrow a^2+bc=1, bc+d^2=1$

$ab+bd=ac+cd=0$

$c\neq 0$ and $b\neq 0 \Rightarrow a+d=0$

$|A|=ad-bc=-a^2-bc=-1$

11. (d) Let $A=\begin{bmatrix} a & b \\ c & d \end{bmatrix}$ then $A^2=I$

$\Rightarrow a^2+bc=1$ and $ab+bd=0$

$ac+cd=0$ and $bc+d^2=1$

From these four relations,

$a^2+bc=bc+d^2 \Rightarrow a^2=d^2$

and $b(a+d)=0=c(a+d) \Rightarrow a=-d$

We can take $a=1, b=0, c=0, d=-1$ as one possible set of values, then $A=\begin{bmatrix} 1 & 0 \\ 0 & -1 \end{bmatrix}$

Clearly $A\neq I$ and $A\neq -I$ and $\det A=-1$

$\therefore$ Statement 1 is true.

Also if $A\neq I$ then $tr(A)=0$

$\therefore$ Statement 2 is false.

12. (a) Given $A=\begin{bmatrix} 5 & 5\alpha & \alpha \\ 0 & \alpha & 5\alpha \\ 0 & 0 & 5 \end{bmatrix}$ and $|A^2|=25$

$\therefore A^2=\begin{bmatrix} 5 & 5\alpha & \alpha \\ 0 & \alpha & 5\alpha \\ 0 & 0 & 5 \end{bmatrix}\begin{bmatrix} 5 & 5\alpha & \alpha \\ 0 & \alpha & 5\alpha \\ 0 & 0 & 5 \end{bmatrix}$

$=\begin{bmatrix} 25 & 25\alpha+5\alpha^2 & 5\alpha+25\alpha^2+5\alpha \\ 0 & \alpha^2 & 5\alpha^2+25\alpha \\ 0 & 0 & 25 \end{bmatrix}$

$\therefore |A^2|=25\ (25\alpha^2)$

$\therefore 25=25\ (25\alpha^2) \Rightarrow |\alpha|=\frac{1}{5}$

13. (b) $\Delta=\begin{vmatrix} 1 & \omega^n & \omega^{2n} \\ \omega^n & \omega^{2n} & 1 \\ \omega^{2n} & 1 & \omega^n \end{vmatrix}$

$=1\left(\omega^{3n}-1\right)-\omega^n\left(\omega^{2n}-\omega^{2n}\right)+\omega^{2n}\left(\omega^n-\omega^{4n}\right)$

$=\omega^{3n}-1-0+\omega^{3n}-\omega^{6n}$

$=1-1+1-1=0\left[\because \omega^{3n}=1\right]$

14. (a) We have

$\frac{1}{2}\begin{vmatrix} k & -3k & 1 \\ 5 & k & 1 \\ -k & 2 & 1 \end{vmatrix}=28$

$\Rightarrow 5k^2+13k-46=0$

or $5k^2+13k+66=0$

Now, $5k^2+13k-46=0$

$\Rightarrow \quad k=\frac{-13\pm\sqrt{1089}}{10}$

$\therefore \quad k=\frac{-23}{5}; k=2$

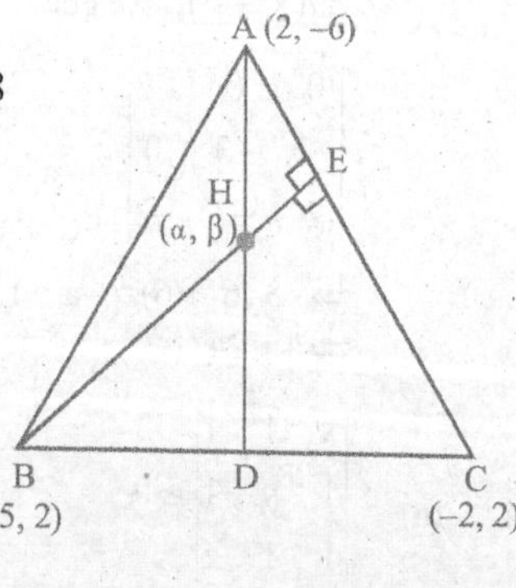

since k is an integer, $\therefore$ k = 2

Also $5k^2 + 13k + 66 = 0$

$$\Rightarrow k = \frac{-13 \pm \sqrt{-1151}}{10}$$

So no real solution exist

For orthocentre

BH $\perp$ AC

$$\therefore \quad \left(\frac{\beta-2}{\alpha-5}\right)\left(\frac{8}{-4}\right) = -1$$

$\Rightarrow \quad \alpha - 2\beta = 1$ ...(a)

Also CH $\perp$ AB

$$\therefore \quad \left(\frac{\beta-2}{\alpha+2}\right)\left(\frac{8}{3}\right) = -1$$

$\Rightarrow \quad 3\alpha + 8\beta = 10$ ... (b)

Solving (a) and (b), we get

$$\alpha = 2, \beta = \frac{1}{2}$$

orthocentre is $\left(2, \frac{1}{2}\right)$

15. (b) Given $2\omega + 1 = z$;

$z = \sqrt{3}i$

$$\Rightarrow \omega = \frac{\sqrt{3}i - 1}{2}$$

$\Rightarrow \omega$ is complex cube root of unity

Applying $R_1 \to R_1 + R_2 + R_3$

$$= \begin{vmatrix} 3 & 0 & 0 \\ 1 & -\omega^2 - 1 & \omega^2 \\ 1 & \omega^2 & \omega \end{vmatrix}$$

$= 3(-1 - \omega - \omega) = -3(1 + 2\omega) = -3z$

$\Rightarrow k = -z$

16. (c) $\begin{vmatrix} \cos x & \sin x & \sin x \\ \sin x & \cos x & \sin x \\ \sin x & \sin x & \cos x \end{vmatrix} = 0$

$R_1 \to R_1 - R_2$

$R_2 \to R_2 - R_3$

$$\begin{vmatrix} \cos x - \sin x & \sin x - \cos x & 0 \\ 0 & \cos x - \sin x & \sin x - \cos x \\ \sin x & \sin x & \cos x \end{vmatrix} = 0$$

$C_2 \to C_2 + C_3$

$$\begin{vmatrix} \cos x - \sin x & \sin x - \cos x & 0 \\ 0 & 0 & \sin x - \cos x \\ \sin x & \sin x & \cos x \end{vmatrix} = 0$$

Expanding using second row

$2 \sin x (\sin x - \cos x)^2 = 0$

$\sin x = 0$ or $\sin x = \cos x$

$$x = 0 \text{ or } x = \frac{\pi}{4}$$

17. (a) Consider

$$\begin{vmatrix} 3 & 1+f(1) & 1+f(2) \\ 1+f(1) & 1+f(2) & 1+f(3) \\ 1+f(2) & 1+f(3) & 1+f(4) \end{vmatrix}$$

$$= \begin{vmatrix} 1+1+1 & 1+\alpha+\beta & 1+\alpha^2+\beta^2 \\ 1+\alpha+\beta & 1+\alpha^2+\beta^2 & 1+\alpha^3+\beta^3 \\ 1+\alpha^2+\beta^2 & 1+\alpha^3+\beta^3 & 1+\alpha^4+\beta^4 \end{vmatrix}$$

$$= \begin{vmatrix} 1 & 1 & 1 \\ 1 & \alpha & \beta \\ 1 & \alpha^2 & \beta^2 \end{vmatrix} \times \begin{vmatrix} 1 & 1 & 1 \\ 1 & \alpha & \beta \\ 1 & \alpha^2 & \beta^2 \end{vmatrix}$$

$$= \begin{vmatrix} 1 & 1 & 1 \\ 1 & \alpha & \beta \\ 1 & \alpha^2 & \beta^2 \end{vmatrix}^2 = [(1-\alpha)(1-\beta)(\alpha-\beta)]^2$$

So, $\boxed{K = 1}$

18. (d) $\sum_{r=1}^{n-1} r = 1 + 2 + 3 + ... + (n-1) = \frac{n(n-1)}{2}$

$\sum_{r=1}^{n-1} (2r-1) = 1 + 3 + 5 + ... + [2(n-1) - 2]$

$= (n-1)^2$

$\sum_{r=1}^{n-1} (3r-2) = 1 + 4 + 7 + .. + (3n - 3 - 2)$

$$= \frac{(n-1)(3n-4)}{2}$$

$$\therefore \sum_{r=1}^{n-1} \Delta_r = \begin{vmatrix} \Sigma r & \Sigma(2r-1) & \Sigma(3r-2) \\ \frac{n}{2} & n-1 & a \\ \frac{n(n-1)}{2} & (n-1)^2 & \frac{(n-1)(3n-4)}{2} \end{vmatrix}$$

$\sum_{r=1}^{n-1} \Delta_r$ consists of $(n-1)$ determinants in L.H.S.

and in R.H.S every constituent of first row consists of (n – 1) elements and hence it can be splitted into sum of $(n-1)$ determinants.

$$\therefore \sum_{r=1}^{n-1} \Delta_r = \begin{vmatrix} \frac{n(n-1)}{2} & (n-1)^2 & \frac{(n-1)(3n-4)}{2} \\ \frac{n}{2} & n-1 & a \\ \frac{n(n-1)}{2} & (n-1)^2 & \frac{(n-1)(3n-4)}{2} \end{vmatrix}$$

$= 0$

($\because$ R_1 and R_3 are identical)

Hence, value of $\sum_{r=1}^{n-1} \Delta_r$ is independent of both 'a' and 'n'.

19. (c) Let $\Delta = \begin{vmatrix} a^2 & b^2 & c^2 \\ (a+\lambda)^2 & (b+\lambda)^2 & (c+\lambda)^2 \\ (a-\lambda)^2 & (b-\lambda)^2 & (c-\lambda)^2 \end{vmatrix}$

Apply $R_2 \to R_2 - R_3$

$$\Delta = \begin{vmatrix} a^2 & b^2 & c^2 \\ (a+\lambda)^2-(a-\lambda)^2 & (b+\lambda)^2-(b-\lambda)^2 & (c+\lambda)^2-(c-\lambda)^2 \\ (a-\lambda)^2 & (b-\lambda)^2 & (c-\lambda)^2 \end{vmatrix}$$

$$= \begin{vmatrix} a^2 & b^2 & c^2 \\ 4a\lambda & 4b\lambda & 4c\lambda \\ (a-\lambda)^2 & (b-\lambda)^2 & (c-\lambda)^2 \end{vmatrix}$$

$(\because (x+y)^2-(x-y)^2 = 4xy)$

Taking out 4 common from R_2

$$= 4\begin{vmatrix} a^2 & b^2 & c^2 \\ a\lambda & b\lambda & c\lambda \\ a^2+\lambda^2-2a\lambda & b^2+\lambda^2-2b\lambda & c^2+\lambda^2-2c\lambda \end{vmatrix}$$

Apply $R_3 \to [R_3 - (R_1 - 2R_2)]$

$$= 4\begin{vmatrix} a^2 & b^2 & c^2 \\ a\lambda & b\lambda & c\lambda \\ \lambda^2 & \lambda^2 & \lambda^2 \end{vmatrix}$$

Taking out λ common from R_2 and λ^2 from R_3.

$$= 4\lambda(\lambda^2)\begin{vmatrix} a^2 & b^2 & c^2 \\ a & b & c \\ 1 & 1 & 1 \end{vmatrix}$$

$$= k\lambda\begin{vmatrix} a^2 & b^2 & c^2 \\ a & b & c \\ 1 & 1 & 1 \end{vmatrix}$$

$\Rightarrow k = 4\lambda^2$

20. (b) $\begin{vmatrix} a & b & c \\ b & c & a \\ c & a & b \end{vmatrix} = \begin{vmatrix} a+b+c & a+b+c & a+b+c \\ b & c & a \\ c & a & b \end{vmatrix}$

$$= (a+b+c)\begin{vmatrix} 1 & 1 & 1 \\ b & c & a \\ c & a & b \end{vmatrix}$$

$$= (a+b+c)\begin{vmatrix} 0 & 0 & 1 \\ b-c & c-a & a \\ c-a & a-b & b \end{vmatrix}$$

$= (a + b + c)\,[ab + bc + ca - a^2 - b^2 - c^2]$

$= -(a + b + c)\,[(a - b)^2 + (b - c)^2 + (c - a)^2]$

Since a, b, c are sides of a scalene triangle, therefore at least two of the a, b, c will be unequal.

$\therefore$ $(a - b)^2 + (b - c)^2 + (c - a)^2 > 0$

Also $a + b + c > 0$

$\therefore$ $-(a + b + c)\,[(a - b)^2 + (b - c)^2 + (c - a)^2] < 0$

21. (c) Let $\Delta = \begin{vmatrix} b^2+c^2 & ab & ac \\ ab & c^2+a^2 & bc \\ ac & bc & a^2+b^2 \end{vmatrix}$

Multiply C_1 by a, C_2 by b and C_3 by c and hence divide by abc.

$$= \frac{1}{abc}\begin{vmatrix} a(b^2+c^2) & ab^2 & ac^2 \\ a^2b & b(c^2+a^2) & bc^2 \\ a^2c & b^2c & c(a^2+b^2) \end{vmatrix}$$

Take out a, b, c common from R_1, R_2 and R_3 respectively.

$$\therefore \Delta = \frac{abc}{abc}\begin{vmatrix} b^2+c^2 & b^2 & c^2 \\ a^2 & c^2+a^2 & c^2 \\ a^2 & b^2 & a^2+b^2 \end{vmatrix}$$

Apply $C_1 \to C_1 - C_2 - C_3$

$$\Delta = \begin{vmatrix} 0 & b^2 & c^2 \\ -2c^2 & c^2+a^2 & c^2 \\ -2b^2 & b^2 & a^2+b^2 \end{vmatrix}$$

$$= -2\begin{vmatrix} 0 & b^2 & c^2 \\ c^2 & c^2+a^2 & c^2 \\ b^2 & b^2 & a^2+b^2 \end{vmatrix}$$

Apply $C_2 - C_1$ and $C_3 - C_1$

$$= -2\begin{vmatrix} 0 & b^2 & c^2 \\ c^2 & a^2 & 0 \\ b^2 & 0 & a^2 \end{vmatrix}$$

$= -2\,[-b^2(c^2a^2) + c^2(-a^2b^2)]$
$= 2a^2b^2c^2 + 2a^2b^2c^2 = 4a^2b^2c^2$
But $\Delta = ka^2b^2c^2 \therefore k = 4$

22. (c) Let $\Delta = \begin{vmatrix} -2a & a+b & a+c \\ b+a & -2b & b+c \\ c+a & b+c & -2c \end{vmatrix}$

Applying $C_1 + C_3$ and $C_2 + C_3$

$$\Delta = \begin{vmatrix} -a+c & 2a+b+c & a+c \\ 2b+a+c & -b+c & b+c \\ a-c & b-c & -2c \end{vmatrix}$$

Now, applying $R_1 + R_3$ and $R_2 + R_3$

$$\Delta = \begin{vmatrix} 0 & 2(a+b) & a-c \\ 2(a+b) & 0 & b-c \\ a-c & b-c & -2c \end{vmatrix}$$

On expanding, we get
$\Delta = -2(a+b)\{-2c\,[2(a+b)]$
$\quad -(a-c)(b-c)\}$
$\quad +(a-c)\,[2(a+b)(b-c)]$
$\Delta = 8c\,(a+b)(a+b)$
$\quad + 4(a+b)(a-c)(b-c)$
$= 4(a+b)\,[2ac + 2bc + ab - bc - ac + c^2]$
$= 4(a+b)\,[ac + bc + ab + c^2]$
$= 4(a+b)\,[c(a+c) + b(a+c)]$
$= 4(a+b)(b+c)(c+a)$
$= \alpha(a+b)(b+c)(c+a)$
Hence, $\alpha = 4$

23. (b) Vertices of triangle in complex form is
$z, iz, z+iz$
In cartesian form vertices are
$(x, y), (-y, x)$ and $(x-y, x+y)$

$$\therefore \text{Area of triangle} = \frac{1}{2}\begin{vmatrix} x & y & 1 \\ -y & x & 1 \\ x-y & x+y & 1 \end{vmatrix}$$

$= \frac{1}{2}[x(x-x-y) - y(-y-x+y) + 1$
$(-yx - y^2 - x^2 + xy)]$

$= \frac{1}{2}[-xy + xy - y^2 - x^2] = \frac{1}{2}(x^2 + y^2)$
($\because$ Area can not be negative)

$= \frac{1}{2}|z|^2 \qquad \left(\because z = x + iy, |z|^2 = x^2 + y^2\right)$

24. (b) Given parabola is $x^2 = 8y$
$\Rightarrow 4a = 8 \Rightarrow a = 2$
To find: Area of ΔABC
$A = (-2a, a) = (-4, 2)$
$B = (2a, a) = (4, 2)$
$C = (0, 0)$

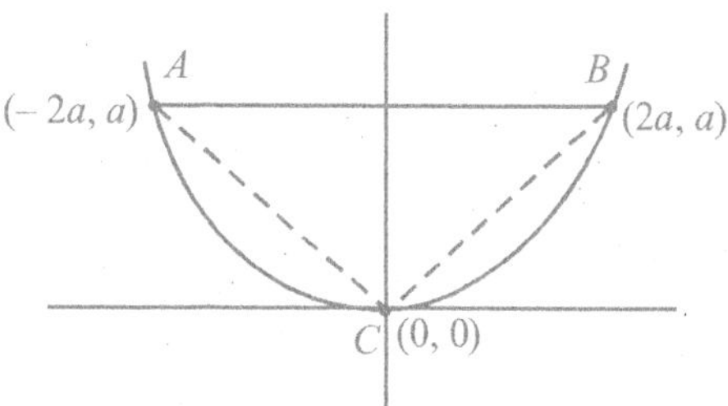

$$\therefore \text{Area} = \frac{1}{2}\begin{vmatrix} -4 & 2 & 1 \\ 4 & 2 & 1 \\ 0 & 0 & 1 \end{vmatrix}$$

$= \frac{1}{2}[-4(2) - 2(4) + 1(0)]$

$= \frac{-16}{2} = -8 \approx 8$ sq. unit

($\because$ area cannot be negative)

25. (b) $\begin{vmatrix} a & a+1 & a-1 \\ -b & b+1 & b-1 \\ c & c-1 & c+1 \end{vmatrix} +$

$$\begin{vmatrix} a+1 & b+1 & c-1 \\ a-1 & b-1 & c+1 \\ (-1)^{n+2}a & (-1)^{n+1}b & (-1)^n c \end{vmatrix} = 0$$

$$\Rightarrow \begin{vmatrix} a & a+1 & a-1 \\ -b & b+1 & b-1 \\ c & c-1 & c+1 \end{vmatrix} + \begin{vmatrix} a+1 & a-1 & (-1)^{n+2}a \\ b+1 & b-1 & (-1)^{n+1}b \\ c-1 & c+1 & (-1)^n c \end{vmatrix} = 0$$

(Taking transpose of second determinant)

$C_1 \Leftrightarrow C_3$

$$\Rightarrow \begin{vmatrix} a & a+1 & a-1 \\ -b & b+1 & b-1 \\ c & c-1 & c+1 \end{vmatrix} - \begin{vmatrix} (-1)^{n+2}a & a-1 & a+1 \\ (-1)^{n+2}(-b) & b-1 & b+1 \\ (-1)^{n+2}c & c+1 & c-1 \end{vmatrix} = 0$$

$C_2 \Leftrightarrow C_3$

$$\Rightarrow \begin{vmatrix} a & a+1 & a-1 \\ -b & b+1 & b-1 \\ c & c-1 & c+1 \end{vmatrix} + (-1)^{n+2} \begin{vmatrix} a & a+1 & a-1 \\ -b & b+1 & b-1 \\ c & c-1 & c+1 \end{vmatrix} = 0$$

$$\Rightarrow \left[1+(-1)^{n+2}\right] \begin{vmatrix} a & a+1 & a-1 \\ -b & b+1 & b-1 \\ c & c-1 & c+1 \end{vmatrix} = 0$$

$C_2 - C_1,\ C_3 - C_1$

$$\Rightarrow \left[1+(-1)^{n+2}\right] \begin{vmatrix} a & 1 & -1 \\ -b & 2b+1 & 2b-1 \\ c & -1 & 1 \end{vmatrix} = 0 \quad R_1 + R_3$$

$$\Rightarrow \left[1+(-1)^{n+2}\right] \begin{vmatrix} a+c & 0 & 0 \\ -b & 2b+1 & 2b-1 \\ c & -1 & 1 \end{vmatrix} = 0$$

$\Rightarrow [1+(-1)^{n+2}](a+c)(2b+1+2b-1)=0$
$\Rightarrow 4b(a+c)[1+(-1)^{n+2}]=0$
$\Rightarrow 1+(-1)^{n+2}=0$ as $b(a+c) \neq 0$
$\Rightarrow n$ should be an odd integer.

26. (d) Given, $D = \begin{vmatrix} 1 & 1 & 1 \\ 1 & 1+x & 1 \\ 1 & 1 & 1+y \end{vmatrix}$

Apply $R_2 \to R_2 - R_1$ and $R \to R_3 - R_1$

$$\therefore D = \begin{vmatrix} 1 & 1 & 1 \\ 0 & x & 0 \\ 0 & 0 & y \end{vmatrix} = xy$$

Hence, D is divisible by both x and y

27. (b) $\because a_1, a_2, a_3, \ldots\ldots$ are in G.P.

$\therefore$ Using $a_n = ar^{n-1}$, we get the given determinant, as

$$\begin{vmatrix} \log ar^{n-1} & \log ar^{n} & \log ar^{n+1} \\ \log ar^{n+2} & \log ar^{n+3} & \log ar^{n+4} \\ \log ar^{n+5} & \log ar^{n+6} & \log ar^{n+7} \end{vmatrix}$$

Operating $C_3 - C_2$ and $C_2 - C_1$ and using

$\log m - \log n = \log \frac{m}{n}$ we get

$$= \begin{vmatrix} \log ar^{n-1} & \log r & \log r \\ \log ar^{n+2} & \log r & \log r \\ \log ar^{n+5} & \log r & \log r \end{vmatrix}$$

$= 0$ (two columns being identical)

28. (d) Applying, $C_1 \to C_1 + C_2 + C_3$ we get

$$f(x) = \begin{vmatrix} 1+(a^2+b^2+c^2+2)x & (1+b^2)x & (1+c^2)x \\ 1+(a^2+b^2+c^2+2)x & 1+b^2x & (1+c^2x) \\ 1+(a^2+b^2+c^2+2)x & (1+b^2)x & 1+c^2x \end{vmatrix}$$

$$= \begin{vmatrix} 1 & (1+b^2)x & (1+c^2)x \\ 1 & 1+b^2x & (1+c^2x) \\ 1 & (1+b^2)x & 1+c^2x \end{vmatrix}$$

[As given that $a^2 + b^2 + c^2 = -2$]

$\therefore a^2 + b^2 + c^2 + 2 = 0$

Applying $R_1 \to R_1 - R_2,\ R_2 \to R_2 - R_3$

$$\therefore f(x) = \begin{vmatrix} 0 & x-1 & 0 \\ 0 & 1-x & x-1 \\ 1 & (1+b^2)x & 1+c^2x \end{vmatrix}$$

$f(x) = (x-1)^2$

Hence degree = 2.

29. (d) Let r be the common ratio, then

$$\begin{vmatrix} \log a_n & \log a_{n+1} & \log a_{n+2} \\ \log a_{n+3} & \log a_{n+4} & \log a_{n+5} \\ \log a_{n+6} & \log a_{n+7} & \log a_{n+8} \end{vmatrix}$$

$$= \begin{vmatrix} \log a_1 r^{n-1} & \log a_1 r^{n} & \log a_1 r^{n+1} \\ \log a_1 r^{n+2} & \log a_1 r^{n+3} & \log a_1 r^{n+4} \\ \log a_1 r^{n+5} & \log a_1 r^{n+6} & \log a_1 r^{n+7} \end{vmatrix}$$

$$= \begin{vmatrix} \log a_1 + (n-1)\log r & \log a_1 + n\log r & \log a_1 + (n+1)\log r \\ \log a_1 + (n+2)\log r & \log a_1 + (n+3)\log r & \log a_1 + (n+4)\log r \\ \log a_1 + (n+5)\log r & \log a_1 + (n+6)\log r & \log a_2 + (n+7)\log r \end{vmatrix}$$

$$= 0 \quad \left[\text{Apply } c_2 \to c_2 - \frac{1}{2}c_1 - \frac{1}{2}c_3\right]$$

30. **(c)** We have $\begin{vmatrix} a & b & ax+b \\ b & c & bx+c \\ ax+b & bx+c & 0 \end{vmatrix}$

By $R_3 \to R_3-(xR_1+R_2)$;

$$= \begin{vmatrix} a & b & ax+b \\ b & c & bx+c \\ 0 & 0 & -(ax^2+2bx+c) \end{vmatrix}$$

$= (ax^2+2bx+c)(b^2-ac) = (+)(-) = -\text{ve}.$

31. **(d)** $l = AR^{p-1} \Rightarrow \log l = \log A + (p-1)\log R$
$m = AR^{q-1} \Rightarrow \log m = \log A + (q-1)\log R$
$n = AR^{r-1} \Rightarrow \log n = \log A + (r-1)\log R$
Now,

$$\begin{vmatrix} \log l & p & 1 \\ \log m & q & 1 \\ \log n & r & 1 \end{vmatrix} = \begin{vmatrix} \log A+(p-1)\log R & p & 1 \\ \log A+(q-1)\log R & q & 1 \\ \log A+(r-1)\log R & r & 1 \end{vmatrix}$$

Operating

$C_1 - (\log R)C_2 + (\log R - \log A)C_3$

$$= \begin{vmatrix} 0 & p & 1 \\ 0 & q & 1 \\ 0 & r & 1 \end{vmatrix} = 0$$

32. **(c)** We have $A = \begin{bmatrix} 2 & -3 \\ -4 & 1 \end{bmatrix}$

$\Rightarrow A^2 = \begin{bmatrix} 16 & -9 \\ -12 & 13 \end{bmatrix}$

$\Rightarrow 3A^2 = \begin{bmatrix} 48 & -27 \\ -36 & 39 \end{bmatrix}$

Also $12A = \begin{bmatrix} 24 & -36 \\ -48 & 12 \end{bmatrix}$

$\therefore 3A^2 + 12A = \begin{bmatrix} 48 & -27 \\ -36 & 39 \end{bmatrix} + \begin{bmatrix} 24 & -36 \\ -48 & 12 \end{bmatrix} = \begin{bmatrix} 72 & -63 \\ -84 & 51 \end{bmatrix}$

$\text{adj}(3A^2+12A) = \begin{bmatrix} 51 & 63 \\ 84 & 72 \end{bmatrix}$

33. **(b)**

34. **(d)** $A(\text{adj } A) = A\,A^T$

$\Rightarrow A^{-1}A\,(\text{adj } A) = A^{-1}A\,A^T$

$\text{adj } A = A^T$

$\Rightarrow \begin{bmatrix} 2 & b \\ -3 & 5a \end{bmatrix} = \begin{bmatrix} 5a & 3 \\ -b & 2 \end{bmatrix}$

$\Rightarrow a = \frac{2}{5}$ and $b = 3$

$\Rightarrow 5a + b = 5$

35. **(a)** $A^2 - 5A = -7I$
$AAA^{-1} - 5AA^{-1} = -7IA^{-1}$
$AI - 5I = -7A^{-1}$
$A - 5I = -7A^{-1}$
$A^{-1} = \frac{1}{7}(5I - A)$

$A^3 - 2A^2 - 3A + I$
$= A(5A - 7I) - 2A^2 - 3A + I$
$= 5A^2 - 7A - 2A^2 - 3A + I$
$= 3A^2 - 10A + I$
$= 3(5A - 7I) - 10A + I$
$= 5A - 20I$
$= 5(A - 4I)$

36. **(a)** $|5.\,\text{adj } A| = 5 \Rightarrow 5^3.\,|A|^{3-1} = 5$

$\Rightarrow 125\,|A|^2 = 5 \Rightarrow |A| = \pm\frac{1}{5}$

37. **(d)** $BB' = B(A^{-1}A')' = B(A')'(A^{-1})'$
$= BA\,(A^{-1})'$
$= (A^{-1}A')(A(A^{-1})')$
$= A^{-1}A.A'.(A^{-1})'$ $\{\text{as } AA' = A'A\}$
$= I(A^{-1}A)' = I.I = I^2 = I$

38. **(a)** Given $A \begin{bmatrix} 1 & 2 & 3 \\ 0 & 2 & 3 \\ 0 & 1 & 1 \end{bmatrix} = \begin{bmatrix} 0 & 0 & 1 \\ 1 & 0 & 0 \\ 0 & 1 & 0 \end{bmatrix}$

Applying $C_1 \leftrightarrow C_3$

$A \begin{bmatrix} 3 & 2 & 1 \\ 3 & 2 & 0 \\ 1 & 1 & 0 \end{bmatrix} = \begin{bmatrix} 1 & 0 & 0 \\ 0 & 0 & 1 \\ 0 & 1 & 0 \end{bmatrix}$

Again Applying $C_2 \leftrightarrow C_3$

$A \begin{bmatrix} 3 & 1 & 2 \\ 3 & 0 & 2 \\ 1 & 0 & 1 \end{bmatrix} = \begin{bmatrix} 1 & 0 & 0 \\ 0 & 1 & 0 \\ 0 & 0 & 1 \end{bmatrix}$

pre-multiplying both sides by A^{-1}

$A^{-1}A \begin{bmatrix} 3 & 1 & 2 \\ 3 & 0 & 2 \\ 1 & 0 & 1 \end{bmatrix} = A^{-1} \begin{bmatrix} 1 & 0 & 0 \\ 0 & 1 & 0 \\ 0 & 0 & 1 \end{bmatrix}$

$I \begin{bmatrix} 3 & 1 & 2 \\ 3 & 0 & 2 \\ 1 & 0 & 1 \end{bmatrix} = A^{-1}\,I = A^{-1}$

($\because A^{-1}A = I$ and I = Identity matrix)

Hence, $A^{-1} = \begin{bmatrix} 3 & 1 & 2 \\ 3 & 0 & 2 \\ 1 & 0 & 1 \end{bmatrix}$

39. (b) $|P| = 1(12-12) - \alpha(4-6) + 3(4-6) = 2\alpha - 6$

Now, adj A = P $\Rightarrow$ |adj A| = |P|

$\Rightarrow |A|^2 = |P|$

$\Rightarrow |P| = 16$

$\Rightarrow 2a - 6 = 16$

$\Rightarrow a = 11$

40. (c) Given $P^3 = Q^3$ ...(1)

and $P^2Q = Q^2P$ ...(2)

Subtracting (1) and (2), we get

$P^3 - P^2Q = Q^3 - Q^2P$

$\Rightarrow P^2(P-Q) + Q^2(P-Q) = 0$

$\Rightarrow (P^2 + Q^2)(P-Q) = 0$

If $|P^2 + Q^2| \neq 0$ then $P^2 + Q^2$ is invertible.

$\Rightarrow P - Q = 0 \Rightarrow P = Q$

Which gives a contradiction ($\because P \neq Q$)

Hence $|P^2 + Q^2| = 0$

41. (d) Let $Au_1 = \begin{pmatrix}1\\0\\0\end{pmatrix}$ and $Au_2 = \begin{pmatrix}0\\1\\0\end{pmatrix}$

Then, $Au_1 + Au_2 = \begin{pmatrix}1\\0\\0\end{pmatrix} + \begin{pmatrix}0\\1\\0\end{pmatrix}$

$\Rightarrow A(u_1 + u_2) = \begin{pmatrix}1\\1\\0\end{pmatrix}$ ...(1)

Also, $A = \begin{pmatrix}1 & 0 & 0\\2 & 1 & 0\\3 & 2 & 1\end{pmatrix}$

$\Rightarrow |A| = 1(1) - 0(2) + 0(4-3) = 1$

We know,

$A^{-1} = \frac{1}{|A|} adjA$

$\Rightarrow A^{-1} = adj(A) \quad (\because |A| = 1)$

Now, from equation (1), we have

$u_1 + u_2 = A^{-1}\begin{pmatrix}1\\1\\0\end{pmatrix}$

$= \begin{bmatrix}1 & 0 & 0\\-2 & 1 & 0\\1 & -2 & 1\end{bmatrix}\begin{pmatrix}1\\1\\0\end{pmatrix} = \begin{bmatrix}1\\-1\\-1\end{bmatrix}$

42. (c) $A = \begin{bmatrix}0 & 0 & a\\0 & b & c\\d & e & f\end{bmatrix}$, $|A| = -abd \neq 0$

$c_{11} = +(bf - ce)$, $c_{12} = -(-cd) = cd$, $c_{13} = +(-bd) = -bd$

$c_{21} = -(-ea) = ae$, $c_{22} = +(-ad) = -ad$, $c_{23} = -(0) = 0$

$c_{31} = +(-ab) = -ab$, $c_{32} = -(0) = 0$, $c_{33} = 0$

$\text{Adj } A = \begin{bmatrix}(bf-ce) & ae & -ab\\cd & -ad & 0\\-bd & 0 & 0\end{bmatrix}$

$A^{-1} = \frac{1}{|A|}(\text{adj } A) = \frac{1}{abd}\begin{bmatrix}bf-ce & ae & -ab\\cd & -ad & 0\\-bd & 0 & 0\end{bmatrix}$

$A^T = \begin{bmatrix}0 & 0 & d\\0 & b & e\\a & c & f\end{bmatrix}$

Now $A^{-1} = A^T$

$\Rightarrow \frac{1}{-abd}\begin{bmatrix}bf-ce & ae & -ab\\cd & -ad & 0\\-bd & 0 & 0\end{bmatrix} = \begin{bmatrix}0 & 0 & d\\0 & b & e\\a & c & f\end{bmatrix}$

$\Rightarrow \begin{bmatrix}bf-ce & ae & -ab\\cd & -ad & 0\\-bd & 0 & 0\end{bmatrix} = \begin{bmatrix}0 & 0 & -abd^2\\0 & -ab^2d & -abde\\-a^2bd & -abcd & -abdf\end{bmatrix}$

$\therefore bf - ce = ae = cd = 0$ ...(i)

$abd^2 = ab,\ ab^2d = ad,\ a^2bd = bd$ ...(ii)

$abde = abcd = abdf = 0$ ...(iii)

From (ii),

$(abd^2).(ab^2d).(a^2bd) = ab.\ ad.\ bd$

$\Rightarrow (abd)^4 - (abd)^2 = 0$

$\Rightarrow (abd)^2[(abd)^2 - 1] = 0$

$\because abd \neq 0,\ \therefore \boxed{abd = \pm 1}$ ...(iv)

From (iii) and (iv),

$\boxed{e = c = f = 0}$ ...(v)

From (i) and (v),

$bf = ae = cd = 0$ ...(vi)

From (iv), (v) and (vi), it is clear that a, b, d can be any non-zero integer such that $abd = \pm 1$

But it is only possible, if $a = b = d = \pm 1$

Hence, there are 2 choices for each a, b and d. there fore, there are 2×2×2 choices for a, b and d. Hence number of required matrices = $2\times2\times2 = (2)^3$

43. **(a)** Let A and B be real matrices such that $A=\begin{bmatrix}\alpha & 0\\ 0 & \beta\end{bmatrix}$

and $B=\begin{bmatrix}0 & \gamma\\ \delta & 0\end{bmatrix}$

Now, $AB=\begin{bmatrix}0 & \alpha\gamma\\ \beta\delta & 0\end{bmatrix}$

and $BA=\begin{bmatrix}0 & \gamma\beta\\ \delta\alpha & 0\end{bmatrix}$

Statement - 1 :

$$AB-BA=\begin{bmatrix}0 & \gamma(\alpha-\beta)\\ \delta(\beta-\alpha) & 0\end{bmatrix}$$

$|AB-BA|=(\alpha-\beta)^2\gamma\delta\neq 0$

$\therefore$ $AB-BA$ is always an invertible matrix.
Hence, statement - 1 is true.
But $AB-BA$ can be identity matrix if $\gamma=-\delta$ or $\delta=-\gamma$
So, statement - 2 is false.

44. **(b)** **For reflexive**

$(A,A)\in R$

$A=P^{-1}AP$ is true,
For $P=I$, which is an invertible matrix.
$\therefore$ R is reflexive.

For symmetry

As $(A,B)\in R$ for matrix P

$A=P^{-1}BP$

$\Rightarrow PAP^{-1}=B$

$\Rightarrow B=PAP^{-1}$

$\Rightarrow B=\left(P^{-1}\right)^{-1}A(P^{-1})$

$\therefore$ $(B,A)\in R$ for matrix P^{-1}
$\therefore$ R is symmetric.

For transitivity

$A=P^{-1}BP$
and $B=P^{-1}CP$

$\Rightarrow A=P^{-1}\left(P^{-1}CP\right)P$

$\Rightarrow A=\left(P^{-1}\right)^2CP^2$

$\Rightarrow A=\left(P^2\right)^{-1}C\left(P^2\right)$

$\therefore$ $(A,C)\in R$ for matrix P^2
$\therefore$ R is transitive.
So R is equivalence

45. **(a)** We know that $|adj\,(adj\,A)|=|A|^{n-2}A$.
$=|A|^0A=A$
Also $|adj\,A|=|A|^{n-1}=|A|^{2-1}=|A|$
$\therefore$ Both the statements are true but statement-2 is not a correct explanation for statement-1 .

46. **(c)** $\because$ All entries of square matrix A are integers, therefore all cofactors should also be integers.
If $\det A=\pm 1$ then A^{-1} exists. Also all entries of A^{-1} are integers.

47. **(d)** Given $A^2-A+I=0$

$A^{-1}A^2-A^{-1}A+A^{-1}.I=A^{-1}.0$

(Multiplying A^{-1} on both sides)

$\Rightarrow A-1+A^{-1}=0$ or $A^{-1}=I-A$.

48. **(a)** Given that $10B=\begin{bmatrix}4 & 2 & 2\\ -5 & 0 & \alpha\\ 1 & -2 & 3\end{bmatrix}$

$$\Rightarrow B=\frac{1}{10}\begin{bmatrix}4 & 2 & 2\\ -5 & 0 & \alpha\\ 1 & -2 & 3\end{bmatrix}$$

Also since, $B=A^{-1}\Rightarrow AB=I$

$$\Rightarrow \frac{1}{10}\begin{bmatrix}1 & -1 & 1\\ 2 & 1 & -3\\ 1 & 1 & 1\end{bmatrix}\begin{bmatrix}4 & 2 & 2\\ -5 & 0 & \alpha\\ 1 & -2 & 3\end{bmatrix}=\begin{bmatrix}1 & 0 & 0\\ 0 & 1 & 0\\ 0 & 0 & 1\end{bmatrix}$$

$$\Rightarrow \frac{1}{10}\begin{bmatrix}10 & 0 & 5-2\\ 0 & 10 & -5+\alpha\\ 0 & 0 & 5+\alpha\end{bmatrix}=\begin{bmatrix}1 & 0 & 0\\ 0 & 1 & 0\\ 0 & 0 & 1\end{bmatrix}$$

$$\Rightarrow \frac{5-\alpha}{10}=0\Rightarrow \alpha=5$$

49. **(a)** $A=\begin{bmatrix}0 & 0 & -1\\ 0 & -1 & 0\\ -1 & 0 & 0\end{bmatrix}$

clearly $A\neq 0$. Also $|A|=-1\neq 0$

$\therefore A^{-1}$ exists, further $(-1)I=\begin{bmatrix}-1 & 0 & 0\\ 0 & -1 & 0\\ 0 & 0 & -1\end{bmatrix}\neq A$

Also $A^2=\begin{bmatrix}0 & 0 & -1\\ 0 & -1 & 0\\ -1 & 0 & 0\end{bmatrix}\begin{bmatrix}0 & 0 & -1\\ 0 & -1 & 0\\ -1 & 0 & 0\end{bmatrix}$

$$=\begin{bmatrix}1 & 0 & 0\\ 0 & 1 & 0\\ 0 & 0 & 1\end{bmatrix}=I$$

50. **(a)** $D=\begin{vmatrix} 1 & 1 & 1 \\ 1 & a & 1 \\ a & b & 1 \end{vmatrix}=0$

$\Rightarrow 1[a-b]-1[1-a]+1[b-a^2]=0 \Rightarrow (a-1)^2=0$

$\Rightarrow a=1$

For a = 1, First two equations are identical

ie. $x+y+z=1$

To have no solution with $x+by+z=0$

$b=1$

So $b=\{1\} \Rightarrow$ It is singleton set.

51. **(b)** Since the given system of linear equations has infinitely many solutions.

$\therefore \begin{vmatrix} 2 & 4 & -\lambda \\ 4 & \lambda & 2 \\ \lambda & 2 & 2 \end{vmatrix}=0$

$\Rightarrow \lambda^3+4\lambda-40=0$

λ has only 1 real root.

52. **(b)** For trivial solution,

$\begin{vmatrix} 1 & \lambda & -1 \\ \lambda & -1 & -1 \\ 1 & 1 & -\lambda \end{vmatrix}=0$

$\Rightarrow -\lambda(\lambda+1)(\lambda-1)=0$

$\Rightarrow \lambda=0,+1,-1$

53. **(a)** $\left.\begin{aligned} 2x_1-2x_2+x_3&=\lambda x_1 \\ 2x_1-3x_2+2x_3&=\lambda x_2 \\ -x_1+2x_2&=\lambda x_3 \end{aligned}\right\}$

$\Rightarrow \quad (2-\lambda)x_1-2x_2+x_3=0$

$2x_1-(3+\lambda)x_2+2x_3=0$

$-x_1+2x_2-\lambda x_3=0$

For non-trivial solution,

$\Delta=0$

i.e. $\begin{vmatrix} 2-\lambda & -2 & 1 \\ 2 & -(3+\lambda) & 2 \\ -1 & 2 & -\lambda \end{vmatrix}=0$

$\Rightarrow (2-\lambda)[\lambda(3+\lambda)-4]+2[-2\lambda+2]+1[4-(3+\lambda)]=0$

$\Rightarrow \lambda^3+\lambda^2-5\lambda+3=0$

$\Rightarrow \lambda=1,1,3$

Hence λ has 2 values.

54. **(b)** Given system of equations can be written as

$(a-1)x-y-z=0$

$-x+(b-1)y-z=0$

$-x-y+(c-1)z=0$

For non-trivial solution, we have

$\begin{vmatrix} a-1 & -1 & -1 \\ -1 & b-1 & -1 \\ -1 & -1 & c-1 \end{vmatrix}=0$

$R_2 \to R_2-R_3$

$\begin{vmatrix} a-1 & -1 & -1 \\ 0 & b & -c \\ -1 & -1 & c-1 \end{vmatrix}=0$

$C_2 \to C_2-C_3$

$\begin{vmatrix} a-1 & 0 & -1 \\ 0 & b+c & -c \\ -1 & -c & c-1 \end{vmatrix}=0$

Apply $R_3 \to R_3-R_1$

$\begin{vmatrix} a-1 & 0 & -1 \\ 0 & b+c & -c \\ -a & -c & c \end{vmatrix}=0$

$\Rightarrow (a-1)[bc+c^2-c^2]-1[a(b+c)]=0$

$\Rightarrow (a-1)[bc]-ab-ac=0$

$\Rightarrow abc-bc-ab-ac=0$

$\Rightarrow ab+bc+ca=abc$

55. **(b)** From the given system, we have

$\frac{k+1}{k}=\frac{8}{k+3}\neq\frac{4k}{3k-1}$

($\because$ System has no solution)

$\Rightarrow k^2+4k+3=8k$

$\Rightarrow k=1,3$

If $k=1$ then $\frac{8}{1+3}\neq\frac{4.1}{2}$ which is false

and if $k=3$ then $\frac{8}{6}\neq\frac{4.3}{9-1}$ which is true, therefore

$k=3$

Hence for only one value of k. System has no solution.

56. **(b)** Given system of equations is homogeneous which is

$x+ay=0$

$y+az=0$

$z+ax=0$

It can be written in matrix form as

$A=\begin{pmatrix} 1 & a & 0 \\ 0 & 1 & a \\ a & 0 & 1 \end{pmatrix}$

Now, $|A|=[1-a(-a^2)]=1+a^3\neq 0$

So, system has only trivial solution.

Now, $|A| = 0$ only when $a = -1$

So, system of equations has infinitely many solutions which is not possible because it is given that system has a unique solution.

Hence set of all real values of 'a' is $R - \{-1\}$.

57. (c) $\Delta_1 = \begin{vmatrix} 1 & \sin\alpha & \cos\alpha \\ 1 & \cos\alpha & \sin\alpha \\ 1 & -\sin\alpha & \cos\alpha \end{vmatrix}$

$= \begin{vmatrix} 0 & \sin\alpha - \cos\alpha & \cos\alpha - \sin\alpha \\ 0 & \cos\alpha + \sin\alpha & \sin\alpha - \cos\alpha \\ 1 & -\sin\alpha & \cos\alpha \end{vmatrix}$

$= (\sin\alpha - \cos\alpha)^2 - (\cos^2\alpha - \sin^2\alpha)$

$= \sin^2\alpha + \cos^2\alpha - 2\sin\alpha \,.\, \cos\alpha - \cos^2\alpha + \sin^2\alpha$

$= 2\sin^2\alpha - 2\sin\alpha \,.\, \cos\alpha$

$= 2\sin\alpha(\sin\alpha - \cos\alpha)$

Now, $\sin\alpha - \cos\alpha = 0$ for only

$\alpha = \frac{\pi}{4}$ in $\left(0, \frac{\pi}{2}\right)$

$\therefore \quad \Delta_1 = 2(\sin\alpha) \times 0 = 0,$

since value of $\sin\alpha$ is finite for $\alpha \in \left(0, \frac{\pi}{2}\right)$

Hence non-trivivial solution for only one value of α in $\left(0, \frac{\pi}{2}\right)$

$\begin{vmatrix} \cos\alpha & \sin\alpha & \cos\alpha \\ \sin\alpha & \cos\alpha & \sin\alpha \\ \cos\alpha & -\sin\alpha & -\cos\alpha \end{vmatrix} = 0$

$\Rightarrow \begin{vmatrix} 0 & \sin\alpha & \cos\alpha \\ 0 & \cos\alpha & \sin\alpha \\ 2\cos\alpha & -\sin\alpha & -\cos\alpha \end{vmatrix} = 0$

$\Rightarrow 2\cos\alpha(\sin^2\alpha - \cos^2\alpha) = 0$

$\therefore \cos\alpha = 0 \quad$ or $\quad \sin^2\alpha - \cos^2\alpha = 0$

But $\cos\alpha = 0$ not possible for any value of $\alpha \in \left(0, \frac{\pi}{2}\right)$

$\therefore \sin^2\alpha - \cos^2\alpha = 0 \Rightarrow \sin\alpha = -\cos\alpha$, which is also not possible for any value of $\alpha \in \left(0, \frac{\pi}{2}\right)$

Hence, there is no solution.

58. (d) Given system of equations can be written in matrix form as $AX = B$ where

$A = \begin{pmatrix} 1 & 2 & 3 \\ 1 & 3 & 5 \\ 2 & 5 & a \end{pmatrix}$ and $B = \begin{pmatrix} 6 \\ 9 \\ b \end{pmatrix}$

Since, system is consistent and has infinitely many solutions

$\therefore$ (adj. A) B = 0

$\Rightarrow \begin{pmatrix} 3a-25 & 15-2a & 1 \\ 10-a & a-6 & -2 \\ -1 & -1 & 1 \end{pmatrix}\begin{pmatrix} 6 \\ 9 \\ b \end{pmatrix} = \begin{pmatrix} 0 \\ 0 \\ 0 \end{pmatrix}$

$\Rightarrow -6 - 9 + b = 0 \Rightarrow b = 15$

and $6(10-a) + 9(a-6) - 2(b) = 0$

$\Rightarrow 60 - 6a + 9a - 54 - 30 = 0$

$\Rightarrow 3a = 24 \Rightarrow a = 8$

Hence, $a = 8, b = 15$.

59. (a) Given system of equations is

$x + ky + 3z = 0$

$3x + ky - 2z = 0$

$2x + 3y - 4z = 0$

Since, system has non-trivial solution

$\therefore \begin{vmatrix} 1 & k & 3 \\ 3 & k & -2 \\ 2 & 3 & -4 \end{vmatrix} = 0$

$\Rightarrow \quad 1(-4k+6) - k(-12+4) + 3(9-2k) = 0$

$\Rightarrow \quad 4k + 33 - 6k = 0 \Rightarrow k = \frac{33}{2}$

Hence, statement - 1 is false.

Statement-2 is the property.

It is a true statement.

60. (d) Given system of equations is

$x + y + z = 6$

$x + 2y + 3z = 10$

$x + 2y + \lambda z = 0$

It has unique solution.

$\therefore \begin{vmatrix} 1 & 1 & 1 \\ 1 & 2 & 3 \\ 1 & 2 & \lambda \end{vmatrix} \neq 0$

$\Rightarrow \quad 1(2\lambda - 6) - 1(\lambda - 3) + 1(2-2) \neq 0$

$\Rightarrow \quad 2\lambda - 6 - \lambda + 3 \neq 0 \Rightarrow \lambda - 3 \neq 0 \Rightarrow \lambda \neq 3$

61. (a) $x - ky + z = 0$

$kx + 3y - kz = 0$

$3x + y - z = 0$

The given system of equations will have non trivial solution, if

$\begin{vmatrix} 1 & -k & 1 \\ k & 3 & -k \\ 3 & 1 & -1 \end{vmatrix} = 0$

$\Rightarrow 1(-3+k)+k(-k+3k)+1(k-9)=0$

$\Rightarrow k-3+2k^2+k-9=0$

$\Rightarrow k^2+k-6=0$

$\Rightarrow k=-3, k=2$

So the equation will have only trivial solution, when $k \in R-\{2,-3\}$

62. (a) $\Delta=0$

$$\Rightarrow \begin{vmatrix} 4 & k & 2 \\ k & 4 & 1 \\ 2 & 2 & 1 \end{vmatrix}=0$$

$\Rightarrow 4(4-2)-k(k-2)+2(2k-8)=0$

$\Rightarrow 8-k^2+2k+4k-16=0$

$k^2-6k+8=0$

$\Rightarrow (k-4)(k-2)=0 \Rightarrow k=4,2$

63. (c) $D=\begin{vmatrix} 1 & 2 & 1 \\ 2 & 3 & 1 \\ 3 & 5 & 2 \end{vmatrix}=0$

$$D_1=\begin{vmatrix} 3 & 2 & 1 \\ 3 & 3 & 1 \\ 1 & 5 & 2 \end{vmatrix} \neq 0$$

$\Rightarrow$ Given system, does not have any solution.

$\Rightarrow$ No solution

64. (d) The given equations are

$-x+cy+bz=0$

$cx-y+az=0$

$bx+ay-z=0$

$\because x, y, z$ are not all zero

$\therefore$ The above system should not have unique (zero) solution

$$\Rightarrow \Delta=0 \Rightarrow \begin{vmatrix} -1 & c & b \\ c & -1 & a \\ b & a & -1 \end{vmatrix}=0$$

$\Rightarrow -1(1-a^2)-c(-c-ab)+b(ac+b)=0$

$\Rightarrow -1+a^2+b^2+c^2+2abc=0$

$\Rightarrow a^2+b^2+c^2+2abc=1$

65. (a) $\alpha x+y+z=\alpha-1$

$x+\alpha y+z=\alpha-1;$

$x+y+z\alpha=\alpha-1$

$$\Delta=\begin{vmatrix} \alpha & 1 & 1 \\ 1 & \alpha & 1 \\ 1 & 1 & \alpha \end{vmatrix}$$

$=\alpha(\alpha^2-1)-1(\alpha-1)+1(1-\alpha)$

$=\alpha(\alpha-1)(\alpha+1)-1(\alpha-1)-1(\alpha-1)$

For infinite solutions, $\Delta=0$

$\Rightarrow (\alpha-1)[\alpha^2+\alpha-1-1]=0$

$\Rightarrow (\alpha-1)[\alpha^2+\alpha-2]=0$

$\Rightarrow (\alpha-1)[\alpha^2+2\alpha-\alpha-2]=0$

$\Rightarrow (\alpha-1)[\alpha(\alpha+2)-1(\alpha+2)]=0$

$(\alpha-1)=0, \alpha+2=0$

$\Rightarrow \alpha=-2, 1;$

But $\alpha \neq 1$.

$\therefore \alpha=-2$

66. (d) For homogeneous system of equations to have non zero solution, $\Delta=0$

$$\begin{vmatrix} 1 & 2a & a \\ 1 & 3b & b \\ 1 & 4c & c \end{vmatrix}=0 \quad C_2 \to C_2-2C_3$$

$$\begin{vmatrix} 1 & 0 & a \\ 1 & b & b \\ 1 & 2c & c \end{vmatrix}=0 \quad R_3 \to R_3-R_2, R_2 \to R_2-R_1$$

On simplification, $\frac{2}{b}=\frac{1}{a}+\frac{1}{c}$

$\therefore a, b, c$ are in Harmonic Progression.

Continuity and Differentiability

TOPIC-1 : Continuity

1. The value of k for which the function

$$f(x)=\begin{cases}\left(\frac{4}{5}\right)^{\frac{\tan 4x}{\tan 5x}}, & 0<x<\frac{\pi}{2}\\ k+\frac{2}{5}, & x=\frac{\pi}{2}\end{cases}$$ is continuous at $x=\frac{\pi}{2}$, is :

[Online April 9, 2017]

(a) $\frac{17}{20}$ (b) $\frac{2}{5}$

(c) $\frac{3}{5}$ (d) $-\frac{2}{5}$

2. Let a, b $\in R, (a \neq 0)$. if the function f defined as

$$f(x)=\begin{cases}\frac{2x^2}{a}, & 0\le x<1\\ a, & 1\le x<\sqrt{2}\\ \frac{2b^2-4b}{x^3}, & \sqrt{2}\le x<\infty\end{cases}$$

is continuous in the interval $[0,\infty)$, then an ordered pair (a, b) is : **[Online April 10, 2016]**

(a) $(-\sqrt{2},1-\sqrt{3})$ (b) $(\sqrt{2},-1+\sqrt{3})$

(c) $(\sqrt{2},1-\sqrt{3})$ (d) $(-\sqrt{2},1+\sqrt{3})$

3. Let k be a non–zero real number. **[Online April 11, 2015]**

$$\text{If } f(x)=\begin{cases}\frac{(e^x-1)}{\sin\left(\frac{x}{k}\right)\log\left(1+\frac{x}{4}\right)}, & x\neq 0\\ 12, & x=0\end{cases}$$

is a continuous function then the value of k is:

(a) 4 (b) 1

(c) 3 (d) 2

4. If the function

$$f(x)=\begin{cases}\frac{\sqrt{2+\cos x}-1}{(\pi-x)^2}, & x\neq\pi\\ k, & x=\pi\end{cases}$$

is continuous at $x=\pi$, then k equals:

[Online April 19, 2014]

(a) 0 (b) $\frac{1}{2}$

(c) 2 (d) $\frac{1}{4}$

5. If f(x) is continuous and $f\left(\frac{9}{2}\right)=\frac{2}{9}$, then $\lim_{x\to 0} f\left(\frac{1-\cos 3x}{x^2}\right)$ is equal to:

[Online April 9, 2014]

(a) $\frac{9}{2}$ (b) $\frac{2}{9}$

(c) 0 (d) $\frac{8}{9}$

6. Consider the function :

$f(x)=[x]+|1-x|,\ -1\le x\le 3$ where $[x]$ is the greatest integer function.

Statement 1 : f is not continuous at $x = 0, 1, 2$ and 3.

Statement 2 : $f(x)=\begin{cases}-x, & -1\le x<0\\ 1-x, & 0\le x<1\\ 1+x, & 1\le x<2\\ 2+x, & 2\le x\le 3\end{cases}$

[Online April 25, 2013]

(a) Statement 1 is true ; Statement 2 is false,

(b) Statement 1 is true; Statement 2 is true; Statement 2 is not correct explanation for Statement 1.

(c) Statement 1 is true; Statement 2 is true; Statement It is a correct explanation for Statement 1.

(d) Statement 1 is false; Statement 2 is true.

7. Let f be a composite function of x defined by $f(u)=\frac{1}{u^2+u-2}, u(x)=\frac{1}{x-1}$.
Then the number of points x where f is discontinuous is : **[Online April 23, 2013]**
(a) 4 (b) 3
(c) 2 (d) 1

8. Let $f(x)=-1+|x-2|$, and $g(x)=1-|x|$; then the set of all points where fog is discontinuous is : **[Online April 22, 2013]**
(a) $\{0,2\}$ (b) $\{0,1,2\}$
(c) $\{0\}$ (d) an empty set

9. If $f: R \to R$ is a function defined by $f(x)=[x]\cos\left(\frac{2x-1}{2}\right)\pi$, where $[x]$ denotes the greatest integer function, then f is. **[2012]**
(a) continuous for every real x.
(b) discontinuous only at $x=0$
(c) discontinuous only at non-zero integral values of x.
(d) continuous only at $x=0$.

10. Let $f:[1,3] \to R$ be a function satisfying $\frac{x}{[x]} \le f(x) \le \sqrt{6-x}$, for all $x \ne 2$ and $f(2)=1$, where R is the set of all real numbers and $[x]$ denotes the largest integer less than or equal to x.
Statement 1: $\lim_{x\to 2^-} f(x)$ exists. **[Online May 19, 2012]**
Statement 2: f is continuous at $x=2$.
(a) Statement 1 is true, Statement 2 is true, Statement 2 is a correct explanation for Statement 1.
(b) Statement 1 is false, Statement 2 is true.
(c) Statement 1 is true, Statement 2 is true, Statement 2 is not a correct explanation for Statement 1.
(d) Statement 1 is true, Statement 2 is false.

11. **Statement 1:** A function $f: R \to R$ is continuous at x_0 if and only if $\lim_{x\to x_0} f(x)$ exists and $\lim_{x\to x_0} f(x)=f(x_0)$
Statement 2: A function $f: R \to R$ is discontinuous at x_0 if and only if, $\lim_{x\to x_0} f(x)$ exists and $\lim_{x\to x_0} f(x) \ne f(x_0)$.
[Online May 12, 2012]
(a) Statement 1 is true, Statement 2 is true, Statement 2 is not a correct explanation of Statement 1.
(b) Statement 1 is false, Statement 2 is true.
(c) Statement 1 is true, Statement 2 is true, Statement 2 is a correct explanation of Statement 1.
(d) Statement 1 is true, Statement 2 is false.

12. Define $f(x)$ as the product of two real functions **[2011RS]**
$$f_1(x)=x, x\in R, \text{and } f_2(x)=\begin{cases}\sin\frac{1}{x}, & if\ x\ne 0\\ 0, & if\ x=0\end{cases}$$
as follows :
$$f(x)=\begin{cases}f_1(x).f_2(x), & if\ x=0\\ 0 & if\ x=0\end{cases}$$
Statement - 1 : $f(x)$ is continuous on R.
Statement - 2 : $f_1(x)$ and $f_2(x)$ are continuous on R.
(a) Statement -1 is true, Statement-2 is true; Statement-2 is a correct explanation for Statement-1.
(b) Statement-1 is true, Statement-2 is true; Statement-2 is NOT a correct explanation for Statement-1
(c) Statement-1 is true, Statement-2 is false
(d) Statement-1 is false, Statement-2 is true

13. The values of p and q for which the function **[2011]**
$$f(x)=\begin{cases}\frac{\sin(p+1)x+\sin x}{x}, & x<0\\ q & ,x=0\\ \frac{\sqrt{x+x^2}-\sqrt{x}}{x^{3/2}} & ,x>0\end{cases}$$
is continuous for all x in R, are
(a) $p=\frac{5}{2}, q=\frac{1}{2}$ (b) $p=-\frac{3}{2}, q=\frac{1}{2}$
(c) $p=\frac{1}{2}, q=\frac{3}{2}$ (d) $p=\frac{1}{2}, q=-\frac{3}{2}$

14. The function $f: R/\{0\} \to R$ given by **[2007]**
$$f(x)=\frac{1}{x}-\frac{2}{e^{2x}-1}$$
can be made continuous at $x=0$ by defining $f(0)$ as
(a) 0 (b) 1
(c) 2 (d) -1

15. Let $f(x)=\frac{1-\tan x}{4x-\pi}, x\ne\frac{\pi}{4}, x\in\left[0,\frac{\pi}{2}\right]$.
If $f(x)$ is continuous in $\left[0,\frac{\pi}{2}\right]$, then $f\left(\frac{\pi}{4}\right)$ is **[2004]**
(a) -1 (b) $\frac{1}{2}$
(c) $-\frac{1}{2}$ (d) 1

16. f is defined in [-5, 5] as **[2002]**
$f(x)=x$ if x is rational
$=-x$ if x is irrational. Then
(a) $f(x)$ is continuous at every x, except $x=0$
(b) $f(x)$ is discontinuous at every x, except $x=0$
(c) $f(x)$ is continuous everywhere
(d) $f(x)$ is discontinuous everywhere

TOPIC-2 : Differentiability

17. If the function

$$f(x) = \begin{cases} -x, & x < 1 \\ a + \cos^{-1}(x+b), & 1 \le x \le 2 \end{cases}$$ is differentiable at

$x = 1$, then $\frac{a}{b}$ is equal to : [Online April 9, 2016]

(a) $\frac{\pi+2}{2}$ (b) $\frac{\pi-2}{2}$

(c) $\frac{-\pi-2}{2}$ (d) $-1-\cos^{-1}(2)$

18. If the function.

$$g(x) = \begin{cases} k\sqrt{x+1}, & 0 \le x \le 3 \\ mx+2, & 3 < x \le 5 \end{cases}$$ is differentiable, then the value

of $k + m$ is : [2015]

(a) $\frac{10}{3}$ (b) 4

(c) 2 (d) $\frac{16}{5}$

19. Let f: $R \to R$ be a function such that $|f(x)| \le x^2$, for all $x \in R$. Then, at $x = 0$, f is: [Online April 19, 2014]

(a) continuous but not differentiable.

(b) continuous as well as differentiable.

(c) neither continuous nor differentiable.

(d) differentiable but not continuous.

20. Let f, g: $R \to R$ be two functions defined by

$$f(x) = \begin{cases} x\sin\left(\frac{1}{x}\right), & x \ne 0 \\ 0, & x = 0 \end{cases}, \text{ and } g(x) = x f(x)$$

Statement I: f is a continuous function at $x = 0$.

Statement II: g is a differentiable function at $x = 0$.

[Online April 12, 2014]

(a) Both statement I and II are false.

(b) Both statement I and II are true.

(c) Statement I is true, statement II is false.

(d) Statement I is false, statement II is true.

21. Consider the function, $f(x) = |x-2| + |x-5|, x \in R$.

Statement-1 : $f'(4) = 0$

Statement-2 : f is continuous in [2,5], differentiable in (2,5) and $f(2) = f(5)$. [2012]

(a) Statement-1 is false, Statement-2 is true.

(b) Statement-1 is true, statement-2 is true; statement-2 is a correct explanation for Statement-1.

(c) Statement-1 is true, statement-2 is true; statement-2 is **not** a correct explanation for Statement-1.

(d) Statement-1 is true, statement-2 is false.

22. If $f(x) = a\,|\sin x| + be^{|x|} + c|x|^3$, where $a, b, c \in R$, is differentiable at $x = 0$, then [Online May 26, 2012]

(a) $a = 0$, b and c are any real numbers

(b) $c = 0, a = 0$, b is any real number

(c) $b = 0, c = 0$, a is any real number

(d) $a = 0, b = 0$, c is any real number

23. If $x + |y| = 2y$, then y as a function of x, at $x = 0$ is [Online May 7, 2012]

(a) differentiable but not continuous

(b) continuous but not differentiable

(c) continuous as well as differentiable

(d) neither continuous nor differentiable

24. If function $f(x)$ is differentiable at $x = a$,

then $\lim_{x \to a} \frac{x^2 f(a) - a^2 f(x)}{x-a}$ is : [2011RS]

(a) $-a^2 f'(a)$

(b) $a\,f(a) - a^2 f'(a)$

(c) $2af(a) - a^2 f'(a)$

(d) $2a\,f(a) + a^2 f'(a)$

25. Let $f(x) = \begin{cases} (x-1)\sin\frac{1}{x-1} & \text{if } x \ne 1 \\ 0 & \text{if } x = 1 \end{cases}$ [2008]

Then which one of the following is true?

(a) f is neither differentiable at $x = 0$ nor at $x = 1$

(b) f is differentiable at $x = 0$ and at $x = 1$

(c) f is differentiable at $x = 0$ but not at $x = 1$

(d) f is differentiable at $x = 1$ but not at $x = 0$

26. Let $f : R \to R$ be a function defined by

$f(x) = \min\{x+1, |x|+1\}$, Then which of the following is true?

(a) $f(x)$ is differentiable everywhere [2007]

(b) $f(x)$ is not differentiable at $x = 0$

(c) $f(x) \ge 1$ for all $x \in R$

(d) $f(x)$ is not differentiable at $x = 1$

27. The set of points where $f(x) = \frac{x}{1+|x|}$ is differentiable is [2006]

(a) $(-\infty, 0) \cup (0, \infty)$

(b) $(-\infty, -1) \cup (-1, \infty)$

(c) $(-\infty, \infty)$

(d) $(0, \infty)$

28. If f is a real valued differentiable function satisfying $|f(x)-f(y)| \leq (x-y)^2, x, y \in R$ and $f(0)=0$, then $f(1)$ equals **[2005]**

(a) -1 (b) 0
(c) 2 (d) 1

29. Suppose $f(x)$ is differentiable at $x = 1$ and $\lim_{h\to 0}\frac{1}{h}f(1+h)=5$, then $f'(1)$ equals **[2005]**

(a) 3 (b) 4
(c) 5 (d) 6

30. If $f(x)=\begin{cases} xe^{-\left(\frac{1}{|x|}+\frac{1}{x}\right)} & , x\neq 0 \\ 0 & , x=0 \end{cases}$ then f(x) is

(a) discontinuous every where **[2003]**
(b) continuous as well as differentiable for all x
(c) continuous for all x but not differentiable at $x=0$
(d) neither differentiable nor continuous at $x=0$

TOPIC-3 : Chain Rule of Differentiation, Differentiation of Explicit & Implicit Functions, Parametric & Composite Functions, Logarithmic & Exponential Functions, Inverse Functions, Differentiation by Trigonometric Substitution

31. If for $x\in\left(0,\frac{1}{4}\right)$, the derivative of $\tan^{-1}\left(\frac{6x\sqrt{x}}{1-9x^3}\right)$ is $\sqrt{x}.g(x)$, then g(x) equals: **[2017]**

(1) $\frac{3}{1+9x^3}$ (2) $\frac{9}{1+9x^3}$
(3) $\frac{3x\sqrt{x}}{1-9x^3}$ (4) $\frac{3x}{1-9x^3}$

32. For $x \in R$, $f(x)=|\log 2-\sin x|$ and $g(x)=f(f(x))$, then : **[2016]**

(a) $g'(0)=-\cos(\log 2)$
(b) g is differentiable at $x=0$ and $g'(0)=-\sin(\log 2)$
(c) g is not differentiable at $x=0$
(d) $g'(0)=\cos(\log 2)$

33. If $f(x)=x^2-x+5$, $x>\frac{1}{2}$, and g(x) is its inverse function, then g′(7) equals: **[Online April 12, 2014]**

(a) $-\frac{1}{3}$ (b) $\frac{1}{13}$
(c) $\frac{1}{3}$ (d) $-\frac{1}{13}$

34. If $y=\sec(\tan^{-1}x)$, then $\frac{dy}{dx}$ at $x=1$ is equal to : **[2013]**

(a) $\frac{1}{\sqrt{2}}$ (b) $\frac{1}{2}$
(c) 1 (d) $\sqrt{2}$

35. If the curves $\frac{x^2}{\alpha}+\frac{y^2}{4}=1$ and $y^3=16x$ intersect at right angles, then a value of α is : **[Online April 23, 2013]**

(a) 2 (b) $\frac{4}{3}$
(c) $\frac{1}{2}$ (d) $\frac{3}{4}$

36. For $a>0$, $t\in\left(0,\frac{\pi}{2}\right)$, let $x=\sqrt{a^{\sin^{-1}t}}$ and $y=\sqrt{a^{\cos^{-1}t}}$, Then, $1+\left(\frac{dy}{dx}\right)^2$ equals : **[Online April 22, 2013]**

(a) $\frac{x^2}{y^2}$ (b) $\frac{y^2}{x^2}$
(c) $\frac{x^2+y^2}{y^2}$ (d) $\frac{x^2+y^2}{x^2}$

37. Let $f(x)=\frac{x^2-x}{x^2+2x}, x\neq 0,-2$. Then $\frac{d}{dx}[f^{-1}(x)]$ (wherever it is defined) is equal to : **[Online April 9, 2013]**

(a) $\frac{-1}{(1-x)^2}$ (b) $\frac{3}{(1-x)^2}$
(c) $\frac{1}{(1-x)^2}$ (d) $\frac{-3}{(1-x)^2}$

38. If $f'(x)=\sin(\log x)$ and $y=f\left(\frac{2x+3}{3-2x}\right)$, then $\frac{dy}{dx}$ equals **[Online May 12, 2012]**

(a) $\sin\left[\log\left(\frac{2x+3}{3-2x}\right)\right]$
(b) $\frac{12}{(3-2x)^2}$
(c) $\frac{12}{(3-2x)^2}\sin\left[\log\left(\frac{2x+3}{3-2x}\right)\right]$
(d) $\frac{12}{(3-2x)^2}\cos\left[\log\left(\frac{2x+3}{3-2x}\right)\right]$

39. Let $f: (-1, 1) \rightarrow R$ be a differentiable function with $f(0) = -1$ and $f'(0) = 1$. Let $g(x) = [f(2f(x) + 2)]^2$. Then $g'(0) =$ **[2010]**

(a) -4 (b) 0
(c) -2 (d) 4

40. Let y be an implicit function of x defined by $x^{2x} - 2x^x \cot y - 1 = 0$. Then $y'(1)$ equals **[2009]**

(a) 1 (b) $\log 2$
(c) $-\log 2$ (d) -1

41. If $x^m . y^n = (x+y)^{m+n}$, then $\frac{dy}{dx}$ is **[2006]**

(a) $\frac{y}{x}$ (b) $\frac{x+y}{xy}$
(c) xy (d) $\frac{x}{y}$

42. If $x = e^{y + e^{y + \cdots \text{to} \infty}}, x > 0$, then $\frac{dy}{dx}$ is **[2004]**

(a) $\frac{1+x}{x}$ (b) $\frac{1}{x}$
(c) $\frac{1-x}{x}$ (d) $\frac{x}{1+x}$

43. Let $f(x)$ be a polynomial function of second degree. If $f(1) = f(-1)$ and a, b, c are in A. P, then $f'(a), f'(b), f'(c)$ are in **[2003]**

(a) Arithmetic -Geometric Progression
(b) A.P
(c) G.P
(d) H.P.

44. If $f(x+y) = f(x).f(y) \forall x.y$ and $f(5) = 2$, $f'(0) = 3$, then $f'(5)$ is **[2002]**

(a) 0 (b) 1
(c) 6 (d) 2

TOPIC-4 : Differentiation of Infinite Series, Successive Differentiation, nth Derivative of Some Standard Functions, Leibnitz's Theorem, Rolle's Theorem, Lagrange's Mean Value Theorem

45. If $2x = y^{\frac{1}{5}} + y^{-\frac{1}{5}}$ = and $(x^2 - 1)\frac{d^2y}{dx^2} + \lambda x \frac{dy}{dx} + ky = 0$, then $\lambda + k$ is equal to : **[Online April 9, 2017]**

(a) -23 (b) -24
(c) 26 (d) -26

46. Let f be a polynomial function such that $f(3x) = f'(x) . f''(x)$, for all $x \in \mathbf{R}$. Then : **[Online April 9, 2017]**

(a) $f(b) + f'(b) = 28$
(b) $f''(b) - f'(b) = 0$
(c) $f''(b) - f'(b) = 4$
(d) $f(b) - f'(b) + f''(b) = 10$

47. If $y = \left[x + \sqrt{x^2 - 1}\right]^{15} + \left[x - \sqrt{x^2 - 1}\right]^{15}$, then $(x^2 - 1)\frac{d^2y}{dx^2} + x\frac{dy}{dx}$ is equal to **[Online April 8, 2017]**

(a) $12y$ (b) $224y^2$
(c) $225y^2$ (d) $225y$

48. If Rolle's theorem holds for the function $f(x)\ 2x^3 + bx^2 + cx$, $x \in [-1, 1]$, at the point $x = \frac{1}{2}$, then $2b + c$ equals : **[Online April 10, 2015]**

(a) -3 (b) -1
(c) 2 (d) 1

49. If f and g are differentiable functions in [0, 1] satisfying $f(0) = 2 = g(1)$, $g(0) = 0$ and $f(1) = 6$, then for some $c \in]0, 1[$ **[2014]**

(a) $f'(c) = g'(c)$ (b) $f'(c) = 2g'(c)$
(c) $2f'(c) = g'(c)$ (d) $2f'(c) = 3g'(c)$

50. Let $f(x) = x|x|$, $g(x) = \sin x$ and $h(x) = (gof)(x)$. Then **[Online April 11, 2014]**

(a) h(x) is not differentiable at $x = 0$.
(b) h(x) is differentiable at $x = 0$, but $h'(x)$ is not continuous at $x = 0$
(c) $h'(x)$ is continuous at $x = 0$ but it is not differentiable at $x = 0$
(d) $h'(x)$ is differentiable at $x = 0$

51. Let for $i = 1, 2, 3$, $p_i(x)$ be a polynomial of degree 2 in x, $p'_i(x)$ and $p''_i(x)$ be the first and second order derivatives of $p_i(x)$ respectively. Let,

$$A(x) = \begin{bmatrix} p_1(x) & p_1'(x) & p_1''(x) \\ p_2(x) & p_2'(x) & p_2''(x) \\ p_3(x) & p_3'(x) & p_3''(x) \end{bmatrix}$$

and $B(x) = [A(x)]^T A(x)$. Then determinant of B(x): **[Online April 11, 2014]**

(a) is a polynomial of degree 6 in x.
(b) is a polynomial of degree 3 in x.
(c) is a polynomial of degree 2 in x.
(d) does not depend on x.

52. If the Rolle's theorem holds for the function $f(x) = 2x^3 + ax^2 + bx$ in the interval $[-1, 1]$ for the point $c = \frac{1}{2}$, then the value of $2a + b$ is: **[Online April 9, 2014]**

(a) 1 (b) -1
(c) 2 (d) -2

53. If $f(x) = \sin(\sin x)$ and $f''(x) + \tan x f'(x) + g(x) = 0$, then $g(x)$ is : **[Online April 23, 2013]**

(a) $\cos^2 x \cos(\sin x)$ (b) $\sin^2 x \cos(\cos x)$
(c) $\sin^2 x \sin(\cos x)$ (d) $\cos^2 x \sin(\sin x)$

54. Consider a quadratic equation $ax^2 + bx + c = 0$, where $2a+3b+6c=0$ and let $g(x)=a\frac{x^3}{3}+b\frac{x^2}{2}+cx$.

[Online May 19, 2012]

Statement 1: The quadratic equation has at least one root in the interval (0, 1).
Statement 2: The Rolle's theorem is applicable to function $g(x)$ on the interval [0, 1].
(a) Statement 1 is false, Statement 2 is true.
(b) Statement 1 is true, Statement 2 is false.
(c) Statement 1 is true, Statement 2 is true, Statement 2 is not a correct explanation for Statement 1.
(d) Statement 1 is true, Statement 2 is true, , Statement 2 is a correct explanation for Statement 1.

55. $\frac{d^2x}{dy^2}$ equals : **[2011]**

(a) $-\left(\frac{d^2y}{dx^2}\right)^{-1}\left(\frac{dy}{dx}\right)^{-3}$

(b) $\left(\frac{d^2y}{dx^2}\right)\left(\frac{dy}{dx}\right)^{-2}$

(c) $-\left(\frac{d^2y}{dx^2}\right)\left(\frac{dy}{dx}\right)^{-3}$

(d) $\left(\frac{d^2y}{dx^2}\right)^{-1}$

56. Let $f(x)=x|x|$ and $g(x)=\sin x$.
Statement-1 : gof is differentiable at $x=0$ and its derivative is continuous at that point.
Statement-2 : gof is twice differentiable at $x=0$. **[2009]**
(a) Statement-1 is true, Statement-2 is true; Statement-2 is not a correct explanation for Statement-1.
(b) Statement-1 is true, Statement-2 is false.
(c) Statement-1 is false, Statement-2 is true.
(d) Statement-1 is true, Statement-2 is true; Statement-2 is a correct explanation for Statement-1.

57. A value of c for which conclusion of Mean Value Theorem holds for the function $f(x)=\log_e x$ on the interval [1, 3] is **[2007]**

(a) $\log_3 e$ (b) $\log_e 3$
(c) $2\log_3 e$ (d) $\frac{1}{2}\log_3 e$

58. Let f be differentiable for all x. If $f(1)=-2$ and $f'(x)\geq 2$ for $x\in[1,6]$, then **[2005]**
(a) $f(6)\geq 8$ (b) $f(6)<8$
(c) $f(6)<5$ (d) $f(6)=5$

59. If the equation $a_nx^n+a_{n-1}x^{n-1}+ .... + a_1x=0$ $a_1\neq 0, n\geq 2$, has a positive root $x=\alpha$, then the equation $na_nx^{n-1}+(n-1)a_{n-1}x^{n-2}+ .... + a_1=0$ has a positive root, which is **[2005]**
(a) greater than α
(b) smaller than α
(c) greater than or equal to α
(d) equal to α

60. If $2a+3b+6c=0$, then at least one root of the equation $ax^2+bx+c=0$ lies in the interval **[2004]**
(a) (1,3) (b) (1,2)
(c) (2,3) (d) (0,1)

61. If $f(x)=x^n$, then the value of **[2003]**

$f(1)-\frac{f'(1)}{1!}+\frac{f''(1)}{2!}-\frac{f'''(1)}{3!}+..........\frac{(-1)^n f^n(1)}{n!}$ is

(a) 1 (b) 2^n
(c) 2^n-1 (d) 0.

62. Let $f(a)=g(a)=k$ and their nth derivatives $f^n(a), g^n(a)$ exist and are not equal for some n. Further if

$$\lim_{x\to a}\frac{f(a)g(x)-f(a)-g(a)f(x)+f(a)}{g(x)-f(x)}=4$$

then the value of k is **[2003]**
(a) 0 (b) 4
(c) 2 (d) 1

63. If $y=(x+\sqrt{1+x^2})^n$, then $(1+x^2)\frac{d^2y}{dx^2}+x\frac{dy}{dx}$ is
(a) n^2y (b) $-n^2y$ **[2002]**
(c) $-y$ (d) $2x^2y$

64. If $2a+3b+6c=0$, $(a, b, c\in R)$ then the quadratic equation $ax^2+bx+c=0$ has **[2002]**
(a) at least one root in [0, 1]
(b) at least one root in [2, 3]
(c) at least one root in [4, 5]
(d) none of these

Hints & Solutions

1. (c) $\lim_{x\to\pi/2} f(x) = f(\pi/2)$

$\Rightarrow \quad k + 2/5 = 1 \Rightarrow k = 1 - \frac{2}{5} \quad \Rightarrow \quad k = \frac{3}{5}$

2. (c) $\frac{2x^2}{a}$ (0 to 1), a (1 to $\sqrt{2}$), $\frac{2b^2-4b}{x^3}$ (beyond $\sqrt{2}$); points marked on the number line: 0, 1, $\sqrt{2}$

Continuity at $x = 1$

$\frac{2}{a} = a \Rightarrow a = \pm\sqrt{2}$

Continuity at $x = \sqrt{2}$ $a = \sqrt{2}$

$a = \frac{2b^2 - 4b}{2\sqrt{2}}$

Put $a = \sqrt{2}$

$2 = b^2 - 2b \qquad \Rightarrow b^2 - 2b - 2 = 0$

$b = \frac{2 \pm \sqrt{4 + 4.2}}{2} = 1 \pm \sqrt{3}$

So, $(a, b) = (\sqrt{2}, 1 - \sqrt{3})$

3. (c) Since f(x) is a continuous function therefore limit of f(x) at $x \to 0$ = value of f(x) at 0.

$\therefore \lim_{x\to 0} f(x) = \lim_{x\to 0} \frac{(e^x - 1)^2}{\sin\left(\frac{x}{k}\right)\log\left(1 + \frac{x}{4}\right)}$

$$= \lim_{x\to 0} \frac{x^2\left(\frac{e^x - 1}{x}\right)^2}{\frac{x}{R}\left[\frac{\sin\left(\frac{x}{R}\right)}{\frac{x}{R}}\right] \cdot \frac{\log\left(1 + \frac{x}{4}\right)}{\left(\frac{x}{4}\right)}} \times \left(\frac{x}{4}\right)$$

$$= \lim_{x\to 0} \frac{x^2\left(\frac{e^x - 1}{x}\right)^2 4k}{\frac{\sin\frac{x}{k}}{\frac{x}{k}} \cdot \frac{\log\left(1 + \frac{x}{4}\right)}{\frac{x}{4}}}$$

on applying limit we get

$4k = 12 \Rightarrow k = 3$

4. (d) Since $f(x) = \frac{\sqrt{2 + \cos x} - 1}{(\pi - x)^2}$ is

Continuous at $x = \pi$

$\therefore$ L.H.L = R.H.L = f (π)

Let $(\pi - x) = \theta$, $\theta \to 0$ when $x \to \pi$

$\therefore \lim_{\theta\to 0} \frac{\sqrt{2 - \cos\theta} - 1}{\theta^2}$

$= \lim_{\theta\to 0} \frac{(2 - \cos\theta) - 1}{\theta^2} \times \frac{1}{\sqrt{2 - \cos\theta} + 1}$

$= \lim_{\theta\to 0} \frac{1 - \cos\theta}{\theta^2} \cdot \frac{1}{2} \qquad (\because \cos 0 = 1)$

$= \frac{1}{2} \lim_{\theta\to 0} \frac{2\sin^2\theta/2}{\theta^2} = \frac{2}{2} \lim_{\theta\to 0} \frac{\sin^2\theta/2}{\frac{\theta^2}{4}.4}$

$= \frac{1}{4} \qquad \left(\because \lim_{x\to 0} \frac{\sin x}{x} = 1\right)$

5. (b) Given that $f\left(\frac{9}{2}\right) = \frac{2}{9}$

$\lim_{x\to 0} f\left(\frac{1 - \cos 3x}{x^2}\right) = \lim_{x\to 0}\left(\frac{x^2}{1 - \cos 3x}\right)$

$= \lim_{x\to 0}\left(\frac{x^2}{2\sin^2\frac{3x}{2}}\right) = \frac{1}{2}\lim_{x\to 0}\left(\frac{\frac{9}{4}.x^2.\frac{4}{9}}{\sin^2\frac{3x}{2}}\right)$

$= \frac{4}{9 \times 2}\lim_{x\to 0}\left(\frac{1}{\frac{\sin^2\frac{3x}{2}}{\left(\frac{3x}{2}\right)^2}}\right)$

$= \frac{2}{9}\left[\frac{\lim_{x\to 0} 1}{\lim_{x\to 0}\frac{\sin^2\frac{3x}{2}}{\left(\frac{3x}{2}\right)^2}}\right] \qquad \left\{\lim_{x\to 0}\frac{\sin x}{x} = 1\right\}$

$= \frac{2}{9}.\left[\frac{1}{1}\right] = \frac{2}{9}$

6. (a) Let $f(x)=[x]+|1-x|,\ -1\le x\le 3$
where $[x]$ = greatest integer function.
f is not continuous at $x=0, 1, 2, 3$
But in statement-2 $f(x)$ is continuous at $x=3$.
Hence, statement-1 is true and 2 is false.

7. (b) $\mu(x)=\dfrac{1}{x-1}$, which is discontinous at $x=1$

$f(u)=\dfrac{1}{u^2+u-2}=\dfrac{1}{(u+2)(u-1)}$,

which is discontinous at $u=-2, 1$

when $u=-2$, then $\dfrac{1}{x-1}=-2 \Rightarrow x=\dfrac{1}{2}$

when $u=1$, then $\dfrac{1}{x-1}=1 \Rightarrow x=2$

Hence given composite function is discontinous at three points, $x=1, \dfrac{1}{2}$ and 2.

8. (d) $fog=f(g(x))=f(1-|x|)$

$=-1+\big|1-|x|-2\big|$

$=-1+\big|-|x|-1\big|=-1+\big||x|+1\big|$

Let $fog=y$

$\therefore y=-1+\big||x|+1\big|$

$\Rightarrow y=\begin{cases}-1+x+1, & x\ge 0\\ -1-x+1, & x<0\end{cases}$

$\Rightarrow y=\begin{cases}x, & x\ge 0\\ -x, & x<0\end{cases}$

LHL at $(x=0)=\lim\limits_{x\to 0}(-x)=0$

RHL at $(x=0)=\lim\limits_{x\to 0}(x)=0$

When $x=0$, then $y=0$
Hence, LHL at $(x=0)$ = RHL at $(x=0)$
= value of y at $(x=0)$
Hence y is continuous at $x=0$.
Clearly at all other point y continuous. Therefore, the set of all points where fog is discontinuous is an empty set.

9. (a) Let $f(x)=[x]\cos\left(\dfrac{2x-1}{2}\right)$

Doubtful points are $x=n,\ n\in I$

L.H.L $=\lim\limits_{x\to n^-}[x]\cos\left(\dfrac{2x-1}{2}\right)\pi$

$=(n-1)\cos\left(\dfrac{2n-1}{2}\right)\pi=0$

($\because$ $[x]$ is the greatest integer function)

R.H.L $=\lim\limits_{x\to n^+}[x]\cos\left(\dfrac{2x-1}{2}\right)\pi$

$=n\cos\left(\dfrac{2n-1}{2}\right)\pi=0$

Now, value of the function at $x=n$ is $f(n)=0$
Since, L.H.L = R.H.L. = $f(n)$

$\therefore$ $f(x)=[x]\cos\left(\dfrac{2x-1}{2}\right)$ is continuous for every real x.

10. (d) Consider $\dfrac{x}{[x]}\le f(x)\le\sqrt{6-x}$

$\Rightarrow \lim\limits_{x\to 2^-}\dfrac{x}{[x]}=\dfrac{2}{1}=2$

$\Rightarrow \lim\limits_{x\to 2^-}\sqrt{6-x}=2$

$\therefore \lim\limits_{x\to 2^-}f(x)=2$ [By Sandwich theorem]

Now $\lim\limits_{x\to 2^+}\dfrac{x}{[x]}=1,\ \lim\limits_{x\to 2^+}\sqrt{6-x}=2$

Hence by Sandwich theorem $\lim\limits_{x\to 2^+}f(x)$ does not exists.
Therefore f is not continuous at $x=2$. Thus statement-1 is true but statement-2 is not true

11. (d) Statement - 1 is true.
It is the definition of continuity.
Statement - 2 is false.

12. (c) $f(x)=\begin{cases}x\sin(1/x), x\ne 0\\ 0\ ;\ x=0\end{cases}$ at $x=0$

LHL $=\lim\limits_{h\to 0^-}\left\{-h\sin\left(-\dfrac{1}{h}\right)\right\}$

$=0\times$ a finite quantity betwen -1 and 1
$=0$

RHL $=\lim\limits_{h\to 0^+}h\sin\dfrac{1}{h}=0$

Also, $f(0)=0$

Thus LHL = RHL = $f(0)$

$\therefore$ $f(x)$ is continuous on R.

$f_2(x)$ is not continuous at $x=0$

13. (b) $\underset{(at\,x=0)}{L.H.L}=\lim\limits_{x\to 0^-}f(x)$

$=\lim\limits_{h\to 0}\dfrac{\sin\{(p+1)(-h)\}-\sin h}{-h}$

$=p+1+1=p+2$

$\underset{(at\,x=0)}{R.H.L}=\lim\limits_{x\to 0^+}f(x)=\lim\limits_{h\to 0}=\dfrac{1}{1+1}=\dfrac{1}{2}$

$f(0)=q\Rightarrow p=-\dfrac{3}{2}, q=\dfrac{1}{2}$

14. **(b)** Given, $f(x)=\dfrac{1}{x}-\dfrac{2}{e^{2x}-1}$

$$\Rightarrow \quad f(0)=\lim_{x\to 0}\frac{1}{x}-\frac{2}{e^{2x}-1}$$

$$=\lim_{x\to 0}\frac{(e^{2x}-1)-2x}{x(e^{2x}-1)} \qquad \left[\frac{0}{0}\text{ form}\right]$$

$\therefore$ using, L'Hospital rule

$$f(0)=\lim_{x\to 0}\frac{4e^{2x}}{2(xe^{2x}2+e^{2x}.1)+e^{2x}.2}$$

$$=\lim_{x\to 0}\frac{4e^{2x}}{4xe^{2x}+2e^{2x}+2e^{2x}} \qquad \left[\frac{0}{0}\text{ form}\right]$$

$$=\lim_{x\to 0}\frac{4e^{2x}}{4(xe^{2x}+e^{2x})}=\frac{4.e^{0}}{4(0+e^{0})}=1$$

15. **(c)** $f(x)=\dfrac{1-\tan x}{4x-\pi}$ is continuous in $\left[0,\dfrac{\pi}{2}\right]$

$$\therefore f\left(\frac{\pi}{4}\right)=\lim_{x\to\frac{\pi}{4}^-} f(x)=\lim_{x\to\frac{\pi}{4}^+} f(x)$$

$$=\lim_{h\to 0} f\left(\frac{\pi}{4}+h\right)$$

$$=\lim_{h\to 0}\frac{1-\tan\left(\frac{\pi}{4}+h\right)}{4\left(\frac{\pi}{4}+h\right)-\pi},\ h>0$$

$$=\lim_{h\to 0}\frac{1-\dfrac{1+\tan h}{1-\tan h}}{4h}$$

$$=\lim_{h\to 0}\frac{-2}{1-\tan h}.\frac{\tan h}{4h}=\frac{-2}{4}=-\frac{1}{2}$$

16. **(b)** Let a is a rational number other than 0, in [–5, 5], then $f(a)=a$ and $\lim_{x\to a} f(x)=-a$

[As in the immediate neighbourhood of a rational number, we find irrational numbers]

$\therefore f(x)$ is not continuous at any rational number

If a is irrational number, then

$f(a)=-a$ and $\lim_{x\to a} f(x)=a$

$\therefore f(x)$ is not continuous at any irrational number clearly

$\lim_{x\to 0} f(x)=f(0)=0$

$\therefore f(x)$ is continuous at $x=0$

17. **(a)** $f(x)=\begin{cases}-x & x<1\\ a+\cos^{-1}(x+b) & 1\le x\le 2\end{cases}$

$f(x)$ is continuous

$\Rightarrow \lim_{x\to 1^-} f(x)=\lim_{x\to 1^+} a+\cos^{-1}(x+b)=f(x)$

$\Rightarrow -1=a+\cos^{-1}(1+b)$

$\cos^{-1}(1+b)=-1-a$ .....(a)

$f(x)$ is differentiate

$\Rightarrow$ LHD = RHD

$$\Rightarrow -1=\frac{-1}{\sqrt{1-(1+b)^2}}$$

$\Rightarrow 1-(1+b)^2=1$

$\Rightarrow b=-1$ .....(b)

From (a) $\Rightarrow \cos^{-1}(0)=-1-a$

$$\therefore \quad -1-a=\frac{\pi}{2}$$

$$a=-1-\frac{\pi}{2}$$

$$a=\frac{-\pi-2}{2} \qquad .....(c)$$

$$\therefore \quad \frac{a}{b}=\frac{\pi+2}{2}$$

18. **(c)** Since g (x) is differentiable, it will be continuous at x = 3

$\therefore \lim_{x\to 3^-} g(x)=\lim_{x\to 3^+} g(x)$

2k = 3m + 2 ...(a)

Also g(x) is differentiable at x = 0

$\therefore \lim_{x\to 3^-} g'(x)=\lim_{x\to 3^+} g'(x)$

$$\frac{k}{2\sqrt{3+1}}=m$$

k = 4m ...(b)

Solving (a) and (b), we get

$$m=\frac{2}{5},\ k=\frac{8}{5}$$

k + m = 2

19. **(b)** Let $|f(x)|\le x^2,\ \forall x\in R$

Now, at $x=0$, $|f(0)|\le 0$

$\Rightarrow f(0)=0$

$$\therefore f'(0)=\lim_{h\to 0}\frac{f(h)-f(0)}{h-0}=\lim_{h\to 0}\frac{f(h)}{h} \qquad ...(1)$$

Now, $\left|\dfrac{f(h)}{h}\right|\le|h|$ $\qquad (\because |f(x)|\le x^2)$

$\Rightarrow -|h| \le \frac{f(h)}{h} \le |h|$

$\Rightarrow \lim_{h \to 0} \frac{f(h)}{h} \to 0$ ...(2)

(using sandwich Theorem)

$\therefore$ from (1) and (2), we get $f'(0) = 0$,

i.e. - $f(x)$ is differentiable, at $x = 0$

Since, differentiability $\Rightarrow$ Continutity

$\therefore |f(x)| \le x^2$, for all $x \in R$ is continuous as well as differentiable at $x = 0$.

20. (b) $f(x) = \begin{cases} x\sin\left(\frac{1}{x}\right), & x \ne 0 \\ 0, & x = 0 \end{cases}$

and $g(x) = x f(x)$

For $f(x)$

$\text{LHL} = \lim_{h \to 0^-} \left\{-h\sin\left(-\frac{1}{h}\right)\right\}$

$= 0 \times$ a finite quantity between -1 and 1

$= 0$

$\text{RHL} = \lim_{h \to 0^+} h\sin\frac{1}{h} = 0$

Also, $f(0) = 0$

Thus LHL = RHL = $f(0)$

$\therefore f(x)$ is continuous at $x = 0$

$g(x) = \begin{cases} x^2 \sin\frac{1}{x}, & x \ne 0 \\ 0, & x = 0 \end{cases}$

For $g(x)$

$\text{LHL} = \lim_{h \to 0^-} \left\{-h^2 \sin\left(\frac{1}{h}\right)\right\}$

$= 0^2 \times$ a finite quantity between -1 and 1

$= 0$

$\text{RHL} = \lim_{h \to 0^+} h^2 \sin\left(\frac{1}{h}\right) = 0$

Also $g(0) = 0$

$\therefore g(x)$ is continuous at $x = 0$

21. (c) $f(x) = |x-2| = \begin{cases} x-2, & x-2 \ge 0 \\ 2-x, & x-2 \le 0 \end{cases}$

$= \begin{cases} x-2, & x \ge 2 \\ 2-x, & x \le 2 \end{cases}$

Similarly,

$f(x) = |x-5| = \begin{cases} x-5, & x \ge 5 \\ 5-x, & x \le 5 \end{cases}$

$\therefore f(x) = |x-2| + |x-5|$

$= \{x-2+5-x = 3, 2 \le x \le 5\}$

Thus $f(x) = 3, 2 \le x \le 5$

$f'(x) = 0, 2 < x < 5$

$f'(4) = 0$

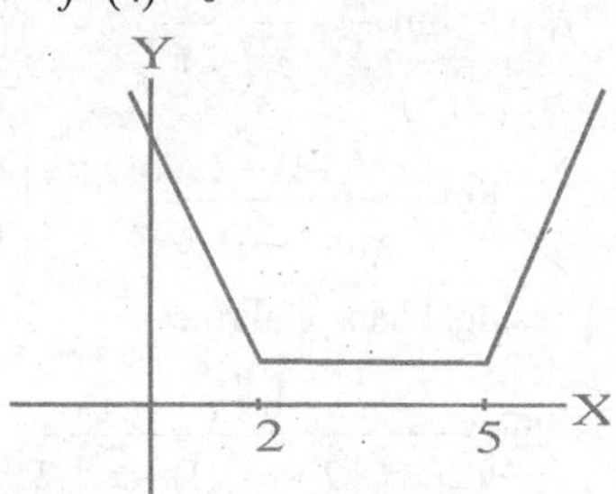

Clearly, statement-2 is also true.

$\because f(2) = 0 + |2-5| = 3$

and $f(5) = |5-2| + 0 = 3$

22. (d) $|\sin x|$ and $e^{|x|}$ are not differentiable at $x = 0$ and $|x|^3$ is differentiable at $x = 0$.

$\therefore$ for $f(x)$ to be differentiable at $x = 0$, we must have $a = 0$, $b = 0$ and c is any real number.

23. (b) Given $x + |y| = 2y$

$\Rightarrow x + y = 2y$ or $x - y = 2y$

$\Rightarrow x = y$ or $x = 3y$

This represent a straight line which passes through origin.

Hence, $x + |y| = 2y$ is continuous at $x = 0$.

Now, we check differentiability at $x = 0$

$x + |y| = 2y \Rightarrow x + y = 2y, y \ge 0$

$x - y = 2y, y < 0$

Thus, $f(x) = \begin{Bmatrix} x, & y < 0 \\ x/3, & y \ge 0 \end{Bmatrix}$

Now, L.H.D. $= \lim_{h \to 0^-} \frac{f(x+h) - f(x)}{-h}$

$= \lim_{h \to 0^-} \frac{x+h-x}{-h} = -1$

R.H.D $= \lim_{h \to 0^+} \frac{f(x+h) - f(x)}{h}$

$= \lim_{h \to 0^+} \frac{\frac{x+h}{3} - \frac{x}{3}}{h} = \lim_{h \to 0^+} \frac{1}{3} = \frac{1}{3}$

Since, L.H.D $\ne$ R.H.D. at $x = 0$

$\therefore$ given function is not differentiable at $x = 0$

24. (c) $\lim_{x \to a} \frac{x^2 f(a) - a^2 f(x)}{x - a}$

$= \lim_{x \to a} \frac{2xf(a) - a^2 f'(x)}{1}$

$= 2af(a) - a^2 f'(a)$

25. **(c)** We have $f(x)=\begin{cases}(x-1)\sin\left(\frac{1}{x-1}\right), & \text{if } x\neq 1\\ 0 & \text{, if } x=1\end{cases}$

$$Rf'(1)=\lim_{h\to 0}\frac{f(1+h)-f(1)}{h}$$

$$=\lim_{h\to 0}\frac{h\sin\frac{1}{h}-0}{h}=\lim_{h\to 0}\sin\frac{1}{h}$$

= a finite number

Let this finite number be l

$$L\,f'(1)=\lim_{h\to 0}\frac{f(1-h)-f(1)}{-h}$$

$$=\lim_{h\to 0}\frac{-h\sin\left(\frac{1}{-h}\right)}{-h}$$

$$=\lim_{h\to 0}\sin\left(\frac{1}{-h}\right)=-\lim_{h\to 0}\sin\left(\frac{1}{h}\right)$$

$= -$ (a finite number) $= -l$

Thus $Rf'(1)\neq Lf'(1)$

$\therefore$ f is not differentiable at $x = 1$

Also, $f'(0)=\left[\sin\frac{1}{(x-1)}-\frac{x-1}{(x-1)^2}\cos\left(\frac{1}{x-1}\right)\right]_{x=0}$

$= -\sin 1+\cos 1$

$\therefore$ f is differentiable at $x = 0$

26. **(a)** $f(x)=\min\{x+1,|x|+1\}\Rightarrow f(x)=x+1\ \forall\ x\in R$

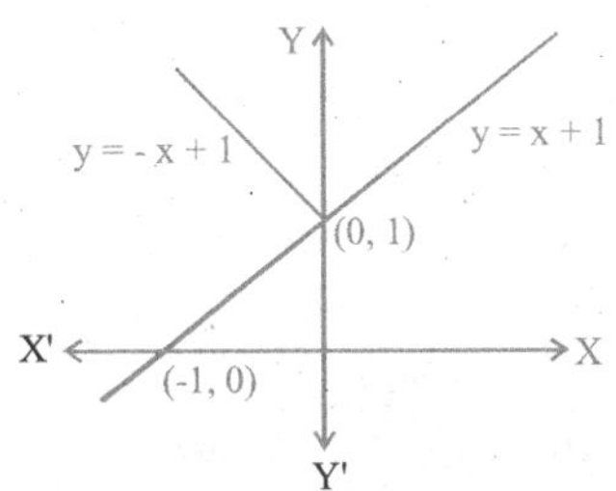

Hence, $f(x)$ is differentiable everywhere for all $x\in R$.

27. **(c)** $f(x)=\begin{cases}\frac{x}{1-x}, & x<0\\ \frac{x}{1+x}, & x\geq 0\end{cases}$

$\Rightarrow f'(x)=\begin{cases}\frac{x}{(1-x)^2}, & x<0\\ \frac{x}{(1+x)^2}, & x\geq 0\end{cases}$

$\therefore$ $f'(x)$ exist at everywhere.

28. **(b)** $f'(x)=\lim_{h\to 0}\frac{f(x+h)-f(x)}{h}$

$$|f'(x)|=\lim_{h\to 0}\left|\frac{f(x+h)-f(x)}{h}\right|\leq\lim_{h\to 0}\left|\frac{(h)^2}{h}\right|$$

$\Rightarrow |f'(x)|\leq 0\ \Rightarrow\ f'(x)=0$

$\Rightarrow f(x)=$ constant

As $f(0)=0$

$\Rightarrow f(1)=0.$

29. **(c)** $f'(1)=\lim_{h\to 0}\frac{f(1+h)-f(1)}{h}$;

As function is differentiable so it is continuous as it is given that $\lim_{h\to 0}\frac{f(1+h)}{h}=5$ and hence $f(1)=0$

Hence $f'(1)=\lim_{h\to 0}\frac{f(1+h)}{h}=5$

30. **(c)** $f(0)=0;\ f(x)=xe^{-\left(\frac{1}{|x|}+\frac{1}{x}\right)}$

R.H.L. $\lim_{h\to 0}(0+h)e^{-2/h}=\lim_{h\to 0}\frac{h}{e^{2/h}}=0$

L.H.L. $\lim_{h\to 0}(0-h)e^{-\left(\frac{1}{h}-\frac{1}{h}\right)}=0$

therefore, $f(x)$ is continuous.

R.H.D $=\lim_{h\to 0}\frac{(0+h)e^{-\left(\frac{1}{h}+\frac{1}{h}\right)}-0}{h}=0$

L.H.D. $=\lim_{h\to 0}\frac{(0-h)e^{-\left(\frac{1}{h}-\frac{1}{h}\right)}-0}{-h}=1$

therefore, L.H.D. $\neq$ R.H.D.

$f(x)$ is not differentiable at $x = 0$.

31. **(b)** Let $F(x)=\tan^{-1}\left(\frac{6x\sqrt{x}}{1-9x^3}\right)$ where $x\in\left(0,\frac{1}{4}\right)$.

$$=\tan^{-1}\left(\frac{2.(3x^{3/2})}{1-(3x^{3/2})^2}\right)=2\tan^{-1}(3x^{3/2})$$

As $3x^{3/2}\in\left(0,\frac{3}{8}\right)$

$$\left[\because 0<x<\frac{1}{4}\Rightarrow 0<x^{3/2}<\frac{1}{8}\Rightarrow 0<3x^{3/2}<\frac{3}{8}\right]$$

So $\frac{dF(x)}{dx}=2\times\frac{1}{1+9x^3}\times 3\times\frac{3}{2}\times x^{1/2}$

$$=\frac{9}{1+9x^3}\sqrt{x}$$

On comparing

$$\therefore g(x)=\frac{9}{1+9x^3}$$

32. **(d)** $g(x) = f(f(x))$

In the neighbourhood of $x = 0$,

$f(x) = |\log 2 - \sin x| = (\log 2 - \sin x)$

$\therefore g(x) = ||\log 2 - \sin| \log 2 - \sin x||$

$= (\log 2 - \sin(\log 2 - \sin x))$

$\therefore g(x)$ is differentiable

and $g'(x) = -\cos(\log 2 - \sin x)(-\cos x)$

$\Rightarrow g'(0) = \cos(\log 2)$

33. **(c)** $f(x) = y = x^2 - x + 5$

$$x^2 - x + \frac{1}{4} - \frac{1}{4} + 5 = y$$

$$\left(x - \frac{1}{2}\right)^2 + \frac{19}{4} = y$$

$$\left(x - \frac{1}{2}\right)^2 = y - \frac{19}{4}$$

$$x - \frac{1}{2} = \pm\sqrt{y - \frac{19}{4}}$$

$$x = \frac{1}{2} \pm \sqrt{y - \frac{19}{4}}$$

As $x > \frac{1}{2}$

$$x = \frac{1}{2} + \sqrt{y - \frac{19}{4}}$$

$$g(x) = \frac{1}{2} + \sqrt{x - \frac{19}{4}}$$

$$g'(x) = \frac{1}{2\sqrt{x - \frac{19}{4}}}$$

$$g'(7) = \frac{1}{2\sqrt{7 - \frac{19}{4}}} = \frac{1}{2\frac{\sqrt{28-19}}{2}} = \frac{1}{3}$$

34. **(a)** Let $y = \sec(\tan^{-1} x)$ and $\tan^{-1} x = \theta$.

$\Rightarrow x = \tan\theta$

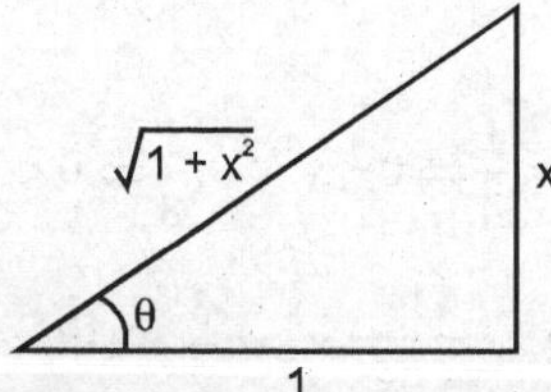

Thus, we have $y = \sec\theta$

$\Rightarrow y = \sqrt{1 + x^2}$ $\quad (\because \sec^2\theta = 1 + \tan^2\theta)$

$$\Rightarrow \frac{dy}{dx} = \frac{1}{2\sqrt{1+x^2}} \cdot 2x$$

At $x = 1$,

$$\frac{dy}{dx} = \frac{1}{\sqrt{2}}.$$

35. **(b)** $\frac{x^2}{\alpha} + \frac{y^2}{4} = 1 \Rightarrow \frac{2x}{\alpha} + \frac{2y}{4} \cdot \frac{dy}{dx} = 0$

$$\Rightarrow \frac{dy}{dx} = \frac{-4x}{\alpha y} \quad \text{...(i)}$$

$$y^3 = 16x \Rightarrow 3y^2 \cdot \frac{dy}{dx} = 16 \Rightarrow \frac{dy}{dx} = \frac{16}{3y^2} \quad \text{...(ii)}$$

Since curves intersects at right angles

$$\therefore \frac{-4x}{\alpha y} \times \frac{16}{3y^2} = -1 \Rightarrow 3\alpha y^3 = 64x$$

$$\Rightarrow \alpha = \frac{64x}{3 \times 16x} = \frac{4}{3}$$

36. **(d)** Let $x = \sqrt{a^{\sin^{-1} t}}$

$\Rightarrow x^2 = a^{\sin^{-1} t} \Rightarrow 2 \log x = \sin^{-1} t \cdot \log a$

$$\Rightarrow \frac{2}{x} = \frac{\log a}{\sqrt{1-t^2}} \cdot \frac{dt}{dx}$$

$$\Rightarrow \frac{2\sqrt{1-t^2}}{x \log a} = \frac{dt}{dx} \quad \text{...(1)}$$

Now, let $y = \sqrt{a^{\cos^{-1} t}}$

$\Rightarrow 2 \log y = \cos^{-1} t . \log a$

$$\Rightarrow \frac{2}{y} \cdot \frac{dy}{dx} = \frac{-\log a}{\sqrt{1-t^2}} \cdot \frac{dt}{dx}$$

$$\Rightarrow \frac{2}{y} \cdot \frac{dy}{dx} = \frac{-\log a}{\sqrt{1-t^2}} \times \frac{2\sqrt{1-t^2}}{x \log a} \quad \text{(from (1))}$$

$$\Rightarrow \frac{dy}{dx} = -\frac{y}{x}$$

Hence, $1 + \left(\frac{dy}{dx}\right)^2 = 1 + \left(\frac{-y}{x}\right)^2 = \frac{x^2 + y^2}{x^2}$

37. **(b)** Let $y = \frac{x^2 - x}{x^2 + 2x}$

$\Rightarrow (x^2 + 2x)y = x^2 - x$

$\Rightarrow x(x+2)y = x(x-1)$

$\Rightarrow x[(x+2)y - (x-1)] = 0$

$\because x \neq 0, \quad \therefore (x+2)y - (x-1) = 0$

$\Rightarrow xy + 2y - x + 1 = 0$

$\Rightarrow x(y-1) = -(2y+1)$

$\therefore \quad x=\frac{2y+1}{1-y} \Rightarrow f^{-1}(x)=\frac{2x+1}{1-x}$

$\frac{d}{dx}(f^{-1}(x))=\frac{2(1-x)-(2x+1)(-1)}{(1-x)^2}$

$=\frac{2-2x+2x+1}{(1-x)^2}=\frac{3}{(1-x)^2}$

38. **(c)** Let $f'(x)=\sin[\log x]$ and $y=f\left(\frac{2x+3}{3-2x}\right)$

Now, $\frac{dy}{dx}=f'\left(\frac{2x+3}{3-2x}\right).\frac{d}{dx}\left(\frac{2x+3}{3-2x}\right)$

$=\sin\left[\log\left(\frac{2x+3}{3-2x}\right)\right]\frac{[(6-4x)-(-4x-6)]}{(3-2x)^2}$

$=\frac{12}{(3-2x)^2}.\sin\left[\log\left(\frac{2x+3}{3-2x}\right)\right]$

39. **(a)** $g'(x)=2\left(f(2f(x)+2)\right)\left(\frac{d}{dx}(f(2f(x)+2))\right)$

$=2f(2f(x)+2)f'(2f(x))+2).(2f'(x))$

$\Rightarrow g'(0)=2f(2f(0)+2).f'(2f(0)+2)$

$.2f'(0)=4f(0)(f'(0))^2=4(-1)(1)^2=-4$

40. **(d)** $x^{2x}-2x^x\cot y-1=0$

$\Rightarrow \; 2\cot y=x^x-x^{-x}$

$\Rightarrow \; 2\cot y=u-\frac{1}{u}$ where $u=x^x$

Differentiating both sides with respect to x, we get

$-2\text{cosec}^2 y\frac{dy}{dx}=\left(1+\frac{1}{u^2}\right)\frac{du}{dx}$

where $u=x^x \Rightarrow \log u=x\log x$

$\Rightarrow \; \frac{1}{u}\frac{du}{dx}=1+\log x$

$\Rightarrow \; \frac{du}{dx}=x^x(1+\log x)$

$\therefore$ We get

$-2\,\text{cosec}^2 y\frac{dy}{dx}=(1+x^{-2x}).x^x(1+\log x)$

$\Rightarrow \; \frac{dy}{dx}=\frac{(x^x+x^{-x})(1+\log x)}{-2(1+\cot^2 y)} \quad \ldots(i)$

Now when $x=1$, $x^{2x}-2x^x\cot y-1=0$, gives

$1-2\cot y-1=0$

$\Rightarrow \; \cot y=0$

$\therefore$ From equation (i), at $x=1$ and $\cot y=0$, we get

$y'(1)=\frac{(1+1)(1+0)}{-2(1+0)}=-1$

41. **(a)** $x^m.y^n=(x+y)^{m+n}$

$\Rightarrow \; m\ln x+n\ln y=(m+n)\ln(x+y)$

Differentiating both sides.

$\therefore \quad \frac{m}{x}+\frac{n}{y}\frac{dy}{dx}=\frac{m+n}{x+y}\left(1+\frac{dy}{dx}\right)$

$\Rightarrow \; \left(\frac{m}{x}-\frac{m+n}{x+y}\right)=\left(\frac{m+n}{x+y}-\frac{n}{y}\right)\frac{dy}{dx}$

$\Rightarrow \; \frac{my-nx}{x(x+y)}=\left(\frac{my-nx}{y(x+y)}\right)\frac{dy}{dx}$

$\Rightarrow \; \frac{dy}{dx}=\frac{y}{x}$

42. **(c)** $x=e^{y+e^{y+\cdots\infty}} \Rightarrow x=e^{y+x}$.

Taking log.

$\log x=y+x \Rightarrow \frac{1}{x}=\frac{dy}{dx}+1$

$\therefore \frac{dy}{dx}=\frac{1}{x}-1=\frac{1-x}{x}$

43. **(b)** $f(x)=ax^2+bx+c$

$f(1)=f(-1)$

$\Rightarrow a+b+c=a-b+c \text{ or } b=0$

$\therefore f(x)=ax^2+c \text{ or } f'(x)=2ax$

Now $f'(a); f'(b)$; and $f'(c)$

are $2a(a); 2a(b); 2a(c)$

i.e. $2a^2, 2ab, 2ac$.

$\Rightarrow$ If a,b,c are in A.P. then $f'(a); f'(b)$ and $f'(c)$ are also in A.P.

44. **(c)** $f(x+y)=f(x)\times f(y)$

Differentiate with respect to x, treating y as constant

$f'(x+y)=f'(x)f(y)$

Putting $x=0$ and $y=x$, we get $f'(x)=f'(0)f(x)$;

$\Rightarrow f'(5)=3f(5)=3\times 2=6.$

45. **(b)** $y^{1/5}+y^{-1/5}=2x$

$\Rightarrow \; \left(\frac{1}{5}y^{-4/5}-\frac{1}{5}y^{-6/5}\right)\frac{dy}{dx}=2$

$\Rightarrow \; y'\left(y^{1/5}-y^{-1/5}\right)=10y$

$\Rightarrow \; y^{1/5}+y^{-1/5}=2x$

$\Rightarrow \; y^{1/5}-y^{-1/5}=\sqrt{4x^2-4}$

$\Rightarrow \; y'\left(2\sqrt{x^2-1}\right)=10y$

$\Rightarrow \; y''\left(2\sqrt{x^2-1}\right)+y'2\frac{2x}{2\sqrt{x^2-1}}=10y'$

$$\Rightarrow \quad y''(x^2-1)+xy' = 5\sqrt{x^2-1}\,(y')$$

$$\Rightarrow \quad \boxed{y''(x^2-1)+xy'-25y=0}$$

$$\lambda = 1, k = -25$$

46. **(b)** Let $f(x) = ax^3 + bx^2 + cx + d$

$\Rightarrow \quad f(3x) = 27ax^3 + 9bx^2 + 3cx + d$

$\Rightarrow \quad f'(x) = 3ax^2 + 2bx + c$

$\Rightarrow \quad f''(x) = 6ax + 2b$

$\Rightarrow \quad f(3x) = f'(x)f''(x)$

$\Rightarrow \quad 27a = 18a^2$

$\Rightarrow \quad a = \frac{3}{2}, b = 0, c = 0, d = 0$

$\Rightarrow \quad f(x) = \frac{3}{2}x^3,$

$f'(x) = \frac{9}{2}x^2,\ f'(x) = 9x$

$\Rightarrow \quad f'(2) = 18$
and $f''(2) = 18$
$\Rightarrow \quad f''(b) - f'(b) = 0$

47. **(d)** $y = \left\{x+\sqrt{x^2-1}\right\}^{15} + \left\{x-\sqrt{x^2-1}\right\}^{15}$

Differentiate w.r.t. 'x'

$$\frac{dy}{dx} = 15\left(x+\sqrt{x^2-1}\right)^{14}\left[1+\frac{x}{\sqrt{x^2-1}}\right]+15\left(x-\sqrt{x^2-1}\right)^{14}\left(1-\frac{x}{\sqrt{x^2-1}}\right)$$

$$\Rightarrow \quad \frac{dy}{dx} = \frac{15}{\sqrt{x^2-1}}.y \qquad \text{....(i)}$$

$$\Rightarrow \quad \sqrt{x^2-1}.\frac{dy}{dx} = 15y$$

Again differentiating both sides w.r.t. x

$$\frac{x}{\sqrt{x^2-1}}.\frac{dy}{dx}+\sqrt{x^2-1}\frac{d^2y}{dx^2} = 15\frac{dy}{dx}$$

$$\Rightarrow \quad x\frac{dy}{dx}+(x^2-1)\frac{d^2y}{dx^2} = 15\sqrt{x^2-1}.\frac{15}{\sqrt{x^2-1}}.y = 225y$$

48. **(b)** Conduction for Rolls theorem
$f(1) = f(-1)$

and $f'\left(\frac{1}{2}\right) = 0$

$c = -2$ and $b = \frac{1}{2}$

$2b + c = -1$

49. **(b)** Since, f and g both are continuous function on [0, 1] and differentiable on (0, 1) then $\exists c \in (0,1)$ such that

$$f'(c) = \frac{f(1)-f(0)}{1} = \frac{6-2}{1} = 4$$

and $g'(c) = \frac{g(1)-g(0)}{1} = \frac{2-0}{1} = 2$

Thus, we get $f'(c) = 2g'(c)$

50. **(c)** Let $f(x) = x|x| = x|x|$, $g(x) = \sin x$
and $h(x) = gof(x) = g[f(x)]$

$$\therefore h(x) = \begin{cases} \sin x^2, & x \ge 0 \\ -\sin x^2, & x < 0 \end{cases}$$

$$\text{Now, } h'(x) = \begin{cases} 2x\cos x^2, & x \ge 0 \\ -2x\cos x^2, & x < 0 \end{cases}$$

Since, L.H.L and R.H.L at $x = 0$ of $h'(x)$ is equal to 0 therefore $h'(x)$ is continuous at $x = 0$
Now, suppose $h'(x)$ is differentiable

$$\therefore h''(x) = \begin{cases} 2(\cos x^2 + 2x^2(-\sin x^2)), & x \ge 0 \\ 2(-\cos x^2 + 2x^2 \sin x^2), & x < 0 \end{cases}$$

Since, L.H.L and R.H.L at $x = 0$ of $h''(x)$ are different therefore $h''(x)$ is not continuous.
$\Rightarrow h''(x)$ is not differentiable
$\Rightarrow$ our assumption is wrong
Hence $h'(x)$ is not differentiable at $x = 0$.

51. **(a)** Let $p_1(x) = a_1x^2 + b_1x + c_1$
$p_2(x) = a_2x^2 + b_2x + c_2$
and $p_3(x) = a_3x^2 + b_3x + c_3$
where $a_1, a_2, a_3, b_1, b_2, b_3, c_1, c_2, c_3$ are real numbers.

$$\therefore A(x) = \begin{bmatrix} a_1x^2+b_1x+c_1 & 2a_1x+b_1 & 2a_1 \\ a_2x^2+b_2x+c_2 & 2a_2x+b_2 & 2a_2 \\ a_3x^2+b_3x+c_3 & 2a_3x+b_3 & 2a_3 \end{bmatrix}$$

$$B(x) = \begin{bmatrix} a_1x^2+b_1x+c_1 & a_2x^2+b_2x+c_2 & a_3x^2+b_3x+c_3 \\ 2a_1x+b_1 & 2a_2x+b_2 & 2a_3x+b_2 \\ 2a_1 & 2a_2 & 2a_3 \end{bmatrix}$$

$$\times \begin{bmatrix} a_1x^2+b_1x+c_1 & 2a_1x+b_1 & 2a_1 \\ a_2x^2+b_2x+c_2 & 2a_2x+b_2 & 2a_2 \\ a_3x^2+b_3x+c_3 & 2a_3x+b_3 & 2a_3 \end{bmatrix}$$

It is clear from the above multiplication, the degree of determinant of $B(x)$ can not be less than 4.

52. (b) $f(x) = 2x^3 + ax^2 + bx$

let, $a = -1, b = 1$

Given that $f(x)$ satisfy Rolle's theorem in interval $[-1, 1]$

$f(x)$ must satisfy two conditions.

(1) $f(a) = f(b)$

(2) $f'(c) = 0$ (c should be between a and b)

$f(a) = f(1) = 2(1)^3 + a(1)^2 + b(1) = 2 + a + b$

$f(b) = f(-1) = 2(-1)^3 + a(-1)^2 + b(-1)$

$= -2 + a - b$

$f(a) = f(b)$

$2 + a + b = -2 + a - b$

$2b = -4$

$b = -2$

(given that $c = \frac{1}{2}$)

$f'(x) = 6x^2 + 2ax + b$

at $x = \frac{1}{2}, f'(x) = 0$

$$0 = 6\left(\frac{1}{2}\right)^2 + 2a\left(\frac{1}{2}\right) + b$$

$$\frac{3}{2} + a + b = 0$$

$$\frac{3}{2} + a - 2 = 0$$

$$a = 2 - \frac{3}{2} = \frac{1}{2}$$

$$2a + b = 2 \times \frac{1}{2} - 2 = 1 - 2 = -1$$

53. (d) $f(x) = \sin(\sin x)$

$\Rightarrow f'(x) = \cos(\sin x) \cdot \cos x$

$\Rightarrow f''(x) = -\sin(\sin x) \cdot \cos^2 x + \cos(\sin x) \cdot (-\sin x)$

$= -\cos^2 x \cdot \sin(\sin x) - \sin x \cdot \cos(\sin x)$

Now $f''(x) + \tan x \cdot f'(x) + g(x) = 0$

$\Rightarrow g(x) = \cos^2 x \cdot \sin(\sin x) + \sin x \cdot \cos(\sin x)$

$- \tan x \cdot \cos x \cdot \cos(\sin x)$

$\Rightarrow g(x) = \cos^2 x \cdot \sin(\sin x)$.

54. (d) Let $g(x) = \frac{ax^3}{3} + b.\frac{x^2}{2} + cx$

$g'(x) = ax^2 + bx + c$

Given: $ax^2 + bx + c = 0$ and $2a + 3b + 6c = 0$

Statement-2:

(*i*) $g(0) = 0$ and $g(1) = \frac{a}{3} + \frac{b}{2} + c = \frac{2a + 3b + 6c}{6}$

$= \frac{0}{6} = 0$

$\Rightarrow g(0) = g(1)$

(*ii*) g is continuous on $[0, 1]$ and differentiable on $(0, 1)$

$\therefore$ By Rolle's theorem $\exists\, k \in (0,1)$ such that $g'(k) = 0$

This holds the statement 2. Also, from statement-2, we can say $ax^2 + bx + c = 0$ has at least one root in $(0, 1)$. Thus statement-1 and 2 both are true and statement-2 is a correct explanation for statement-1.

55. (c) $$\frac{d^2x}{dy^2} = \frac{d}{dy}\left(\frac{dx}{dy}\right) = \frac{d}{dx}\left(\frac{dx}{dy}\right)\frac{dx}{dy}$$

$$= \frac{d}{dx}\left(\frac{1}{dy/dx}\right)\frac{dx}{dy}$$

$$= -\frac{1}{\left(\frac{dy}{dx}\right)^2} \cdot \frac{d^2y}{dx^2} \cdot \frac{1}{\frac{dy}{dx}}$$

$$= -\frac{1}{\left(\frac{dy}{dx}\right)^3} \frac{d^2y}{dx^2}$$

56. (b) Given that $f(x) = x|x|$ and $g(x) = \sin x$

So that

$gof(x) = g(f(x)) = g(x|x|) = \sin x|x|$

$$= \begin{cases} \sin(-x^2), & \text{if } x < 0 \\ \sin(x^2), & \text{if } x \geq 0 \end{cases}$$

$$= \begin{cases} -\sin x^2, & \text{if } x < 0 \\ \sin x^2, & \text{if } x \geq 0 \end{cases}$$

$$\therefore (gof)'(x) = \begin{cases} -2x\cos x^2, & \text{if } x < 0 \\ 2x\cos x^2, & \text{if } x \geq 0 \end{cases}$$

Here we observe

$L(gof)'(0) = 0 = R(gof)'(0)$

$\Rightarrow$ gof is differentiable at $x = 0$

and $(gof)'$ is continuous at $x = 0$

Now $(gof)''(x)$

$$= \begin{cases} -2\cos x^2 + 4x^2\sin x^2, x < 0 \\ 2\cos x^2 - 4x^2\sin x^2, x \geq 0 \end{cases}$$

Here

$L(gof)''(0) = -2$ and $R(gof)''(0) = 2$

$\because$ $L(gof)''(0) \neq R(gof)''(0)$

$\Rightarrow$ $gof(x)$ is not twice differentiable at $x = 0$.

$\therefore$ Statement - 1 is true but statement -2 is false.

57. (c) Using Lagrange's Mean Value Theorem

Let $f(x)$ be a function defined on $[a, b]$

then, $f'(c) = \frac{f(b) - f(a)}{b - a}$ ....(i)

$c \in [a, b]$

$\therefore$ Given $f(x) = \log_e x \therefore f'(x) = \frac{1}{x}$

$\therefore$ equation (i) become

$$\frac{1}{c} = \frac{f(3) - f(1)}{3 - 1}$$

$$\Rightarrow \frac{1}{c} = \frac{\log_e 3 - \log_e 1}{2} = \frac{\log_e 3}{2}$$

$$\Rightarrow c = \frac{2}{\log_e 3} \Rightarrow c = 2\log_3 e$$

58. (a) As $f(1)=-2$ & $f'(x) \geq 2 \ \forall \ x \in [1, 6]$

Applying Lagrange's mean value theorem

$$\frac{f(6)-f(1)}{5} = f'(c) \geq 2$$

$\Rightarrow \ f(6) \geq 10+f(1)$

$\Rightarrow \ f(6) \geq 10-2 \Rightarrow \ f(6) \geq 8.$

59. (b) Let $f(x)=a_n x^n + a_{n-1}x^{n-1} + \ldots\ldots + a_1 x = 0$

The other given equation,

$n a_n x^{n-1} + (n-1)\, a_{n-1} x^{n-2} + \ldots + a_1 = 0 = f'(x)$

Given $a_1 \neq 0 \Rightarrow f(0)=0$

Again $f(x)$ has root α, $\Rightarrow f(\alpha)=0$

$\therefore \quad f(0)=f(\alpha)$

$\therefore \quad$ By Rolle's theorem $f'(x)=0$ has root between $(0, \alpha)$

Hence $f'(x)$ has a positive root smaller than α.

60. (d) Let us define a function

$$f(x)=\frac{ax^3}{3}+\frac{bx^2}{2}+cx$$

Being polynomial, it is continuous and differentiable, also,

$f(0)=0$ and $f(1)=\frac{a}{3}+\frac{b}{2}+c$

$\Rightarrow f(1)=\frac{2a+3b+6c}{6}=0$ (given)

$\therefore f(0)=f(1)$

$\therefore f(x)$ satisfies all conditions of Rolle's theorem therefore $f'(x)=0$ has a root in (0, 1)

i.e. $ax^2+bx+c=0$ has at lease one root in (0, 1)

61. (d) $f(x)=x^n \Rightarrow f(1)=1$

$f'(x)=nx^{n-1} \Rightarrow f'(1)=n$

$f''(x)=n(n-1)x^{n-2} \Rightarrow f''(1)=n(n-1)$

....

.... $f^n(x)=n! \Rightarrow f^n(1)=n!$

$$=1-\frac{n}{1!}+\frac{n(n-1)}{2!}-\frac{n(n-1)(n-2)}{3!}+\ldots+(-1)^n\frac{n!}{n!}$$

$$= {}^nC_0 - {}^nC_1 + {}^nC_2 - {}^nC_3 + \ldots + (-1)^n\, {}^nC_n = 0$$

62. (b) $\lim\limits_{x\to a}\frac{f(a)g'(x)-g(a)f'(x)}{g'(x)-f'(x)}=4$

(By L' Hospital rule)

$\lim\limits_{x\to a}\frac{k\,g'(x)-k\,f'(x)}{g'(x)-f'(x)}=4 \qquad \therefore k=4.$

63. (a) $y=(x+\sqrt{1+x^2})^n$

$$\frac{dy}{dx}=n(x+\sqrt{1+x^2})^{n-1}\left(1+\frac{1}{2}(1+x^2)^{-1/2}.\,2x\right);$$

$$\frac{dy}{dx}=n(x+\sqrt{1+x^2})^{n-1}\frac{(\sqrt{1+x^2}+x)}{\sqrt{1+x^2}}$$

$$=\frac{n(\sqrt{1+x^2}+x)^n}{\sqrt{1+x^2}}$$

or $\sqrt{1+x^2}\,\frac{dy}{dx}=ny$ or $\sqrt{1+x^2}\,y_1=ny$

$(y_1=\frac{dy}{dx})$ Squaring, $(1+x^2)y_1^2=n^2y^2$

Differentiating, $(1+x^2)2y_1y_2+y_1^2.2x=n^2.2yy_1$

or $(1+x^2)y_2+xy_1=n^2y$

64. (a) Let $f(x)=\frac{ax^3}{3}+\frac{bx^2}{2}+cx$

$\Rightarrow f(0)=0$ and

$f(1)=\frac{a}{3}+\frac{b}{2}+c=\frac{2a+3b+6c}{6}=0$

Also $f(x)$ is continuous and differentiable in [0, 1] and [0, 1[. So by Rolle's theorem, $f'(x)=0$.

i.e $ax^2+bx+c=0$ has at least one root in [0, 1].

Applications of Derivatives

TOPIC-1 : Rate of Change of Quantities

1. If the volume of a spherical ball is increasing at the rate of 4π cc/sec, then the rate of increase of its radius (in cm/sec), when the volume is $288\ \pi$ cc, **[Online April 19, 2014]**

(a) $\frac{1}{6}$ (b) $\frac{1}{9}$

(c) $\frac{1}{36}$ (d) $\frac{1}{24}$

2. Two ships A and B are sailing straight away from a fixed point O along routes such that $\angle AOB$ is always 120°. At a certain instance, OA = 8 km, OB = 6 km and the ship A is sailing at the rate of 20 km/hr while the ship B sailing at the rate of 30 km/hr. Then the distance between A and B is changing at the rate (in km/hr): **[Online April 11, 2014]**

(a) $\frac{260}{\sqrt{37}}$ (b) $\frac{260}{37}$

(c) $\frac{80}{\sqrt{37}}$ (d) $\frac{80}{37}$

3. A spherical balloon is being inflated at the rate of 35cc/min. The rate of increase in the surface area (in cm^2/min.) of the balloon when its diameter is 14 cm, is : **[Online April 25, 2013]**

(a) 10 (b) $\sqrt{10}$

(c) 100 (d) $10\sqrt{10}$

4. If the surface area of a sphere of radius r is increasing uniformly at the rate 8 cm^2/s, then the rate of change of its volume is : **[Online April 9, 2013]**

(a) constant

(b) proportional to $\sqrt{r}$

(c) proportional to r^2

(d) proportional to r

5. A spherical balloon is filled with 4500π cubic meters of helium gas. If a leak in the balloon causes the gas to escape at the rate of 72π cubic meters per minute, then the rate (in meters per minute) at which the radius of the balloon decreases 49 minutes after the leakage began is:

(a) $\frac{9}{7}$ (b) $\frac{7}{9}$ **[2012]**

(c) $\frac{2}{9}$ (d) $\frac{9}{2}$

6. If a metallic circular plate of radius 50 cm is heated so that its radius increases at the rate of 1 mm per hour, then the rate at which, the area of the plate increases (in cm^2/hour) is **[Online May 26, 2012]**

(a) 5π (b) 10π

(c) 100π (d) 50π

7. The weight W of a certain stock of fish is given by $W = nw$, where n is the size of stock and w is the average weight of a fish. If n and w change with time t as $n = 2t^2 + 3$ and $w = t^2 - t + 2$, then the rate of change of W with respect to t at $t = 1$ is **[Online May 19, 2012]**

(a) 1 (b) 8

(c) 13 (d) 5

8. Consider a rectangle whose length is increasing at the uniform rate of 2 *m/sec*, breadth is decreasing at the uniform rate of 3 *m/sec* and the area is decreasing at the uniform rate of 5 m^2/sec. If after some time the breadth of the rectangle is 2 m then the length of the rectangle is **[Online May 12, 2012]**

(a) 2m (b) 4m

(c) 1m (d) 3m

9. If a circular iron sheet of radius 30 cm is heated such that its area increases at the uniform rate of 6π cm^2/hr, then the rate (in mm/hr) at which the radius of the circular sheet increases is **[Online May 7, 2012]**

(a) 1.0 (b) 0.1

(c) 1.1 (d) 2.0

10. Two points A and B move from rest along a straight line with constant acceleration f and f' respectively. If A takes m sec. more than B and describes 'n' units more than B in acquiring the same speed then **[2005]**

(a) $(f - f')m^2 = ff'n$

(b) $(f + f')m^2 = ff'n$

(c) $\frac{1}{2}(f + f')m = ff'n^2$

(d) $(f' - f)n = \frac{1}{2}ff'm^2$

11. A lizard, at an initial distance of 21 cm behind an insect, moves from rest with an acceleration of 2 cm/s^2 and pursues the insect which is crawling uniformly along a straight line at a speed of 20 cm/s. Then the lizard will catch the insect after **[2005]**
(a) 20 *s* (b) 1 *s*
(c) 21 *s* (d) 24 *s*

12. A spherical iron ball 10 cm in radius is coated with a layer of ice of uniform thickness that melts at a rate of 50 cm^3/min. When the thickness of ice is 5 cm, then the rate at which the thickness of ice decreases is **[2005]**
(a) $\frac{1}{36\pi}$ cm/min. (b) $\frac{1}{18\pi}$ cm/min.
(c) $\frac{1}{54\pi}$ cm/min. (d) $\frac{5}{6\pi}$ cm/min

13. A point on the parabola $y^2 = 18x$ at which the ordinate increases at twice the rate of the abscissa is **[2004]**
(a) $\left(\frac{9}{8}, \frac{9}{2}\right)$ (b) $(2, -4)$
(c) $\left(\frac{-9}{8}, \frac{9}{2}\right)$ (d) $(2, 4)$

TOPIC-2 : Increasing & Decreasing Functions

14. The function f defined by $f(x) = x^3 - 3x^2 + 5x + 7$, is: **[Online April 9, 2017]**
(a) increasing in R.
(b) decreasing in R.
(c) decreasing in $(0, \infty)$ and increasing in $(-\infty, 0)$.
(d) increasing in $(0, \infty)$ and decreasing in $(-\infty, 0)$.

15. Let $f(x) = \sin^4 x + \cos^4 x$. Then f is an increasing function in the interval :
(a) $\left]\frac{5\pi}{8}, \frac{3\pi}{4}\right]$ (b) $\left]\frac{\pi}{2}, \frac{5\pi}{8}\right]$
(c) $\left]\frac{\pi}{4}, \frac{\pi}{2}\right]$ (d) $\left]0, \frac{\pi}{4}\right]$

16. Let f and g be two differentiable functions on R such that $f'(x) > 0$ and $g'(x) < 0$ for all $x \in R$. Then for all x: **[Online April 12, 2014]**
(a) $f(g(x)) > f(g(x-1))$ (b) $f(g(x)) > f(g(x+1))$
(c) $g(f(x)) > g(f(x-1))$ (d) $g(f(x)) < g(f(x+1))$

17. The real number k for which the equation, $2x^3 + 3x + k = 0$ has two distinct real roots in [0, 1] **[2013]**
(a) lies between 1 and 2
(b) lies between 2 and 3
(c) lies between .1 and 0
(d) does not exist.

18. **Statement-1:** The function $x^2(e^x + e^{-x})$ is increasing for all $x > 0$.
Statement-2: The functions x^2e^x and x^2e^{-x} are increasing for all $x > 0$ and the sum of two increasing functions in any interval (a, b) is an increasing function in (a, b). **[Online April 22, 2013]**
(a) Statement-1 is false; Statement-2 is true.
(b) Statement-1 is true; Statement-2 is true; Statement-2 is **not** a correct explanation for Statement-1.
(c) Statement-1 is true; Statement-2 is false.
(d) Statement-1 is true; Statement-2 is true; Statement-2 is a correct explanation for statement-1.

19. **Statement-1:** The equation $x \log x = 2 - x$ is satisfied by at least one value of x lying between 1 and 2.
Statement-2: The function $f(x) = x \log x$ is an increasing function in [1, 2] and $g(x) = 2 - x$ is a decreasing function in [1, 2] and the graphs represented by these functions intersect at a point in [1, 2] **[Online April 9, 2013]**
(a) Statement-1 is true; Statement-2 is true; Statement-2 is a correct explanation for Statement-1.
(b) Statement-1 is true; Statement-2 is true; Statement-2 is **not** correct explanation for Statement-1.
(c) Statement-1 is false, Statement-2 is true.
(d) Statement-1 is true, Statement-2 is false.

20. If $f(x) = xe^{x(1-x)}$, $x \in R$, then $f(x)$ is **[Online May 12, 2012]**
(a) decreasing on [–1/2, 1]
(b) decreasing on R
(c) increasing on [–1/2, 1]
(d) increasing on R

21. For real x, let $f(x) = x^3 + 5x + 1$, then **[2009]**
(a) f is onto R but not one-one
(b) f is one-one and onto R
(c) f is neither one-one nor onto R
(d) f is one-one but not onto R

22. How many real solutions does the equation $x^7 + 14x^5 + 16x^3 + 30x - 560 = 0$ have? **[2008]**
(a) 7 (b) 1
(c) 3 (d) 5

23. The function $f(x) = \tan^{-1}(\sin x + \cos x)$ is an increasing function in **[2007]**
(a) $\left(0, \frac{\pi}{2}\right)$ (b) $\left(-\frac{\pi}{2}, \frac{\pi}{2}\right)$
(c) $\left(\frac{\pi}{4}, \frac{\pi}{2}\right)$ (d) $\left(-\frac{\pi}{2}, \frac{\pi}{4}\right)$

24. A function is matched below against an interval where it is supposed to be increasing. Which of the following pairs is incorrectly matched? **[2005]**

	Interval	*Function*
(a)	$(-\infty, \infty)$	$x^3 - 3x^2 + 3x + 3$
(b)	$[2, \infty)$	$2x^3 - 3x^2 - 12x + 6$

(c) $\left(-\infty, \frac{1}{3}\right]$ $3x^2 - 2x + 1$

(d) $(-\infty, -4)$ $x^3 + 6x^2 + 6$

TOPIC-3 : Tangents & Normals

25. The normal to the curve $y(x-2)(x-3) = x+6$ at the point where the curve intersects the y-axis passes through the point: **[2017]**

(a) $\left(\frac{1}{2}, \frac{1}{3}\right)$ (b) $\left(-\frac{1}{2}, -\frac{1}{2}\right)$

(c) $\left(\frac{1}{2}, \frac{1}{2}\right)$ (d) $\left(\frac{1}{2}, -\frac{1}{3}\right)$

26. The eccentricity of an ellipse whose centre is at the origin is $\frac{1}{2}$. If one of its directices is $x = -4$, then the equation of the normal to it at $\left(1, \frac{3}{2}\right)$ is: **[2017]**

(a) $x + 2y = 4$ (b) $2y - x = 2$
(c) $4x - 2y = 1$ (d) $4x + 2y = 7$

27. A tangent to the curve, $y = f(x)$ at $P(x, y)$ meets x-axis at A and y-axis at B. If AP : BP = 1 : 3 and $f(a) = 1$, then the curve also passes through the point : **[Online April 9, 2017]**

(a) $\left(\frac{1}{3}, 24\right)$ (b) $\left(\frac{1}{2}, 4\right)$

(c) $\left(2, \frac{1}{8}\right)$ (d) $\left(3, \frac{1}{28}\right)$

28. The tangent at the point (2, –2) to the curve, $x^2y^2 - 2x = 4(1-y)$ does not pass through the point : **[Online April 8, 2017]**

(a) $\left(4, \frac{1}{3}\right)$ (b) $(8, 5)$

(c) $(-4, -9)$ (d) $(-2, -7)$

29. Consider

$$f(x) = \tan^{-1}\left(\sqrt{\frac{1+\sin x}{1-\sin x}}\right), x \in \left(0, \frac{\pi}{2}\right).$$ **[2016]**

A normal to $y = f(x)$ at $x = \frac{\pi}{6}$ also passes through the point :

(a) $\left(\frac{\pi}{6}, 0\right)$ (b) $\left(\frac{\pi}{4}, 0\right)$

(c) $(0, 0)$ (d) $\left(0, \frac{2\pi}{3}\right)$

30. Let C be a curve given by $y(x) = 1 + \sqrt{4x-3}, x > \frac{3}{4}$. If P is a point on C, such that the tangent at P has slope $\frac{2}{3}$, then a point through which the normal at P passes, is : **[Online April 10, 2016]**

(a) (1, 7) (b) (3, –4)
(c) (4, –3) (d) (2, 3)

31. If the tangent at a point P, with parameter t, on the curve $x = 4t^2 + 3, y = 8t^3 - 1, t \in R$, meets the curve again at a point Q, then the coordinates of Q are : **[Online April 9, 2016]**

(a) $(16t^2 + 3, -64t^3 - 1)$ (b) $(4t^2 + 3, -8t^3 - 2)$
(c) $(t^2 + 3, t^3 - 1)$ (d) $(t^2 + 3, -t^3 - 1)$

32. The normal to the curve, $x^2 + 2xy - 3y^2 = 0$, at (1, 1) **[2015]**

(a) meets the curve again in the third quadrant.
(b) meets the curve again in the fourth quadrant.
(c) does not meet the curve again.
(d) meets the curve again in the second quadrant.

33. The equation of a normal to the curve,

$\sin y = x \sin\left(\frac{\pi}{3} + y\right)$ at $x = 0$, is :

[Online April 11, 2015]

(a) $2x - \sqrt{3}y = 0$ (b) $2x + \sqrt{3}y = 0$

(c) $2y - \sqrt{3}x = 0$ (d) $2y + \sqrt{3}x = 0$

34. If the tangent to the conic, $y - 6 = x^2$ at (2, 10) touches the circle,
$x^2 + y^2 + 8x - 2y = k$ (for some fixed k) at a point (α, β); then (α, β) is : **[Online April 10, 2015]**

(a) $\left(-\frac{7}{17}, \frac{6}{17}\right)$ (b) $\left(-\frac{4}{17}, \frac{1}{17}\right)$

(c) $\left(-\frac{6}{17}, \frac{10}{17}\right)$ (d) $\left(-\frac{8}{17}, \frac{2}{17}\right)$

35. The distance, from the origin, of the normal to the curve,

$x = 2\cos t + 2t \sin t, y = 2\sin t - 2t\cos t$ at $t = \frac{\pi}{4}$, is :

[Online April 10, 2015]

(a) 2 (b) 4
(c) $\sqrt{2}$ (d) $2\sqrt{2}$

36. For the curve $y = 3\sin\theta\cos\theta$, $x = e^{\theta}\sin\theta$, $0 \le \theta \le \pi$, the tangent is parallel to x-axis when θ is:

[Online April 11, 2014]

(a) $\frac{3\pi}{4}$ (b) $\frac{\pi}{2}$

(c) $\frac{\pi}{4}$ (d) $\frac{\pi}{6}$

37. If an equation of a tangent to the curve, $y-\cos(x+f), -1\ -1\leq x\leq 1+\pi$, is $x+2y=k$ then k is equal to : [Online April 25, 2013]
(a) 1 (b) 2
(c) $\frac{\pi}{4}$ (d) $\frac{\pi}{2}$

38. The equation of the normal to the parabola, $x^2=8y$ at $x=4$ is [Online May 19, 2012]
(a) $x+2y=0$ (b) $x+y=2$
(c) $x-2y=0$ (d) $x+y=6$

39. The equation of the tangent to the curve $y=x+\frac{4}{x^2}$, that is parallel to the x-axis, is [2010]
(a) $y=1$ (b) $y=2$
(c) $y=3$ (d) $y=0$

40. Angle between the tangents to the curve $y=x^2-5x+6$ at the points (2, 0) and (3, 0) is [2006]
(a) π (b) $\frac{\pi}{2}$
(c) $\frac{\pi}{6}$ (d) $\frac{\pi}{4}$

41. The normal to the curve [2005]
$x=a(\cos\theta+\theta\sin\theta), y=a(\sin\theta-\theta\cos\theta)$ at any point θ is such that
(a) it passes through the origin
(b) it makes an angle $\frac{\pi}{2}+\theta$ with the x- axis
(c) it passes through $\left(a\frac{\pi}{2},-a\right)$
(d) It is at a constant distance from the origin

42. The normal to the curve $x=a(1+\cos\theta), y=a\sin\theta$ at 'θ' always passes through the fixed point [2004]
(a) (a, a) (b) $(0, a)$
(c) $(0,0)$ (d) $(a,0)$

43. A function $y=f(x)$ has a second order derivative $f''(x)=6(x-1)$. If its graph passes through the point (2,1) and at that point the tangent to the graph is $y=3x-5$, then the function is [2004]
(a) $(x+1)^2$ (b) $(x-1)^3$
(c) $(x+1)^3$ (d) $(x-1)^2$

TOPIC-4 : Approximations, Maxima & Minima

44. Twenty metres of wire is available for fencing off a flower-bed in the form of a circular sector. Then the maximum area (in sq. m) of the flower-bed, is : [2017]
(a) 30 (b) 12.5
(c) 10 (d) 25

45. A wire of length 2 units is cut into two parts which are bent respectively to form a square of side = x units and a circle of radius = r units. If the sum of the areas of the square and the circle so formed is minimum, then: [2016]
(a) $x=2r$ (b) $2x=r$
(c) $2x=(\pi+4)r$ (d) $(4-\pi)x=\pi r$

46. The minimum distance of a point on the curve $y=x^2-4$ from the origin is : [Online April 9, 2016]
(a) $\frac{\sqrt{15}}{2}$ (b) $\sqrt{\frac{19}{2}}$
(c) $\sqrt{\frac{15}{2}}$ (d) $\frac{\sqrt{19}}{2}$

47. Let k and K be the minimum and the maximum values of the function $f(x)=\frac{(1+x)^{0.6}}{1+x^{0.6}}$ in [0, 1] respectively, then the ordered pair (k, K) is equal to : [Online April 11, 2015]
(a) $(2^{-0.4}, 1)$ (b) $(2^{-0.4}, 2^{0.6})$
(c) $(2^{-0.6}, 1)$ (d) $(1, 2^{0.6})$

48. From the top of a 64 metres high tower, a stone is thrown upwards vertically with the velocity of 48 m/s. The greatest height (in metres) attained by the stone, assuming the value of the gravitational acceleration $g = 32\ m\ s^2$, is: [Online April 11, 2015]
(a) 128 (b) 88
(c) 112 (d) 100

49. If $x=-1$ and $x=2$ are extreme points of $f(x)=\alpha\log|x|+\beta x^2+x$ then [2014]
(a) $\alpha=2, \beta=-\frac{1}{2}$ (b) $\alpha=2, \beta=\frac{1}{2}$
(c) $\alpha=-6, \beta=\frac{1}{2}$ (d) $\alpha=-6, \beta=-\frac{1}{2}$

50. The minimum area of a triangle formed by any tangent to the ellipse $\frac{x^2}{16}+\frac{y^2}{81}=1$ and the co-ordinate axes is: [Online April 12, 2014]
(a) 12 (b) 18
(c) 26 (d) 36

51. The volume of the largest possible right circular cylinder that can be inscribed in a sphere of radius = $\sqrt{3}$ is: [Online April 11, 2014]
(a) $\frac{4}{3}\sqrt{3}\pi$ (b) $\frac{8}{3}\sqrt{3}\pi$
(c) 4π (d) 2π

52. The cost of running a bus from A to B, is ₹$\left(av+\frac{b}{v}\right)$, where v km/h is the average speed of the bus. When the bus travels at 30 km/h, the cost comes out to be ₹ 75 while at 40 km/h, it is ₹ 65. Then the most economical speed (in km/ h) of the bus is : **[Online April 23, 2013]**

(a) 45 (b) 50
(c) 60 (d) 40

53. The maximum area of a right angled triangle with hypotenuse h is : **[Online April 22, 2013]**

(a) $\frac{h^2}{2\sqrt{2}}$ (b) $\frac{h^2}{2}$
(c) $\frac{h^2}{\sqrt{2}}$ (d) $\frac{h^2}{4}$

54. Let $a, b \in R$ be such that the function f given by $f(x) = ln|x| + bx^2 + ax, x \neq 0$ has extreme values at $x = -1$ and $x = 2$

Statement-1 : f has local maximum at $x = -1$ and *at* $x = 2$.

Statement-2 : $a = \frac{1}{2}$ and $b = \frac{-1}{4}$ **[2012]**

(a) Statement-1 is false, Statement-2 is true.
(b) Statement-1 is true, statement-2 is true; statement-2 is a correct explanation for Statement-1.
(c) Statement-1 is true, statement-2 is true; statement-2 is **not** a correct explanation for Statement-1.
(d) Statement-1 is true, statement-2 is false.

55. A line is drawn through the point (1,2) to meet the coordinate axes at P and Q such that it forms a triangle OPQ, where O is the origin. If the area of the triangle OPQ is least, then the slope of the line PQ is : **[2012]**

(a) $-\frac{1}{4}$ (b) -4
(c) -2 (d) $-\frac{1}{2}$

56. Let $f: (-\infty, \infty) \to (-\infty, \infty)$ be defined by $f(x) = x^3 + 1$. **[Online May 26, 2012]**

Statement 1: The function f has a local extremum at $x = 0$

Statement 2: The function f is continuous and differentiable on $(-\infty, \infty)$ and $f'(0) = 0$

(a) Statement 1 is true, Statement 2 is false.
(b) Statement 1 is true, Statement 2 is true, Statement 2 is a correct explanation for Statement 1.
(c) Statement 1 is true, Statement 2 is true, Statement 2 is not the correct explanation for Statement 1.
(d) Statement 1 is false, Statement 2 is true.

57. Let f be a function defined by - **[2011RS]**

$$f(x) = \begin{cases} \frac{\tan x}{x}, & x \neq 0 \\ 1, & x = 0 \end{cases}$$

Statement - 1 : $x = 0$ is point of minima of f

Statement - 2 : $f'(0) = 0$.

(a) Statement-1 is true, statement-2 is true; statement-2 is a correct explanation for statement-1.
(b) Statement-1 is true, statement-2 is true; statement-2 is NOT a correct explanation for statement-1.
(c) Statement-1 is true, statement-2 is false.
(d) Statement-1 is false, statement-2 is true.

58. For $x \in \left(0, \frac{5\pi}{2}\right)$, define $f(x) = \int_0^x \sqrt{t} \sin t \, dt$. Then f has **[2011]**

(a) local minimum at π and 2π
(b) local minimum at π and local maximum at 2π
(c) local maximum at π and local minimum at 2π
(d) local maximum at π and 2π

59. Let f : R $\to$ R be a continuous function defined by

$$f(x) = \frac{1}{e^x + 2e^{-x}}$$ **[2010]**

Statement -1 : $f(c) = \frac{1}{3}$, for some $c \in$ R.

Statement -2 : $0 < f(x) \leq \frac{1}{2\sqrt{2}}$, for all $x \in$ R

(a) Statement -1 is true, Statement -2 is true ; Statement -2 is **not** a correct explanation for Statement -1.
(b) Statement -1 is true, Statement -2 is false.
(c) Statement -1 is false, Statement -2 is true .
(d) Statement - 1 is true, Statement 2 is true ; Statement -2 is a correct explanation for Statement -1.

60. Let f: R $\to$ R be defined by

$$f(x) = \begin{cases} k-2x, & if \ x \leq -1 \\ 2x+3, & if \ x > -1 \end{cases}$$

If f has a local minimum at $x = -1$, then a possible value of k is **[2010]**

(a) 0 (b) $-\frac{1}{2}$
(c) -1 (d) 1

61. Given P(x) = $x^4 + ax^3 + bx^2 + cx + d$ such that $x = 0$ is the only real root of P' (x) = 0. If P(–1) < P(1), then in the interval [–1, 1]: **[2009]**

(a) P(–1) is not minimum but P(1) is the maximum of P
(b) P(–1) is the minimum but P(1) is not the maximum of P
(c) Neither P(–1) is the minimum nor P(1) is the maximum of P
(d) P(–1) is the minimum and P(1) is the maximum of P

62. Suppose the cubic $x^3 - px + q$ has three distinct real roots where $p > 0$ and $q > 0$. Then which one of the following holds? **[2008]**

(a) The cubic has minima at $\sqrt{\frac{p}{3}}$ and maxima at $-\sqrt{\frac{p}{3}}$

(b) The cubic has minima at $-\sqrt{\frac{p}{3}}$ and maxima at $\sqrt{\frac{p}{3}}$

(c) The cubic has minima at both $\sqrt{\frac{p}{3}}$ and $-\sqrt{\frac{p}{3}}$

(d) The cubic has maxima at both $\sqrt{\frac{p}{3}}$ and $-\sqrt{\frac{p}{3}}$

63. The function $f(x)=\frac{x}{2}+\frac{2}{x}$ has a local minimum at **[2006]**

(a) $x=2$ (b) $x=-2$
(c) $x=0$ (d) $x=1$

64. The real number x when added to its inverse gives the minimum value of the sum at x equal to

(a) –2 (b) 2 **[2003]**
(c) 1 (d) –1

65. If the function $f(x)=2x^3-9ax^2+12a^2x+1$, where $a>0$, attains its maximum and minimum at p and q respectively such that $p^2=q$, then a equals **[2003]**

(a) $\frac{1}{2}$ (b) 3
(c) 1 (d) 2

66. The maximum distance from origin of a point on the curve $x=a\sin t-b\sin\left(\frac{at}{b}\right)$, $y=a\cos t-b\cos\left(\frac{at}{b}\right)$, both $a, b>0$ is

(a) $a-b$ (b) $a+b$ **[2002]**
(c) $\sqrt{a^2+b^2}$ (d) $\sqrt{a^2-b^2}$

Hints & Solutions

1. (c) Volume of sphere $V = \frac{4}{3}\pi r^3$ ...(1)

$$\frac{dv}{dt} = \frac{4}{3}.3\pi r^2.\frac{dr}{dt}$$

$$4\pi = 4\pi r^2.\frac{dr}{dt}$$

$$\frac{1}{r^2} = \frac{dr}{dt}$$

Since, V = 288π, therefore from (1), we have

$$288\pi = \frac{4}{3}\pi(r^3) \Rightarrow \frac{288\times 3}{4} = r^3$$

$\Rightarrow 216 = r^3$

$\Rightarrow r = 6$

Hence, $\frac{dr}{dt} = \frac{1}{36}$.

2. (a)

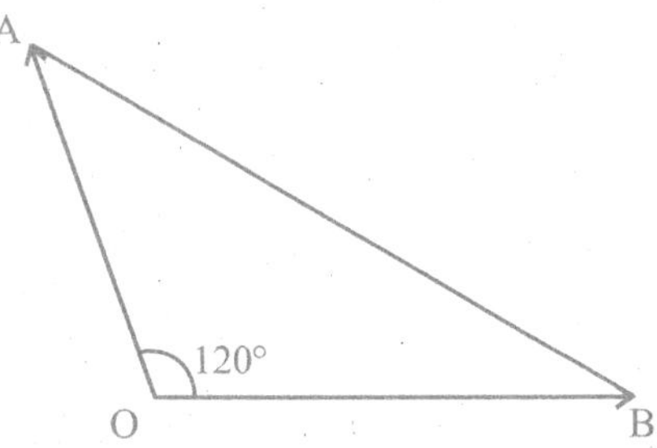

Let OA = x km, OB = y km, AB = R

$(AB)^2 = (OA)^2 + (OB)^2 - 2\,(OA)\,(OB)\cos 120°$

$$R^2 = x^2 + y^2 - 2xy\left(-\frac{1}{2}\right) = x^2 + y^2 + xy \quad ...(1)$$

R at x = 6 km, and y = 8 km

$$R = \sqrt{6^2 + 8^2 + 6\times 8} = 2\sqrt{37}$$

Differentiating equation (1) with respect to t

$$2R\frac{dR}{dt} = 2x\frac{dx}{dt} + 2y\frac{dy}{dt} + \left(x\frac{dy}{dt} + y\frac{dx}{dt}\right)$$

$$= \frac{1}{2R}[2\times 8\times 20 + 2\times 6\times 30 + (8\times 30 + 6\times 20)]$$

$$\frac{dR}{dt} = \frac{1}{2\times 2\sqrt{37}}[1040] = \frac{260}{\sqrt{37}}$$

3. (a) Volume of sphere $V = \frac{4}{3}\pi r^3$

$$\frac{dV}{dt} = \frac{4}{3}.\pi.3r^2.\frac{dr}{dt}$$

$$35 = 4\pi r^2.\frac{dr}{dt} \text{ or } \frac{dr}{dt} = \frac{35}{4\pi r^2} \quad ...(1)$$

Surface area of sphere = S = $4\pi r^2$

$$\frac{dS}{dt} = 4\pi\times 2r\times\frac{dr}{dt} = 8\pi r.\frac{dr}{dt}$$

$$\frac{dS}{dt} = \frac{70}{r} \quad \text{(By using (1))}$$

Now, diameter = 14 cm, $r = 7$

$$\therefore \frac{dS}{dt} = 10$$

4. (d) $V = \frac{4}{3}\pi r^3 \Rightarrow \frac{dV}{dt} = 4\pi r^2.\frac{dr}{dt}$ ...(i)

$$S = 4\pi r^2 \Rightarrow \frac{dS}{dt} = 8\pi r.\frac{dr}{dt}$$

$$\Rightarrow 8 = 8\pi r\frac{dr}{dt} \Rightarrow \frac{dr}{dt} = \frac{1}{\pi r}$$

Putting the value of $\frac{dr}{dt}$ in (i), we get

$$\frac{dV}{dt} = 4\pi r^2\times\frac{1}{\pi r} = 4r$$

$\Rightarrow \frac{dV}{dt}$ is proportional to r.

5. (c) Volume of spherical balloon

$$= V = \frac{4}{3}\pi r^3$$

$$\Rightarrow 4500\pi = \frac{4\pi r^3}{3}$$

($\because$ Given, volume = $4500\pi m^3$)

Differentiate both the side, w.r.t 't' we get,

$$\frac{dV}{dt} = 4\pi r^2\left(\frac{dr}{dt}\right)$$

Now, it is given that $\frac{dV}{dt} = 72\pi$

$\therefore$ After 49 min,

Volume = $(4500 - 49\times 72)\pi$

$= (4500 - 3528)\pi = 972\pi\, m^3$

$\Rightarrow \quad V = 972\pi m^3$

$\therefore\ 972\pi = \frac{4}{3}\pi r^3$

$\Rightarrow \quad r^3 = 3 \times 243 = 3 \times 3^5 = 3^6 = (3^2)^3$

$\Rightarrow \quad r = 9$

Also, we have $\frac{dV}{dt} = 72\pi$

$\therefore \quad 72\pi = 4\pi \times 9 \times 9\left(\frac{dr}{dt}\right) \Rightarrow \frac{dr}{dt} = \left(\frac{2}{9}\right)$

6. (b) Let $A = \pi r^2$ be area of metalic circular plate of $r = 50$ cm.

Also, given $\frac{dr}{dt} = 1\text{mm} = \frac{1}{10}\text{cm}$

$\therefore A = \pi r^2$

$\Rightarrow \quad \frac{dA}{dt} = 2\pi r\frac{dr}{dt} = 2\pi.50.\frac{1}{10} = 10\pi$

Hence, area of plate increases in 10π cm²/hour.

7. (c) Let W = nw

$\Rightarrow \quad \frac{dW}{dt} = n\frac{dw}{dt} + w.\frac{dn}{dt}$ ...(1)

Given : $w = t^2 - t + 2$ and $n = 2t^2 + 3$

$\Rightarrow \quad \frac{dw}{dt} = 2t - 1$ and $\frac{dn}{dt} = 4t$

$\therefore$ Equation (1)

$\Rightarrow \frac{dw}{dt} = (2t^2 + 3)(2t - 1) + (t^2 - t + 2)(4t)$

Thus, $\left.\frac{dW}{dt}\right|_{t=1} = (2 + 3)(2 - 1) + (2)(4)$

$= 5(1) + 8 = 13$

8. (d) Let A be the area, b be the breadth and ℓ be the length of the rectangle.

Given : $\frac{dA}{dt} = -5,\ \frac{d\ell}{dt} = 2,\ \frac{db}{dt} = -3$

We know, $A = \ell \times b$

$\Rightarrow \quad \frac{dA}{dt} = \ell.\frac{db}{dt} + b.\frac{d\ell}{dt} = -3\ell + 2b$

$\Rightarrow -5 = -3\ell + 2b.$

When $b = 2$, we have

$-5 = -3\ell + 4 \Rightarrow \ell = \frac{9}{3} = 3m$

9. (b) Let $A = \pi r^2$.

$\frac{dA}{dt} = 2\pi r.\frac{dr}{dt}$

$6\pi = 2\pi(30).\frac{dr}{dt}$

$\Rightarrow \quad \frac{3}{30} = \frac{dr}{dt} \Rightarrow \frac{dr}{dt} = \frac{1}{10} = 0.1$

Thus, the rate at which the radius of the circular sheet increases is 0.1

10. (d)

A: u=0, f, t+m, s+n → v

B: u=0, f′, t, s → v

As per question if point B moves s distance in t time then point A moves $(s + n)$ distance in time $(t + m)$ after which both have same velocity v.

Then using equation $v = u + at$ we get

$v = f(t+m) = f't \Rightarrow t = \frac{f\,m}{f'-f}$ ....(1)

Using equation $v^2 = u^2 + 2$, as we get

$v^2 = 2f(s+n) = 2f's \quad \Rightarrow s = \frac{f\,n}{f'-f}$ ....(2)

Also for point B using the eqn $s = ut + \frac{1}{2}at^2$, we get

$s = \frac{1}{2}f't^2$

Substituting values of t and s from equations (1) and (2) in the above relation, we get

$\frac{f\,n}{f'-f} = \frac{1}{2}f'\frac{f^2m^2}{(f'-f)^2}$

$\Rightarrow (f'-f)n = \frac{1}{2}ff'm^2$

11. (c) Let the lizard catches the insect after time t then distance covered by lizard = 21cm + distance covered by insect

$\Rightarrow \frac{1}{2}ft^2 = 4 \times t + 21$

$\Rightarrow \frac{1}{2} \times 2 \times t^2 = 20 \times t + 21$

$\Rightarrow t^2 - 20t - 21 = 0$

$\Rightarrow t = 21$ sec

12. (b) Given that

$\frac{dv}{dt} = 50$ cm³/min $\Rightarrow \frac{d}{dt}\left(\frac{4}{3}\pi r^3\right) = 50$

$\Rightarrow \quad 4\pi r^2\frac{dr}{dt} = 50$

$\Rightarrow \quad \frac{dr}{dt} = \frac{50}{4\pi(15)^2} = \frac{1}{18\pi}$ cm/min

(here $r = 10+5$)

13. (a) $y^2 = 18x \Rightarrow 2y\frac{dy}{dx} = 18 \Rightarrow \frac{dy}{dx} = \frac{9}{y}$

Given $\frac{dy}{dx} = 2 \Rightarrow \frac{9}{y} = 2 \Rightarrow y = \frac{9}{2}$

Putting in $y^2 = 18x \Rightarrow x = \frac{9}{8}$

$\therefore$ Required point is $\left(\frac{9}{8}, \frac{9}{2}\right)$

14. (a) $f(x) = x^3 - 3x^2 + 5x + 7$

For increasing

$f'(x) = 3x^2 - 6x + 5 > 0$

$\Rightarrow x \in R$

For decreasing

$f'(x) = 3x^2 - 6x + 5 < 0$

15. (c) $f(x) = \sin^4 x + \cos^4 x$

$f'(x) = 4\sin^3 x \cos x + 4\cos^3 x(-\sin x)$

$= 4\sin x \cos x (\sin^2 x - \cos^2 x)$

$= -2\sin 2x \cos 2x$

$= -\sin 4x$

$f(x)$ is increasing when $f'(x) > 0$

$\Rightarrow -\sin 4x > 0$

$\Rightarrow \sin 4x < 0$

$\Rightarrow x \in \left(\frac{\pi}{4}, \frac{\pi}{2}\right]$

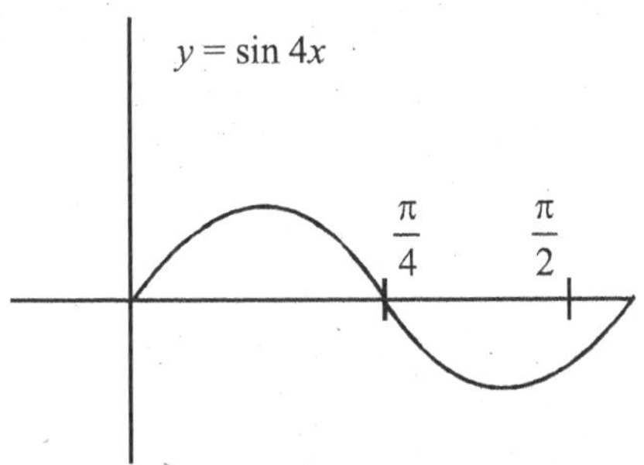

16. (b) Since $f'(x) > 0$ and $g'(x) < 0$, therefore $f(x)$ is increasing function and $g(x)$ is decreasing function.

$\Rightarrow f(x+1) > f(x)$ and $g(x+1) < g(x)$

$\Rightarrow g[f(x+1)] < g[f(x)]$ and $f[g(x+1)] < f[g(x)]$

Hence option (b) is correct.

17. (d) $f(x) = 2x^3 + 3x + k$

$f'(x) = 6x^2 + 3 > 0 \ \forall x \in R \quad (\because \ x^2 > 0)$

$\Rightarrow f(x)$ is strictly increasing function

$\Rightarrow f(x) = 0$ has only one real root, so two roots are not possible.

18. (c) Let $y = x^2 . e^{-x}$

For increasing function,

$\frac{dy}{dx} > 0 \Rightarrow x[(2-x)e^{-x}] > 0$

$\because x > 0, \therefore (2-x)e^{-x} > 0$

$\Rightarrow (2-x)\frac{1}{e^x} > 0$

For $0 < x < 2$, $(2-x) < 0$

$\therefore \frac{1}{e^x} < 0$, but it is not possible

Hence the statement-2 is false.

19. (a) $f(x) = x\log x, f(1) = 0, f(2) = 4$

$g(x) = 2 - x, g(1) = 1, g(2) = 0$

$\log 10 > \log 4 \Rightarrow 1 > \log 4$

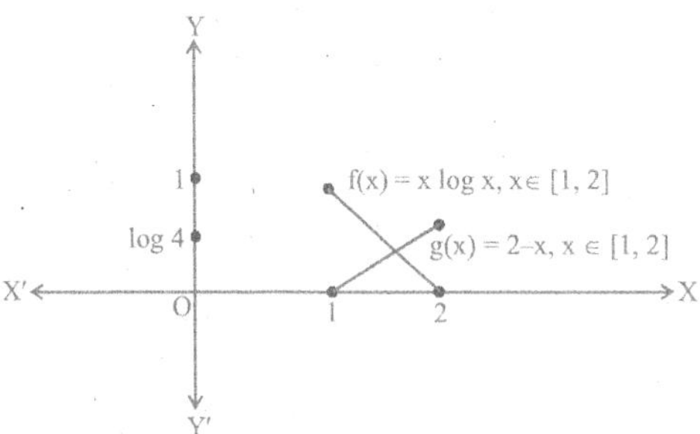

Thus statement -1 and 2 both are true and statement-2 is a correct explanation of statement 1.

20. (c) $f(x) = xe^{x(1-x)}, x \in R$

$f'(x) = e^{x(1-x)}.\left[1 + x - 2x^2\right]$

$= -e^{x(1-x)}.\left[2x^2 - x - 1\right] = -2e^{x(1-x)}.\left[\left(x+\frac{1}{2}\right)(x-1)\right]$

$f'(x) = -2e^{x(1-x)}.A$

where $A = \left(x + \frac{1}{2}\right)(x-1)$

Now, exponential function is always +ve and $f'(x)$ will be opposite to the sign of A which is –ve in $\left[-\frac{1}{2}, 1\right]$

Hence, $f'(x)$ is +ve in $\left[-\frac{1}{2}, 1\right]$

$\therefore f(x)$ is increasing on $\left[-\frac{1}{2}, 1\right]$

21. (b) Given that $f(x) = x^3 + 5x + 1$

$\therefore f'(x) = 3x^2 + 5 > 0, \quad \forall x \in R$

$\Rightarrow f(x)$ is strictly increasing on R

$\Rightarrow f(x)$ is one one

$\therefore$ Being a polynomial $f(x)$ is continuous and increasing.

on R with $\lim\limits_{x \to \infty} f(x) = -\infty$

and $\lim\limits_{x \to \infty} f(x) = \infty$

$\therefore$ Range of $f = (-\infty, \infty) = R$

Hence f is onto also. So, f is one one and onto R.

22. **(b)** Let $f(x) = x^7 + 14x^5 + 16x^3 + 30x - 560$

$\Rightarrow f'(x) = 7x^6 + 70x^4 + 48x^2 + 30 > 0, \forall\ x \in R$

$\Rightarrow f$ is an increasing function on R

Also $\lim_{x\to\infty} f(x) = \infty$ and $\lim_{x\to-\infty} f(x) = -\infty$

$\Rightarrow$ The curve $y = f(x)$ crosses x-axis only once.

$\therefore f(x) = 0$ has exactly one real root.

23. **(d)** Given $f(x) = \tan^{-1}(\sin x + \cos x)$

$$f'(x) = \frac{1}{1 + (\sin x + \cos x)^2}.(\cos x - \sin x)$$

$$= \frac{\sqrt{2}.\left(\frac{1}{\sqrt{2}}\cos x - \frac{1}{\sqrt{2}}\sin x\right)}{1 + (\sin x + \cos x)^2}$$

$$= \frac{\left(\cos\frac{\pi}{4}.\cos x - \sin\frac{\pi}{4}.\sin x\right)}{1 + (\sin x + \cos x)^2}$$

$$\therefore \quad f'(x) = \frac{\sqrt{2}\cos\left(x + \frac{\pi}{4}\right)}{1 + (\sin x + \cos x)^2}$$

if $f'(x) > 0$ then $f(x)$ is increasing function.

Hence $f(x)$ is increasing, if $-\frac{\pi}{2} < x + \frac{\pi}{4} < \frac{\pi}{2}$

$\Rightarrow \ -\frac{3\pi}{4} < x < \frac{\pi}{4}$

Hence, $f(x)$ is increasing when $n \in \left(-\frac{\pi}{2}, \frac{\pi}{4}\right)$

24. **(c)** Clearly function $f(x) = 3x^2 - 2x + 1$ is increasing when

$f'(x) = 6x - 2 \geq 0$

$\Rightarrow \quad x \in [1/3, \infty)$

$\therefore f(x)$ is incorrectly matched with $\left(-\infty, \frac{1}{3}\right]$

25. **(c)** We have $y = \dfrac{x+6}{(x-2)(x-3)}$

At y-axis, $x = 0 \Rightarrow y = 1$

On differentiating, we get

$$\frac{dy}{dx} = \frac{(x^2 - 5x + 6)(1) - (x+6)(2x-5)}{(x^2 - 5x + 6)^2}$$

$\dfrac{dy}{dx} = 1$ at point (0, 1)

$\therefore$ Slope of normal $= -1$

Now equation of normal is $y - 1 = -1(x - 0)$

$\Rightarrow y - 1 = -x$

$x + y = 1$

$\therefore \left(\frac{1}{2}, \frac{1}{2}\right)$ satisfy it.

26. **(c)** Eccentricity of ellipse $= \frac{1}{2}$

Now, $-\frac{a}{e} = -4 \Rightarrow a = 4 \times \frac{1}{2} = 2 \Rightarrow a = 2$

We have $b^2 = a^2(1 - e^2) = a^2\left(1 - \frac{1}{4}\right) = 4 \times \frac{3}{4} = 3$

$\therefore$ Equation of ellipse is

$$\frac{x^2}{4} + \frac{y^2}{3} = 1$$

Now differentiating, we get

$\Rightarrow \frac{x}{2} + \frac{2y}{3} \times y' = 0 \Rightarrow y' = -\frac{3x}{4y}$

$y'\Big|_{(1,3/2)} = -\frac{3}{4} \times \frac{2}{3} = -\frac{1}{2}$

Slope of normal $= 2$

$\therefore$ Equation of normal at $\left(1, \frac{3}{2}\right)$ is

$y - \frac{3}{2} = 2(x - 1) \Rightarrow 2y - 3 = 4x - 4$

$\therefore 4x - 2y = 1$

27. **(c)**

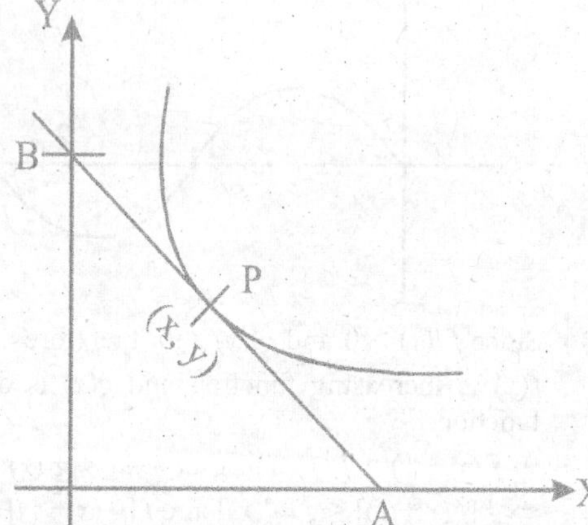

Let $y = f(x)$ be a curve

slope of tangent $= f'(x)$

Equation of tangent $(Y - y) = f'(x)(X - x)$

Put $Y = 0$

$\Rightarrow \quad X = \left(x - \frac{y}{f'(x)}\right)$

Put $X = 0$

$\Rightarrow \quad Y = y - x f'(x)$

$\Rightarrow \quad A = \left(x - \frac{y}{f'(x)}, 0\right)$

and $B = (0, y - x f'(x))$

$\therefore \quad AP : PB = 1 : 3$

$\Rightarrow \quad x = \frac{3}{4}\left(x - \frac{y}{f'(x)}\right)$

$\Rightarrow \quad x = \frac{-3y}{f'(x)}$

$\Rightarrow \quad \frac{dy}{dx} = \frac{-3y}{x}$

$\frac{dy}{y} = \frac{-3\,dx}{x}$

$\Rightarrow \quad y = \frac{C}{x^3}$

$\because \quad f(a) = 1$

$\Rightarrow \quad C = 1$

$\therefore \quad y = \frac{1}{x^3}$ is required curve

and $\left(2, \frac{1}{8}\right)$ passing through

$y = \frac{1}{x^3}$

28. (d)

$x^2y^2 - 2x = 4 - 4y$

Differentiate w.r.t. 'x'

$2xy^2 + 2y \,.\, x^2 \,.\, \frac{dy}{dx} - 2 = -4 \,.\, \frac{dy}{dx}$

$\Rightarrow \quad \frac{dy}{dx}(2y \,.\, x^2 + 4) = 2 - 2x \,.\, y^2$

$\Rightarrow \quad \left.\frac{dy}{dx}\right|_{2,-2} = \frac{2 - 2 \times 2 \times 4}{2(-2) \times 4 + 4} = \frac{-14}{-12} = \frac{7}{6}$

$\therefore$ Equation of tangent is

$(y + 2) = \frac{7}{6}(x - 2)$ *or* $7x - 6y = 26$

$\therefore \quad$ (–2, –7) does not passes through the required tangent.

29. (d) $f(x) = \tan^{-1}\left(\sqrt{\frac{1 + \sin x}{1 - \sin x}}\right)$

$= \tan^{-1}\left(\sqrt{\frac{\left(\sin\frac{x}{2} + \cos\frac{x}{2}\right)^2}{\left(\sin\frac{x}{x} - \cos\frac{x}{2}\right)^2}}\right) = \tan^{-1}\left(\frac{1 + \tan\frac{x}{2}}{1 - \tan\frac{x}{2}}\right)$

$= \tan^{-1}\left(\tan\left(\frac{\pi}{4} + \frac{x}{2}\right)\right)$

$\Rightarrow \quad y = \frac{\pi}{4} + \frac{x}{2}$

$\Rightarrow \quad \frac{dy}{dx} = \frac{1}{2}$

Slope of normal $= \frac{-1}{\left(\frac{dy}{dx}\right)} = -2$

At $\left(\frac{\pi}{6}, \frac{\pi}{4} + \frac{\pi}{12}\right)$

$y - \left(\frac{\pi}{4} + \frac{\pi}{12}\right) = -2\left(x - \frac{\pi}{6}\right)$

$y - \frac{4\pi}{12} = -2x + \frac{2\pi}{6}$

$y - \frac{\pi}{3} = -2x + \frac{\pi}{3}$

$y = -2x + \frac{2\pi}{3}$

This equation is satisfied only by the point $\left(0, \frac{2\pi}{3}\right)$

30. (a) $\frac{dy}{dx} = \frac{1}{2\sqrt{4x - 3}} \times 4 = \frac{2}{3}$

$\Rightarrow \quad 4x - 3 = 9$

$\Rightarrow \quad x = 3$

So, $y = 4$

Equation of normal at $P(3, 4)$ is

$y - 4 = -\frac{3}{2}(x - 3)$

i.e. $2y - 8 = -3x + 9$

$\Rightarrow \quad 3x + 2y - 17 = 0$

This line is satisfied by the point (1, 7)

31. (d) $P(4t^2 + 3, 8t^3 - 1)$

$\frac{dy/dt}{dt/dt} = \frac{dy}{dx} = 3t$ (slope of tangent at P)

Let $Q = (4\lambda^2 + 3, 8\lambda^3 - 1)$

slope of PQ $= 3t$

$\frac{8t^3 - 8\lambda^3}{4t^2 - 4\lambda^2} = 3t$

$\Rightarrow \quad t^3 - 3\lambda^2 t + 2\lambda^3 = 0$

$(t - \lambda) \,.\, (t^2 + t\lambda - 2\lambda^2) = 0$

$(t - \lambda)^2 \,.\, (t + 2\lambda) = 0$

$t = \lambda$ (or) $\lambda = \frac{-t}{2}$

$\therefore \quad Q\,[t^2 + 3, -t^3 - 1]$.

32. (b) Given curve is

$x^2+2xy-3y^2=0$ ...(a)

Differentiate w.r.t. x, $2x+2x\frac{dy}{dx}+2y-6y\frac{dy}{dx}=0$

$\left(\frac{dy}{dx}\right)_{(1,1)}=1$

Equation of normal at (1, 1) is

$y=2-x$ ...(b)

Solving eq. (a) and (b), we get

$x=1,3$

Point of intersection (1, 1), (3, –1)

Normal cuts the curve again in 4th quadrant.

33. (b) Given curve is $\sin y = x\sin\left(\frac{\pi}{3}+y\right)$

Diff with respect to x, we get

$\cos y\frac{dy}{dx}=\sin\left(\frac{\pi}{3}+y\right)+x\cos\left(\frac{\pi}{3}+y\right)\frac{dy}{dx}$

$\Rightarrow \frac{dy}{dx}=\frac{\sin\left(\frac{\pi}{3}+y\right)}{\cos y - x\cos\left(\frac{\pi}{3}+y\right)}$

$\frac{dy}{dx}$ at $(0, 0)=\frac{\sqrt{3}}{2}$

$\Rightarrow$ Equation of normal is $y-0$

$=-\frac{2}{\sqrt{3}}(x-0)$

$\Rightarrow 2x+\sqrt{3}\,y=0$

34. (d) $x^2-y+6=0$

$2x-\frac{dy}{dx}=0\Rightarrow\frac{dy}{dx}=2x$

$\left.\frac{dy}{dx}\right|_{(x,y)=(2,10)}=4$

equation of tangent

$y-10=4(x-z)$

$4x-y+z=0$

tangent passes through (α,β)

$4\alpha-\beta+z=0\Rightarrow\beta=4\alpha+z$ ...(a)

and $2x+2yy'+8-2y'=0$

$y'=\frac{2x+8}{2-2y}=\frac{2\alpha+8}{2-2\beta}=4$ ...(b)

from (a) and (b)

$\alpha=\frac{-8}{17},\beta=\frac{2}{17}$

$\left(\frac{-8}{17},\frac{2}{17}\right)$

35. (a) Given that

$x=2\cos t+2t\sin t$

so, $\frac{dx}{dt}=-2\sin t+2[t\cos t+\sin t]$

$\frac{dy}{dt}=2\cos t-2[-t\sin t+\cos t]$

$\frac{dy}{dx}=2t\sin t$ ...(ii)

$\frac{dy}{dx}=\frac{2t\sin t}{2t\cos t}$

$\frac{dy}{dx}=\tan t$

$\left(\frac{dy}{dx}\right)_{t=\pi/4}=1$

so the slope of the normal is – 1

At $t=\pi/4\ x=\sqrt{2}+\frac{\pi}{2\sqrt{2}}$ and

$y=\sqrt{2}-\pi/2\sqrt{2}$

the equation of normal is

$\left[y-\left(\sqrt{2}-\pi/2\sqrt{2}\right)\right]=-1\left[\left(x-\left(\sqrt{2}+\pi/2\sqrt{2}\right)\right)\right]$

$y-\sqrt{2}+\frac{\pi}{2\sqrt{2}}=-x+\sqrt{2}+\pi/2\sqrt{2}$

$x+y=2\sqrt{2}$ so the distance from the origin is 2

36. (c) Given, $y=3\sin\theta.\cos\theta$

$\frac{dy}{d\theta}=3[\sin\theta(-\sin\theta)+\cos\theta(\cos\theta)]$

$\frac{dy}{d\theta}=3[\cos^2\theta-\sin^2\theta]=3\cos 2\theta$ ...(1)

and $x=e^{\theta}\sin\theta$

$\frac{dx}{d\theta}=e^{\theta}\cos\theta+\sin\theta\,e^{\theta}$

$\frac{dx}{d\theta}=e^{\theta}(\sin\theta+\cos\theta)$ ...(2)

Dividing (1) by (2)

$\frac{dy}{dx}=\frac{3\cos 2\theta}{e^{\theta}(\sin\theta+\cos\theta)}=\frac{3(\cos^2\theta-\sin^2\theta)}{e^{\theta}(\sin\theta+\cos\theta)}$

$\frac{dy}{dx}=\frac{3(\cos\theta+\sin\theta)(\cos\theta-\sin\theta)}{e^{\theta}(\sin\theta+\cos\theta)}$

$\frac{dy}{dx}=\frac{3(\cos\theta-\sin\theta)}{e^{\theta}}$

Given tangent is parallel to x-axis then $\frac{dy}{dx} = 0$

$0 = \frac{3(\cos\theta - \sin\theta)}{e^{\theta}}$

or $\cos\theta - \sin\theta = 0 \Rightarrow \cos\theta = \sin\theta$

$\Rightarrow \tan\theta = 1 \Rightarrow \tan\theta = \frac{\tan\pi}{4} \Rightarrow \theta = \frac{\pi}{4}$

37. **(d)** Let $y = \cos(x+y)$

$\Rightarrow \frac{dy}{dx} = -\sin(x+y)\left(1+\frac{dy}{dx}\right)$ ...(1)

Now, given equation of tangent is
$x + 2y = k$

$\Rightarrow \text{Slope} = \frac{-1}{2}$

So, $\frac{dy}{dx} = \frac{-1}{2}$ put this value in (1), we get

$\frac{-1}{2} = -\sin(x+y)\left(1-\frac{1}{2}\right)$

$\Rightarrow \sin(x+y) = 1$

$\Rightarrow x + y = \frac{\pi}{2} \Rightarrow y = \frac{\pi}{2} - x$

Now, $\frac{\pi}{2} - x = \cos(x+y)$

$\Rightarrow x = \frac{\pi}{2}$ and $y = 0$

Thus $x + 2y = k \Rightarrow \frac{\pi}{2} = k$

38. **(d)** $x^2 = 8y$ ...(i)
When, $x = 4$, then $y = 2$

Now $\frac{dy}{dx} = \frac{2x}{8} = \frac{x}{4}, \left.\frac{dy}{dx}\right]_{x=4} = 1$

Slope of normal $= -\frac{1}{\frac{dy}{dx}} = -1$

Euqation of normal at $x = 4$ is
$y - 2 = -1(x-4)$
$\Rightarrow y = -x + 4 + 2 = -x + 6$
$\Rightarrow x + y = 6$

39. **(c)** Since tangent is parallel to x-axis,

$\therefore \frac{dy}{dx} = 0 \Rightarrow 1 - \frac{8}{x^3} = 0 \Rightarrow x = 2 \Rightarrow y = 3$

Equation of tangent is $y - 3 = 0(x-2)$
$\Rightarrow y = 3$

40. **(b)** $\frac{dy}{dx} = 2x - 5 \therefore m_1 = (2x-5)_{(2,0)} = -1$,

$m_2 = (2x-5)_{(3,0)} = 1 \Rightarrow m_1 m_2 = -1$

i.e. the tangents are perpendicular to each other.

41. **(d)** $x = a(\cos\theta + \theta\sin\theta)$

$\Rightarrow \frac{dx}{d\theta} = a(-\sin\theta + \sin\theta + \theta\cos\theta)$

$\Rightarrow \frac{dx}{d\theta} = a\theta\cos\theta$ .....(1)

$y = a(\sin\theta - \theta\cos\theta)$

$\frac{dy}{d\theta} = a[\cos\theta - \cos\theta + \theta\sin\theta]$

$\Rightarrow \frac{dy}{d\theta} = a\theta\sin\theta$ .....(2)

From equations (1) and (2) we get

$\frac{dy}{dx} = \tan\theta \Rightarrow$ Slope of normal $= -\cot\theta$

Equation of normal at 'θ' is $y - a(\sin\theta - \theta\cos\theta)$
$= -\cot\theta\ (x - a(\cos\theta + \theta\sin\theta))$

$\Rightarrow y\sin\theta - a\sin^2\theta + a\theta\cos\theta\sin\theta$

$= -x\cos\theta + a\cos^2\theta + a\theta\sin\theta\cos\theta$

$\Rightarrow x\cos\theta + y\sin\theta = a$

Clearly this is an equation of straight line which is at a constant distance 'a' from origin.

42. **(d)** $\frac{dx}{d\theta} = -a\sin\theta$ and $\frac{dy}{d\theta} = a\cos\theta$

$\therefore \frac{dy}{dx} = -\cot\theta.$

$\therefore$ The slope of the normal at $\theta = \tan\theta$
$\therefore$ The equation of the normal at θ is

$y - a\sin\theta = \tan\theta(x - a - a\cos\theta)$

$\Rightarrow y\cos\theta - a\sin\theta\cos\theta = x\sin\theta - a\sin\theta - a\sin\theta\cos\theta$

$\Rightarrow x\sin\theta - y\cos\theta = a\sin\theta$
$\Rightarrow y = (x-a)\tan\theta$
which always passes through $(a, 0)$

43. **(b)** $f''(x) = 6(x-1)$. Inegrating, we get

$f'(x) = 3x^2 - 6x + c$

Slope at $(2, 1) = f'(2) = c = 3$
[$\because$ slope of tangent at (2,1) is 3]

$\therefore f'(x) = 3x^2 - 6x + 3 = 3(x-1)^2$

Inegrating again, we get $f(x) = (x-1)^3 + D$

The curve passes through (2, 1)

$\Rightarrow 1=(2-1)^3+D \Rightarrow D=0$

$\therefore f(x)=(x-1)^3$

44. (d) We have

Total length $= r+r+r\theta=20$

$\Rightarrow 2r+r\theta=20$

$\Rightarrow \theta=\dfrac{20-2r}{r}$ ...(a)

$A=\text{Area}=\dfrac{\theta}{2\pi}\times\pi r^2=\dfrac{1}{2}r^2\theta=\dfrac{1}{2}r^2\left(\dfrac{20-2r}{r}\right)$

$A=10r-r^2$

For A to be maximum

$\dfrac{dA}{dr}=0 \Rightarrow 10-2r=0$

$\Rightarrow r=5$

$\dfrac{d^2A}{dr^2}=-2<0$

$\therefore$ For $r=5$ A is maximum

From (a)

$\theta=\dfrac{20-2(5)}{5}=\dfrac{10}{5}=2$

$A=\dfrac{2}{2\pi}\times\pi(5)^2=25$ sq. m.

45. (a) $4x+2\pi r=2 \Rightarrow 2x+\pi r=1$

$S=x^2+\pi r^2$

$S=\left(\dfrac{1-\pi r}{2}\right)^2+\pi r^2$

$\dfrac{dS}{dr}=2\left(\dfrac{1-\pi r}{2}\right)\left(\dfrac{-\pi}{2}\right)+2\pi r$

$\Rightarrow \dfrac{-\pi}{2}+\dfrac{\pi^2 r}{2}+2\pi r=0 \Rightarrow r=\dfrac{1}{\pi+4}$

$\Rightarrow x=\dfrac{2}{\pi+4} \Rightarrow x=2r$

46. (a) $D=\sqrt{\alpha^2+(\alpha^2-4)^2}$

$D^2=\alpha^2+\alpha^4+16-8\alpha^2$

$=\alpha^4-7\alpha^2+16$

$\dfrac{dD^2}{d\alpha}=4\alpha^3-14\alpha=0$

$2\alpha(2\alpha^2-7)=0$

$\alpha^2=\dfrac{7}{2}$

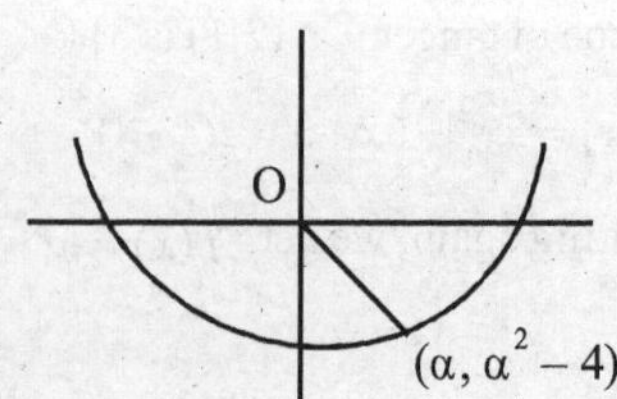

$D^2=\dfrac{49}{4}-\dfrac{49}{2}+16=-\dfrac{49}{4}+16=\dfrac{15}{4}$

$D=\dfrac{\sqrt{15}}{2}$

47. (a) Let $f(x)=\dfrac{(1+x)^{\frac{3}{5}}}{1+x^{\frac{3}{5}}}$ and $x\in[0,1]$

$\Rightarrow f'(x)=\dfrac{(1+x^{\frac{3}{5}})\frac{3}{5}(1+x)^{-\frac{2}{5}}-\frac{3}{5}(1+x)^{\frac{3}{5}}(x^{\frac{-2}{5}})}{(1+x^{\frac{3}{5}})^2}$

$=\dfrac{3}{5}\left[\left(1+x^{\frac{3}{5}}\right)(1+x)^{-\frac{2}{5}}-(1+x)^{\frac{3}{5}}x^{\frac{-2}{5}}\right]$

$=\dfrac{3}{5}\left[\dfrac{1+x^{\frac{3}{5}}}{(1+x)^{\frac{2}{5}}}-\dfrac{(1+x)^{\frac{3}{5}}}{x^{\frac{2}{5}}}\right]$

$=\dfrac{x^{\frac{2}{5}}+x-1-x}{x^{\frac{2}{5}}(1+x)^{\frac{2}{5}}}=\dfrac{x^{\frac{2}{5}}-1}{x^{\frac{2}{5}}(1+x)^{\frac{2}{5}}}<0$

Also, $f(0)=1 \Rightarrow f(x)\in[2^{-0.4}, 1]$

$f(a)=2^{-0.4}$

48. (d) Let 'u' be the velocity

$\therefore u=48$ m/s, Given, $g=32$

At maximum height $v=0$

Now, we know $v^2=u^2-2gh$

$\Rightarrow 0=(48)^2-2(32)h \Rightarrow h=36$

Maximum height $=36+64=100$ mt

49. (a) Let $f(x)=\alpha\log|x|+\beta x^2+x$

Differentiate both side,

$f'(x)=\dfrac{\alpha}{x}+2\beta x+1$

Since $x=-1$ and $x=2$ are extreme points therefore $f'(x)=0$ at these points.

Put $x=-1$ and $x=2$ in $f'(x)$, we get

$-\alpha-2\beta+1=0 \Rightarrow \alpha+2\beta=1$ ...(i)

$\dfrac{\alpha}{2}+4\beta+1=0 \Rightarrow \alpha+8\beta=-2$ ...(ii)

On solving (i) and (ii), we get

$6\beta=-3 \Rightarrow \beta=-\dfrac{1}{2}$ $\therefore \alpha=2$

50. (d)

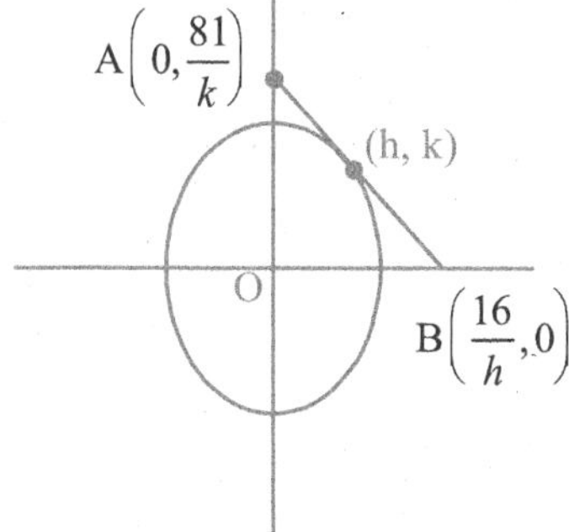

Let (h, k) be the point on ellipse through which tangent is passing.

Equation of tangent at (h, k) = $\frac{xh}{16} + \frac{yk}{81} = 1$

at $y = 0$, $x = \frac{16}{h}$

at $x = 0$, $y = \frac{81}{k}$

Area of AOB = $\frac{1}{2} \times \left(\frac{16}{h}\right) \times \left(\frac{81}{k}\right) = \frac{648}{hk}$

$$A^2 = \frac{(648)^2}{h^2k^2} \quad ...(1)$$

(h, k) must satisfy equation of ellipse

$$\frac{h^2}{16} + \frac{k^2}{81} = 1$$

$$h^2 = \frac{16}{81}(81 - k^2)$$

Putting value of h^2 in equation (1)

$$A^2 = \frac{81(648)^2}{16 \times k^2(81 - k^2)} = \frac{\alpha}{81k^2 - k^4}$$

differentiating w.r. to k

$$2AA' = \alpha\left(\frac{-1}{81k^2 - k^4}\right)(162k - 4k^3)$$

$2AA' = -2A\,(81k - 4k^3) \Rightarrow A' = -81k - 4k^3$

Put $A' = 0$

$\Rightarrow$ $162k - 4k^3 = 0$, $k\,(162 - 4k^2) = 0$

$\Rightarrow$ $k = 0$, $k = \pm\frac{9}{\sqrt{2}}$

$A'' = -(81 - 12k^2)$

For both value of k, $A'' = 405 > 0$

Area will be minimum for $k = \pm\frac{9}{\sqrt{2}}$

$$h^2 = \frac{16}{81}(81 - k^2) = 8$$

$$h = \pm 2\sqrt{2}$$

Area of triangle AOB = $\frac{648 \times \sqrt{2}}{2\sqrt{2} \times 9}$ = 36 sq unit

51. (c) Given, radius of sphere = $\sqrt{3}$

Now, In ΔOAB, by Pythagoras theorem

$(OA)^2 = (OB)^2 + (AB)^2$

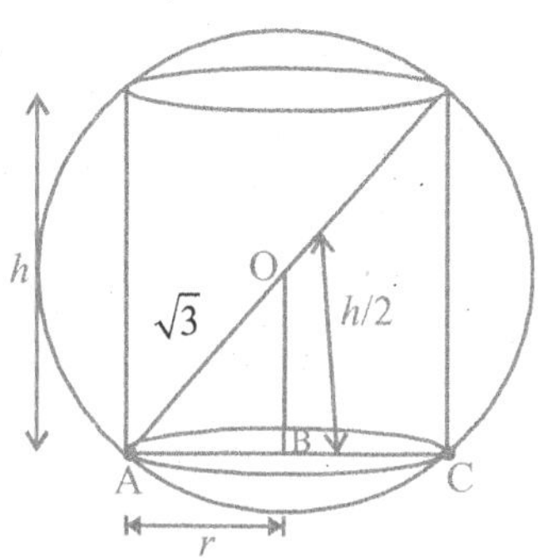

$$(\sqrt{3})^2 = \left(\frac{h}{2}\right)^2 + r^2$$

$$3 = \frac{h^2}{4} + r^2 \Rightarrow \boxed{r^2 = 3 - \frac{h^2}{4}} \quad ...(1)$$

Now, volume of cylinder = $\pi r^2 h$

$$V = \pi\left(3 - \frac{h^2}{4}\right)h \quad \text{(using eq. (1))}$$

$$V = 3\pi h - \frac{\pi h^3}{4} \quad ...(2)$$

Now, for largest possible right circular cylinder the volume must be maximum

$\therefore$ For maximum volume, $\frac{dV}{dh} = 0$

Now, Differentiating eq. (2) w.r.t. h

$$\frac{dV}{dh} = 3\pi - \frac{3}{4}\pi h^2$$

or $3\pi - \frac{3}{4}\pi h^2 = 0 \Rightarrow 3\pi = \frac{3}{4}\pi h^2$

$\Rightarrow h^2 = 4 \Rightarrow h = 2$

Now, volume (V) of the cylinder

$$= \pi\left(3 - \frac{h^2}{4}\right)h = \pi(6 - 2) = 4\pi$$

52. (c) Let cost $C = av + \frac{b}{v}$

According to given question,

$$30a+\frac{b}{30}=75 \quad \ldots\text{(i)}$$

$$40a+\frac{b}{40}=65 \quad \ldots\text{(ii)}$$

On solving (i) and (ii), we get

$$a=\frac{1}{2} \text{ and } b=1800$$

Now, $C=av+\frac{b}{v}$

$$\Rightarrow \frac{dC}{dv}=a-\frac{b}{v^2}$$

$$\frac{dC}{dv}=0 \Rightarrow a-\frac{b}{v^2}=0$$

$$\Rightarrow v=\sqrt{\frac{b}{a}}=\sqrt{3600}$$

$$\Rightarrow v=60 \text{ kmph}$$

53. **(d)** Let base = b

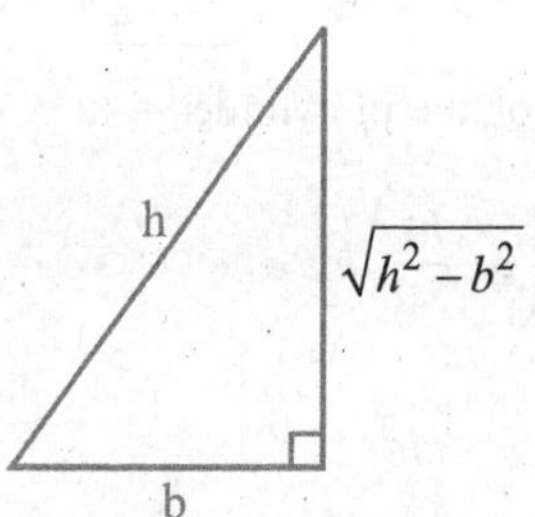

Altitude (or perpendicular) = $\sqrt{h^2-b^2}$

Area, A= $\frac{1}{2}$ × base × altitude

$$=\frac{1}{2}\times b\times\sqrt{h^2-b^2}$$

$$\Rightarrow \frac{dA}{db}=\frac{1}{2}\left[\sqrt{h^2-b^2}+b.\frac{-2b}{2\sqrt{h^2-b^2}}\right]$$

$$=\frac{1}{2}\left[\frac{h^2-2b^2}{\sqrt{h^2-b^2}}\right]$$

Put $\frac{dA}{db}=0, \Rightarrow b=\frac{h}{\sqrt{2}}$

Maximum area $=\frac{1}{2}\times\frac{h}{\sqrt{2}}\times\sqrt{h^2-\frac{h^2}{2}}=\frac{h^2}{4}$

54. **(b)** Given, $f(x)=ln|x|+bx^2+ax$

$$\therefore f'(x)=\frac{1}{x}+2bx+a$$

At $x=-1$, $f'(x)=-1-2b+a=0$

$$\Rightarrow a-2b=1 \quad \ldots\text{(i)}$$

At $x=2$, $f'(x)=\frac{1}{2}+4b+a=0$

$$\Rightarrow a+4b=-\frac{1}{2} \quad \ldots\text{(ii)}$$

On solving (i) and (ii) we get $a=\frac{1}{2}, b=-\frac{1}{4}$

Thus, $f'(x)=\frac{1}{x}-\frac{x}{2}+\frac{1}{2}=\frac{2-x^2+x}{2x}$

$$=\frac{-x^2+x+2}{2x}=\frac{-\left(x^2-x-2\right)}{2x}$$

$$=\frac{-(x+1)(x-2)}{2x}$$

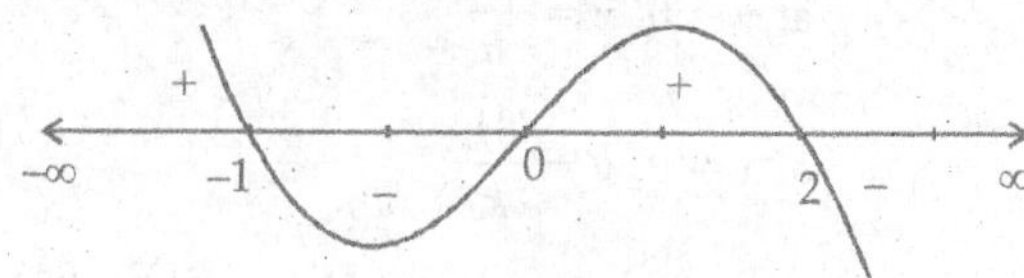

So maxima at $x=-1, 2$

55. **(c)** Equation of a line passing through (x_1, y_1) having slope m is given by $y-y_1=m(x-x_1)$

Since the line PQ is passing through (1,2) therefore its equation is $(y-2)=m(x-1)$

where m is the slope of the line PQ.

Now, point $P(x,0)$ will also satisfy the equation of PQ

$\therefore \; y-2=m(x-1) \Rightarrow 0-2=m(x-1)$

$$\Rightarrow -2=m(x-1) \Rightarrow x-1=\frac{-2}{m}$$

$$\Rightarrow x=\frac{-2}{m}+1$$

Also, $OP=\sqrt{(x-0)^2+(0-0)^2}=x$

$$=\frac{-2}{m}+1$$

Similarly, point $Q(0,y)$ will satisfy equation of PQ

$\therefore \; y-2=m(x-1)$

$\Rightarrow y-2=m(-1)$

$\Rightarrow y=2-m$ and $OQ=y=2-m$

Area of $\Delta POQ=\frac{1}{2}(OP)(OQ)$

$$=\frac{1}{2}\left(1-\frac{2}{m}\right)(2-m)$$

($\because$ Area of $\Delta=\frac{1}{2}\times$base$\times$height)

$$=\frac{1}{2}\left[2-m-\frac{4}{m}+2\right]=\frac{1}{2}\left[4-\left(m+\frac{4}{m}\right)\right]$$

$= 2 - \frac{m}{2} - \frac{2}{m}$

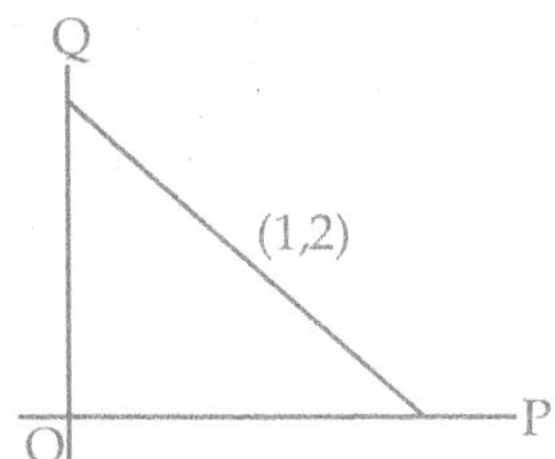

Let Area $= f(m) = 2 - \frac{m}{2} - \frac{2}{m}$

Now, $f'(m) = \frac{-1}{2} + \frac{2}{m^2}$

Put $f'(m) = 0$

$\Rightarrow m^2 = 4 \Rightarrow m = \pm 2$

Now, $f''(m) = \frac{-4}{m^3}$

$f''(m)\big|_{m=2} = -\frac{1}{2} < 0$

$f''(m)\big|_{m=-2} = \frac{1}{2} > 0$

Area will be least at $m = -2$

Hence, slope of PQ is -2.

56. (d) Let $f : (-\infty, \infty) \to (-\infty, \infty)$ be defined by $f(x) = x^3 + 1$.

Clearly, $f(x)$ is symmetric along $y = 1$ and it has neither maxima nor minima.

$\therefore$ Statement - 1 is false.

Hence, option (d) is correct.

57. (b) $f(x) = \begin{cases} \frac{\tan x}{x}, & x \neq 0 \\ 1, & x = 0 \end{cases}$

In right neighbourhood of '0'

$\tan x > x$

$\frac{\tan x}{x} > 1$

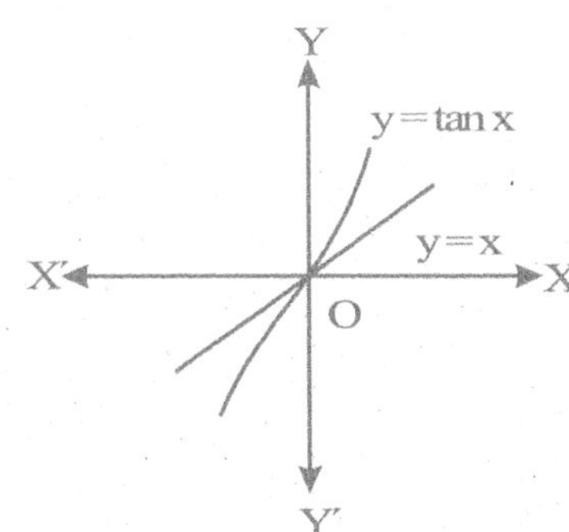

In left neighbourhood of '0'

$\tan x < x$

$\frac{\tan x}{x} > 1$ as $(\tan x < 0)$

at $x = 0$, $f(x) = 1$

$\Rightarrow$ $x = 0$ is the point of minima

So Statement 1 is true.

Statement 2 obvious.

58. (c) $f'(x) = \sqrt{x}\sin x$

$f'(x) = 0$

$\Rightarrow x = 0$ or $\sin x = 0$

$\Rightarrow x = 2\pi, \pi$

$f''(x) = \sqrt{x}\cos x + \frac{1}{2\sqrt{x}}\sin x$

$= \frac{1}{2\sqrt{x}}(2x\cos x + \sin x)$

At $x = \pi$, $f''(x) < 0$

Hence, local maxima at $x = \pi$

At $x = 2\pi$, $f''(x) > 0$

Hence local minima at $x = 2\pi$

59. (d) $f(x) = \frac{1}{e^x + 2e^{-x}} = \frac{e^x}{e^{2x} + 2}$

$f'(x) = \frac{(e^{2x} + 2)e^x - 2e^{2x}.e^x}{(e^{2x} + 2)^2}$

$f'(x) = 0 \Rightarrow e^{2x} + 2 = 2e^{2x}$

$e^{2x} = 2 \Rightarrow e^x = \sqrt{2}$

maximum $f(x) = \frac{\sqrt{2}}{4} = \frac{1}{2\sqrt{2}}$

$0 < f(x) \leq \frac{1}{2\sqrt{2}} \quad \forall x \in R$

Since $0 < \frac{1}{3} < \frac{1}{2\sqrt{2}} \Rightarrow$ for some $c \in R$

$f(c) = \frac{1}{3}$

60. (c)

$f(x) = \begin{cases} k - 2x, & \text{if } x \leq -1 \\ 2x + 3, & \text{if } x > -1 \end{cases}$

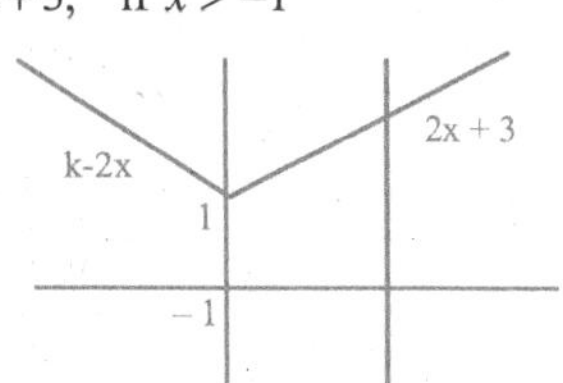

This is true where k = – 1

61. **(a)** We have $P(x) = x^4 + ax^3 + bx^2 + cx + d$

$\Rightarrow P'(x) = 4x^3 + 3ax^2 + 2bx + c$

But $P'(0) = 0 \Rightarrow c = 0$

$\therefore P(x) = x^4 + ax^3 + bx^2 + d$

As given that $P(-1) < P(a)$

$\Rightarrow 1 - a + b + d < 1 + a + b + d$

$\Rightarrow a > 0$

Now $P'(x) = 4x^3 + 3ax^2 + 2bx = x(4x^2 + 3ax + 2b)$

As $P'(x) = 0$, there is only one solution $x = 0$, therefore $4x^2 + 3ax + 2b = 0$ should not have any real roots i.e. $D < 0$

$\Rightarrow 9a^2 - 32b < 0 \quad \Rightarrow \quad b > \dfrac{9a^2}{32} > 0$

Hence $a, b > 0 \Rightarrow P'(x) = 4x^3 + 3ax^2 + 2bx > 0$

$\forall x > 0$

$\therefore$ $P(x)$ is an increasing function on $(0,1)$

$\therefore$ $P(0) < P(a)$

Similarly we can prove $P(x)$ is decreasing on $(-1, 0)$

$\therefore$ $P(-1) > P(0)$

So we can conclude that

Max $P(x) = P(1)$ and Min $P(x) = P(0)$

$\Rightarrow$ $P(-1)$ is not minimum but $P(1)$ is the maximum of P.

62. **(a)** Let $y = x^3 - px + q \Rightarrow \dfrac{dy}{dx} = 3x^2 - p$

For $\dfrac{dy}{dx} = 0 \Rightarrow 3x^2 - p = 0$

$\Rightarrow x = \pm\sqrt{\dfrac{p}{3}}$

$\dfrac{d^2y}{dx^2} = 6x$

$\left.\dfrac{d^2y}{dx^2}\right|_{x=\sqrt{\frac{p}{3}}} = +ve$ and $\left.\dfrac{d^2y}{dx^2}\right|_{x=-\sqrt{\frac{p}{3}}} = -ve$

$\therefore$ y has minima at $x = \sqrt{\dfrac{p}{3}}$ and maxima at $x = -\sqrt{\dfrac{p}{3}}$

63. **(a)** $\dfrac{x}{2} + \dfrac{2}{x}$ is of the form $y + \dfrac{1}{y}$ where $y + \dfrac{1}{y} \geq 2$ and equality holds for $y = 1$

$\therefore$ Min value of function occurs at $\dfrac{x}{2} = 1$ i.e., at $x = 2$

64. **(c)** $y = x + \dfrac{1}{x}$ or $\dfrac{dy}{dx} = 1 - \dfrac{1}{x^2}$

For max. or min., $1 - \dfrac{1}{x^2} = 0 \Rightarrow x = \pm 1$

$\dfrac{d^2y}{dx^2} = \dfrac{2}{x^3} \Rightarrow \left(\dfrac{d^2y}{dx^2}\right)_{x=2} = 2$ (+ve minima)

$\therefore x = 1$

65. **(d)** $f(x) = 2x^3 - 9ax^2 + 12a^2x + 1$

$f'(x) = 6x^2 - 18ax + 12a^2$; $f''(x) = 12x - 18a$

For max. or min.

$6x^2 - 18ax + 12a^2 = 0 \Rightarrow x^2 - 3ax + 2a^2 = 0$

$\Rightarrow x = a$ or $x = 2a$. At $x = a$ max. and at $x = 2a$ min

$\therefore p = a$ and $q = 2a$

As per question $p^2 = q$

$\therefore a^2 = 2a \Rightarrow a = 2$ or $a = 0$

but $a > 0$, therefore, $a = 2$.

66. **(b)** Distance of origin from $(x, y) = \sqrt{x^2 + y^2}$

$= \sqrt{a^2 + b^2 - 2ab\cos\left(t - \dfrac{at}{b}\right)}$;

$\leq \sqrt{a^2 + b^2 + 2ab}$

$\left[\left\{\cos\left(t - \dfrac{at}{b}\right)\right\}_{\min} = -1\right]$

$= a + b$

$\therefore$ Maximum distance from origin $= a + b$

Integrals

TOPIC-1 : Standard Integrals, Integration by Substitution, Integration by Parts

1. If $f\left(\frac{3x-4}{3x+4}\right)=x+2,\ x\neq-\frac{4}{3}$, and $\int f(x)\,dx = \text{A}\log|1-x|+\text{B}x+\text{C}$, then the ordered pair (A, B) is equal to : **[Online April 9, 2017]**
(where C is a constant of integration)

(a) $\left(\frac{8}{3},\frac{2}{3}\right)$ (b) $\left(-\frac{8}{3},\frac{2}{3}\right)$

(c) $\left(-\frac{8}{3},-\frac{2}{3}\right)$ (d) $\left(\frac{8}{3},-\frac{2}{3}\right)$

2. The integral $\int\sqrt{1+2\cot x(\operatorname{cosec} x+\cot x)}\,dx \quad \left(0<x<\frac{\pi}{2}\right)$ is equal to : **[Online April 8, 2017]**
(where C is a constant of integration)

(a) $2\log\left|\sin\frac{x}{2}\right|+C$ (b) $4\log\left|\sin\frac{x}{2}\right|+C$

(c) $2\log\left|\cos\frac{x}{2}\right|+C$ (d) $4\log\left|\cos\frac{x}{2}\right|+C$

3. If $\int\frac{dx}{\cos^3 x\sqrt{2\sin 2x}}=(\tan x)^A+C(\tan x)^B+k$, where k is a constant of integration, then A + B + C equals : **[Online April 9, 2016]**

(a) $\frac{16}{5}$ (b) $\frac{27}{10}$

(c) $\frac{7}{10}$ (d) $\frac{21}{5}$

4. If $\int\frac{\log(t+\sqrt{1+t^2})}{\sqrt{1+t^2}}dt=\frac{1}{2}(g(t))^2+C$, where C is a constant, then g(b) is equal to : **[Online April 11, 2015]**

(a) $\frac{1}{\sqrt{5}}\log(2+\sqrt{5})$ (b) $\frac{1}{2}\log(2+\sqrt{5})$

(c) $2\log(2+\sqrt{5})$ (d) $\log(2+\sqrt{5})$

5. The integral $\int\left(1+x-\frac{1}{x}\right)e^{x+\frac{1}{x}}dx$ is equal to **[2014]**

(a) $(x+1)e^{x+\frac{1}{x}}+c$ (b) $-xe^{x+\frac{1}{x}}+c$

(c) $(x-1)e^{x+\frac{1}{x}}+c$ (d) $xe^{x+\frac{1}{x}}+c$

6. The integral $\int\frac{\sin^2 x\cos^2 x}{\left(\sin^3 x+\cos^3 x\right)^2}dx$ is equal to: **[Online April 12, 2014]**

(a) $\frac{1}{\left(1+\cot^3 x\right)}+c$ (b) $-\frac{1}{3\left(1+\tan^3 x\right)}+c$

(c) $\frac{\sin^3 x}{\left(1+\cos^3 x\right)}+c$ (d) $-\frac{\cos^3 x}{3\left(1+\sin^3 x\right)}+c$

7. The integral $\int x\cos^{-1}\left(\frac{1-x^2}{1+x^2}\right)dx\ (x>0)$ is equal to: **[Online April 11, 2014]**

(a) $-x+(1+x^2)\tan^{-1}x+c$
(b) $x-(1+x^2)\cot^{-1}x+c$
(c) $-x+(1+x^2)\cot^{-1}x+c$
(d) $x-(1+x^2)\tan^{-1}x+c$

8. $\int\frac{\sin^8 x-\cos^8 x}{\left(1-2\sin^2 x\cos^2 x\right)}dx$ is equal to: **[Online April 9, 2014]**

(a) $\frac{1}{2}\sin 2x+c$ (b) $-\frac{1}{2}\sin 2x+c$

(c) $-\frac{1}{2}\sin x+c$ (d) $-\sin^2 x+c$

9. If $\int f(x)dx = \psi(x)$, then $\int x^5 f(x^3)dx$ is equal to **[2013]**

(a) $\frac{1}{3}\left[x^3\psi(x^3) - \int x^2\psi(x^3)dx\right] + C$

(b) $\frac{1}{3}x^3\psi(x^3) - 3\int x^3\psi(x^3)dx + C$

(c) $\frac{1}{3}x^3\psi(x^3) - \int x^2\psi(x^3)dx + C$

(d) $\frac{1}{3}\left[x^3\psi(x^3) - \int x^3\psi(x^3)dx\right] + C$

10. If the integral

$\int \frac{\cos 8x + 1}{\cot 2x - \tan 2x} dx = A\cos 8x + k,$

where k is an arbitrary constant, then A is equal to : **[Online April 25, 2013]**

(a) $-\frac{1}{16}$ (b) $\frac{1}{16}$

(c) $\frac{1}{8}$ (d) $-\frac{1}{8}$

11. If the $\int \frac{5\tan x}{\tan x - 2} dx = x + a\ln|\sin x - 2\cos x| + k$, then a is equal to : **[2012]**

(a) -1 (b) -2

(c) 1 (d) 2

12. If $f(x) = \int \left(\frac{x^2 + \sin^2 x}{1 + x^2}\right)\sec^2 x\, dx$ and $f(0) = 0$, then $f(1)$ equals **[Online May 19, 2012]**

(a) $\tan 1 - \frac{\pi}{4}$ (b) $\tan 1 + 1$

(c) $\frac{\pi}{4}$ (d) $1 - \frac{\pi}{4}$

13. The integral of $\frac{x^2 - x}{x^3 - x^2 + x - 1}$ w.r.t. x is **[Online May 12, 2012]**

(a) $\frac{1}{2}\log\left(x^2 + 1\right) + C$

(b) $\frac{1}{2}\log\left|x^2 - 1\right| + C$

(c) $\log\left(x^2 + 1\right) + C$

(d) $\log\left|x^2 - 1\right| + C$

14. Let $f(x)$ be an indefinite integral of $\cos^3 x$.

Statement 1: $f(x)$ is a periodic function of period π.

Statement 2: $\cos^3 x$ is a periodic function. **[Online May 7, 2012]**

(a) Statement 1 is true, Statement 2 is false.

(b) Both the Statements are true, but Statement 2 is not the correct explanation of Statement 1.

(c) Both the Statements are true, and Statement 2 is correct explanation of Statement 1.

(d) Statement 1 is false, Statement 2 is true.

15. The value of $\sqrt{2}\int \frac{\sin x\, dx}{\sin\left(x - \frac{\pi}{4}\right)}$ is **[2008]**

(a) $x + \log\left|\cos\left(x - \frac{\pi}{4}\right)\right| + c$

(b) $x - \log\left|\sin\left(x - \frac{\pi}{4}\right)\right| + c$

(c) $x + \log\left|\sin\left(x - \frac{\pi}{4}\right)\right| + c$

(d) $x - \log\left|\cos\left(x - \frac{\pi}{4}\right)\right| + c$

16. $\int \frac{dx}{\cos x + \sqrt{3}\sin x}$ equals **[2007]**

(a) $\log\tan\left(\frac{x}{2} + \frac{\pi}{12}\right) + C$

(b) $\log\tan\left(\frac{x}{2} - \frac{\pi}{12}\right) + C$

(c) $\frac{1}{2}\log\tan\left(\frac{x}{2} + \frac{\pi}{12}\right) + C$

(d) $\frac{1}{2}\log\tan\left(\frac{x}{2} - \frac{\pi}{12}\right) + C$

17. $\int \frac{dx}{\cos x - \sin x}$ is equal to **[2004]**

(a) $\frac{1}{\sqrt{2}}\log\left|\tan\left(\frac{x}{2} + \frac{3\pi}{8}\right)\right| + C$

(b) $\frac{1}{\sqrt{2}}\log\left|\cot\left(\frac{x}{2}\right)\right| + C$

(c) $\frac{1}{\sqrt{2}}\log\left|\tan\left(\frac{x}{2} - \frac{3\pi}{8}\right)\right| + C$

(d) $\frac{1}{\sqrt{2}}\log\left|\tan\left(\frac{x}{2} - \frac{\pi}{8}\right)\right| + C$

18. If $\int \frac{\sin x}{\sin(x - \alpha)} dx = Ax + B\log\sin(x - \alpha), + C$, then value of (A, B) is **[2004]**

(a) $(-\cos\alpha, \sin\alpha)$ (b) $(\cos\alpha, \sin\alpha)$

(c) $(-\sin\alpha, \cos\alpha)$ (d) $(\sin\alpha, \cos\alpha)$

19. $f(x)$ and $g(x)$ are two differentiable functions on [0, 2] such that $f''(x)-g''(x)=0,\ f'(1)=2g'(1)=4f(2)=3g(2)=9$ then $f(x)-g(x)$ at $x=3/2$ is **[2002]**

(a) 0 (b) 2
(c) 10 (d) 5

TOPIC-2 : Integration of the Forms: ∫ex(f(x) + f′(x))dx, ∫ekx(df(x) + f′(x))dx, Integration by Partial Fractions, Integration of Some Special Irrational Algebraic Functions, Integration of Different Expressions of e^x

20. The integral $\int \frac{dx}{(1+\sqrt{x})\sqrt{x-x^2}}$ is equal to : (where C is a constant of integration) **[Online April 10, 2016]**

(a) $-2\sqrt{\frac{1+\sqrt{x}}{1-\sqrt{x}}}+C$ (b) $-\sqrt{\frac{1-\sqrt{x}}{1+\sqrt{x}}}+C$

(c) $-2\sqrt{\frac{1-\sqrt{x}}{1+\sqrt{x}}}+C$ (d) $2\sqrt{\frac{1+\sqrt{x}}{1-\sqrt{x}}}+C$

21. The integral $\int \frac{dx}{x^2(x^4+1)^{3/4}}$ equals : **[2015]**

(a) $-(x^4+1)^{\frac{1}{4}}+c$ (b) $-\left(\frac{x^4+1}{x^4}\right)^{\frac{1}{4}}+c$

(c) $\left(\frac{x^4+1}{x^4}\right)^{\frac{1}{4}}+c$ (d) $(x^4+1)^{\frac{1}{4}}+c$

22. The integral $\int \frac{dx}{(x+1)^{\frac{3}{4}}(x-2)^{\frac{5}{4}}}$ is equal to : **[Online April 10, 2015]**

(a) $-\frac{4}{3}\left(\frac{x+1}{x-2}\right)^{\frac{1}{4}}+C$ (b) $4\left(\frac{x+1}{x-2}\right)^{\frac{1}{4}}+C$

(c) $4\left(\frac{x-2}{x+1}\right)^{\frac{1}{4}}+C$ (d) $-\frac{4}{3}\left(\frac{x-2}{x+1}\right)^{\frac{1}{4}}+C$

23. If m is a non-zero number and

$$\int \frac{x^{5m-1}+2x^{4m-1}}{\left(x^{2m}+x^m+1\right)^3}dx=f(x)+c,$$

then f(x) is: **[Online April 19, 2014]**

(a) $\frac{x^{5m}}{2m\left(x^{2m}+x^m+1\right)^2}$ (b) $\frac{x^{4m}}{2m\left(x^{2m}+x^m+1\right)^2}$

(c) $\frac{2m\left(x^{5m}+x^{4m}\right)}{\left(x^{2m}+x^m+1\right)^2}$ (d) $\frac{\left(x^{5m}-x^{4m}\right)}{2m\left(x^{2m}+x^m+1\right)^2}$

24. The integral $\int \frac{xdx}{2-x^2+\sqrt{2-x^2}}$ equals : **[Online April 23, 2013]**

(a) $\log\left|1+\sqrt{2+x^2}\right|+c$

(b) $-\log\left|1+\sqrt{2-x^2}\right|+c$

(c) $-x\log\left|1-\sqrt{2-x^2}\right|+c$

(d) $x\log\left|1-\sqrt{2+x^2}\right|+c$

25. If $\int \frac{x^2-x+1}{x^2+1}e^{\cot^{-1}x}dx=A(x)e^{\cot^{-1}x}+C$, then $A(x)$ is equal to : **[Online April 22, 2013]**

(a) $-x$ (b) x
(c) $\sqrt{1-x}$ (d) $\sqrt{1+x}$

26. If $\int \frac{dx}{x+x^7}=p(x)$ then, $\int \frac{x^6}{x+x^7}dx$ is equal to: **[Online April 9, 2013]**

(a) $\ln|x|-p(x)+c$ (b) $\ln|x|+p(x)+c$
(c) $x-p(x)+c$ (d) $x+p(x)+c$

27. $\int\left\{\frac{(\log x-1)}{1+(\log x)^2}\right\}^2dx$ is equal to **[2005]**

(a) $\frac{\log x}{(\log x)^2+1}+C$ (b) $\frac{x}{x^2+1}+C$

(c) $\frac{xe^x}{1+x^2}+C$ (d) $\frac{x}{(\log x)^2+1}+C$

TOPIC-3 : Evaluation of Definite Integral by Substitution, Properties of Definite Integrals

28. The integral $\int_{\frac{\pi}{4}}^{\frac{3\pi}{4}} \frac{dx}{1+\cos x}$ is equal to : **[2017]**

(a) –1 (b) –2
(c) 2 (d) 4

29. Let $I_n=\int \tan^n x\,dx,(n>1)$. $I_4+I_6=a\tan^5x+bx^5+C$, where C is constant of integration, then the ordered pair (a, b) is equal to : **[2017]**

(a) $\left(-\frac{1}{5},0\right)$ (b) $\left(-\frac{1}{5},1\right)$

(c) $\left(\frac{1}{5},0\right)$ (d) $\left(\frac{1}{5},-1\right)$

30. If $\int_1^2 \frac{dx}{(x^2-2x+4)^{\frac{3}{2}}} = \frac{k}{k+5}$ then k is equal to : **[Online April 9, 2017]**

(a) 1 (b) 2
(c) 3 (d) 4

31. The integral $\int_{\frac{\pi}{12}}^{\frac{\pi}{4}} \frac{8\cos 2x}{(\tan x+\cot x)^3} dx$ equals : **[Online April 8, 2017]**

(a) $\frac{15}{128}$ (b) $\frac{15}{64}$
(c) $\frac{13}{32}$ (d) $\frac{15}{256}$

32. The integral $\int \frac{2x^{12}+5x^9}{\left(x^5+x^3+1\right)^3} dx$ is equal to : **[2016]**

(a) $\frac{x^5}{2\left(x^5+x^3+1\right)^2}+C$ (b) $\frac{-x^{10}}{2\left(x^5+x^3+1\right)^2}+C$
(c) $\frac{-x^5}{\left(x^5+x^3+1\right)^2}+C$ (d) $\frac{x^{10}}{2\left(x^5+x^3+1\right)^2}+C$

33. For $x \in R, x \neq 0$, if y(x) is a differentiable function such that $x\int_1^x y(t)dt = (x+1)\int_1^x ty(t)dt$, then y(x) equals :
(where C is a constant) **[Online April 10, 2016]**

(a) $Cx^3 e^{\frac{1}{x}}$ (b) $\frac{C}{x^2}e^{-\frac{1}{x}}$
(c) $\frac{C}{x}e^{-\frac{1}{x}}$ (d) $\frac{C}{x^3}e^{-\frac{1}{x}}$

34. The value of the integral
$\int_4^{10} \frac{[x^2]dx}{[x^2-28x+196]+[x^2]}$, where [x] denotes the greatest integer less than or equal to x, is : **[Online April 10, 2016]**

(a) $\frac{1}{3}$ (b) 6
(c) 7 (d) 3

35. If $2\int_0^1 \tan^{-1}x\,dx = \int_0^1 \cot^{-1}(1-x+x^2)dx$, then $\int_0^1 \tan^{-1}(1-x+x^2)dx$ is equal to : **[Online April 9, 2016]**

(a) $\frac{\pi}{2}+\log 2$ (b) log2
(c) $\frac{\pi}{2}-\log 4$ (d) log4

36. The integral **[2015]**
$\int_2^4 \frac{\log x^2}{\log x^2+\log(36-12x+x^2)}dx$ is equal to :

(a) 1 (b) 6
(c) 2 (d) 4

37. Let f : R → R be a function such that f(2 – x) = f(2 + x) and f(4 – x) = f(4 + x), for all $x \in R$ and $\int_0^2 f(x)\,dx = 5$.

Then the value of $\int_{10}^{50} f(x)\,dx$ is : **[Online April 11, 2015]**

(a) 125 (b) 80
(c) 100 (d) 200

38. Let f : (–1, 1) → R be a continuous function. If $\int_0^{\sin x} f(t)dt = \frac{\sqrt{3}}{2}x$, then $f\left(\frac{\sqrt{3}}{2}\right)$ is equal to : **[Online April 11, 2015]**

(a) $\frac{1}{2}$ (b) $\frac{\sqrt{3}}{2}$
(c) $\sqrt{\frac{3}{2}}$ (d) $\sqrt{3}$

39. For $x > 0$, let $f(x) = \int_1^x \frac{\log t}{1+t}dt$. Then $f(x)+f\left(\frac{1}{x}\right)$ is equal to: **[Online April 10, 2015]**

(a) $\frac{1}{4}(\log x)^2$ (b) log x
(c) $\frac{1}{2}(\log x)^2$ (d) $\frac{1}{4}\log x^2$

40. The integral $\int_0^{\pi} \sqrt{1+4\sin^2\frac{x}{2}-4\sin\frac{x}{2}}\,dx$ equals: **[2014]**

(a) $4\sqrt{3}-4$ (b) $4\sqrt{3}-4-\frac{\pi}{3}$
(c) $\pi-4$ (d) $\frac{2\pi}{3}-4-4\sqrt{3}$

41. Let function F be defined as $F(x)=\int_1^x \frac{e^t}{t}dt, x>0$ then the value of the integral $\int_1^x \frac{e^t}{t+a}dt$, where $a>0$, is: **[Online April 19, 2014]**

(a) $e^a\left[F(x)-F(1+a)\right]$

(b) $e^{-a}\left[F(x+a)-F(a)\right]$

(c) $e^a\left[F(x+a)-F(1+a)\right]$

(d) $e^{-a}\left[F(x+a)-F(1+a)\right]$

42. If for a continuous function f(x), $\int_{-\pi}^{t}(f(x)+x)dx=\pi^2-t^2$, for all $t\geq-\pi$, then $f\left(-\frac{\pi}{3}\right)$ is equal to: **[Online April 12, 2014]**

(a) π (b) $\frac{\pi}{2}$

(c) $\frac{\pi}{3}$ (d) $\frac{\pi}{6}$

43. If [ ] denotes the greatest integer function, then the integral $\int_0^\pi [\cos x]dx$ is equal to: **[Online April 12, 2014]**

(a) $\frac{\pi}{2}$ (b) 0

(c) –1 (d) $-\frac{\pi}{2}$

44. If for $n\geq1$, $P_n=\int_1^e(\log x)^n dx$, then $P_{10}-90P_8$ is equal to: **[Online April 11, 2014]**

(a) –9 (b) 10e

(c) –9 e (d) 10

45. The integral $\int_0^{\frac{1}{2}}\frac{\ln(1+2x)}{1+4x^2}dx$, equals: **[Online April 9, 2014]**

(a) $\frac{\pi}{4}\ln2$ (b) $\frac{\pi}{8}\ln2$

(c) $\frac{\pi}{16}\ln2$ (d) $\frac{\pi}{32}\ln2$

46. The intercepts on *x*-axis made by tangents to the curve, $y=\int_0^x|t|\,dt, x\in R$, which are parallel to the line $y=2x$, are equal to: **[2013]**

(a) ±1 (b) ±2

(c) ±3 (d) ±4

47. **Statement-1 :** The value of the integral $\int_{\pi/6}^{\pi/3}\frac{dx}{1+\sqrt{\tan x}}$ is equal to $\pi/6$

Statement-2 : $\int_a^b f(x)dx=\int_a^b f(a+b-x)dx.$ **[2013]**

(a) Statement-1 is true; Statement-2 is true; Statement-2 is a correct explanation for Statement-1.

(b) Statement-1 is true; Statement-2 is true; Statement-2 is not a correct explanation for Statement-1.

(c) Statement-1 is true; Statement-2 is false.

(d) Statement-1 is false; Statement-2 is true.

48. For $0\leq x\leq\frac{\pi}{2}$, the value of

$\int_0^{\sin^2 x}\sin^{-1}(\sqrt{t})dt+\int_0^{\cos^2 x}\cos^{-1}(\sqrt{t})\,dt$ equals : **[Online April 25, 2013]**

(a) $\frac{\pi}{4}$ (b) 0

(c) 1 (d) $-\frac{\pi}{4}$

49. The value of $\int_{-\pi/2}^{\pi/2}\frac{\sin^2 x}{1+2^x}dx$ is : **[Online April 23, 2013]**

(a) π (b) $\frac{\pi}{2}$

(c) 4π (d) $\frac{\pi}{4}$

50. The integral $\int_{7\pi/4}^{7\pi/3}\sqrt{\tan^2 x}\,dx$ is equal to : **[Online April 22, 2013]**

(a) $\log 2\sqrt{2}$ (b) $\log 2$

(c) $2\log 2$ (d) $\log\sqrt{2}$

51. If $x=\int_0^y\frac{dt}{\sqrt{1+t^2}}$, then $\frac{d^2y}{dx^2}$ is equal to : **[Online April 9, 2013]**

(a) y (b) $\sqrt{1+y^2}$

(c) $\frac{x}{\sqrt{1+y^2}}$ (d) y^2

52. If $g(x)=\int_0^x\cos 4t\,dt$, then $g(x+\pi)$ equals **[2012]**

(a) $\frac{g(x)}{g(\pi)}$ (b) $g(x)+g(\pi)$

(c) $g(x)-g(\pi)$ (d) $g(x).g(\pi)$

53. If $[x]$ is the greatest integer $\leq x$, then the value of the integral $\int_{-0.9}^{0.9}\left(\left[x^2\right]+\log\left(\frac{2-x}{2+x}\right)\right)dx$ is **[Online May 26, 2012]**

(a) 0.486 (b) 0.243
(c) 1.8 (d) 0

54. The value of the integral $\int_0^{0.9}\left[x-2[x]\right]dx$, where [.] denotes the greatest integer function is **[Online May 19, 2012]**

(a) 0.9 (b) 1.8
(c) −0.9 (d) 0

55. If $\frac{d}{dx}G(x)=\frac{e^{\tan x}}{x}$, $x\in(0,\pi/2)$, then $\int_{1/4}^{1/2}\frac{2}{x}.e^{\tan(\pi x^2)}dx$ is equal to **[Online May 12, 2012]**

(a) $G(\pi/4)-G(\pi/16)$
(b) $2[G(\pi/4)-G(\pi/16)]$
(c) $\pi[G(1/2)-G(1/4)]$
(d) $G(1/\sqrt{2})-G(1/2)$

56. If $\int_e^x t\,f(t)\,dt=\sin x-x\cos x-\frac{x^2}{2}$, for all $x\in R-\{0\}$, then the value of $f\left(\frac{\pi}{6}\right)$ is **[Online May 7, 2012]**

(a) 1/2 (b) 1
(c) 0 (d) −1/2

57. Let [.] denote the greatest integer function then the value of $\int_0^{1.5}x\left[x^2\right]dx$ is :. **[2011 RS]**

(a) 0 (b) $\frac{3}{2}$
(c) $\frac{3}{4}$ (d) $\frac{5}{4}$

58. The value of $\int_0^1\frac{8\log(1+x)}{1+x^2}dx$ is **[2011]**

(a) $\frac{\pi}{8}\log 2$ (b) $\frac{\pi}{2}\log 2$
(c) $\log 2$ (d) $\pi\log 2$

59. Let $p(x)$ be a function defined on **R** such that $p'(x)=p'(1-x)$, for all $x\in[0,1]$, $p(0)=1$ and $p(1)=41$. Then $\int_0^1 p(x)\,dx$ equals **[2010]**

(a) 21 (b) 41
(c) 42 (d) $\sqrt{41}$

60. $\int_0^{\pi}[\cot x]dx$, where [.] denotes the greatest integer function, is equal to : **[2009]**

(a) 1 (b) −1
(c) $-\frac{\pi}{2}$ (d) $\frac{\pi}{2}$

61. Let $I=\int_0^1\frac{\sin x}{\sqrt{x}}dx$ and $J=\int_0^1\frac{\cos x}{\sqrt{x}}dx$. Then which one of the following is true? **[2008]**

(a) $I>\frac{2}{3}$ and $J>2$ (b) $I<\frac{2}{3}$ and $J<2$
(c) $I<\frac{2}{3}$ and $J>2$ (d) $I>\frac{2}{3}$ and $J<2$

62. The solution for x of the equation $\int_{\sqrt{2}}^{x}\frac{dt}{t\sqrt{t^2-1}}=\frac{\pi}{2}$ is **[2007]**

(a) $\frac{\sqrt{3}}{2}$ (b) $2\sqrt{2}$
(c) 2 (d) None of these

63. Let $F(x)=f(x)+f\left(\frac{1}{x}\right)$, where $f(x)=\int_l^x\frac{\log t}{1+t}dt$, Then $F(e)$ equals **[2007]**

(a) 1 (b) 2
(c) 1/2 (d) 0,

64. The value of $\int_1^a[x]f'(x)dx$, $a>1$ where $[x]$ denotes the greatest integer not exceeding x is **[2006]**

(a) $af(a)-\{f(1)+f(2)+............f([a])\}$
(b) $[a]f(a)-\{f(1)+f(2)+............f([a])\}$
(c) $[a]f([a])-\{f(1)+f(2)+............f(a)\}$
(d) $af([a])-\{f(1)+f(2)+............f(a)\}$

65. $\int_{-\frac{3\pi}{2}}^{-\frac{\pi}{2}}[(x+\pi)^3+\cos^2(x+3\pi)]dx$ is equal to

(a) $\frac{\pi^4}{32}$ (b) $\frac{\pi^4}{32}+\frac{\pi}{2}$ **[2006]**
(c) $\frac{\pi}{2}$ (d) $\frac{\pi}{4}-1$

66. $\int_0^{\pi}xf(\sin x)dx$ is equal to **[2006]**

(a) $\pi\int_0^{\pi}f(\cos x)dx$ (b) $\pi\int_0^{\pi}f(\sin x)dx$

(c) $\frac{\pi}{2}\int_0^{\pi/2} f(\sin x)dx$ (d) $\pi\int_0^{\pi/2} f(\cos x)dx$

67. The value of integral, $\int_3^6 \frac{\sqrt{x}}{\sqrt{9-x}+\sqrt{x}}dx$ is

(a) $\frac{1}{2}$ (b) $\frac{3}{2}$ **[2006]**
(c) 2 (d) 1

68. The value of $\int_{-\pi}^{\pi} \frac{\cos^2 x}{1+a^x}dx$, a > 0, is **[2005]**

(a) $a\pi$ (b) $\frac{\pi}{2}$
(c) $\frac{\pi}{a}$ (d) 2π

69. If $I_1 = \int_0^1 2^{x^2}dx$, $I_2 = \int_0^1 2^{x^3}dx$, $I_3 = \int_1^2 2^{x^2}dx$ and $I_4 = \int_1^2 2^{x^3}dx$ then **[2005]**

(a) $I_2 > I_1$ (b) $I_1 > I_2$
(c) $I_3 = I_4$ (d) $I_3 > I_4$

70. Let $f: R \to R$ be a differentiable function having $f(2) = 6$, $f'(2) = \left(\frac{1}{48}\right)$. Then $\lim_{x\to 2}\int_6^{f(x)} \frac{4t^3}{x-2}dt$ equals **[2005]**

(a) 24 (b) 36
(c) 12 (d) 18

71. If $f(x) = \frac{e^x}{1+e^x}$, $I_1 = \int_{f(-a)}^{f(a)} xg\{x(1-x)\}dx$ and $I_2 = \int_{f(-a)}^{f(a)} g\{x(1-x)\}dx$, then the value of $\frac{I_2}{I_1}$ is **[2004]**

(a) 1 (b) –3
(c) –1 (d) 2

72. If $\int_0^{\pi} xf(\sin x)dx = A\int_0^{\pi/2} f(\sin x)dx$, then A is

(a) 2π (b) π **[2004]**
(c) $\frac{\pi}{4}$ (d) 0

73. The value of $I = \int_0^{\pi/2} \frac{(\sin x+\cos x)^2}{\sqrt{1+\sin 2x}}dx$ is

(a) 3 (b) 1 **[2004]**
(c) 2 (d) 0

74. The value of $\int_{-2}^{3} |1-x^2|dx$ is **[2004]**

(a) $\frac{1}{3}$ (b) $\frac{14}{3}$
(c) $\frac{7}{3}$ (d) $\frac{28}{3}$

75. The value of the integral $I = \int_0^1 x(1-x)^n dx$ is

(a) $\frac{1}{n+1}+\frac{1}{n+2}$ (b) $\frac{1}{n+1}$ **[2003]**
(c) $\frac{1}{n+2}$ (d) $\frac{1}{n+1}-\frac{1}{n+2}$.

76. Let $f(x)$ be a function satisfying $f'(x) = f(x)$ with $f(0)=1$ and $g(x)$ be a function that satisfies $f(x) + g(x) = x^2$. Then the value of the integral $\int_0^1 f(x)g(x)dx$, is **[2003]**

(a) $e+\frac{e^2}{2}+\frac{5}{2}$ (b) $e-\frac{e^2}{2}-\frac{5}{2}$
(c) $e+\frac{e^2}{2}-\frac{3}{2}$ (d) $e-\frac{e^2}{2}-\frac{3}{2}$.

77. If $f(a+b-x) = f(x)$ then $\int_a^b xf(x)dx$ is equal to

(a) $\frac{a+b}{2}\int_a^b f(a+b+x)dx$ **[2003]**

(b) $\frac{a+b}{2}\int_a^b f(b-x)dx$

(c) $\frac{a+b}{2}\int_a^b f(x)dx$

(d) $\frac{b-a}{2}\int_a^b f(x)dx$.

78. The value of $\lim_{x\to 0}\frac{\int_0^{x^2}\sec^2 t\,dt}{x\sin x}$ is **[2003]**

(a) 0 (b) 3
(c) 2 (d) 1

79. If $f(y)=e^y$, $g(y)=y;\ y>0$ and

$$F(t)=\int_0^t f(t-y)g(y)\,dy,$$ then **[2003]**

(a) $F(t)=te^{-t}$

(b) $F(t)=1-te^{-t}(1+t)$

(c) $F(t)=e^t-(1+t)$

(d) $F(t)=te^t$.

80. $\int_{-\pi}^{\pi}\frac{2x(1+\sin x)}{1+\cos^2 x}dx$ is **[2002]**

(a) $\frac{\pi^2}{4}$ (b) π^2

(c) zero (d) $\frac{\pi}{2}$

81. $\int_0^2[x^2]dx$ is **[2002]**

(a) $2-\sqrt{2}$ (b) $2+\sqrt{2}$

(c) $\sqrt{2}-1$ (d) $-\sqrt{2}-\sqrt{3}+5$

82. $I_n=\int_0^{\pi/4}\tan^n x\,dx$ then $\lim_{n\to\infty} n[I_n+I_{n+2}]$ equals

(a) $\frac{1}{2}$ (b) 1 **[2002]**

(c) ∞ (d) zero

83. $\int_0^{10\pi}|\sin x|\,dx$ is **[2002]**

(a) 20 (b) 8

(c) 10 (d) 18

TOPIC-4 : Reduction Formulae for Definite Integration, Gamma & Beta Function, Walli's Formula, Summation of Series by Integration

84. If $\lim_{n\to\infty}\frac{1^a+2^a+.........+n^a}{(n+1)^{a-1}[(na+2)+.....(na+n)]}=\frac{1}{60}$

for some positive real number a, then a is equal to : **[Online April 9, 2017]**

(a) 7 (b) 8

(c) $\frac{15}{2}$ (d) $\frac{17}{2}$

85. $\lim_{n\to\infty}\left(\frac{(n+1)(n+2)...3n}{n^{2n}}\right)^{\frac{1}{n}}$ is equal to: **[2016]**

(a) $\frac{9}{e^2}$ (b) $3\log 3-2$

(c) $\frac{18}{e^4}$ (d) $\frac{27}{e^2}$

86. $f(x)=\int\frac{dx}{\sin^6 x}$ is a polynomial of degree **[Online May 26, 2012]**

(a) 5 in $\cot x$ (b) 5 in $\tan x$

(c) 3 in $\tan x$ (d) 3 in $\cot x$

87. $\underset{n\to\infty}{\text{Lim}}\left[\frac{1}{n^2}\sec^2\frac{1}{n^2}+\frac{2}{n^2}\sec^2\frac{4}{n^2}............+\frac{1}{n}\sec^2 1\right]$

equals **[2005]**

(a) $\frac{1}{2}\sec 1$ (b) $\frac{1}{2}$ cosec 1

(c) $\tan 1$ (d) $\frac{1}{2}\tan 1$

88. $\underset{n\to\infty}{Lim}\sum_{r=1}^{n}\frac{1}{n}e^{\frac{r}{n}}$ is **[2004]**

(a) $e+1$ (b) $e-1$

(c) $1-e$ (d) e

89. $\lim_{n\to\infty}\frac{1+2^4+3^4+...n^4}{n^5}-\lim_{n\to\infty}\frac{1+2^3+3^3+...n^3}{n^5}$ **[2003]**

(a) $\frac{1}{5}$ (b) $\frac{1}{30}$

(c) Zero (d) $\frac{1}{4}$

90. $\lim_{n\to\infty}\frac{1^p+2^p+3^p+.....+n^p}{n^{p+1}}$ is **[2002]**

(a) $\frac{1}{p+1}$ (b) $\frac{1}{1-p}$

(c) $\frac{1}{p}-\frac{1}{p-1}$ (d) $\frac{1}{p+2}$

Hints & Solutions

1. (b) $f\left(\frac{3x-4}{3x+4}\right)=x+2,\ x\neq-\frac{4}{3}$

Consider $\frac{3x-4}{3x+4}=t$

$\Rightarrow 3x-4=3tx+4t$

$\Rightarrow x=\frac{4t+4}{3-3t}+2$

$\Rightarrow f(t)=\frac{10-2t}{3-3t}$

$\Rightarrow f(x)=\frac{2x-10}{3x-3}$

$\therefore \int f(x)dx=\int\frac{2x-10}{3x-3}dx$

$=\int\frac{2x}{3x-3}dx-10\int\frac{dx}{3x-3}$

$=\frac{2}{3}\int\frac{x-1}{x-1}dx+\frac{2}{3}\int\frac{dx}{x-1}-\frac{10}{3}\int\frac{dx}{x-1}$

$=\frac{2x}{3}-\frac{8}{3}\ln(x-1)+C$

Here, $A=-\frac{8}{3}, B=\frac{2}{3}$

$\therefore (A,B)=\left(-\frac{8}{3},\frac{2}{3}\right)$

2. (a) Let, $I=\int\sqrt{1+2\cot x\operatorname{cosec} x+2\cot^2 x}\,.dx$

$\Rightarrow I=\int\sqrt{\frac{\sin^2 x+2\cos x+2\cos^2 x}{\sin^2 x}}\,.dx$

$\Rightarrow I=\int\sqrt{\frac{1+2\cos x+\cos^2 x}{\sin x}}\,.dx$

$\Rightarrow I=\int\left|\frac{1+\cos x}{\sin x}\right|.dx$

$\Rightarrow I=\int|\operatorname{cosec} x+\cot x|\,.dx$

$\Rightarrow I=\log|\operatorname{cosec} x-\cot x|+\log|\sin x|+C$

$\Rightarrow I=\log|1-\cos x|+C$

$\Rightarrow I=\log\left|2\sin^2\frac{x}{2}\right|+C$

$\Rightarrow I=\log\left|\sin^2\frac{x}{2}\right|+\log 2+C$

$\Rightarrow I=2\log\left|\sin\frac{x}{2}\right|+C_1$

3. (a) $\int\frac{dx}{\cos^3 x\sqrt{4\sin x\cos x}}=\int\frac{dx}{2\cos^4 x\sqrt{\tan x}}$

Let $\tan x=t^2\Rightarrow\sec^2 x=1+t^4$

$\sec^2 x\,dx=2t\,dt$

$=\int\frac{\sec^4 x\,dx}{2\sqrt{\tan x}}=\int\frac{\sec^2 x(\sec^2 x\,dx)}{2\sqrt{\tan x}}$

$=\int\frac{(1+t^4)2t\,dt}{2t}=\int(1+t^4)\,dt$

$=t+\frac{t^5}{5}+k$

$=\sqrt{\tan x}+\frac{1}{5}\tan^{5/2}x+k\left[t=\sqrt{\tan x}\right]$

$A=\frac{1}{2}, B=\frac{5}{2}, C=\frac{1}{5}$

$A+B+C=\frac{16}{5}$

4. (d) Let $I=\int\frac{\log(t+\sqrt{1+t^2})}{\sqrt{1+t^2}}dt$

put $u=\log(t+\sqrt{1+t^2})$

$du=\frac{1}{t+\sqrt{1+t^2}}.\left[\frac{t+\sqrt{1+t^2}}{\sqrt{1+t^2}}\right]=\frac{1}{\sqrt{1+t^2}}dt$

$\therefore I=\int u\,du=\frac{u^2}{2}+c$

Since $I=\frac{1}{2}[g(t)]^2+c$

$\therefore g(t)=\log\,(t+\sqrt{1+t^2})$

Put t = 2

g (b) = log $(2+\sqrt{5})$

5. (d) Let $I=\int\left(1+x-\frac{1}{x}\right)e^{x+1/x}dx$

$$=\int e^{x+1/x}dx+\int\left(x-\frac{1}{x}\right)e^{x+1/x}dx$$

$$=x.e^{x+1/x}-\int x\left(1-\frac{1}{x^2}\right)e^{x+1/x}dx+\int\left(x-\frac{1}{x}\right)e^{x+1/x}dx$$

$$=x.e^{x+\frac{1}{x}}-\int\left(x-\frac{1}{x}\right)e^{x+1/x}dx+\int\left(x-\frac{1}{x}\right)e^{x+1/x}dx$$

$$=xe^{x+\frac{1}{x}}+C$$

6. (b) Let $I=\int\frac{\sin^2 x\cos^2 x}{(\sin^3 x+\cos^3 x)^2}dx$

$$I=\int\left(\frac{\sin x.\cos x}{\sin^3 x+\cos^3 x}\right)^2 dx$$

$$I=\int\left(\frac{\sin x.\cancel{\cos x}}{\cancel{\cos^3} x\,(1+\tan^3 x)}\right)^2 dx$$

$$=\int\left(\frac{\sin x.\sec^2 x}{(1+\tan^3 x)}\right)^2 dx$$

Put $1+\tan^3 x=t$

$$dt=3\tan^2 x\sec^2 x\,dx \text{ or } dx=\frac{dt}{3\tan^2 x\sec^2 x}$$

$$\therefore I=\int\frac{\sin^2 x.\sec^4 x}{t^2}\times\frac{dt}{3\tan^2 x\sec^2 x}$$

$$I=\frac{1}{3}\int\frac{\sin^2 x.\sec^4 x}{t^2}\times\frac{dt}{\frac{\sin^2 x}{\cos^2 x}\times\sec^2 x}$$

$$=\frac{1}{3}\int\frac{\cancel{\sin^2 x.\sec^4 x}}{t^2}\times\frac{dt}{\cancel{\sin^2 x\sec^4 x}}$$

$$\therefore I=\frac{1}{3}\int\frac{dt}{t^2}=\frac{1}{3}\int t^{-2}dt$$

$$I=\frac{1}{3}\left[\frac{t^{-2+1}}{-2+1}\right]+c=\frac{-1}{3}\left[\frac{1}{t}\right]+c$$

or $I=-\frac{1}{3(1+\tan^3 x)}+c$

7. (a) Let $I=\int x\cos^{-1}\left(\frac{1-x^2}{1+x^2}\right)dx$

$$\therefore I=2\int \underset{\text{II}}{x}.\underset{\text{I}}{\tan^{-1}x}\,dx$$

Applying Integration by parts

$$I=2\left[\tan^{-1}x\int xdx-\int\left(\frac{d}{dx}(\tan^{-1}x)\int xdx\right)dx\right]$$

$$I=2\left[\frac{x^2}{2}\tan^{-1}x-\int\frac{1}{1+x^2}\times\frac{x^2}{2}dx\right]+c$$

$$I=2\left[\frac{x^2}{2}\tan^{-1}x-\frac{1}{2}\int\frac{x^2+1-1}{x^2+1}dx\right]+c$$

$$I=2\left[\frac{x^2}{2}\tan^{-1}x-\frac{1}{2}\int\frac{\cancel{x^2+1}}{\cancel{x^2+1}}dx+\frac{1}{2}\int\frac{1}{1+x^2}dx\right]+c$$

$$I=2\left[\frac{x^2}{2}\tan^{-1}x-\frac{1}{2}\int 1.dx+\frac{1}{2}\tan^{-1}x\right]+c$$

$$I=2\left[\frac{x^2}{2}\tan^{-1}x-\frac{x}{2}+\frac{1}{2}\tan^{-1}x\right]+c$$

$$I=x^2\tan^{-1}x+\tan^{-1}x-x+c$$

or $\boxed{I=-x+(x^2+1)\tan^{-1}x+c}$

8. (b) Let $I=\int\frac{\sin^8 x-\cos^8 x}{1-2\sin^2 x\cos^2 x}dx$

$$=\int\frac{(\sin^4 x)^2-(\cos^4 x)^2}{1-2\sin^2 x\cos^2 x}dx$$

$$=\int\frac{(\sin^4 x+\cos^4 x)(\sin^4 x-\cos^4 x)}{1-2\sin^2 x\cos^2 x}dx$$

$$=\int\frac{[(\sin^2 x+\cos^2 x)^2-2\sin^2 x\cos^2 x]\,[(\sin^2 x+\cos^2 x][\sin^2 x-\cos^2 x]}{1-2\sin^2 x\cos^2 x}dx$$

$$=-\int\cos 2x\,dx=\frac{-\sin 2x}{2}+c=-\frac{1}{2}\sin 2x+c$$

9. (c) Let $\int f(x)dx=\psi(x)$

Let $I=\int x^5 f(x^3)dx$

put $x^3=t$

$\Rightarrow\ 3x^2dx = dt$

$$I = \frac{1}{3}\int 3\cdot x^2\cdot x^3\cdot f(x^3)\cdot dx$$

$$= \frac{1}{3}\int tf(t)dt = \frac{1}{3}\left[t\int f(t)dt - \int f(t)dt\right]$$

$$= \frac{1}{3}\left[t\psi(t) - \int \psi(t)dt\right]$$

$$= \frac{1}{3}\left[x^3\psi(x^3) - 3\int x^2\psi(x^3)dx\right] + c$$

$$= \frac{1}{3}x^3\psi(x^3) - \int x^2\psi(x^3)dx + c$$

10. (a) Let $I = \int \dfrac{\cos 8x + 1}{\cot 2x - \tan 2x}dx$

Now, $D^r = \cot 2x - \tan 2x = \dfrac{\cos 2x}{\sin 2x} - \dfrac{\sin 2x}{\cos 2x}$

$$= \frac{\cos^2 2x - \sin^2 2x}{\sin 2x \cos 2x} = \frac{2\cos 4x}{\sin 4x}$$

$$\therefore\ I = \int \frac{2\cos^2 4x}{\frac{2\cos 4x}{\sin 4x}}dx = \int \frac{2\cos^2 4x . \sin 4x}{2\cos 4x}dx$$

$$= \frac{1}{2}\int \sin 8x\, dx = -\frac{1}{2}\frac{\cos 8x}{8} + k$$

$$= -\frac{1}{16}.\cos 8x + k$$

Now, $-\dfrac{1}{16}.\cos 8x + k = A\cos 8x + k$

$\Rightarrow A = -\dfrac{1}{16}$

11. (d) $\displaystyle\int \frac{5\tan x}{\tan x - 2}dx = \int \frac{5\frac{\sin x}{\cos x}}{\frac{\sin x}{\cos x} - 2}dx$

$$= \int\left(\frac{5\sin x}{\cos x}\times\frac{\cos x}{\sin x - 2\cos x}\right)dx$$

$$= \int \frac{5\sin x\, dx}{\sin x - 2\cos x}$$

$$= \int\left(\frac{4\sin x + \sin x + 2\cos x - 2\cos x}{\sin x - 2\cos x}\right)dx$$

$$= \int \frac{(\sin x - 2\cos x) + (4\sin x + 2\cos x)}{\sin x - 2\cos x}dx$$

$$= \int \frac{(\sin x - 2\cos x) + 2(\cos x + 2\sin x)}{(\sin x - 2\cos x)}dx$$

$$= \int \frac{\sin x - 2\cos x}{\sin x - 2\cos x}dx + 2\int\left(\frac{\cos x + 2\sin x}{\sin x - 2\cos x}\right)dx$$

$$= \int dx + 2\int \frac{\cos x + 2\sin x}{\sin x - 2\cos x}dx$$

$= I_1 + I_2$

where

$I_1 = \int dx$ and $I_2 = 2\int \dfrac{\cos x + 2\sin x}{\sin x - 2\cos x}dx$

put $\sin x - 2\cos x = t$

$\Rightarrow\ (\cos x + 2\sin x)\, dx = dt$

$\therefore\ I_2 = 2\int \dfrac{dt}{t} = 2\ln t + C$

$= 2\ ln\ (\sin x - 2\cos x) + C$

Hence,

$I_1 + I_2 = \int dx + 2\ln(\sin x - 2\cos x) + c$

$= x + 2ln\ |(\sin x - 2\cos x)| + k \Rightarrow a = 2$

12. (a) Let $f(x) = \displaystyle\int\left(\frac{x^2 + \sin^2 x}{1 + x^2}\right)\sec^2 x\, dx$

$$= \int \frac{x^2\sec^2 x + \frac{\sin^2 x}{\cos^2 x}}{1 + x^2}dx$$

$$= \int \frac{x^2\sec^2 x + \tan^2 x}{1 + x^2}dx$$

$$= \int \frac{x^2\left(1 + \tan^2 x\right) + \tan^2 x}{1 + x^2}dx$$

$$= \int \frac{x^2 + \tan^2 x(1 + x^2)}{1 + x^2}dx$$

$$= \int \frac{x^2}{1 + x^2}dx + \int \tan^2 x\, dx$$

$$= \int \frac{x^2 + 1 - 1}{1 + x^2}dx + \int\left(\sec^2 x - 1\right)dx$$

$$= \int 1\, dx - \int \frac{dx}{1 + x^2} + \int sec^2 x dx - \int dx$$

$= -\tan^{-1}x + \tan x + c$

Given: $f(0) = 0$

$\Rightarrow f(0) = -\tan^{-1}0 + \tan 0 + c$

$\Rightarrow c = 0$

$\therefore f(x) = -\tan^{-1}x + \tan x$

Now,

$f(1) = -\tan^{-1}(1) + \tan 1 = \tan 1 - \dfrac{\pi}{4}$

13. (a) Let $I = \displaystyle\int \frac{x^2 - x}{x^3 - x^2 + x - 1}dx$

$$= \int \frac{x(x-1)}{x^2(x-1) + (x-1)}dx = \int \frac{x\, dx}{x^2 + 1}$$

$$= \frac{1}{2}\int \frac{2x\, dx}{\left(x^2 + 1\right)}$$

Let $x^2 + 1 = t \Rightarrow 2x\, dx = dt$

$\therefore\ I = \frac{1}{2}\int \frac{dt}{t} = \frac{1}{2}\log t + c$

$= \frac{1}{2}\log\left(x^2+1\right)+c$

where 'c' is the constant of integration.

14. **(d)** Statement - 2: $\cos^3 x$ is a periodic function.
It is a true statement.
Statement - 1

Given $f(x) = \int \cos^3 x\,dx$

$= \int\left(\frac{\cos 3x}{4}+\frac{3\cos x}{4}\right)dx$

$= \frac{1}{4}\frac{\sin 3x}{3}+\frac{3}{4}\sin x$

$= \frac{1}{12}\sin 3x+\frac{3}{4}\sin x$

Now, period of $\frac{1}{12}\sin 3x = \frac{2\pi}{3}$

Period of $\frac{3}{4}\sin x = 2\pi$

Hence period of $f(x) = \frac{\text{L.C.M.}(2\pi, 2\pi)}{\text{HCF of }(1,3)}$

$= \frac{2\pi}{1} = 2\pi$

Thus, $f(x)$ is a periodic function of period 2π.
Hence, Statement - 1 is false.

15. **(c)** Let $I = \sqrt{2}\int \frac{\sin x\,dx}{\sin\left(x-\frac{\pi}{4}\right)}$ put $x-\frac{\pi}{4}=t$

$\Rightarrow\ dx = dt \Rightarrow I = \sqrt{2}\int \frac{\sin\left(t+\frac{\pi}{4}\right)}{\sin t}dt$

$= \frac{\sqrt{2}}{\sqrt{2}}\int\left(\frac{\sin t+\cos t}{\sin t}\right)dt$

$\Rightarrow\ I = \int(1+\cot t)dt = t+\log|\sin t|+c_1$

$= x-\frac{\pi}{4}+\log\left|\sin\left(x-\frac{\pi}{4}\right)\right|+c_1$

$= x+\log\left|\sin\left(x-\frac{\pi}{4}\right)\right|+c\ \left(\text{where } c = c_1-\frac{\pi}{4}\right)$

16. **(c)** $I = \int \frac{dx}{\cos x+\sqrt{3}\sin x}$

$\Rightarrow\ I = \int \frac{dx}{2\left[\frac{1}{2}\cos x+\frac{\sqrt{3}}{2}\sin x\right]}$

$= \frac{1}{2}\int \frac{dx}{\left[\sin\frac{\pi}{6}\cos x+\cos\frac{\pi}{6}\sin x\right]}$

$= \frac{1}{2}.\int \frac{dx}{\sin\left(x+\frac{\pi}{6}\right)}$

$\Rightarrow\ I = \frac{1}{2}.\int \operatorname{cosec}\left(x+\frac{\pi}{6}\right)dx$

But we know that

$\int \operatorname{cosec} x\,dx = \log|(\tan x/2)|+C$

$\therefore\ I = \frac{1}{2}.\log\tan\left(\frac{x}{2}+\frac{\pi}{12}\right)+C$

17. **(a)** $\int \frac{dx}{\cos x-\sin x} = \int \frac{dx}{\sqrt{2}\cos\left(x+\frac{\pi}{4}\right)}$

$= \frac{1}{\sqrt{2}}\int \sec\left(x+\frac{\pi}{4}\right)dx$

$= \frac{1}{\sqrt{2}}\log\left|\tan\left(\frac{\pi}{4}+\frac{x}{2}+\frac{\pi}{8}\right)\right|+C$

$\left[\because \int \sec x\,dx = \log\left|\tan\left(\frac{\pi}{4}+\frac{x}{2}\right)\right|\right]$

$= \frac{1}{\sqrt{2}}\log\left|\tan\left(\frac{x}{2}+\frac{3\pi}{8}\right)\right|+C$

18. **(b)** $\int \frac{\sin x}{\sin(x-\alpha)}dx = \int \frac{\sin(x-\alpha+\alpha)}{\sin(x-\alpha)}dx$

$= \int \frac{\sin(x-\alpha)\cos\alpha+\cos(x-\alpha)\sin\alpha}{\sin(x-\alpha)}dx$

$= \int\{\cos\alpha+\sin\alpha\cot(x-\alpha)\}dx$

$= (\cos\alpha)x+(\sin\alpha)\log\sin(x-\alpha)+C$

$\therefore\ A = \cos\alpha,\ B = \sin\alpha$

19. **(d)** $\because f''(x)-g''(x)=0$

Integrating, $f'(x)-g'(x)=c;$

$\Rightarrow f'(1)-g'(1)=c \Rightarrow 4-2=c \Rightarrow c=2.$

$\therefore\ f'(x)-g'(x)=2;$

Integrating, $f(x)-g(x)=2x+c_1$

$\Rightarrow f(2)-g(2)=4+c_1 \Rightarrow 9-3=4+c_1;$

$\Rightarrow c_1=2 \qquad \therefore f(x)-g(x)=2x+2$

At $x=3/2, f(x)-g(x)=3+2=5.$

20. (c) $I=\int\frac{dx}{(1+\sqrt{x}).\sqrt{x}\sqrt{1-x}}$

Put $1+\sqrt{x}=t\Rightarrow\frac{1}{2\sqrt{x}}\,dx=dt$

$\Rightarrow\ I=\int\frac{2dt}{t\sqrt{2t-t^2}}$

Again put $t=\frac{1}{z}\Rightarrow dt=\frac{-1}{z^2}dz$

$\Rightarrow\ I=2\int\frac{\frac{-1}{z^2}dz}{\frac{1}{z}\sqrt{\frac{2}{z}-\frac{1}{z^2}}}=2\int\frac{-dz}{\sqrt{2z-1}}=-2\sqrt{2z-1}+c$

$=-2\sqrt{\frac{2}{t}-1}+c=-2\sqrt{\frac{2-t}{t}}+c=-2\sqrt{\frac{1-\sqrt{x}}{1+\sqrt{x}}}+c$

21. (b) $\mathrm{I}=\int\frac{dx}{x^2(x^4+1)^{3/4}}=\int\frac{dx}{x^3(1+x^{-4})^{3/4}}$

Let $x^{-4}=y$

$\Rightarrow -4x^{-3}\,dx=dy$

$\Rightarrow dx=\frac{-1}{4}x^3dy$

$\therefore\ \mathrm{I}=\frac{-1}{4}\int\frac{x^3dy}{x^3(1+y)^{3/4}}=\frac{-1}{4}\int\frac{dy}{(1+y)^{3/4}}$

$=\frac{-1}{4}\times4(1+y)^{1/4}=-(1+x^{-4})^{1/4}+C$

$=-\left(\frac{x^4+1}{x^4}\right)^{1/4}+C$

22. (b) $\int\frac{dx}{(x+1)^{3/4}(x-2)^{5/4}}$

$\int\frac{dx}{\left(\frac{x+1}{x-2}\right)^{3/4}(x-2)^2}$

put $\frac{x+1}{x-2}=t$

$\frac{-3}{(x-2)^2}=\frac{dt}{dx}$

$\frac{dx}{(x-2)^2}=-\frac{dt}{3}$

$=\frac{-1}{3}\int\frac{dt}{t^{3/4}}=-\frac{1}{3}\int t^{\frac{-3}{4}}dt$

$=\frac{1}{3}\left[\frac{t^{\frac{-3}{4}+1}}{\frac{-3}{4}+1}\right]$

$=\frac{-4}{3}\left[\frac{x+1}{x-2}\right]^{1/4}+c$

23. (b) $\int\frac{x^{5m-1}+2x^{4m-1}}{(x^{2m}+x^m+1)^3}dx$

$=\int\frac{x^{5m-1}+2x^{4m-1}}{x^{6m}(1+x^{-m}+x^{-2m})^3}dx$

$=\int\frac{x^{-m-1}+2x^{-2m-1}}{(1+x^{-m}+x^{-2m})^3}dx$

Put $t=1+x^{-m}+x^{-2m}$

$\therefore\ \frac{dt}{dx}=-mx^{-m-1}-2mx^{-2m-1}$

$\Rightarrow\ \frac{dt}{-m}=(x^{-m-1}+2x^{-2m-1})dx$

$\therefore\ \int\frac{x^{5m-1}+2x^{4m-1}}{(x^{2m}+x^m+1)^3}dx=\frac{1}{-m}\int t^{-3}dt=\frac{1}{2mt^2}+C$

$=\frac{1}{2m(1+x^{-m}+x^{-2m})^2}+C$

$=\frac{x^{4m}}{2m(x^{2m}+x^m+1)^2}+C$

$\therefore\ f(x)=\frac{x^{4m}}{2m(x^{2m}+x^m+1)^2}$

24. (b) $\mathrm{I}=\int\frac{x\,dx}{2-x^2+\sqrt{2-x^2}}$

Put $t=\sqrt{2-x^2},\ \frac{dt}{dx}=\frac{1}{2\sqrt{2-x^2}}.(-2x)$

$\Rightarrow -t\,dt=x\,dx$

$\therefore\ \mathrm{I}=\int\frac{(-t)\,dt}{t^2+t}=-\int\frac{1}{t+1}dt=-\log|t+1|$

$=-\log\left|\sqrt{2-x^2}+1\right|+c$

25. (b) Let $\mathrm{I}=\int\frac{x^2-x+1}{x^2+1}.e^{\cot^{-1}x}\,dx$

Put $x=\cot t\Rightarrow -\mathrm{cosec}^2\,t\,dt=dx$

Now, $1 + \cot^2 t = \operatorname{cosec}^2 t$

$$\therefore \quad I = \int \frac{e^t(\cot^2 t - \cot t + 1)}{(1+\cot^2 t)}(-\operatorname{cosec}^2 t)\, dt$$

$$= -\int e^t(\operatorname{cosec}^2 t - \cot t)\, dt$$

$$= \int e^t(\cot t - \operatorname{cosec}^2 t)\, dt$$

$$= e^t \cot t + C$$

$$= e^{\cot^{-1} x}(x) + C \equiv A(x) . e^{\cot^{-1} x} + C$$

$$\Rightarrow A(x) = x$$

26. **(a)** $\int \frac{x^6}{x+x^7} dx = \int \frac{x^6}{x(1+x^6)} dx$

$$= \int \frac{(1+x^6)-1}{x(1+x^6)} dx$$

$$= \int \frac{1}{x} dx - \int \frac{1}{x+x^7} dx$$

$$= \ln|x| - p(x) + c$$

27. **(d)** $\int \frac{(\log x - 1)^2}{(1+(\log x)^2)^2} dx = \int \frac{1+(\log x)^2 - 2\log x}{\left[1+(\log x)^2\right]^2} dx$

$$= \int \left[\frac{1}{(1+(\log x)^2)} - \frac{2\log x}{(1+(\log x)^2)^2}\right] dx$$

$$= \int \left[\frac{e^t}{1+t^2} - \frac{2t\, e^t}{(1+t^2)^2}\right] dt \quad \text{put } \log x = t$$

$$\Rightarrow dx = e^t\, dt$$

$$= \int e^t \left[\frac{1}{1+t^2} - \frac{2t}{(1+t^2)^2}\right] dt$$

[Which is of the form $\int e^x (f(x) + f'(x))\, dx$]

$$= \frac{e^t}{1+t^2} + c = \frac{x}{1+(\log x)^2} + c$$

28. **(c)** $I = \int_{\pi/4}^{3\pi/4} \frac{dx}{1+\cos x}$ ...(i)

$I = \int_{\pi/4}^{3\pi/4} \frac{dx}{1-\cos x}$ ...(ii)

Using $\int_a^b f(x)dx = \int_a^b f(a+b-x)\, dx$

Adding (i) and (ii)

$$2I = \int_{\pi/4}^{3\pi/4} \frac{2}{\sin^2 x} dx$$

$$I = \int_{\pi/4}^{3\pi/4} \operatorname{cosec}^2 x\, dx$$

$$I = -(\cot x)_{\pi/4}^{3\pi/4} = -\left[\cot\frac{3\pi}{4} - \cot\frac{\pi}{4}\right] = 2$$

29. **(c)** $I_n = \int \tan^n x\, dx, n > 1$

Let $I = I_4 + I_6$

$= \int (\tan^4 x + \tan^6 x) dx = \int \tan^4 x \sec^2 x\, dx$

Let $\tan x = t$

$\Rightarrow \sec^2 x\, dx = dt$

$\therefore I = \int t^4 dt$

$$= \frac{t^5}{5} + C$$

$= \frac{1}{5}\tan^5 x + C \Rightarrow$ On comparing, we have

$$a = \frac{1}{5}, b = 0$$

30. **(a)** Let $I = \int_1^2 \frac{dx}{\left((x-1)^2+3\right)^{3/2}}$

Let; $x - 1 = \sqrt{3}\tan\theta$

$\Rightarrow \quad dx = \sqrt{3}\sec^2 . d\theta$

$$\Rightarrow I = \int_0^{\pi/6} \frac{\sqrt{3}\sec^2\theta\, d\theta}{\left(\left(\sqrt{3}\tan\theta\right)^2 + \left(\sqrt{3}\right)^2\right)^{3/2}}$$

$$= \frac{1}{3}\int_0^{\pi/6} \frac{\sec^2\theta}{\sec^3\theta} d\theta$$

$$= \frac{1}{3}\int_0^{\pi/6} \cos\theta\, d\theta$$

$$= \frac{1}{3}[\sin\theta]_0^{\pi/6}$$

$$= \frac{1}{3} \times \frac{1}{2} = \frac{1}{6}$$

$= \frac{1}{6} = \frac{k}{k+5} \Rightarrow k+5 = 6k$

$\Rightarrow \boxed{k=1}$

31. (a) $\int_{\pi/12}^{\pi/4} \frac{\cos 2x}{\left(\frac{1}{\sin 2x}\right)^3} = \int_{\pi/12}^{\pi/4} \cos 2x \times \sin 2x \, . \sin^2(2x)\, dx$

$= \frac{1}{4}\int_{\pi/12}^{\pi/4} \sin 4x \, . (1 - \cos 4x)\, dx$

$= \frac{1}{4}\left[\int_{\pi/12}^{\pi/4} \sin 4x - \frac{1}{2}\int_{\pi/12}^{\pi/4} \sin 8x\right]$

$= \frac{1}{4}\left[-\frac{\cos 4x}{4} + \frac{\cos 8x}{16}\right]_{\pi/12}^{\pi/4} = \frac{1}{4}\left[\frac{15}{32}\right] = \frac{15}{128}$

32. (d) $\int \frac{2x^{12} + 5x^9}{(x^5 + x^3 + 1)^3} dx$

Dividing by x^{15} in numerator and denominator

$\int \frac{\frac{2}{x^3} + \frac{5}{x^6} dx}{\left(1 + \frac{1}{x^2} + \frac{1}{x^5}\right)^3}$

Substitute $1 + \frac{1}{x^2} + \frac{1}{x^5} = t$

$\Rightarrow \left(\frac{-2}{x^3} - \frac{5}{x^6}\right) dx = dt$

$\Rightarrow \left(\frac{2}{x^3} + \frac{5}{x^6}\right) dx = -dt$

This gives,

$\int \frac{\frac{2}{x^3} + \frac{5}{x^6} dx}{\left(1 + \frac{1}{x^2} + \frac{1}{x^5}\right)^3} = \int \frac{-dt}{t^3}$

$= \frac{1}{2t^2} + C$

$= \frac{1}{2\left(1 + \frac{1}{x^2} + \frac{1}{x^5}\right)^2} + C$

$= \frac{x^{10}}{2(x^5 + x^3 + 1)^2} + C$

33. (d) $x\int_1^x y(t)\,dt = x\int_1^x ty(t)\,dt + \int_1^x ty(t)\,dt$

Differentiate *w.r.* to *x*.

$\int_1^x y(t)dt + x[y(x) - y(1)]$

$= \int_1^x ty(t)dt + x[xy(x) - y(1)] + xy(x) - y(1)$

$\int_1^x y(t)dt = \int_1^x ty(t)dt + x^2 y(x) - y(1)$

Diff. again *w.r.* to *x*

$y(x) - y(a) = xy(x) - y(a) + 2x\,y(x) + x^2 y^1(x)$

$(1 - 3x)\, y(x) = x^2 y^1(x)$

$\frac{y^1(x)}{y(x)} = \frac{1-3x}{x^2}$

$\frac{1}{y}\frac{dy}{dx} = \frac{1-3x}{x^2} \Rightarrow \ln y = -\frac{1}{x} - 3\ln x$

$\ln(yx^3) = -\frac{1}{x}$

$yx^3 = -e^{-1/x}$

$y = \frac{e^{-\frac{1}{x}}}{x^3}$ or $y = \frac{ce^{-\frac{1}{x}}}{x^3}$

34. (d) $I = \int_4^{10} \frac{[x^2]}{[x^2 - 28x + 196] + [x^2]} dx$ .....(a)

Use $\int_a^b f(a+b-x)\,dx = \int_a^b f(x)\,dx$

$I = \int_4^{10} \frac{[(x-14)^2]}{[x^2] + [(x-14)^2]} dx$ .....(b)

(a) + (b)

$2I = \int_4^{10} \frac{[(x-14)^2] + [x^2]}{[x^2] + [(x-14)^2]} dx$

$2I = \int_4^{10} dx \Rightarrow 2I = 6 \Rightarrow I = 3$

35. (b) $2\int_0^1 \tan^{-1} x\,dx = \int_0^1\left(\frac{\pi}{2} - \tan^{-1}(1-x+x^2)\right)dx$

$2\int_0^1 \tan^{-1} x\,dx = \int_0^1 \frac{\pi}{2}dx - \int_0^1 \tan^{-1}(1-x+x^2)\,dx$

$\int_0^1 \tan^{-1}(1-x+x^2)\,dx = \frac{\pi}{2} - 2\int_0^1 \tan^{-1} x dx$ .....(a)

Let

$I_1 = \int_0^1 \tan^{-1} x dx$

$= \left[(\tan^{-1} x)x\right]_0^1 - \int_0^1 \frac{1}{1+x^2} x\,dx$

$= \frac{\pi}{4} - \int_0^1 \frac{x}{1+x^2}\,dx$

$= \frac{\pi}{4} - \frac{1}{2}\log 2$

By equation (a)

$\frac{\pi}{2} - 2\left[\frac{\pi}{4} - \frac{1}{2}\log 2\right] = \log 2$

36. (a) $I = \int_2^4 \frac{\log x^2}{\log x^2 + \log(36-12x+x^2)}dx$

$I = \int_2^4 \frac{\log x^2}{\log x^2 + \log(6-x)^2}dx$ ...(i)

$I = \int_2^4 \frac{\log(6-x)^2}{\log(6-x)^2 + \log x^2}dx$ ...(ii)

Adding (i) and (ii)

$2I = \int_2^4 dx = [x]_2^4 = 2$

$I = 1$

37. (c) Let $f : R \to R$ be a function such that $f(2-x) = f(e+x)$
Put $x = 2 + x$ we get
$f(-x) = f(4+x) = f(4-x)$
$\Rightarrow f(x) = f(x+4)$
Hence period is 4

Consider $\int_{10}^{50} f(x)dx = 10\int_{10}^{14} f(x)dx = 10[5+5] = 100$

38. (d) Let $f: (-1, 1) \to R$ be a continuous function

Let $\int_0^{\sin x} f(t)dt = \frac{\sqrt{3}}{2}x$

$f(\sin x).\frac{d}{dx}(\sin x) = \frac{\sqrt{3}}{2}$

$\Rightarrow f(\sin x).\cos x = \frac{\sqrt{3}}{2}$

put $x = \frac{\pi}{3}$

$f\left(\sin\frac{\pi}{3}\right).\cos\frac{\pi}{3} = \frac{\sqrt{3}}{2}$

$f\left(\frac{\sqrt{3}}{2}\right).\frac{1}{2} = \frac{\sqrt{3}}{2}$

$f\left(\frac{\sqrt{3}}{2}\right) = \sqrt{3}$

39. (c) $f\left(\frac{1}{x}\right) = \int_1^{1/x} \frac{\ln t}{1+t}dt$

Let $t = \frac{1}{z}$

$dt = -\frac{1}{z^2}dz$

$f(x) = \int_1^x \frac{\ln z}{z(z+1)}dz$

$f(x) + f\left(\frac{1}{x}\right) = \int_1^x \frac{\ln x}{z}dz$

$= \left[\frac{(\ln z)^2}{2}\right]_1^x = \frac{(\ln x)^2}{2}$

40. (b) Let $I = \int_0^{\pi}\sqrt{1+4\sin^2\frac{x}{2} - 4\sin\frac{x}{2}}dx$

$= \int_0^{\pi}\left|2\sin\frac{x}{2} - 1\right|dx$

$= \int_0^{\pi/3}\left(1 - 2\sin\frac{x}{2}\right)dx + \int_{\pi/3}^{\pi}\left(2\sin\frac{x}{2} - 1\right)dx$

$\left[\because \sin\frac{x}{2} = \frac{1}{2} \Rightarrow \frac{x}{2} = \frac{\pi}{6}\right.$

$\left.\Rightarrow x = \frac{\pi}{3}, \frac{x}{2} = \frac{5\pi}{6} \Rightarrow x = \frac{5\pi}{3}\right]$

$$= \left[x + 4\cos\frac{x}{2}\right]_0^{\pi/3} + \left[-4\cos\frac{x}{2} - x\right]_{\pi/3}^{\pi}$$

$$= \frac{\pi}{3} + 4\frac{\sqrt{3}}{2} - 4 + \left(0 - \pi + 4\frac{\sqrt{3}}{2} + \frac{\pi}{3}\right)$$

$$= 4\sqrt{3} - 4 - \frac{\pi}{3}$$

41. (d) $F(x) = \int_1^x \frac{e^t}{t} dt,\ x > 0$

Let $I = \int_1^x \frac{e^t}{t+a} dt$

Put $t + a = z \Rightarrow t = z - a;\ dt = dz$
for $t = 1,\ z = 1 + a$
for $t = x,\ z = x + a$

$$\therefore I = \int_{1+a}^{x+a} \frac{e^{z-a}}{z} dz$$

$$= e^{-a}\int_{1+a}^{x+a} \frac{e^z}{z} dz \equiv e^{-a}\int_{1+a}^{x+a} \frac{e^t}{t} dt$$

$$I = e^{-a}\left[\int_{1+a}^{1} \frac{e^t}{t} dt + \int_1^{x+a} \frac{e^t}{t} dt\right]$$

$$= e^{-a}\left[-\int_1^{1+a} \frac{e^t}{t} dt + \int_1^{x+a} \frac{e^t}{t} dt\right]$$

$$= e^{-a}[-F(1+a) + F(x+a)]$$

(By the definition of F(x))

$$= e^{-a}[F(x+a) - F(1+a)]$$

42. (a) Let $\int_{-\pi}^{t} (f(x) + x)dx = \pi^2 - t^2$

$$\Rightarrow \int_{-\pi}^{t} f(x)dx + \int_{-\pi}^{t} xdx = \pi^2 - t^2$$

$$\Rightarrow \int_{-\pi}^{t} f(x)dx + \left(\frac{t^2}{2} - \frac{\pi^2}{2}\right) = \pi^2 - t^2$$

$$\Rightarrow \int_{-\pi}^{t} f(x)dx = \frac{3}{2}(\pi^2 - t^2)$$

differentiating with respect to t

$$\frac{d}{dt}\left[\int_{-\pi}^{t} f(x)dx\right] = \frac{3}{2}\frac{d}{dt}(\pi^2 - t^2)$$

$$f(t).\frac{dt}{dt} - f(-\pi)\frac{d}{dt}(-\pi) = -3t$$

$$f(t) = -3t$$

$$f\left(-\frac{\pi}{3}\right) = -3\left(-\frac{\pi}{3}\right) = \pi$$

43. (d) Let $I = \int_0^{\pi} [\cos x]dx$ ...(1)

$$I = \int_0^{\pi} [\cos(\pi - x)]dx = \int_0^{\pi} [-\cos x]dx \quad ...(2)$$

On adding (1) and (2), we get

$$2I = \int_0^{\pi}[\cos x]dx + \int_0^{\pi}[-\cos x]dx$$

$$2I = \int_0^{\pi} [\cos x] + [-\cos x]dx$$

$$2I = \int_0^{\pi} -1dx \quad (\because [x] + [-x] = -1 \text{ if } x \notin Z)$$

$$2I = -x|_0^{\pi} = -\pi$$

$$\Rightarrow I = \frac{-\pi}{2}$$

44. (c) $P_n = \int_1^{e} (\log x)^n dx$

put $\log x = t$ then $x = e^t$ and $dx = e^t\ dt$
Also, when $x = 1$, then $t = \log 1 = 0$
and when $x = e$, then $t = \log_e e = 1$

$$\therefore P_n = \int_0^1 t^n.e^t\,dt$$

$$\therefore P_{10} = \int_0^1 t^{10}e^t dt \text{ and } P_8 = \int_0^1 t^8 e^t dt$$

$$\text{Now, } P_{10} - 90P_8 = \int_0^1 \underset{\text{I}}{t^{10}}\ \underset{\text{II}}{e^t}\,dt - 90\int_0^1 t^8 e^t dt$$

$$P_{10} - 90\ P_8 = \left[t^{10}e^t\right]_0^1 - 10\int_0^1 t^9 e^t dt - 90\int_0^1 t^8 e^t dt$$

$$P_{10} - 90\ P_8$$

$$= e - 10\left[t^9\int_0^1 e^t dt - \int_0^1 \frac{d}{dt}(t^9)\int e^t dt\right] - 90\int_0^1 t^8 e^t dt$$

$$P_{10} - 90\ P_8 = e - 10\left[e - 9\int_0^1 t^8 e^t dt\right] - 90\int_0^1 t^8 e^t dt$$

$$P_{10} - 90\ P_8 = e - 10e + 90\int t^8 \cancel{e^t}\,dt - 90\int_0^1 t^8 \cancel{e^t}\,dt$$

$$\therefore P_{10} - 90P_8 = -9e$$

45. **(c)** Let $I = \int_0^{1/2} \frac{\ln(1+2x)}{1+4x^2}dx$ or $\int_0^{1/2} \frac{\ln(1+2x)}{1+(2x)^2}dx$

Put $2x = \tan\theta$

$\therefore \frac{2dx}{d\theta} = \sec^2\theta$ or $dx = \frac{\sec^2\theta d\theta}{2}$

also when $x = 0 \Rightarrow \theta = 0$

and when $x = \frac{1}{2} \Rightarrow \theta = 45°$ or $\frac{\pi}{4}$

$$\therefore I = \int_0^{\frac{\pi}{4}} \frac{\ln(1+\tan\theta)}{1+\tan^2\theta} \times \frac{\sec^2\theta d\theta}{2}$$

$$I = \frac{1}{2}\int_0^{\frac{\pi}{4}} \frac{\ln(1+\tan\theta)}{1+\tan^2\theta} \times \sec^2\theta d\theta$$

$(\because 1 + \tan^2\theta = \sec^2\theta)$

$$I = \frac{1}{2}\int_0^{\frac{\pi}{4}} \ln(1+\tan\theta)d\theta \quad ...(1)$$

$$I = \frac{1}{2}\int_0^{\frac{\pi}{4}} \ln\left[1+\tan\left(\frac{\pi}{4}-\theta\right)\right]d\theta$$

(Using the property of definite integral)

$$I = \frac{1}{2}\int_0^{\frac{\pi}{4}} \ln\left[1+\frac{\tan\frac{\pi}{4}-\tan\theta}{1+\tan\frac{\pi}{4}\times\tan\theta}\right]d\theta$$

$$I = \frac{1}{2}\int_0^{\frac{\pi}{4}} \ln\left[1+\frac{1-\tan\theta}{1+\tan\theta}\right]d\theta$$

$$I = \frac{1}{2}\int_0^{\frac{\pi}{4}} \ln\left[\frac{1+\cancel{\tan\theta}+1-\cancel{\tan\theta}}{1+\tan\theta}\right]d\theta$$

$$I = \frac{1}{2}\int_0^{\frac{\pi}{4}} \ln\left[\frac{2}{1+\tan\theta}\right]d\theta$$

$$I = \frac{1}{2}\int_0^{\frac{\pi}{4}} [\ln 2 - \ln(1+\tan\theta)]d\theta$$

$$I = \frac{1}{2}\int_0^{\frac{\pi}{4}} \ln 2 . d\theta - \frac{1}{2}\int_0^{\frac{\pi}{4}} \ln(1+\tan\theta)d\theta$$

$$I = \frac{1}{2}\ln 2\theta\Big|_0^{\pi/4} - I \quad \text{(from eq. (1))}$$

$$I + I = \frac{1}{2}\ln 2\left(\frac{\pi}{4}-0\right)$$

$$2I = \frac{1}{2}\times\frac{\pi}{4}\times\ln 2$$

$$2I = \frac{\pi}{8}\ln 2 \text{ or } I = \frac{\pi}{16}\ln 2$$

46. **(a)** Since, $y = \int_0^x |t|dt, x \in R$

therefore $\frac{dy}{dx} = |x|$

But from $y = 2x$, $\frac{dy}{dx} = 2$

$\Rightarrow |x| = 2 \Rightarrow x = \pm 2$

Points $y = \int_0^{\pm 2} |t|dt = \pm 2$

$\therefore$ equation of tangent is

$y - 2 = 2(x-2)$ or $y + 2 = 2(x+2)$

$\Rightarrow$ x-intercept $= \pm 1$.

47. **(d)** Let $I = \int_{\pi/6}^{\pi/3} \frac{dx}{1+\sqrt{\tan x}}$

$$= \int_{\pi/6}^{\pi/3} \frac{dx}{1+\sqrt{\tan\left(\frac{\pi}{2}-x\right)}}$$

$$= \int_{\pi/6}^{\pi/3} \frac{\sqrt{\tan x}\,dx}{1+\sqrt{\tan x}} \quad ...(1)$$

Also, given

$$I = \int_{\pi/6}^{\pi/3} \frac{\sqrt{\tan x}\,dx}{1+\sqrt{\tan x}} \quad ...(2)$$

By adding (1) and (2), we get

$$2I = \int_{\pi/6}^{\pi/3} dx$$

$$\Rightarrow I = \frac{1}{2}\left[\frac{\pi}{3}-\frac{\pi}{6}\right] = \frac{\pi}{12},$$

statement-1 is false

$$\int_a^b f(x)dx = \int_a^b f(a+b-x)dx$$

It is fundamental property.

48. **(a)** Consider

$$\int_0^{\sin^2 x} \sin^{-1}(\sqrt{t})\, dt + \int_0^{\cos^2 x} \cos^{-1}(\sqrt{t})\, dt$$

Let $I = f(x)$ after integrating and putting the limits.

$$f'(x) = \sin^{-1}\sqrt{\sin^2 x}\,(2\sin x\cos x) - 0$$

$$+\cos^{-1}\sqrt{\cos^2 x}\,(-2\cos x\sin x) - 0$$

$\therefore f'(x) = 0 \Rightarrow f(x) = C$ (constant)

Now, we find $f(x)$ at $x = \frac{\pi}{4}$

$$\therefore\ I = \int_0^{1/2} \sin^{-1}\sqrt{t}\, dt + \int_0^{1/2} \cos^{-1}\sqrt{t}\, dt$$

$$= \int_0^{1/2} (\sin^{-1}\sqrt{t} + \cos^{-1}\sqrt{t})\, dt$$

$$= \int_0^{1/2} \frac{\pi}{2}\, dt = \frac{\pi}{4} = C$$

$$\therefore\ f(x) = \frac{\pi}{4}$$

$\therefore$ Required integration $= \frac{\pi}{4}$

49. (d) $I = \int_{-\pi/2}^{\pi/2} \frac{\sin^2 x}{1+2^x}\, dx$ ...(i)

$\Rightarrow I = \int_{-\pi/2}^{\pi/2} \frac{\sin^2 x}{1+2^{-x}}\, dx$, by replacing x by $\left(\frac{\pi}{2} - \frac{\pi}{2} - x\right)$

$\Rightarrow I = \int_{-\pi/2}^{\pi/2} \frac{2^x . \sin^2 x}{1+2^x}\, dx$ ...(ii)

Adding equations (i) and (ii), we get

$$2I = \int_{-\pi/2}^{\pi/2} \sin^2 x\, dx = \frac{1}{2}\int_{-\pi/2}^{\pi/2} (1-\cos 2x)\, dx$$

$$\Rightarrow I = \frac{1}{4}\left[x + \frac{\sin 2x}{2}\right]_{-\pi/2}^{\pi/2}$$

$$= \frac{1}{4}\left[\left(\frac{\pi}{2} + \frac{\sin \pi}{2}\right) - \left(-\frac{\pi}{2} + \frac{\sin(-\pi)}{2}\right)\right]$$

$$\Rightarrow I = \frac{1}{4}\left[\frac{\pi}{2} + \frac{\pi}{2}\right] = \frac{\pi}{4}$$

50. (d) Let $I = \int_{7\pi/4}^{7\pi/3} \sqrt{\tan^2 x}\, dx$

$$= \int_{7\pi/4}^{7\pi/3} \tan x\, dx = -\log\cos x\Big|_{7\pi/4}^{7\pi/3}$$

$$= -\left[\log\cos\frac{7\pi}{3} - \log\cos\frac{7\pi}{4}\right]$$

$$= \log\cos\frac{7\pi}{4} - \log\cos\frac{7\pi}{3}$$

$$= \log\left[\frac{\cos\frac{7\pi}{4}}{\cos\frac{7\pi}{3}}\right] = \log\left[\frac{\cos\left(2\pi - \frac{\pi}{4}\right)}{\cos\left(2\pi + \frac{\pi}{3}\right)}\right]$$

$$= \log\left(\frac{\cos\frac{\pi}{4}}{\cos\frac{\pi}{3}}\right) = \log\left(\frac{\frac{1}{\sqrt{2}}}{\frac{1}{2}}\right)$$

$$= \log\left(\frac{2}{\sqrt{2}}\right) = \log\sqrt{2}.$$

51. (a) $x = \int_0^y \frac{dt}{\sqrt{1+t^2}}$

$$\Rightarrow 1 = \frac{1}{\sqrt{1+y^2}} \cdot \frac{dy}{dx}$$

$$\left[\because \text{ If } I(x) = \int_{\phi(x)}^{\psi(x)} f(t)\, dt, \text{ then } \frac{dI(x)}{dx} = f\{\psi(x)\} . \left\{\frac{d}{dx}\psi(x)\right\} - f\{\phi(x)\} . \left\{\frac{d}{dx}\phi(x)\right\}\right]$$

$$\frac{dy}{dx} = \sqrt{1-y^2}$$

$$\Rightarrow \frac{d^2y}{dx^2} = \frac{1}{2\sqrt{1+y^2}} . 2y . \frac{dy}{dx} = \frac{y}{\sqrt{1+y^2}} . \sqrt{1+y^2} = y$$

52. (b, c) $g(x+\pi) = \int_0^{x+\pi} \cos 4t\, dt$

$$= \int_0^x \cos 4t\, dt + \int_x^{\pi+x} \cos 4t\, dt = g(x) + \int_0^{\pi} \cos 4t\, dt$$

(from graph of cos 4t, it is clear that

$$\int_x^{\pi+x} \cos 4t\, dt = \int_0^{\pi} \cos 4t\, dt$$

$= g(x) + g(\pi) = g(x) - g(\pi)$

($\because$ from graph of cos 4t, $g(\pi) = 0$)

53. (d) $\int_{-0.9}^{0.9} \left\{[x^2] + \log\left(\frac{2-x}{2+x}\right)\right\} dx$

$$= \int_{-0.9}^{0.9} [x^2]dx + \int_{-0.9}^{0.9} \log\left(\frac{2-x}{2+x}\right) dx$$

$$= 0 + \int_{-0.9}^{0.9} \log\left(\frac{2-x}{2+x}\right) dx$$

Put $x = -x \Rightarrow f(x) = \log\frac{2-x}{2+x}$

and $f(-x) = \log\frac{2+x}{2-x}$

$$= -\log\frac{(2-x)}{2+x} = -f(x)$$

So, it is an odd function, hence
Required integral = 0.

54. (d) Since $\int_0^a [x] = 0$ where $0 \le a \le 1$

$$\therefore \int_0^{0.9} [x - 2[x]]dx = 0$$

55. (a) Let $\frac{d}{dx}G(x) = \frac{e^{\tan x}}{x}, x \in \left(0, \frac{\pi}{2}\right)$

Now, $I = \int_{1/4}^{1/2} \frac{2}{x} e^{\tan \pi x^2} .dx$

$$= \int_{1/4}^{1/2} \frac{2\pi x}{\pi x^2} e^{\tan \pi x^2} .dx$$

Let $\pi x^2 = t \Rightarrow 2\pi x\, dx = dt$

When $x = \frac{1}{2}, t = \frac{\pi}{4}$ and $x = \frac{1}{4}, t = \frac{\pi}{16}$

$$\therefore I = \int_{\pi/16}^{\pi/4} \frac{e^{\tan t}}{t} dt = G(t)\Big|_{\frac{\pi}{16}}^{\frac{\pi}{4}}$$

$$= G\left(\frac{\pi}{4}\right) - G\left(\frac{\pi}{16}\right)$$

56. (d) Let $\int_e^x t\, f(t)\, dt = \sin x - x\cos x - \frac{x^2}{2}$

By using Leibnitz rule, we get

$$\frac{d}{dx}\left[\int_e^x t\, f(t)\, dt\right] = \frac{d}{dx}\left[\sin x - x\cos x - \frac{x^2}{2}\right]$$

$$\Rightarrow x f(x) - e f(e).\, 0 = x \sin x - x$$

Now, put $x = \frac{\pi}{6}$, we get

$$\frac{\pi}{6}.f\left(\frac{\pi}{6}\right) = \frac{\pi}{6}.\sin\frac{\pi}{6} - \frac{\pi}{6}$$

$$\Rightarrow f\left(\frac{\pi}{6}\right) = \sin\frac{\pi}{6} - 1 = \frac{1}{2} - 1 = -\frac{1}{2}$$

57. (c) $\int_0^{1.5} x\left[x^2\right]dx = \int_0^1 x[x^2]dx + \int_1^{\sqrt{2}} x\left[x^2\right]dx + \int_{\sqrt{2}}^{1.5} x\left[x^2\right]dx$

$$= \int_0^1 x.0\, dx + \int_1^{\sqrt{2}} x dx + \int_{\sqrt{2}}^{1.5} 2x dx$$

$$= 0 + \left[\frac{x^2}{2}\right]_1^{\sqrt{2}} + \left[x^2\right]_{\sqrt{2}}^{1.5}$$

$$= \frac{1}{2}(2-1) + (2.25-2) = \frac{1}{2} + 0.25$$

$$= \frac{1}{2} + \frac{1}{4} = \frac{3}{4}$$

58. (d) $I = \int_0^1 \frac{8\log(1+x)}{1+x^2} dx$

Put $x = \tan\theta$,

$$\therefore \frac{dx}{d\theta} = \sec^2\theta \Rightarrow dx = \sec^2\theta d\theta$$

$$\therefore I = 8\int_0^{\pi/4} \frac{\log(1+\tan\theta)}{1+\tan^2\theta}.\sec^2\theta d\theta$$

$$I = 8\int_0^{\pi/4} \log(1+\tan\theta)d\theta \quad ...(i)$$

$$= 8\int_0^{\pi/4} \log\left[1+\tan\left(\frac{\pi}{4}-\theta\right)\right]d\theta$$

$$= 8\int_0^{\pi/4} \log\left[1+\frac{1-\tan\theta}{1+\tan\theta}\right]d\theta$$

$$= 8\int_0^{\pi/4} \log\left[\frac{2}{1+\tan\theta}\right]d\theta$$

$$= 8\int_0^{\pi/4} [\log 2 - \log(1+\tan\theta)]d\theta$$

$$I = 8.(\log 2)[x]_0^{\pi/4} - 8\int_0^{\pi/4} \log(1+\tan\theta)d\theta$$

$I = 8.\frac{\pi}{4}.\log 2 - I$ [From equation (i)]

$\Rightarrow 2I = 2\pi \log 2$

$\therefore I = \pi \log 2$

59. **(a)** $p'(x) = p'(1-x)$

$\Rightarrow p(x) = -p(1-x) + c$

at $x = 0$

$p(0) = -p(1) + c \Rightarrow 42 = c$

Now, $p(x) = -p(1-x) + 42$

$\Rightarrow p(x) + p(1-x) = 42$

$\Rightarrow I = \int_0^1 p(x)dx$ ...(i)

$\Rightarrow I = \int_0^1 p(1-x)dx$ ...(ii)

on adding (i) and (ii),

$2I = \int_0^1 (42)\,dx \Rightarrow I = 21$

60. **(c)** Let $I = \int_0^{\pi} [\cot x]\, dx$ ....(1)

$= \int_0^{\pi} [\cot(\pi - x)]\, dx = \int_0^{\pi} [-\cot x]\, dx$ ....(2)

Adding two values of I in eq^n s (1) & (2),
We get

$2I = \int_0^{\pi} ([\cot x] + [-\cot x])\, dx$

$= \int_0^{\pi} (-1) dx$

$[\because [x] + [-x] = -1,$ if $x \notin z$ and $[x] + [-x] = 0,$ if $x \in z]$

$= [-x]_0^{\pi} = -\pi$

$\Rightarrow I = -\frac{\pi}{2}$

61. **(b)** We know that $\frac{\sin x}{x} < 1$, for $x \in (0, 1)$

$\Rightarrow \frac{\sin x}{\sqrt{x}} < \sqrt{x}$ on $x \in (0, 1)$

$\Rightarrow \int_0^1 \frac{\sin x}{\sqrt{x}} dx < \int_0^1 \sqrt{x} dx = \left[\frac{2x^{3/2}}{3}\right]_0^1$

$\Rightarrow \int_0^1 \frac{\sin x}{\sqrt{x}} dx < \frac{2}{3} \Rightarrow I < \frac{2}{3}$

Also $\frac{\cos x}{\sqrt{x}} < \frac{1}{\sqrt{x}}$ for $x \in (0, 1)$

$\Rightarrow \int_0^1 \frac{\cos x}{\sqrt{x}} dx < \int_0^1 x^{-1/2} dx = \left[2\sqrt{x}\right]_0^1 = 2$

$\Rightarrow \int_0^1 \frac{\cos x}{\sqrt{x}} dx < 2 \Rightarrow J < 2$

62. **(d)** $\int_{\sqrt{2}}^{x} \frac{dt}{t\sqrt{t^2 - 1}} = \frac{\pi}{2}$

$\therefore \left[\sec^{-1} t\right]_{\sqrt{2}}^{x} = \frac{\pi}{2}$ $\left[\because \int \frac{dx}{x\sqrt{x^2 - 1}} = \sec^{-1} x\right]$

$\Rightarrow \sec^{-1} x - \sec^{-1}\sqrt{2} = \frac{\pi}{2}$

$\Rightarrow \sec^{-1} x - \frac{\pi}{4} = \frac{\pi}{2} \Rightarrow \sec^{-1} x = \frac{\pi}{2} + \frac{\pi}{4}$

$\Rightarrow \sec^{-1} x = \frac{3\pi}{4} \Rightarrow x = \sec\frac{3\pi}{4}$

$\Rightarrow x = -\sqrt{2}$

63. **(c)** Given $F(x) = f(x) + f\left(\frac{1}{x}\right)$, where

$f(x) = \int_1^x \frac{\log t}{1+t} dt$

$\therefore F(e) = f(e) + f\left(\frac{1}{e}\right)$

$\Rightarrow F(e) = \int_1^e \frac{\log t}{1+t} dt + \int_1^{1/e} \frac{\log t}{1+t} dt$ ....(A)

Now for solving, $I = \int_1^{1/e} \frac{\log t}{1+t} dt$

$\therefore$ Put $\frac{1}{t} = z \Rightarrow -\frac{1}{t^2} dt = dz \Rightarrow dt = -\frac{dz}{z^2}$

and limit for $t = 1 \Rightarrow z = 1$ and for $t = 1/e \Rightarrow z = e$

$\therefore I = \int_1^e \frac{\log\left(\frac{1}{z}\right)}{1 + \frac{1}{z}} \left(-\frac{dz}{z^2}\right)$

$= \int_1^e \frac{(\log 1 - \log z).z}{z+1} \left(-\frac{dz}{z^2}\right)$

$= \int_1^e -\frac{\log z}{(z+1)} \left(-\frac{dz}{z}\right)$ $[\because \log 1 = 0]$

$= \int_1^e \frac{\log z}{z(z+1)} dz$

$\therefore I = \int_1^e \frac{\log t}{t(t+1)} dt$

[By property $\int_a^b f(t)dt = \int_a^b f(x)dx$]

Equation (A) becomes

$$F(e) = \int_1^e \frac{\log t}{1+t}dt + \int_1^e \frac{\log t}{t(1+t)}dt$$

$$= \int_1^e \frac{t.\log t + \log t}{t(1+t)}dt = \int_1^e \frac{(\log t)(t+1)}{t(1+t)}dt$$

$$\Rightarrow F(e) = \int_1^e \frac{\log t}{t}dt$$

Let $\log t = x$ $\quad\therefore \frac{1}{t}dt = dx$

[for limit $t = 1, x = 0$ and $t = e, x = \log e = 1$]

$$\therefore F(e) = \int_0^1 x\,dx \quad F(e) = \left[\frac{x^2}{2}\right]_0^1$$

$$\Rightarrow F(e) = \frac{1}{2}$$

64. (b) Let $a = k + h$ where k is an integer such that $[a] = k$ and $0 \le h < 1$

$$\therefore \int_1^a [x]f'(x)dx = \int_1^2 1f'(x)dx + \int_2^3 2f'(x)dx + \ldots$$

$$\int_{k-1}^{k} (k-1)dx + \int_k^{k+h} kf'(x)dx$$

$$= \{f(2)-f(1)\} + 2\{f(3)-f(2)\} + 3\{f(4)-f(3)\} + \ldots\ldots + (k-1)\{f(k)-f(k-1)\} + k\{f(k+h) - f(k)\}$$

$$= -f(1) - f(2) - f(3) \ldots\ldots - f(k) + kf(k+h)$$

$$= [a]f(a) - \{f(1) + f(2) + f(3) + \ldots f([a])\}$$

65. (c) $$I = \int_{-\frac{3\pi}{2}}^{-\frac{\pi}{2}} [(x+\pi)^3 + \cos^2(x+3\pi)]dx$$

Put $x + \pi = t$

$$I = \int_{-\frac{\pi}{2}}^{\frac{\pi}{2}} [t^3 + \cos^2 t]dt = 2\int_{-\frac{\pi}{2}}^{\frac{\pi}{2}} \cos^2 t dt$$

[using the property of even and odd function]

$$= \int_0^{\frac{\pi}{2}} (1 + \cos 2t)dt = \frac{\pi}{2} + 0$$

66. (d) $$I = \int_0^{\pi} xf(\sin x)dx = \int_0^{\pi} (\pi - x)f(\sin x)dx$$

$$= \pi\int_0^{\pi} f(\sin x)dx - I$$

$$\Rightarrow 2I = \pi\int_0^{\pi} f(\sin x)dx$$

$$I = \frac{\pi}{2}\int_0^{\pi} f(\sin x)dx = \pi\int_0^{\pi/2} f(\sin x)dx$$

$$= \pi\int_0^{\pi/2} f(\cos x)dx$$

67. (b) $$I = \int_3^6 \frac{\sqrt{x}}{\sqrt{9-x}+\sqrt{x}}dx \quad \ldots(1)$$

$$I = \int_3^6 \frac{\sqrt{9-x}}{\sqrt{9-x}+\sqrt{x}}dx \quad \ldots(2)$$

[using $\int_a^b f(x)dx = \int_a^b f(a+b-x)dx$]

Adding equation (1) and (2)

$$2I = \int_3^6 dx = 3 \Rightarrow I = \frac{3}{2}$$

68. (b) Let $I = \int_{-\pi}^{\pi} \frac{\cos^2 x}{1+a^x}dx$ ....(1)

$$= \int_{-\pi}^{\pi} \frac{\cos^2(-x)}{1+a^{-x}}dx$$

$$\left[\text{Using} \int_a^b f(x)dx = \int_a^b f(a+b-x)dx\right]$$

$$= \int_{-\pi}^{\pi} \frac{\cos^2 x}{1+a^x}dx \quad \ldots(2)$$

Adding equations (1) and (2) we get

$$2I = \int_{-\pi}^{\pi} \cos^2 x\left(\frac{1+a^x}{1+a^x}\right)dx = \int_{-\pi}^{\pi} \cos^2 x\,dx$$

$$= 2\int_0^{\pi} \cos^2 x\,dx$$

$$= 2\times 2\int_0^{\frac{\pi}{2}} \cos^2 x\, dx = 4\int_0^{\frac{\pi}{2}} \sin^2 x\, dx$$

$$\Rightarrow I = 2\int_0^{\frac{\pi}{2}} \sin^2 x\, dx = 2\int_0^{\frac{\pi}{2}} \left(1-\cos^2 x\right)dx$$

$$\Rightarrow I = 2\int_0^{\frac{\pi}{2}} dx - 2\int_0^{\frac{\pi}{2}} \cos^2 x\, dx$$

$$\Rightarrow I + I = 2\left(\frac{\pi}{2}\right) = \pi \Rightarrow \mathrm{I} = \frac{\pi}{2}$$

69. **(b)** $I_1 = \int_0^1 2^{x^2} dx,\ I_2 = \int_0^1 2^{x^3} dx,$

$$I_3 = \int_0^1 2^{x^2} dx,\ I_4 = \int_0^1 2^{x^3} dx\ \forall 0 < x < 1,\ x^2 > x^3$$

$$\Rightarrow \int_0^1 2^{x^2} dx > \int_0^1 2^{x^3} dx \Rightarrow I_1 > I_2$$

70. **(d)** $\lim\limits_{x\to 2} \int_0^{f(x)} \frac{4t^3}{x-2} dt = \lim\limits_{x\to 0} \frac{\int_0^{f(x)} 4t^3\, dt}{x-2}$

Applying L Hospital rule

$$\lim_{x\to 2} \frac{[4f(x)^3 f'(x)]}{1} = 4(f(2))^3 f'(2)$$

$$= 4\times 6^3 \times \frac{1}{48} = 18$$

71. **(d)** $f(x) = \frac{e^x}{1+e^x} \Rightarrow f(-x) = \frac{e^{-x}}{1+e^{-x}} = \frac{1}{e^x+1}$

$$\therefore f(x) + f(-x) = 1\ \forall\ x$$

$$\text{Now } I_1 = \int_{f(-a)}^{f(a)} xg\{x(1-x)\}dx$$

$$= \int_{f(-a)}^{f(a)} (1-x)g\{x(1-x)\}dx$$

$$\left[\text{using} \int_a^b f(x)\, dx\ a = \int_a^b f(a+b-x)\, dx\right]$$

$$= I_2 - I_1 \Rightarrow 2I_1 = I_2$$

72. **(b)** Let $I = \int_0^{\pi} xf(\sin x)dx = \int_0^{\pi} (\pi - x)f(\sin x)dx$

$$\therefore 2I = \pi\int_2^{\pi} f(\sin x)dx = \pi.2\int_0^{\frac{\pi}{2}} f(\sin x)dx$$

$$\therefore I = \pi\int_0^{\frac{\pi}{2}} f(\sin x)dx \Rightarrow A = \pi$$

73. **(c)** $I = \int_0^{\frac{\pi}{2}} \frac{(\sin x + \cos x)^2}{\sqrt{1+\sin 2x}} dx$

We know $[(\sin x + \cos x)^2 = 1 + \sin 2x]$, so

$$I = \int_0^{\frac{\pi}{2}} \frac{(\sin x + \cos x)^2}{(\sin x + \cos x)} dx$$

$$= \int_0^{\frac{\pi}{2}} (\sin x + \cos x)dx \left[\because \sin x + \cos x > 0\ if\ 0 < x < \frac{\pi}{2}\right]$$

or $I = \left[-\cos x + \sin x\right]_0^{\frac{\pi}{2}} = 2$

74. **(d)** $\int_{-2}^{3} |1-x^2|\, dx = \int_{-2}^{3} |x^2-1|\, dx$

$$\text{Now } |x^2-1| = \begin{cases} x^2-1 & if \quad x \le -1 \\ 1-x^2 & if \quad -1 \le x \le 1 \\ x^2-1 & if \quad x \ge 1 \end{cases}$$

$$\therefore \text{Integral is} \int_{-2}^{-1} (x^2-1)dx + \int_{-1}^{1} (1-x^2)dx + \int_{1}^{3} (x^2-1)dx$$

$$= \left[\frac{x^3}{3} - x\right]_{-2}^{-1} + \left[x - \frac{x^3}{3}\right]_{-1}^{1} + \left[\frac{x^3}{3} - x\right]_{1}^{3}$$

$$= \left(-\frac{1}{3}+1\right) - \left(-\frac{8}{3}+2\right) + \left(2-\frac{2}{3}\right) + \left(\frac{27}{3}-3\right) - \left(\frac{1}{3}-1\right)$$

$$= \frac{2}{3} + \frac{2}{3} + \frac{4}{3} + 6 + \frac{2}{3} = \frac{28}{3}$$

75. (d) $I=\int_0^1 x(1-x)^n\,dx=\int_0^1(1-x)(1-1+x)^n\,dx$

$=\int_0^1(1-x)x^n dx=\left[\frac{x^{n+1}}{n+1}-\frac{x^{n+2}}{n+2}\right]_0^1$

$=\frac{1}{n+1}-\frac{1}{n+2}$

76. (d) Given $f'(x)=f(x)\Rightarrow\frac{f'(x)}{f(x)}=1$

Integrating

$\log f(x)=x+c\Rightarrow f(x)=e^{x+c}$

$f(0)=1\Rightarrow f(x)=e^x$

$\therefore\int_0^1 f(x)g(x)dx=\int_0^1 e^x(x^2-e^x)dx$

$=\int_0^1 x^2e^x dx-\int_0^1 e^{2x}dx$

$=\left[x^2e^x\right]_0^1-2\left[xe^x-e^x\right]_0^1-\frac{1}{2}\left[e^{2x}\right]_0^1$

$=e-\left[\frac{e^2}{2}-\frac{1}{2}\right]-2[e-e+1]=e-\frac{e^2}{2}-\frac{3}{2}$

77. (c) $I=\int_a^b xf(x)dx=\int_a^b(a+b-x)f(a+b-x)dx$

$=(a+b)\int_a^b f(a+b-x)dx-\int_a^b xf(a+b-x)dx$

$=(a+b)\int_a^b f(x)\,dx-\int_a^b xf(x)dx$

[$\because$ given that $f(a+b-x)=f(x)$]

$2I=(a+b)\int_a^b f(x)dx$

$\Rightarrow\quad I=\frac{(a+b)}{2}\int_a^b f(x)dx$

78. (d) $\lim_{x\to0}\frac{\frac{d}{dx}\int_0^{x^2}\sec^2 t\,dt}{\frac{d}{dx}(x\sin x)}=\lim_{x\to0}\frac{\sec^2 x^2.2x}{\sin x+x\cos x}$

(by L' Hospital rule)

$\lim_{x\to0}\frac{2\sec^2 x^2}{\left(\frac{\sin x}{x}+\cos x\right)}=\frac{2\times1}{1+1}=1$

79. (c) $F(t)=\int_0^t f(t-y)g(y)dy$

$=\int_0^t e^{t-y}y\,dy=e^t\int_0^t e^{-y}y\,dy$

$=e^t\left[-ye^{-y}-e^{-y}\right]_0^t=-e^t\left[ye^{-y}+e^{-y}\right]_0^t$

$=-e^t\left[te^{-t}+e^{-t}-0-1\right]=-e^t\left[\frac{t+1-e^t}{e^t}\right]$

$=e^t-(1+t)$

80. (b) $\int_{-\pi}^{\pi}\frac{2x\,(1+\sin x)}{1+\cos^2 x}dx$

$=\int_{-\pi}^{\pi}\frac{2x\,dx}{1+\cos^2 x}+2\int_{-\pi}^{\pi}\frac{x\sin x}{1+\cos^2 x}dx$

$=0+4\int_0^{\pi}\frac{x\sin x\,dx}{1+\cos^2 x}$; $\left[\because\int_{-a}^{a}f(x)\,dx=0\right.$

if f(x) is odd

$=2\int_0^a f(x)\,dx$ if $f(x)$ is even.

$I=4\int_0^{\pi}\frac{(\pi-x)\sin(\pi-x)}{1+\cos^2(\pi-x)}dx$

$I=4\int_0^{\pi}\frac{(\pi-x)\sin x}{1+\cos^2 x}dx$

$\Rightarrow I=4\pi\int_0^{\pi}\frac{\sin x\,dx}{1+\cos^2 x}-4\int\frac{x\sin x\,dx}{1+\cos^2 x}$

$\Rightarrow\ 2I=4\pi\int_0^{\pi}\frac{\sin x}{1+\cos^2 x}dx$

put $\cos x=t\ \Rightarrow-\sin x\,dx=dt$

$\therefore\ I=-2\pi\int_1^{-1}\frac{1}{1+t^2}dt=2\pi\int_{-1}^{1}\frac{1}{1+t^2}dt$

$=2\pi\left[\tan^{-1}t\right]_{-1}^{1}$

$=2\pi\left[\tan^{-1}1-\tan^{-1}(-1)\right]$

$$= 2\pi\left[\frac{\pi}{4} - \left(\frac{-\pi}{4}\right)\right] = 2\pi.\frac{\pi}{2} = \pi^2$$

81. (d) $\int_0^2 [x^2]dx = \int_0^1 [x^2]dx + \int_1^{\sqrt{2}} [x^2]dx + \int_{\sqrt{2}}^{\sqrt{3}} [x^2] + \int_{\sqrt{3}}^{2} [x^2]dx$

$$= \int_0^1 0dx + \int_1^{\sqrt{2}} 1dx + \int_{\sqrt{2}}^{\sqrt{3}} 2dx + \int_{\sqrt{3}}^{2} 3dx$$

$$= [x]_1^{\sqrt{2}} + [2x]_{\sqrt{2}}^{\sqrt{3}} + [3x]_{\sqrt{3}}^{2}$$

$$= \sqrt{2} - 1 + 2\sqrt{3} - 2\sqrt{2} + 6 - 3\sqrt{3}$$

$$= 5 - \sqrt{3} - \sqrt{2}$$

82. (b) $I_n + I_{n+2} = \int_0^{\pi/4} \tan^n x(1+\tan^2 x)dx$

$$= \int_0^{\pi/4} \tan^n x \sec^2 x\, dx = \left[\frac{\tan^{n+1} x}{n+1}\right]_0^{\pi/4}$$

$$= \frac{1-0}{n+1} = \frac{1}{n+1}$$

$$\therefore I_n + I_{n+2} = \frac{1}{n+1} \Rightarrow \lim_{n\to\infty} n[I_n + I_{n+2}]$$

$$= \lim_{n\to\infty} n.\frac{1}{n+1} = \lim_{n\to\infty}\frac{n}{n+1} = \lim_{n\to\infty}\frac{n}{n\left(1+\frac{1}{n}\right)} = 1$$

83. (a) $I = \int_0^{10\pi} |\sin x|\, dx = 10\int_0^{\pi} |\sin x|\, dx = 10\int_0^{\pi} \sin x\, dx$

[$\because$ $|\sin x|$ is periodic with period π and $\sin x > 0$ if $0 < x < \pi$]

$$I = 20\int_0^{\pi/2} \sin x\, dx = 20[-\cos x]_0^{\pi/2} = 20$$

84. (a) $\lim_{n\to\infty} \dfrac{\frac{1}{(a+1)}.n^{a+1} + a_1 n^a + a_2 n^{a-1} + ...}{(n+1)^{a-1}.n^2\left(a + \frac{1+\frac{1}{n}}{2}\right)} = \dfrac{1}{60}$

$$\Rightarrow \lim_{n\to\infty} \frac{\left(\frac{1}{n}\right)^a + \left(\frac{2}{n}\right)^a + ... + \left(\frac{n}{n}\right)^a}{(n+1)^{a-1}\left[n^2 a + \frac{n(n+1)}{2}\right]} = \frac{1}{60}$$

$$= \frac{\lim_{n\to\infty}\frac{1}{n}\sum_{r=1}^{n}\left(\frac{r}{n}\right)^a}{\left(1+\frac{1}{n}\right)^{a-1}\left[a + \frac{1}{2}\left(1+\frac{1}{n}\right)\right]} = \frac{1}{60}$$

$$= \frac{\int_0^1 x^a dx}{\left(a+\frac{1}{2}\right)} = \frac{1}{60} = \frac{\frac{1}{a+1}}{a+\frac{1}{2}} = \frac{1}{60}$$

$$\Rightarrow \frac{\frac{1}{a+1}}{\left(a+\frac{1}{2}\right)} = \frac{1}{60} \Rightarrow (a+1)(2a+1) = 120$$

$$\Rightarrow 2a^2 + 3a - 119 = 0$$

$$\Rightarrow 2a^2 + 17a - 14a - 119 = 0$$

$$\Rightarrow (a-7)(2a+17) = 0$$

$$\Rightarrow a = 7, -\frac{17}{2}$$

85. (d) $y = \lim_{n\to\infty}\left(\frac{(n+1)(n+2)...3n}{n^{2n}}\right)^{\frac{1}{n}}$

$$\ln y = \lim_{n\to\infty}\frac{1}{n}\ln\left(1+\frac{1}{n}\right)\left(1+\frac{2}{n}\right)....\left(1+\frac{2n}{n}\right)$$

$$\ln y = \lim_{n\to\infty}\frac{1}{n}\left[\ln\left(1+\frac{1}{n}\right) + \ln\left(1+\frac{2}{n}\right) + ... + \ln\left(1+\frac{2n}{n}\right)\right]$$

$$= \lim_{n\to\infty}\frac{1}{n}\sum_{r=1}^{2n}\ln\left(1+\frac{r}{n}\right) = \int_0^2 \ln(1+x)dx$$

Let $1 + x = t \Rightarrow dx = dt$

when $x = 0,\ t = 1$

$x = 2,\ t = 3$

$$\ln y = \int_1^3 \ln t\, d\,t = [t\ln t - t]_1^3 = \ln\left(\frac{3^3}{e^2}\right) = \ln\left(\frac{27}{e^2}\right)$$

$$\Rightarrow y = \frac{27}{e^2}$$

86. (a) Let $f(x) = \int \frac{dx}{\sin^6 x}$

$$f(x) = \int \operatorname{cosec}^6 x\, dx$$

From reduction formula, we have

$I_n = \int \operatorname{cosec}^n x\,dx$

$= -\dfrac{\operatorname{cosec}^{n-2} x \cot x}{n-1} + \dfrac{n-2}{n-1} I_{n-2}$

$\therefore f(x) = -\dfrac{\operatorname{cosec}^4 x \cot x}{5} + \dfrac{4}{5}\left[\dfrac{-\operatorname{cosec}^2 x \cot x}{3} + \dfrac{2}{3} I_2\right]$

$= -\dfrac{\operatorname{cosec}^4 x \cot x}{5} - \dfrac{4}{15}\operatorname{cosec}^2 x.\cot x + \dfrac{8}{15}[-\cot x]$

$= \dfrac{-(1+\cot^2 x)^2.\cot x}{5} - \dfrac{4}{15}(1+\cot^2 x)\cot x$

$-\dfrac{8}{15}(-\cot x)$ $(\because \operatorname{cosec}^2 x = 1+\cot^2 x)$

$= \dfrac{-1}{5}\left[1+\cot^4 x + 2\cot^2 x\right]\cot x - \dfrac{4}{15}\left[\cot x + \cot^3 x\right]$

$-\dfrac{8}{15}\cot x$

$= \dfrac{-1}{5}[\cot x + \cot^5 x + 2\cot^3 x]\dfrac{-4}{15}\cot x - \dfrac{4}{15}\cot^3 x - \dfrac{8}{15}\cot x$

$= \dfrac{-15}{15}\cot x - \dfrac{\cot^5 x}{5} - \dfrac{10}{15}\cot^3 x$

$= \dfrac{-\cot^5 x}{5} - \dfrac{2}{3}\cot^3 x - \cot x$

It is a polynomial of degree 5 in cot x.

87. (d) $\lim_{n\to\infty}\left[\begin{matrix}\dfrac{1}{n^2}\sec^2\dfrac{1}{n^2} + \dfrac{2}{n^2}\sec^2\dfrac{4}{n^2} \\ +\dfrac{3}{n^2}\sec^2\dfrac{9}{n^2} + ... + \dfrac{1}{n}\sec^2 1\end{matrix}\right]$ is equal to

$\lim_{n\to\infty}\dfrac{r}{n^2}\sec^2\dfrac{r^2}{n^2} = \lim_{n\to\infty}\dfrac{1}{n}.\dfrac{r}{n}\sec^2\dfrac{r^2}{n^2}$

$\Rightarrow$ Given limit is equal to value of integral

$\int_0^1 x\sec^2 x^2 dx$

or $\dfrac{1}{2}\int_0^1 2x\sec\ x^2 dx = \dfrac{1}{2}\int_0^1 \sec^2 t dt$ [put $x^2 = t$]

$= \dfrac{1}{2}(\tan t)_0^1 = \dfrac{1}{2}\tan 1$.

88. (b) $\lim_{n\to\infty}\sum_{r=1}^{n}\dfrac{1}{n}e^{\frac{r}{n}}$ [Using definite integrals as limit of sum]

$= \int_0^1 e^x dx = e - 1$

89. (a) $\lim_{n\to\infty}\dfrac{1^4+2^4+3^4+.......n^4}{n^5} -$

$\lim_{n\to\infty}\dfrac{1^3+2^3+3^3+.......+n^3}{n^5}$

$= \lim_{n\to\infty}\dfrac{1}{n}\sum_{r=1}^{n}\left(\dfrac{r}{n}\right)^4 - \lim_{n\to\infty}\dfrac{1}{n}.\lim_{n\to\infty}\dfrac{1}{n}\left(\dfrac{r}{n}\right)^3$

$= \int_0^1 x^4\,dx - \lim_{n\to\infty}\dfrac{1}{n}\times\int_0^1 x^3\,dx = \left[\dfrac{x^5}{5}\right]_0^1 - 0 = \dfrac{1}{5}$

90. (a) We have $\lim_{n\to\infty}\dfrac{1^p+2^p+....+n^p}{n^{p+1}}$;

$\lim_{n\to\infty}\sum_{r=1}^{n}\dfrac{r^p}{n^p\cdot n} = \int_0^1 x^p dx = \left[\dfrac{x^{p+1}}{p+1}\right]_0^1 = \dfrac{1}{p+1}$

Applications of Integrals

TOPIC-1 : Area of the Region Bounded by a Curve & X-axis Between two Ordinates, Area of the Region Bounded by a Curve & Y-axis Between two Abscissa

1. Let $f: [-2, 3] \to [0, \infty)$ be a continuous function such that $f(1-x) = f(x)$ for all $x \in [-2, 3]$.
If R_1 is the numerical value of the area of the region bounded by $y = f(x)$, $x = -2$, $x = 3$ and the axis of x and

$R_2 = \int_{-2}^{3} x f(x)\, dx$, then : **[Online April 25, 2013]**

(a) $3R_1 = 2R_2$ (b) $2R_1 = 3R_2$
(c) $R_1 = R_2$ (d) $R_1 = 2R_2$

2. Let $f(x)$ be a non – negative continuous function such that the area bounded by the curve $y = f(x)$, x - axis and the ordinates $x = \frac{\pi}{4}$ and $x = \beta > \frac{\pi}{4}$ is $\left(\beta \sin\beta + \frac{\pi}{4}\cos\beta + \sqrt{2}\beta\right)$. Then $f\left(\frac{\pi}{2}\right)$ is **[2005]**

(a) $\left(\frac{\pi}{4} + \sqrt{2} - 1\right)$ (b) $\left(\frac{\pi}{4} - \sqrt{2} + 1\right)$

(c) $\left(1 - \frac{\pi}{4} - \sqrt{2}\right)$ (d) $\left(1 - \frac{\pi}{4} + \sqrt{2}\right)$

3. The area enclosed between the curve $y = \log_e(x+e)$ and the coordinate axes is **[2005]**

(a) 1 (b) 2
(c) 3 (d) 4

4. If $y = f(x)$ makes +ve intercept of 2 and 0 unit on x and y axes and encloses an area of 3/4 square unit with the axes then $\int_0^2 x f'(x)\, dx$ is

(a) 3/2 (b) 1 **[2002]**
(c) 5/4 (d) –3/4

TOPIC-2 : Different Cases of Area Bounded Between the Curves

5. The area (in sq. units) of the region $\{(x, y) : x \geq 0, x + y \leq 3, x^2 \leq 4y \text{ and } y \leq 1 + \sqrt{x}\}$ is : **[2017]**

(a) $\frac{5}{2}$ (b) $\frac{59}{12}$

(c) $\frac{3}{2}$ (d) $\frac{7}{3}$

6. The area (in sq. units) of the smaller portion enclosed between the curves, $x^2 + y^2 = 4$ and $y^2 = 3x$, is : **[Online April 8, 2017]**

(a) $\frac{1}{2\sqrt{3}} + \frac{\pi}{3}$ (b) $\frac{1}{\sqrt{3}} + \frac{2\pi}{3}$

(c) $\frac{1}{2\sqrt{3}} + \frac{2\pi}{3}$ (d) $\frac{1}{\sqrt{3}} + \frac{4\pi}{3}$

7. The area (in sq. units) of the region $\{(x, y) : y^2 \geq 2x$ and $x^2 + y^2 \leq 4x, x \geq 0, y \geq 0\}$ is : **[2016]**

(a) $\pi - \frac{4\sqrt{2}}{3}$ (b) $\frac{\pi}{2} - \frac{2\sqrt{2}}{3}$

(c) $\pi - \frac{4}{3}$ (d) $\pi - \frac{8}{3}$

8. The area (in sq. units) of the region described by
$A = \{(x, y) | y \geq x^2 - 5x + 4, x + y \geq 1, y \leq 0\}$ is: **[Online April 9, 2016]**

(a) $\frac{19}{6}$ (b) $\frac{17}{6}$

(c) $\frac{7}{2}$ (d) $\frac{13}{6}$

9. The area (in sq. units) of the region described by $\{(x, y) : y^2 \leq 2x \text{ and } y \geq 4x - 1\}$ is **[2015]**

(a) $\frac{15}{64}$ (b) $\frac{9}{32}$

(c) $\frac{7}{32}$ (d) $\frac{5}{64}$

10. The area (in square units) of the region bounded by the curves $y + 2x^2 = 0$ and $y + 3x^2 = 1$, is equal to : **[Online April 10, 2015]**

(a) $\frac{3}{5}$ (b) $\frac{1}{3}$

(c) $\frac{4}{3}$ (d) $\frac{3}{4}$

11. The area of the region described by

$A = \{(x, y) : x^2 + y^2 \le 1 \text{ and } y^2 \le 1 - x\}$ is: **[2014]**

(a) $\frac{\pi}{2} - \frac{2}{3}$ (b) $\frac{\pi}{2} + \frac{2}{3}$

(c) $\frac{\pi}{2} + \frac{4}{3}$ (d) $\frac{\pi}{2} - \frac{4}{3}$

12. The area of the region above the x-axis bounded by the curve y = tan x, $0 \le x \le \frac{\pi}{2}$ and the tangent to the curve at $x = \frac{\pi}{4}$ is: **[Online April 19, 2014]**

(a) $\frac{1}{2}\left(\log 2 - \frac{1}{2}\right)$ (b) $\frac{1}{2}\left(\log 2 + \frac{1}{2}\right)$

(c) $\frac{1}{2}(1 - \log 2)$ (d) $\frac{1}{2}(1 + \log 2)$

13. Let A = {(x, y): $y^2 \le 4x$, $y - 2x \ge -4$}. The area (in square units) of the region A is: **[Online April 9, 2014]**

(a) 8 (b) 9

(c) 10 (d) 11

14. The area (in square units) bounded by the curves $y = \sqrt{x}$, $2y - x + 3 = 0$, x-axis, and lying in the first quadrant is : **[2013]**

(a) 9 (b) 36

(c) 18 (d) $\frac{27}{4}$

15. The area under the curve $y = |\cos x - \sin x|$, $0 \le x \le \frac{\pi}{2}$, and above x-axis is : **[Online April 23, 2013]**

(a) $2\sqrt{2}$ (b) $2\sqrt{2} - 2$

(c) $2\sqrt{2} + 2$ (d) 0

16. The area of the region (in sq. units), in the first quadrant bounded by the parabola $y = 9x^2$ and the lines $x = 0, y = 1$ and $y = 4$, is : **[Online April 22, 2013]**

(a) 7/9 (b) 14/3

(c) 7/3 (d) 14/9

17. The area bounded by the curve $y = \ln(x)$ and the lines $y = 0, y = \ln(3)$ and $x = 0$ is equal to : **[Online April 9, 2013]**

(a) 3 (b) $3 \ln(3) - 2$

(c) $3 \ln(3) + 2$ (d) 2

18. The area between the parabolas $x^2 = \frac{y}{4}$ and $x^2 = 9y$ and the straight line $y = 2$ is : **[2012]**

(a) $20\sqrt{2}$ (b) $\frac{10\sqrt{2}}{3}$

(c) $\frac{20\sqrt{2}}{3}$ (d) $10\sqrt{2}$

19. The area bounded by the parabola $y^2 = 4x$ and the line $2x - 3y + 4 = 0$, in square unit, is **[Online May 26, 2012]**

(a) $\frac{2}{5}$ (b) $\frac{1}{3}$

(c) 1 (d) $\frac{1}{2}$

20. The area of the region bounded by the curve $y = x^3$, and the lines, $y = 8$, and $x = 0$, is **[Online May 19, 2012]**

(a) 8 (b) 12

(c) 10 (d) 16

21. If a straight line $y - x = 2$ divides the region $x^2 + y^2 \le 4$ into two parts, then the ratio of the area of the smaller part to the area of the greater part is **[Online May 12, 2012]**

(a) $3\pi - 8 : \pi + 8$ (b) $\pi - 3 : 3\pi + 3$

(c) $3\pi - 4 : \pi + 4$ (d) $\pi - 2 : 3\pi + 2$

22. The area enclosed by the curves $y = x^2$, $y = x^3$, $x = 0$ and $x = p$, where $p > 1$, is 1/6. The p equals **[Online May 12, 2012]**

(a) 8/3 (b) 16/3

(c) 2 (d) 4/3

23. The parabola $y^2 = x$ divides the circle $x^2 + y^2 = 2$ into two parts whose areas are in the ratio **[Online May 7, 2012]**

(a) $9\pi + 2 : 3\pi - 2$ (b) $9\pi - 2 : 3\pi + 2$

(c) $7\pi - 2 : 2\pi - 3$ (d) $7\pi + 2 : 3\pi + 2$

24. The area bounded by the curves **[2011 RS]**

$y^2 = 4x$ and $x^2 = 4y$ is:

(a) $\frac{32}{3}$ sq units (b) $\frac{16}{3}$ sq units

(c) $\frac{8}{3}$ sq. units (d) 0 sq. units

25. The area of the region enclosed by the curves $y = x$, $x = e$, $y = \frac{1}{x}$ and the positive x-axis is **[2011]**

(a) 1 square unit (b) $\frac{3}{2}$ square units

(c) $\frac{5}{2}$ square units (d) $\frac{1}{2}$ square unit

26. The area bounded by the curves $y = \cos x$ and $y = \sin x$ between the ordinates $x = 0$ and $x = \frac{3\pi}{2}$ is **[2010]**

(a) $4\sqrt{2}+2$ (b) $4\sqrt{2}-1$

(c) $4\sqrt{2}+1$ (d) $4\sqrt{2}-2$

27. The area of the region bounded by the parabola $(y-2)^2 = x-1$, the tangent of the parabola at the point (2, 3) and the x-axis is: **[2009]**

(a) 6 (b) 9

(c) 12 (d) 3

28. The area of the plane region bounded by the curves $x + 2y^2 = 0$ and $x + 3y^2 = 1$ is equal to **[2008]**

(a) $\frac{5}{3}$ (b) $\frac{1}{3}$

(c) $\frac{2}{3}$ (d) $\frac{4}{3}$

29. The area enclosed between the curves $y^2 = x$ and $y = |x|$ is **[2007]**

(a) 1/6 (b) 1/3

(c) 2/3 (d) 1

30. The parabolas $y^2 = 4x$ and $x^2 = 4y$ divide the square region bounded by the lines $x = 4$, $y = 4$ and the coordinate axes. If S_1, S_2, S_3 are respectively the areas of these parts numbered from top to bottom; then $S_1 : S_2 : S_3$ is **[2005]**

(a) 1 : 2 : 1 (b) 1 : 2 : 3

(c) 2 : 1 : 2 (d) 1 : 1 : 1

31. The area of the region bounded by the curves $y = |x-2|, x = 1, x = 3$ and the x-axis is **[2004]**

(a) 4 (b) 2

(c) 3 (d) 1

32. The area of the region bounded by the curves $y = |x-1|$ *and* $y = 3-|x|$ is **[2003]**

(a) 6 sq. units (b) 2 sq. units

(c) 3 sq. units (d) 4 sq. units.

33. The area bounded by the curves $y = \ln x$, $y = \ln |x|$, $y = |\ln x|$ and $y = |\ln |x||$ is **[2002]**

(a) 4sq. units (b) 6 sq. units

(c) 10 sq. units (d) none of these

Hints & Solutions

1. (d) We have

$$R_2 = \int_{-2}^{3} x\, f(x)\, dx = \int_{-2}^{3} (1-x)\, f(1-x)\, dx$$

$$\left[\text{Using} \int_a^b f(x)\, dx = \int_a^b f(a+b-x)\, dx\right]$$

$$\Rightarrow R_2 = \int_{-2}^{3} (1-x)\, f(x)\, dx$$

$$(\because f(x) = f(1-x) \text{ on } [-2, 3])$$

$$\therefore R_2 + R_2 = \int_{-2}^{3} x\, f(x)\, dx + \int_{-2}^{3} (1-x)\, f(x)\, dx$$

$$= \int_{-2}^{3} f(x)\, dx = R_1$$

$$\Rightarrow 2R_2 = R_1$$

2. (d) Given that $\int_{\pi/4}^{\beta} f(x)dx = \beta \sin\beta + \frac{\pi}{4}\cos\beta + \sqrt{2}\beta$

Differentiating w. r . t β

$$f(\beta) = \beta \cos\beta + \sin\beta - \frac{\pi}{4}\sin\beta + \sqrt{2}$$

$$f\left(\frac{\pi}{2}\right) = \left(1 - \frac{\pi}{4}\right)\sin\frac{\pi}{2} + \sqrt{2} = 1 - \frac{\pi}{4} + \sqrt{2}$$

3. (a) The graph of the curve $y = \log_e(x+e)$ is as shown in the fig.

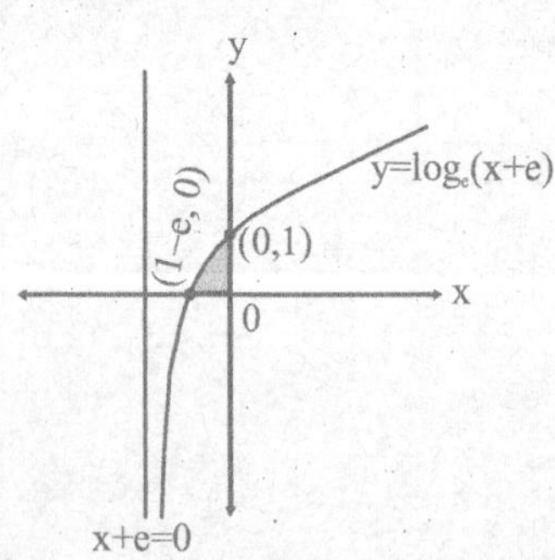

Required area $A = \int_{1-e}^{0} y dx = \int_{1-e}^{0} \log_e(x+e)dx$

put $x + e = t \Rightarrow dx = dt$ also At $x = 1 - e, t = 1$

4. (d) We have $\int_0^2 f(x)dx = \frac{3}{4}$; Now,

$$\int_0^2 xf'(x)dx = x\int_0^2 f'(x)dx - \int_0^2 f(x)dx$$

$$= [x\, f(x)]_0^2 - \frac{3}{4} = 2f(2) - \frac{3}{4}$$

$$= 0 - \frac{3}{4}\ (\because f(2) = 0) = -\frac{3}{4}.$$

5. (a)

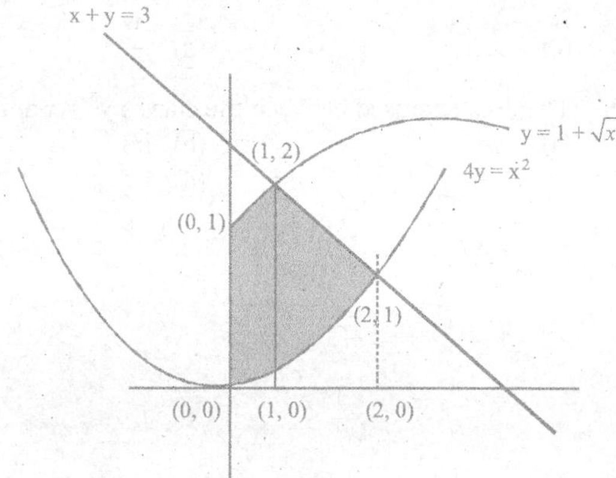

Area of shaded region

$$= \int_0^1 (1+\sqrt{x})dx + \int_1^2 (3-x)dx - \int_0^2 \frac{x^2}{4}dx$$

$$= x]_0^1 + \left.\frac{x^{\frac{3}{2}}}{\frac{3}{2}}\right]_0^1 + 3x]_1^2 - \left.\frac{x^2}{2}\right]_1^2 - \left.\frac{x^3}{12}\right]_0^2 = \frac{5}{2}\text{sq.units}$$

6. (d)

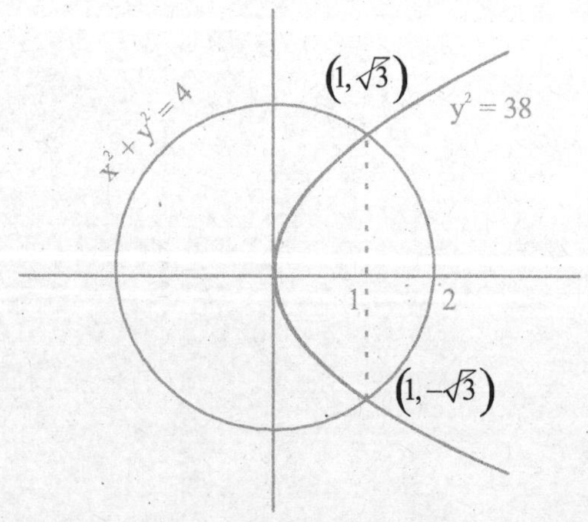

From the equations we get;

$x^2+3x-4=0$

$\Rightarrow (x+4)(x-1)=0$

$\Rightarrow x=-4, x=1$

when $x=1,\ y=\sqrt{3}$

$$\text{Area}=\int_0^1\left(\int_0^1 \sqrt{3}.\sqrt{x}\,dx+\int_1^2\sqrt{4-x^2}\,.dx\right)\times 2$$

$$=\left(\sqrt{3}\left(\frac{x^{3/2}}{3/2}\right)_0^1+\left(\frac{x}{2}\sqrt{4-x^2}+2\sin^{-1}\frac{x}{2}\right)_1^2\right)\times 2$$

$$=\left(\sqrt{3}\left(\frac{2}{3}\right)+\left\{2.\frac{\pi}{2}-\left(\frac{\sqrt{3}}{2}+\frac{\pi}{3}\right)\right\}\right)\times 2$$

$$=\left(\frac{2}{\sqrt{3}}-\frac{\sqrt{3}}{2}+\frac{2\pi}{3}\right)\times 2$$

$$=\left(\frac{1}{2\sqrt{3}}+\frac{2\pi}{3}\right)\times 2=\frac{1}{\sqrt{3}}+\frac{4\pi}{3}$$

7. (d)

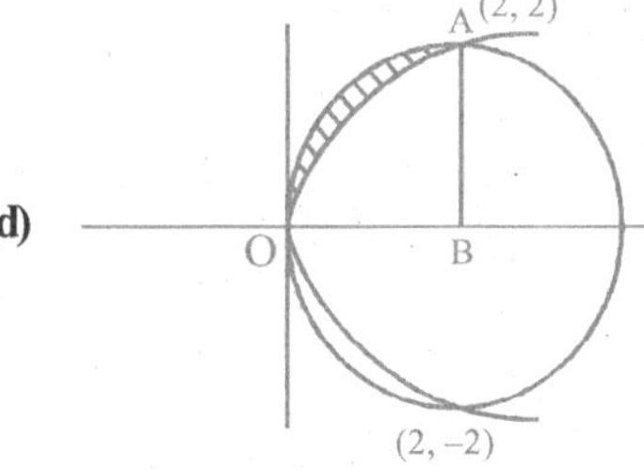

Points of intersection of the two curves are (0, 0), (2, 2) and (2, –2)

Area = Area (OAB) – area under parabola (0 to 2)

$$=\frac{\pi\times(2)^2}{4}-\int_0^2\sqrt{2}\sqrt{x}\,dx$$

$$=\pi-\frac{8}{3}$$

8. (a)

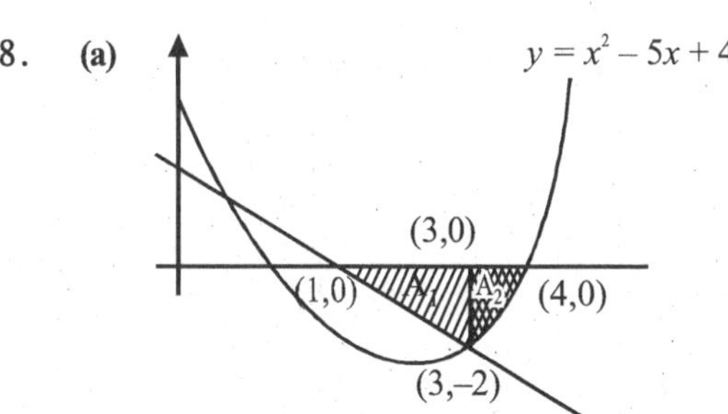

Required area $= A_1 + A_2$

$$=\frac{1}{2}\times 2\times 2+\left|\int_3^4(x^2-5x+4)\,dx\right|$$

$$=2+\frac{7}{6}=\frac{19}{6}\text{ sq. units}$$

9. (b) Required area

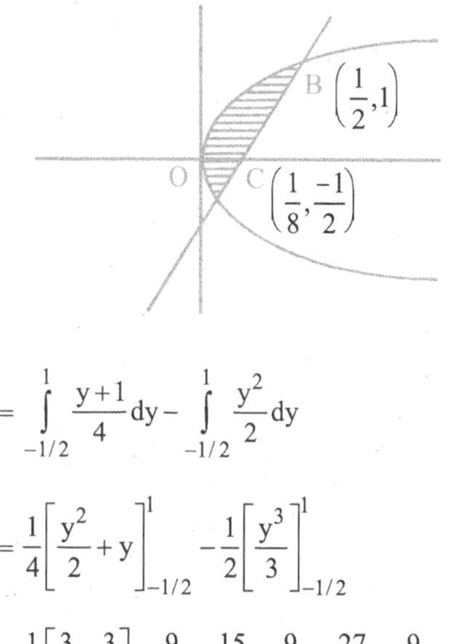

$$=\int_{-1/2}^{1}\frac{y+1}{4}dy-\int_{-1/2}^{1}\frac{y^2}{2}dy$$

$$=\frac{1}{4}\left[\frac{y^2}{2}+y\right]_{-1/2}^{1}-\frac{1}{2}\left[\frac{y^3}{3}\right]_{-1/2}^{1}$$

$$=\frac{1}{4}\left[\frac{3}{2}+\frac{3}{8}\right]-\frac{9}{48}=\frac{15}{32}-\frac{9}{48}=\frac{27}{96}=\frac{9}{32}$$

10. (c) Solving

$y=2x^2=0$

$y=3x^2=1$

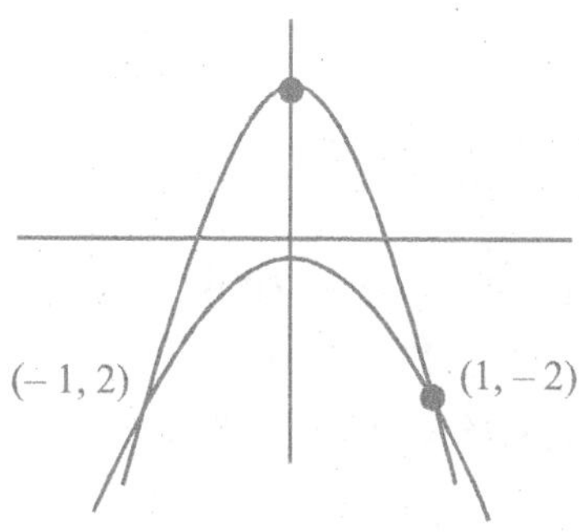

Point of intersection (1, – 2) and (– 1, – 2)

$$\text{Area}=2\int_0^1\left(\left(1-3x^2\right)-\left(-2x^2\right)\right)dx$$

$$2\int_0^1\left(1-x^2\right)dx=2\left(x-\frac{x^3}{3}\right)_0^1=\frac{4}{3}$$

$= 15 - 6 = 9$ sq units

11. (c) Given curves are $x^2+y^2=1$ and $y^2=1-x$.

Intersecting points are $x=0, 1$

Area of shaded portion is the required area.

So, Required Area = Area of semi-circle + Area bounded by parabola

$$= \frac{\pi r^2}{2} + 2\int_0^1 \sqrt{1-x}dx$$

$$= \frac{\pi}{2} + 2\int_0^1 \sqrt{1-x}\,dx \quad (\because \text{ radius of circle} = 1)$$

$$= \frac{\pi}{2} + 2\left[\frac{(1-x)^{3/2}}{-3/2}\right]_0^1$$

$$= \frac{\pi}{2} - \frac{4}{3}(-1) = \frac{\pi}{2} + \frac{4}{3} \text{ Sq. unit}$$

12. **(a)** The given curve is $y = \tan x$ ...(1)

when $x = \frac{\pi}{4}$, $y = 1$

Equation of tangent at P is

$$y - 1 = \left(\sec^2 \frac{\pi}{4}\right)\left(x - \frac{\pi}{4}\right)$$

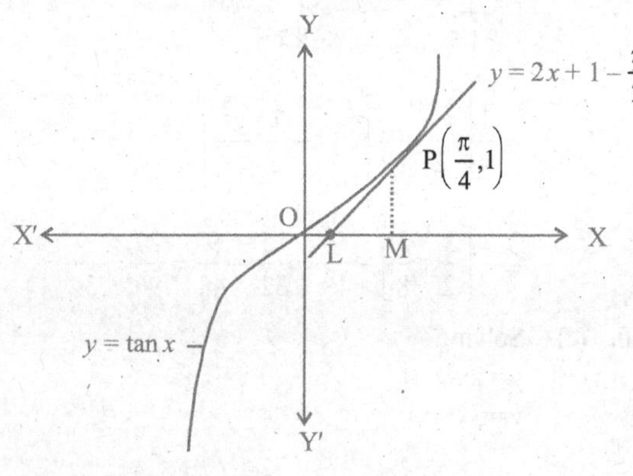

or $y = 2x + 1 - \frac{\pi}{2}$ ...(2)

Area of shaded region

= area of OPMO – ar (ΔPLM)

$$= \int_0^{\frac{\pi}{4}} \tan x\, dx - \frac{1}{2}(\text{OM} - \text{OL})\text{PM}$$

$$= [\log \sec x]_0^{\frac{\pi}{4}} - \frac{1}{2}\left\{\frac{\pi}{4} - \frac{\pi - 2}{4}\right\} \times 1$$

$$= \frac{1}{2}\left[\log 2 - \frac{1}{2}\right] \text{ sq unit}$$

13. **(b)** Area of shaded portion

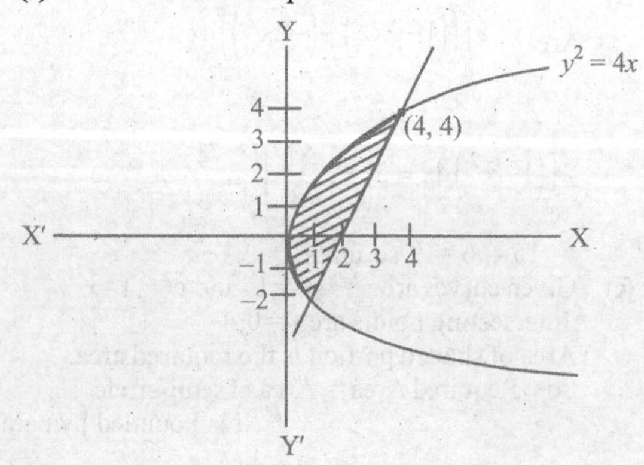

$$= \left|\int_2^4 \left(\frac{y+4}{2}\right) dy\right| - \left|\int_{-2}^4 \frac{y^2}{4} dy\right|$$

$$= \left|\frac{1}{2}\left[\frac{y^2}{2} + 4y\right]_{-2}^4\right| - \left|\frac{1}{4}\left[\frac{y^3}{3}\right]_{-2}^4\right|$$

$$= \left|\frac{1}{2}[\{8+16\} - \{2-8\}]\right| - \left|\frac{1}{4}\left\{\frac{64}{3} + \frac{8}{3}\right\}\right|$$

14. **(a)** Given curves are

$y = \sqrt{x}$ ...(1)

and $2y - x + 3 = 0$ ...(2)

On solving both we get $y = -1, 3$

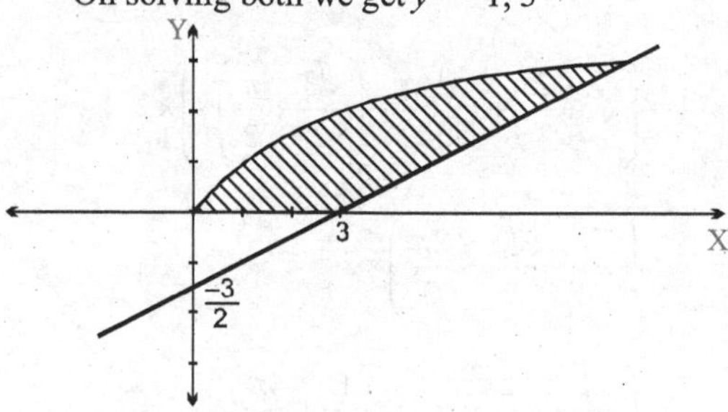

$$\text{Required area} = \int_0^3 \left\{(2y+3) - y^2\right\} dy$$

$$= y^2 + 3y - \frac{y^3}{3}\Big|_0^3 = 9.$$

15. **(b)** $y = |\cos x - \sin x|$

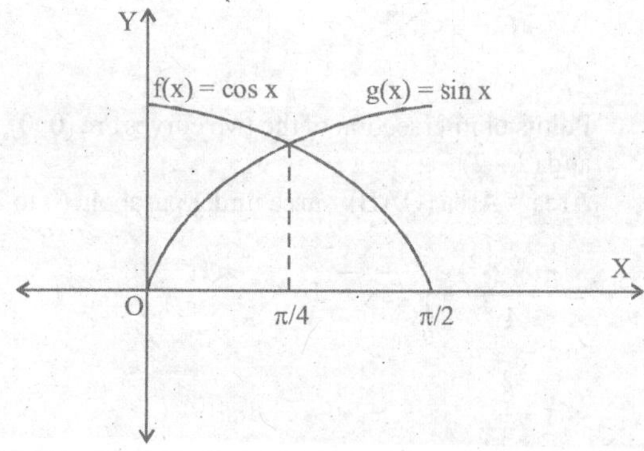

$$\text{Required area} = 2\int_0^{\pi/4} (\cos x - \sin x)\, dx$$

$$= 2\left[\sin x + \cos x\right]_0^{\pi/4}$$

$$= 2\left[\frac{2}{\sqrt{2}} - 1\right] = (2\sqrt{2} - 2) \text{ sq. units}$$

16. **(d)** $\text{Required area} = \int_{y=1}^{4} \sqrt{\frac{y}{9}}\, dy$

$$=\frac{1}{3}\int_{y=1}^{4} y^{1/2}\,dy=\frac{1}{3}\times\frac{2}{3}\left(y^{3/2}\right)\Big|_1^4$$

$$=\frac{2}{9}[(4^{1/2})^3-(1^{1/2})^3]=\frac{2}{9}[8-1]$$

$$=\frac{2}{9}\times 7=\frac{14}{9}\text{ sq. units.}$$

17. **(d)** To find the point of intersection of curves $y=\ln(x)$ and $y=\ln(3)$, put $\ln(x)=\ln(3)$

$\Rightarrow$ $\ln(x)-\ln(3)=0$

$\Rightarrow$ $\ln(x)-\ln(3)=\ln(1)$

$\Rightarrow$ $\frac{x}{3}=1,\ \Rightarrow x=3$

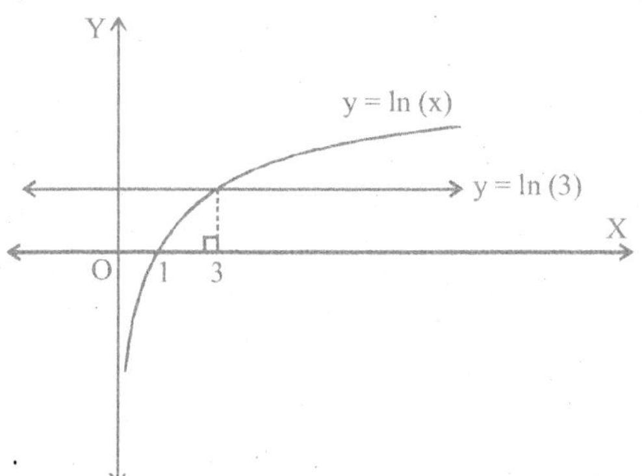

$$\text{Required area}=\int_0^3 \ln(3)\,dx-\int_1^3 \ln(x)\,dx$$

$$=[x\ln(3)]_0^3-[x\ln(x)-x]_1^3=2$$

18. **(c)** Given curves $x^2=\frac{y}{4}$ and $x^2=9y$ are the parabolas whose equations can be written as $y=4x^2$ and $y=\frac{1}{9}x^2$.

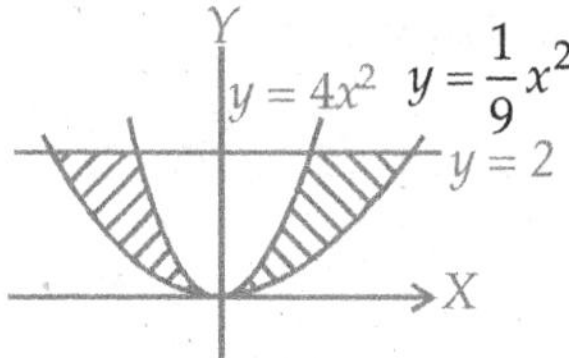

Also, given $y=2$.
Now, shaded portion shows the required area which is symmetric.

$$\therefore\quad \text{Area}=2\int_0^2\left(\sqrt{9y}-\sqrt{\frac{y}{4}}\right)dy$$

$$\text{Area}=2\int_0^2\left(3\sqrt{y}-\frac{\sqrt{y}}{2}\right)dy$$

$$=2\left[\frac{3.y^{\frac{1}{2}+1}}{\frac{1}{2}+1}-\frac{1}{2}.\frac{y^{\frac{1}{2}+1}}{\frac{1}{2}+1}\right]_0^2$$

$$=2\left[\frac{2}{3}\times 3.y^{\frac{3}{2}}-\frac{1}{2}\times\frac{2}{3}.y^{\frac{3}{2}}\right]_0^2$$

$$=2\left[2y^{\frac{3}{2}}-\frac{1}{3}y^{\frac{3}{2}}\right]=2\times\frac{5}{3}y^{\frac{3}{2}}\Big|_0^2$$

$$=2.\frac{5}{3}2\sqrt{2}=\frac{20\sqrt{2}}{3}$$

19. **(b)** Intersecting points are $x=1, 4$

$$\therefore\ \text{Required area}=\int_1^4\left[2\sqrt{x}-\left(\frac{2x+4}{3}\right)\right]dx$$

$$=\frac{2x^{3/2}}{3/2}\Big|_1^4-\frac{2x^2}{3\times 2}\Big|_1^4-\frac{4}{3}x\Big|_1^4$$

$$=\frac{4}{3}\left(4^{3/2}-1^{3/2}\right)-\frac{1}{3}(16-1)-\left[\frac{4}{3}(4)-\frac{4}{3}\right]$$

$$=\frac{4}{3}(7)-5-4=\frac{28}{3}-9=\frac{28-27}{3}=\frac{1}{3}$$

20. **(b)** Required Area $=\int_{y=0}^{8} y^{1/3}dy$

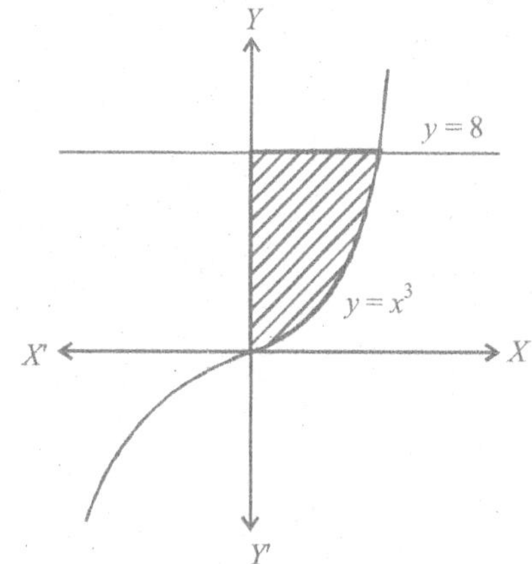

$$=\frac{y^{1/3+1}}{\frac{1}{3}+1}\Bigg|_0^8=\frac{3}{4}\left(y^{4/3}\right)\Big|_0^8$$

$$=\frac{3}{4}\left[(8)^{4/3}-0\right]=\frac{3}{4}\left[2^4\right]=\frac{3}{4}\times 16=12\text{ sq. unit.}$$

21. **(d)** Let I be the smaller portion and II be the greater portion of the given figure then,

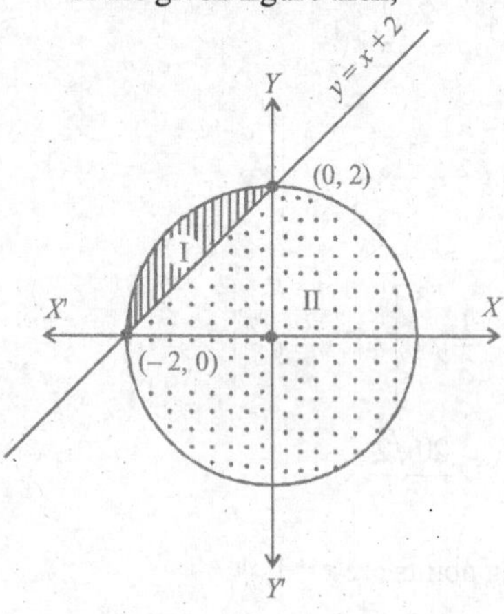

Area of $I = \int_{-2}^{0} \left[\sqrt{4-x^2} - (x+2)\right] dx$

$= \left[\frac{x}{2}\sqrt{4-x^2} + \frac{4}{2}\sin^{-1}\left(\frac{x}{2}\right)\right]_{-2}^{0} - \left[\frac{x^2}{2} + 2x\right]_{-2}^{0}$

$= \left[2\sin^{-1}(-1)\right] - \left[-\frac{4}{2} + 4\right] = 2 \times \frac{\pi}{2} - 2 = \pi - 2$

Now, area of II = Area of circle − area of I.

$= 4\pi - (\pi - 2)$

$= 3\pi + 2$

Hence, required ratio $= \frac{\text{area of I}}{\text{area of II}} = \frac{\pi - 2}{3\pi + 2}$

22. **(d)** Given curves are $y = x^2$ and $y = x^3$

Also, $x = 0$ and $x = p, p > 1$

Now, intersecting point is (1, 1)

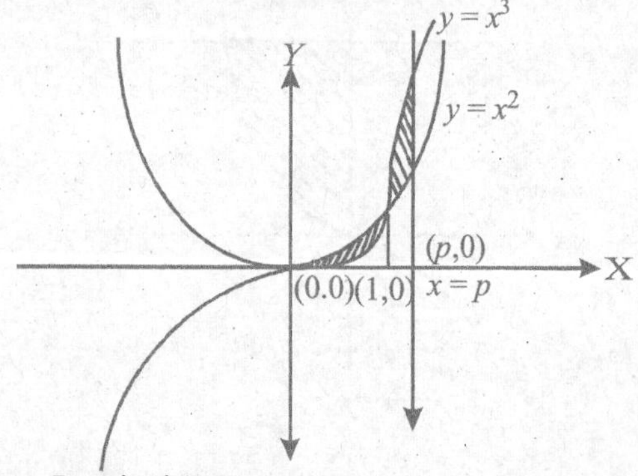

Required Area

$= \int_{0}^{1} \left(x^2 - x^3\right) dx + \int_{1}^{p} \left(x^3 - x^2\right) dx$

$\frac{1}{6} = \left.\frac{x^3}{3} - \frac{x^4}{4}\right|_{0}^{1} + \left.\frac{x^4}{4} - \frac{x^3}{3}\right|_{1}^{p}$

$\Rightarrow \frac{1}{6} = \left(\frac{1}{3} - \frac{1}{4}\right) + \left(\frac{p^4}{4} - \frac{p^3}{3} - \frac{1}{4} + \frac{1}{3}\right)$

$\Rightarrow \frac{1}{6} - \frac{1}{3} + \frac{1}{4} + \frac{1}{4} - \frac{1}{3} = \frac{3p^4 - 4p^3}{12}$

$\Rightarrow \frac{p^3(3p-4)}{12} = 0 \Rightarrow p^3(3p-4) = 0$

$\Rightarrow p = 0$ or $\frac{4}{3}$

Since, it is given that $p > 1$

$\therefore$ p can not be zero.

Hence, $p = \frac{4}{3}$

23. **(b)**

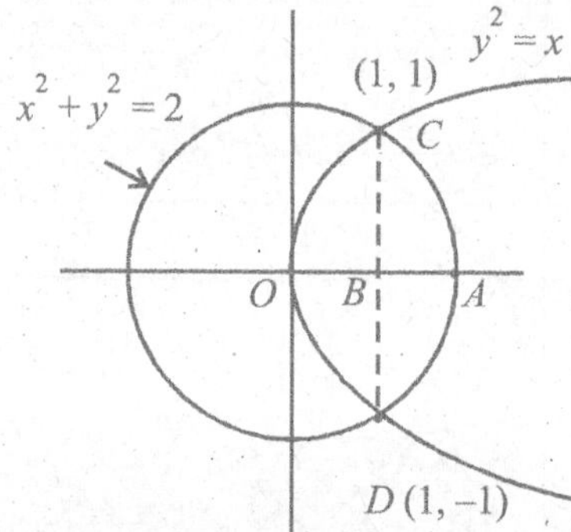

Area of circle $= \pi\left(\sqrt{2}\right)^2 = 2\pi$

Area of $OCADO = 2\{\text{Area of } OCAO\}$

$= 2\ \{\text{area of } OCB + \text{area of } BCA\}$

$= 2\int_{0}^{1} y_p dx + 2\int_{1}^{\sqrt{2}} y_c dx$

where $y_p = \sqrt{x}$ and $y_c = \sqrt{2-x^2}$

$\therefore$ Required Area

$= 2\int_{0}^{1} \sqrt{x}\, dx + 2\int_{1}^{\sqrt{2}} \sqrt{2-x^2}\, dx$

$= 2\left[\frac{2}{3}.1 - 0\right] + 2\left[\frac{x\sqrt{2-x^2}}{2} + \sin^{-1}\frac{x}{\sqrt{2}}\right]_{1}^{\sqrt{2}}$

$= \frac{4}{3} + 2\left\{\frac{\pi}{2} - \frac{\pi}{4} - \frac{1}{2}\right\} = \frac{4}{3} + 2\left\{\frac{\pi}{4} - \frac{1}{2}\right\} = \frac{3\pi + 2}{6}$

Bigger area $= 2\pi - \frac{3\pi + 2}{6} = \frac{9\pi - 2}{6}$

$\therefore$ Required Ratio $= \frac{9\pi - 2}{3\pi + 2}$ i.e., $9\pi - 2 : 3\pi + 2$

24. **(b)**

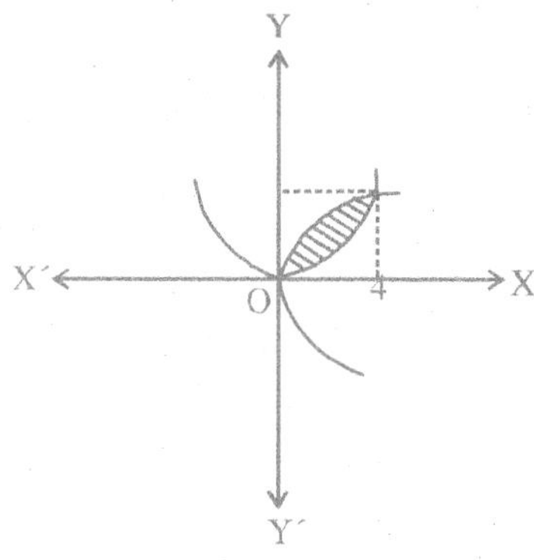

$$\text{Area} = \int_0^4 \left(2\sqrt{x} - \frac{x^2}{4}\right)dx$$

$$= \left[2\left(\frac{x^{3/2}}{3/2}\right) - \frac{x^3}{12}\right]_0^4 = \frac{4}{3}\times 8 - \frac{64}{12}$$

$$= \frac{32}{3} - 16 = \frac{16}{3} \text{ sq. units}$$

25. **(b)** Area of required region $AOBC$

$$= \int_0^1 x dx + \int_1^e \frac{1}{x} dx$$

$$= \frac{1}{2} + 1 = \frac{3}{2} \text{ sq. units}$$

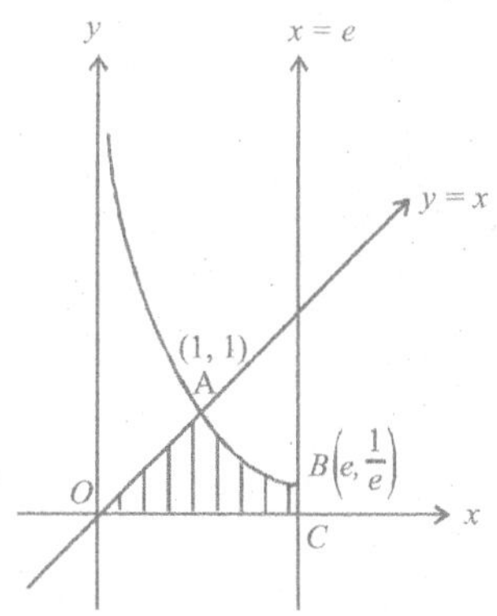

26. **(d)**

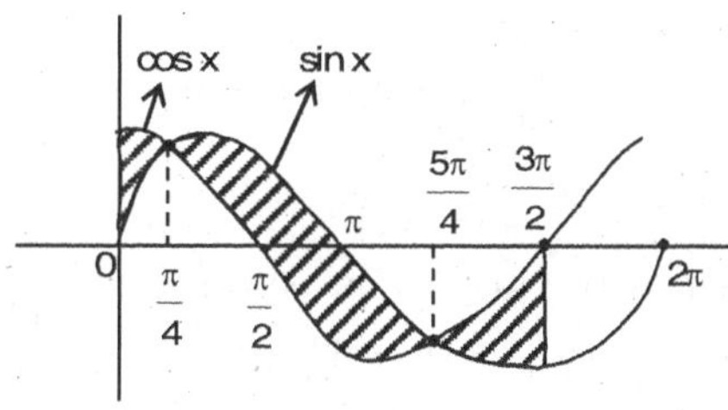

Area above x-axis = Area below x-axis

∴ Required area

$$= 2\left[\int_0^{\frac{\pi}{4}} (\cos x - \sin x)dx + \int_{\frac{\pi}{4}}^{\frac{\pi}{2}} (\sin x - \cos x)dx + \int_{\frac{\pi}{2}}^{\pi} \sin x \, dx\right]$$

$$= 4\sqrt{2} - 2$$

27. **(b)** The given parabola is $(y-2)^2 = x-1$

Vertex (1, 2) and it meets x –axis at (5, 0)

Also it gives $y^2 - 4y - x + 5 = 0$

So, that equation of tangent to the parabola at (2, 3) is

$$y.3 - 2(y+3) - \frac{1}{2}(x+2) + 5 = 0$$

or $x - 2y + 4 = 0$

which meets x-axis at (– 4, 0).

In the figure shaded area is the required area.

Let us draw PD perpendicular to y – axis.

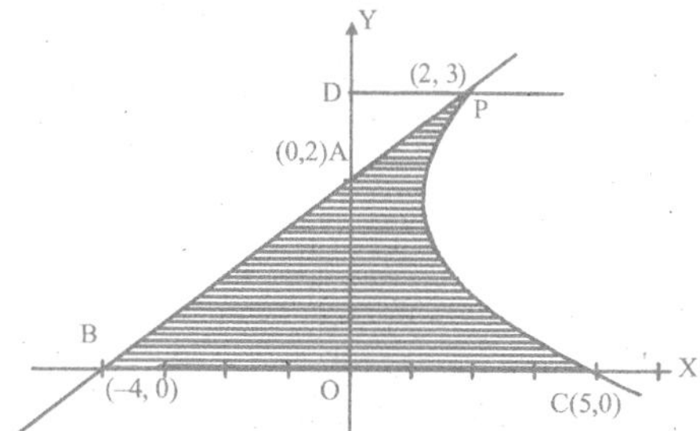

Then required area = Ar ΔBOA + Ar (OCPD) – Ar (ΔAPD)

$$= \frac{1}{2}\times 4\times 2 + \int_0^3 xdy - \frac{1}{2}\times 2\times 1$$

$$= 3 + \int_0^3 (y-2)^2 + 1 \, dy$$

$$= 3 + \left[\frac{(y-2)^3}{3} + y\right]_0^3$$

$$= 3 + \left[\frac{1}{3} + 3 + \frac{8}{3}\right] = 3 + 6 = 9 \text{ Sq. units}$$

28. **(d)** $x + 2y^2 = 0 \Rightarrow y^2 = -\frac{x}{2}$

[Left handed parabola with vertex at (0, 0)]

$$x + 3y^2 = 1 \Rightarrow y^2 = -\frac{1}{3}(x-1)$$

[Left handed parabola with vertex at (1, 0)]

Solving the two equations we get the points of intersection as (–2, 1), (–2, –1)

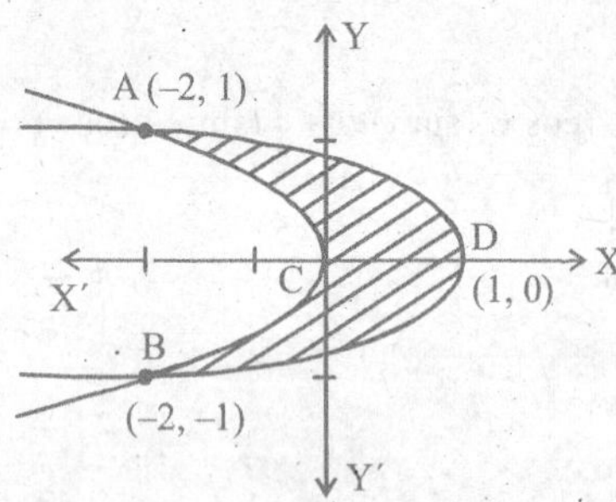

The required area is ACBDA, given by

$$=\left|\int_{-1}^{1}(1-3y^2-2y^2)dy\right|=\left|\left[y-\frac{5y^3}{3}\right]_{-1}^{1}\right|$$

$$=\left|\left(1-\frac{5}{3}\right)-\left(-1+\frac{5}{3}\right)\right|=2\times\frac{2}{3}=\frac{4}{3}\text{ sq. units.}$$

29. (a) The area enclosed between the curves $y^2 = x$ and $y = |x|$

From the figure, area lies between $y^2 = x$ and $y = x$

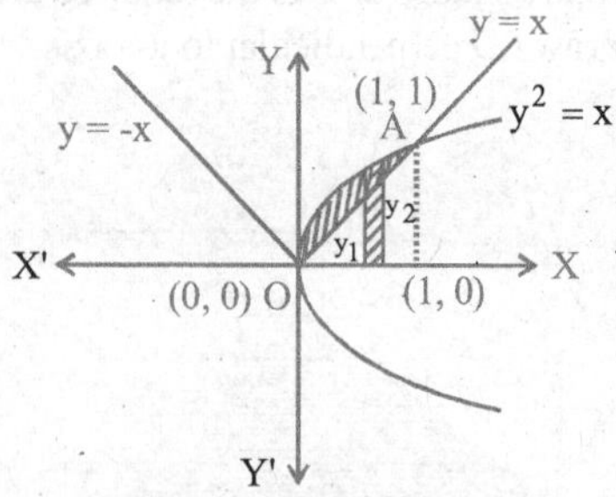

$\therefore$ Required area $= \int_0^1 (y_2 - y_1)dx$

$$= \int_0^1 (\sqrt{x}-x)dx = \left[\frac{x^{3/2}}{3/2}-\frac{x^2}{2}\right]_0^1$$

$$\therefore \text{Required area} = \frac{2}{3}\left[x^{3/2}\right]_0^1 - \frac{1}{2}\left[x^2\right]_0^1 = \frac{2}{3}-\frac{1}{2}=\frac{1}{6}$$

30. (d) Intersection points of $x^2 = 4y$ and $y^2 = 4x$ are (0, 0) and (4, 4). The graph is as shown in the figure.

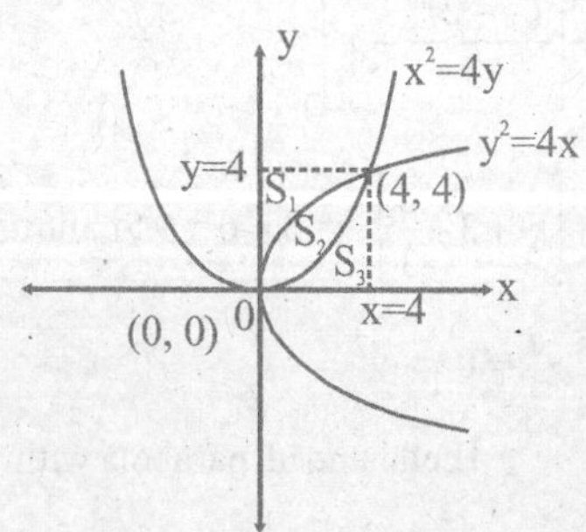

By symmetry, we observe

$$S_1 = S_3 = \int_0^4 y\,dx = \int_0^4 \frac{x^2}{4}dx = \left[\frac{x^3}{12}\right]_0^4 = \frac{16}{3}\ sq.\ units$$

Also

$$S_2 = \int_0^4 \left(2\sqrt{x}-\frac{x^2}{4}\right)dx = \left[\frac{2x^{\frac{3}{2}}}{\frac{3}{2}}-\frac{x^3}{12}\right]_0^4$$

$$=\frac{4}{3}\times 8-\frac{16}{3}=\frac{16}{3}\text{ sq. units}$$

$$\therefore S_1 : S_2 : S_3 = 1:1:1$$

31. (d) The required area is shown by shaded region

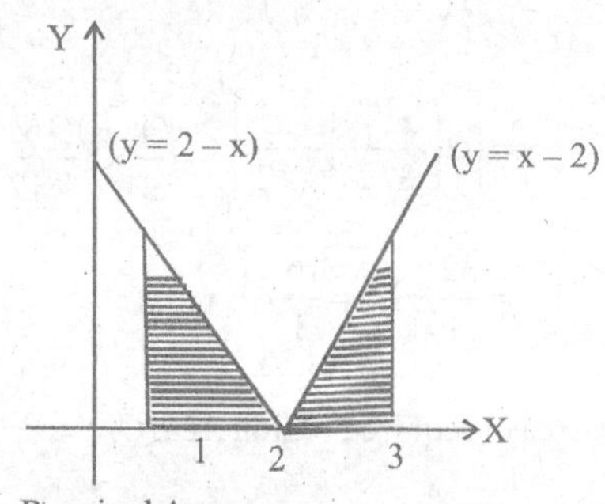

Required Area

$$A=\int_1^3 |x-2|dx = 2\int_2^3 (x-2)dx$$

$$=2\left[\frac{x^2}{2}-2x\right]_2^3 = 1$$

32. (d)

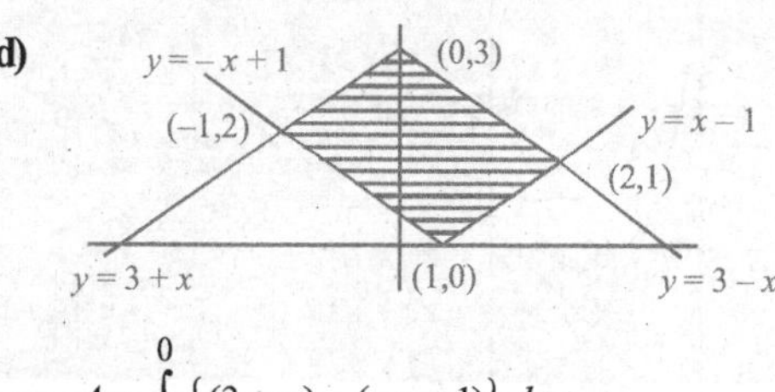

$$A=\int_{-1}^{0}\{(3+x)-(-x+1)\}dx+$$

$$\int_0^1\{(3-x)-(-x+1)\}dx+\int_1^2\{(3-x)-(x-1)\}dx$$

$$=\int_{-1}^{0}(2+2x)dx+\int_0^1 2dx+\int_1^2(4-2x)dx$$

$$=\left[2x-x^2\right]_{-1}^{0}+\left[2x\right]_0^1+\left[4x-x^2\right]_1^2$$

$$=0-(-2+1)+(2-0)+(8-4)-(4-1)$$

$$=1+2+4-3=4\ sq.\ units$$

33. **(a)** First we draw each curve as separate graph

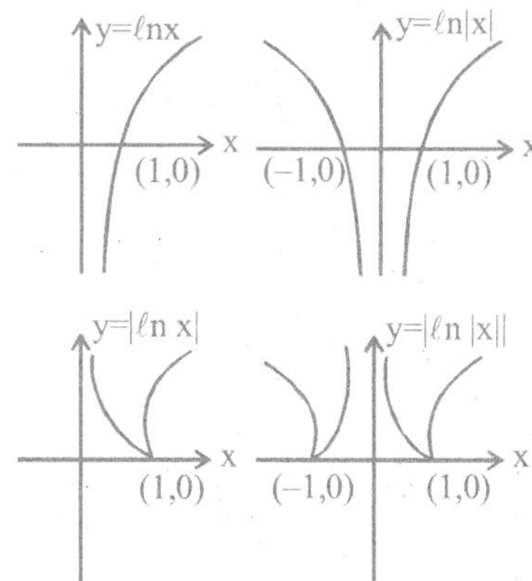

NOTE Graph of $y = |f(x)|$ can be obtained from the graph of the curve $y = f(x)$ by drawing the mirror image of the portion of the graph below x-axis, with respect to x-axis.

Clearly the bounded area is as shown in the following figure.

Required area $= 4\int_0^1 (-\ell nx)dx$

$= -4\left[x\ \ell n\ x - x\right]_0^1 = 4$ sq. units

Differential Equations

TOPIC-1 : Ordinary Differential Equations, Order & Degree of Differential Equations, Formation of Differential Equations

1. If the differential equation representing the family of all circles touching x-axis at the origin is

$\left(x^2 - y^2\right)\frac{dy}{dx} = g(x)y$, then g(x) equals:

[Online April 9, 2014]

(a) $\frac{1}{2}x$ (b) $2x^2$

(c) $2x$ (d) $\frac{1}{2}x^2$

2. **Statement-1:** The slope of the tangent at any point P on a parabola, whose axis is the axis of x and vertex is at the origin, is inversely proportional to the ordinate of the point P.

Statement-2: The system of parabolas $y^2 = 4ax$ satisfies a differential equation of degree 1 and order 1.

[Online April 9, 2013]

(a) Statement-1 is true; Statement-2 is true; Statement-2 is a correct explanation for statement-1.

(b) Statement-1 is true; Statement-2 is true; Statement-2 is **not** a correct explanation for statement-1.

(c) Statement-1 is true; Statement-2 is false.

(d) Statement-1 is false; Statement-2 is true.

3. **Statement 1:** The degrees of the differential equations $\frac{dy}{dx} + y^2 = x$ and $\frac{d^2y}{dx^2} + y = \sin x$ are equal.

Statement 2: The degree of a differential equation, when it is a polynomial equation in derivatives, is the highest positive integral power of the highest order derivative involved in the differential equation, otherwise degree is not defined.

[Online May 12, 2012]

(a) Statement 1 is true, Statement 2 is true, Statement 2 is not a correct explanation of Statement 1.

(b) Statement 1 is false, Statement 2 is true.

(c) Statement 1 is true, Statement 2 is false.

(d) Statement 1 is true, Statement 2 is true; Statement 2 is a correct explanation of Statement 1.

4. The differential equation which represents the family of curves $y = c_1 e^{c_2 x}$, where c_1, and c_2 are arbitrary constants, is **[2009]**

(a) $y'' = y'y$ (b) $yy'' = y'$

(c) $yy'' = (y')^2$ (d) $y' = y^2$

5. The differential equation of the family of circles with fixed radius 5 units and centre on the line $y = 2$ is **[2009]**

(a) $(x-2)y'^2 = 25 - (y-2)^2$

(b) $(y-2)y'^2 = 25 - (y-2)^2$

(c) $(y-2)^2 y'^2 = 25 - (y-2)^2$

(d) $(x-2)^2 y'^2 = 25 - (y-2)^2$

6. The differential equation of all circles passing through the origin and having their centres on the x-axis is **[2007]**

(a) $y^2 = x^2 + 2xy\frac{dy}{dx}$ (b) $y^2 = x^2 - 2xy\frac{dy}{dx}$

(c) $x^2 = y^2 + xy\frac{dy}{dx}$ (d) $x^2 = y^2 + 3xy\frac{dy}{dx}$

7. The differential equation whose solution is $Ax^2 + By^2 = 1$ where A and B are arbitrary constants is of **[2006]**

(a) second order and second degree

(b) first order and second degree

(c) first order and first degree

(d) second order and first degree

8. The differential equation representing the family of curves $y^2 = 2c(x + \sqrt{c})$, where $c > 0$, is a parameter, is of order and degree as follows : **[2005]**

(a) order 1, degree 2 (b) order 1, degree 1

(c) order 1, degree 3 (d) order 2, degree 2

9. The differential equation for the family of circle $x^2 + y^2 - 2ay = 0$, where a is an arbitrary constant is **[2004]**

(a) $(x^2 + y^2)y' = 2xy$

(b) $2(x^2 + y^2)y' = xy$

(c) $(x^2 - y^2)y' = 2xy$

(d) $2(x^2 - y^2)y' = xy$

10. The degree and order of the differential equation of the family of all parabolas whose axis is x - axis, are respectively. [2003]

(a) 2, 3 (b) 2, 1
(c) 1, 2 (d) 3, 2.

11. The order and degree of the differential equation $\left(1+3\frac{dy}{dx}\right)^{2/3}=4\frac{d^3y}{dx^3}$ are [2002]

(a) $(1, \frac{2}{3})$ (b) (3, 1)
(c) (3, 3) (d) (1, 2)

TOPIC-2 : General & Particular Solution of Differential Equation, Solution of Differential Equation by the Method of Separation of Variables, Solution of Homogeneous Differential Equations

12. If $(2+\sin x)\frac{dy}{dx}+(y+1)\cos x=0$ and $y(0)=1$, then $y\left(\frac{\pi}{2}\right)$ is equal to : [2017]

(a) $\frac{4}{3}$ (b) $\frac{1}{3}$
(c) $-\frac{2}{3}$ (d) $-\frac{1}{3}$

13. If a curve $y=f(x)$ passes through the point $(1,-1)$ and satisfies the differential equation, $y(1+xy)\,dx=x\,dy$, then $f\left(-\frac{1}{2}\right)$ is equal to : [2016]

(a) $\frac{2}{5}$ (b) $\frac{4}{5}$
(c) $-\frac{2}{5}$ (d) $-\frac{4}{5}$

14. If f(x) is a differentiable function in the interval ($(0,\infty)$ such that $f(a)=1$ and $\lim\limits_{t\to x}\frac{t^2f(x)-x^2f(t)}{t-x}=1$, for each $x>0$, then $f\left(\frac{3}{2}\right)$ is equal to : [Online April 9, 2016]

(a) $\frac{23}{18}$ (b) $\frac{13}{6}$
(c) $\frac{25}{9}$ (d) $\frac{31}{18}$

15. The solution of the differential equation $ydx-(x+2y^2)dy=0$ is $x=f(y)$. If $f(-1)=1$, then f(a) is equal to : [Online April 11, 2015]

(a) 4 (b) 3
(c) 1 (d) 2

16. If $y(x)$ is the solution of the differential equation $(x+2)\frac{dy}{dx}=x^2+4x-9, x\neq-2$ and $y(0)=0$, then $y(-4)$ is equal to : [Online April 10, 2015]

(a) 0 (b) 2
(c) 1 (d) –1

17. Let the population of rabbits surviving at time t be governed by the differential equation $\frac{dp(t)}{dt}=\frac{1}{2}p(t)-200$. If $p(0)=100$, then $p(t)$ equals: [2014]

(a) $600-500\,e^{t/2}$ (b) $400-300\,e^{-t/2}$
(c) $400-300\,e^{t/2}$ (d) $300-200\,e^{-t/2}$

18. If the general solution of the differential equation $y'=\frac{y}{x}+\Phi\left(\frac{x}{y}\right)$, for some function Φ, is given by $y\ln|cx|=x$, where c is an arbitrary constant, then $\Phi(2)$ is equal to: [Online April 11, 2014]

(a) 4 (b) $\frac{1}{4}$
(c) –4 (d) $-\frac{1}{4}$

19. At present, a firm is manufacturing 2000 items. It is estimated that the rate of change of production P w.r.t. additional number of workers x is given by $\frac{dP}{dx}=100-12\sqrt{x}$. If the firm employs 25 more workers, then the new level of production of items is [2013]

(a) 2500 (b) 3000
(c) 3500 (d) 4500

20. If a curve passes through the point $\left(2,\frac{7}{2}\right)$ and has slope $\left(1-\frac{1}{x^2}\right)$ at any point (x, y) on it, then the ordinate of the point on the curve whose abscissa is – 2 is : [Online April 23, 2013]

(a) $-\frac{3}{2}$ (b) $\frac{3}{2}$
(c) $\frac{5}{2}$ (d) $-\frac{5}{2}$

21. Consider the differential equation :

$$\frac{dy}{dx}=\frac{y^3}{2\left(xy^2-x^2\right)}$$ **[Online April 22, 2013]**

Statement-1: The substitution $z=y^2$ transforms the above equation into a first order homogenous differential equation.
Statement-2: The solution of this differential equation is $y^2e^{-y^2/x}=C$.

(a) Both statements are false.
(b) Statement-1 is true and statement-2 is false.
(c) Statement-1 is false and statement-2 is true.
(d) Both statements are true.

22. The population $p(t)$ at time t of a certain mouse species satisfies the differential equation $\frac{dp(t)}{dt}=0.5\,p(t)-450$. If $p(0)=850$, then the time at which the population becomes zero is : **[2012]**

(a) $2\ln 18$ (b) $\ln 9$
(c) $\frac{1}{2}\ln 18$ (d) $\ln 18$

23. Let $y(x)$ be a solution of $\frac{(2+\sin x)}{(1+y)}\frac{dy}{dx}=\cos x$. If $y(0)=2$, then $y\left(\frac{\pi}{2}\right)$ equals **[Online May 7, 2012]**

(a) $\frac{5}{2}$ (b) 2
(c) $\frac{7}{2}$ (d) 3

24. The curve that passes through the point (2, 3), and has the property that the segment of any tangent to it lying between the coordinate axes is bisected by the point of contact is given by : **[2011RS]**

(a) $2y-3x=0$ (b) $y=\frac{6}{x}$
(c) $x^2+y^2=13$ (d) $\left(\frac{x}{2}\right)^2+\left(\frac{y}{3}\right)^2=2$

25. Let I be the purchase value of an equipment and $V(t)$ be the value after it has been used for t years. The value $V(t)$ depreciates at a rate given by differential equation $\frac{dV(t)}{dt}=-k(T-t)$, where $k>0$ is a constant and T is the total life in years of the equipment. Then the scrap value $V(T)$ of the equipment is **[2011]**

(a) $I-\frac{kT^2}{2}$ (b) $I-\frac{k(T-t)^2}{2}$
(c) e^{-kT} (d) $T^2-\frac{1}{k}$

26. If $\frac{dy}{dx}=y+3>0$ and $y(0)=2$, then $y(\ln 2)$ is equal to : **[2011]**

(a) 5 (b) 13
(c) -2 (d) 7

27. The solution of the differential equation $\frac{dy}{dy}=\frac{x+y}{x}$ satisfying the condition $y(1)=1$ is **[2008]**

(a) $y=\ln x+x$ (b) $y=x\ln x+x^2$
(c) $y=xe^{(x-1)}$ (d) $y=x\ln x+x$

28. The normal to a curve at $P(x, y)$ meets the x-axis at G. If the distance of G from the origin is twice the abscissa of P, then the curve is a **[2007]**

(a) circle (b) hyperbola
(c) ellipse (d) parabola.

29. If $x\frac{dy}{dx}=y(\log y-\log x+1)$, then the solution of the equation is **[2005]**

(a) $y\log\left(\frac{x}{y}\right)=cx$ (b) $x\log\left(\frac{y}{x}\right)=cy$
(c) $\log\left(\frac{y}{x}\right)=cx$ (d) $\log\left(\frac{x}{y}\right)=cy$

30. The solution of the equation $\frac{d^2y}{dx^2}=e^{-2x}$ **[2002]**

(a) $\frac{e^{-2x}}{4}$ (b) $\frac{e^{-2x}}{4}+cx+d$
(c) $\frac{1}{4}e^{-2x}+cx^2+d$ (d) $\frac{1}{4}e^{-4x}+cx+d$

TOPIC-3: Linear Differential Equation of First Order. Differential Equation of the form: $\frac{d^2y}{dx^2}=F(x)$, Solution by Inspection Method

31. The curve satisfying the differential equation, $ydx-(x+3y^2)dy=0$ and passing through the point (1, 1), also passes through the point : **[Online April 8, 2017]**

(a) $\left(\frac{1}{4},-\frac{1}{2}\right)$ (b) $\left(-\frac{1}{3},\frac{1}{3}\right)$
(c) $\left(\frac{1}{3},-\frac{1}{3}\right)$ (d) $\left(\frac{1}{4},\frac{1}{2}\right)$

32. The solution of the differential equaiton $\frac{dy}{dx}+\frac{y}{2}\sec x=\frac{\tan x}{2y}$, where $0\le x<\frac{\pi}{2}$, and $y(0)=1$, is given by : **[Online April 10, 2016]**

(a) $y^2=1+\frac{x}{\sec x+\tan x}$ (b) $y=1+\frac{x}{\sec x+\tan x}$

(c) $y=1-\frac{x}{\sec x+\tan x}$ (d) $y^2=1-\frac{x}{\sec x+\tan x}$

33. Let y(x) be the solution of the differential equation $(x\log x)\frac{dy}{dx}+y=2x\log x,(x\ge 1)$. Then y (e) is equal to: **[2015]**

(a) 2 (b) 2e
(c) e (d) 0

34. If $\frac{dy}{dx}+y\tan x=\sin 2x$ and $y(0)=1$, then $y(\pi)$ is equal to: **[Online April 19, 2014]**

(a) 1 (b) –1
(c) –5 (d) 5

35. The general solution of the differential equation, $\sin 2x\left(\frac{dy}{dx}-\sqrt{\tan x}\right)-y=0$, is: **[Online April 12, 2014]**

(a) $y\sqrt{\tan x}=x+c$ (b) $y\sqrt{\cot x}=\tan x+c$

(c) $y\sqrt{\tan x}=\cot x+c$ (d) $y\sqrt{\cot x}=x+c$

36. The equation of the curve passing through the origin and satisfying the differential equation $(1+x^2)\frac{dy}{dx}+2xy=4x^2$ is **[Online April 25, 2013]**

(a) $(1+x^2)y=x^3$ (b) $3(1+x^2)y=2x^3$

(c) $(1+x^2)y=3x^3$ (d) $3(1+x^2)y=4x^3$

37. The integrating factor of the differential equation $\left(x^2-1\right)\frac{dy}{dx}+2xy=x$ is **[Online May 26, 2012]**

(a) $\frac{1}{x^2-1}$ (b) x^2-1

(c) $\frac{x^2-1}{x}$ (d) $\frac{x}{x^2-1}$

38. The general solution of the differential equation $\frac{dy}{dx}+\frac{2}{x}y=x^2$ is **[Online May 19, 2012]**

(a) $y=cx^{-3}-\frac{x^2}{4}$ (b) $y=cx^3-\frac{x^2}{4}$

(c) $y=cx^2+\frac{x^3}{5}$ (d) $y=cx^{-2}+\frac{x^3}{5}$

39. Consider the differential equation **[2011RS]**

$y^2dx+\left(x-\frac{1}{y}\right)dy=0$. If $y(1)=1$, then x is given by :

(a) $4-\frac{2}{y}-\frac{e^{\frac{1}{y}}}{e}$ (b) $3-\frac{1}{y}+\frac{e^{\frac{1}{y}}}{e}$

(c) $1+\frac{1}{y}-\frac{e^{\frac{1}{y}}}{e}$ (d) $1-\frac{1}{y}+\frac{e^{\frac{1}{y}}}{e}$

40. Solution of the differential equation $\cos x\,dy=y(\sin x-y)\,dx,\ 0<x<\frac{\pi}{2}$ is **[2010]**

(a) $y\sec x=\tan x+c$
(b) $y\tan x=\sec x+c$
(c) $\tan x=(\sec x+c)y$
(d) $\sec x=(\tan x+c)y$

41. Solution of the differential equation $ydx+(x+x^2y)dy=0$ is **[2004]**

(a) $\log y=Cx$ (b) $-\frac{1}{xy}+\log y=C$

(c) $\frac{1}{xy}+\log y=C$ (d) $-\frac{1}{xy}=C$

42. The solution of the differential equation $(1+y^2)+(x-e^{\tan^{-1}y})\frac{dy}{dx}=0$, is **[2003]**

(a) $xe^{2\tan^{-1}y}=e^{\tan^{-1}y}+k$

(b) $(x-2)=ke^{2\tan^{-1}y}$

(c) $2xe^{\tan^{-1}y}=e^{2\tan^{-1}y}+k$

(d) $xe^{\tan^{-1}y}=\tan^{-1}y+k$

Hints & Solutions

1. **(c)** Since family of all circles touching x-axis at the origin

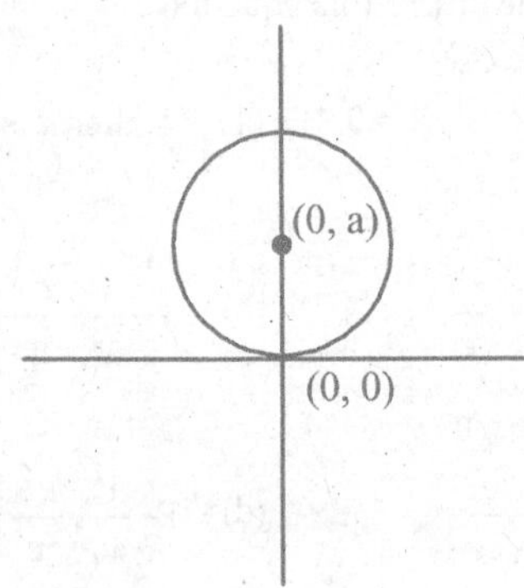

$\therefore$ Eqn is $(x)^2 + (y - a)^2 = a^2$
where $(0, a)$ is the centre of circle.

$\Rightarrow x^2 + y^2 + a^2 - 2ay = a^2$

$\Rightarrow x^2 + y^2 - 2ay = 0$ ...(1)

Differentiate both side w.r.t 'x', we get

$$2x + 2y\frac{dy}{dx} - 2a\frac{dy}{dx} = 0$$

$$\Rightarrow x + y\frac{dy}{dx} - a\frac{dy}{dx} = 0$$

$$\Rightarrow \frac{x + y\frac{dy}{dx}}{\frac{dy}{dx}} = a$$

Put value of 'a' in eqn (1), we get

$$x^2 + y^2 - 2y\left[\frac{y\frac{dy}{dx} + x}{\frac{dy}{dx}}\right] = 0$$

$$\Rightarrow (x^2 + y^2)\frac{dy}{dx} - 2y^2\frac{dy}{dx} - 2xy = 0$$

$$\Rightarrow (x^2 + y^2 - 2y^2)\frac{dy}{dx} = 2xy$$

$$\Rightarrow (x^2 - y^2)\frac{dy}{dx} = 2xy \equiv g(x)y$$

Hence, $g(x) = 2x$

2. **(b)** Statement - 1 : $y^2 = \pm 4ax$

$$\Rightarrow \frac{dy}{dx} = \pm 2a.\frac{1}{y} \Rightarrow \frac{dy}{dx} \propto \frac{1}{y}$$

Statement - 2 : $y^2 = 4ax \Rightarrow 2y\frac{dy}{dx} = 4a$

Thus both statements are true but statement-2 is not a correct explanation for statement-1.

3. **(d)** **Statement - 1**

Given differential equations are $\frac{dy}{dx} + y^2 = x$ and

$$\frac{d^2y}{dx^2} + y = \sin x$$

Their degrees are 1.
Both have equal degree.
Also, Statement - 2 is the correct explanation for Statement - 1.

4. **(c)** We have $y = c_1e^{c_2x}$

$$\Rightarrow y' = c_1c_2\, e^{c_2x} = c_2y$$

$$\Rightarrow \frac{y''}{y} = c_2 \Rightarrow \frac{y''y - (y')^2}{y^2} = 0$$

$$\Rightarrow y''y = (y')^2$$

5. **(c)** Let the centre of the circle be $(h, 2)$
$\therefore$ Equation of circle is
$(x - h)^2 + (y - 2)^2 = 25$ ...(1)
Differentiating with respect to x, we get

$$2(x - h) + 2(y - 2)\frac{dy}{dx} = 0$$

$$\Rightarrow x - h = -(y - 2)\frac{dy}{dx}$$

Substituting in equation (1) we get

$$(y - 2)^2\left(\frac{dy}{dx}\right)^2 + (y - 2)^2 = 25$$

$$\Rightarrow (y - 2)^2\,(y')^2 = 25 - (y - 2)^2$$

6. **(a)** General equation of circles passing through origin and having their centres on the x-axis is
$x^2 + y^2 + 2gx = 0$ ...(i)
On differentiating w.r.t x, we get

$$2x + 2y.\frac{dy}{dx} + 2g = 0 \Rightarrow g = -\left(x + y\frac{dy}{dx}\right)$$

$\therefore$ equation (i) be

$$x^2+y^2+2\left\{-\left(x+y\frac{dy}{dx}\right)\right\}.x=0$$

$$\Rightarrow x^2+y^2-2x^2-2x\frac{dy}{dx}.y=0$$

$$\Rightarrow y^2=x^2+2xy\frac{dy}{dx}$$

7. (d) $Ax^2+By^2=1$ ....(1)

$$Ax+By\frac{dy}{dx}=0 \quad \text{..........(2)}$$

$$A+By\frac{d^2y}{dx^2}+B\left(\frac{dy}{dx}\right)^2=0 \quad \text{........(3)}$$

From (2) and (3)

$$x\left\{-By\frac{d^2y}{dx^2}-B\left(\frac{dy}{dx}\right)^2\right\}+By\frac{dy}{dx}=0$$

Dividing both sides by –B, we get

$$xy\frac{d^2y}{dx^2}+x\left(\frac{dy}{dx}\right)^2-y\frac{dy}{dx}=0$$

Which is a DE of order 2 and degree 1.

8. (c) $y^2=2c(x+\sqrt{c})$ .... (i)

$2yy'=2c.1$ or $yy'=c$ .... (ii)

$\Rightarrow \; y^2=2yy'(x+\sqrt{yy'})$

[On putting value of c from (ii) in (i)]

On simplifying, we get

$(y-2xy')^2=4yy'^3$ .... (iii)

Hence equation (iii) is of order 1 and degree 3.

9. (c) $x^2+y^2-2ay=0$ ....(1)

Differentiate,

$$2x+2y\frac{dy}{dx}-2a\frac{dy}{dx}=0 \Rightarrow a=\frac{x+yy'}{y'}$$

Put in (1), $x^2+y^2-2\left(\frac{x+yy'}{y'}\right)y=0$

$$\Rightarrow (x^2+y^2)y'-2xy-2y^2y'=0$$

$$\Rightarrow (x^2-y^2)y'=2xy$$

10. (c) $y^2=4a(x-h),\; 2yy_1=4a \Rightarrow yy_1=2a$

Differentiating, $\Rightarrow y_1{}^2+yy_2=0$

Degree $=1$, order $=2$.

11. (c) $\left(1+3\frac{dy}{dx}\right)^2=\left(\frac{4d^3y}{dx^3}\right)^3$

$$\Rightarrow \left(1+3\frac{dy}{dx}\right)^2=16\left(\frac{d^3y}{dx^3}\right)^3$$

12. (b) We have $(2+\sin x)\frac{dy}{dx}+(y+1)\cos x=0$

$$\Rightarrow \frac{d}{dx}(2+\sin x)(y+1)=0$$

On integrating, we get

$(2+\sin x)(y+1)=C$

At $x=0, y=1$ we have

$(2+\sin 0)(1+1)=C$

$\Rightarrow C=4$

$$\Rightarrow y+1=\frac{4}{2+\sin x}$$

$$y=\frac{4}{2+\sin x}-1$$

Now $y\left(\frac{\pi}{2}\right)=\frac{4}{2+\sin\frac{\pi}{2}}-1$

$$=\frac{4}{3}-1=\frac{1}{3}$$

13. (b) $y(1+xy)dx=xdy$

$$\frac{xdy-ydx}{y^2}=xdx$$

$$\Rightarrow \int -d\left(\frac{x}{y}\right)=\int xdx$$

$$-\frac{x}{y}=\frac{x^2}{2}+C \text{ as } y(a)=-1 \Rightarrow C=\frac{1}{2}$$

Hence, $y=\frac{-2x}{x^2+1} \Rightarrow f\left(\frac{-1}{2}\right)=\frac{4}{5}$

14. (d) Let $L=\lim\limits_{t\to x}\frac{t^2f(x)-x^2f(t)}{t-x}=1$

Applying L.H. rule

$$L=\lim_{t\to x}\frac{2tf(x)-x^2f'(t)}{1}=1$$

$2xf(x)-x^2f'(x)=1$

solving above differential equation, we get

$$f(x)=\frac{2}{3}x^2+\frac{1}{3x}$$

Put $x=\frac{3}{2}$

$$f\left(\frac{3}{2}\right)=\frac{2}{3}\times\left(\frac{3}{2}\right)^2+\frac{1}{3}\times\frac{2}{3}$$

$$=\frac{3}{2}+\frac{2}{9}=\frac{27+4}{18}=\frac{31}{18}$$

15. (b) Given differential equation is

$y dx-(x+2y^2)dy=0$

$\Rightarrow y dx - x dy - 2y^2 dy = 0$

$$\Rightarrow \frac{y dx - x dy}{y^2}=2dy$$

$$\Rightarrow d\left(\frac{x}{y}\right)=2dy$$

Integrate both the side

$$\Rightarrow \frac{x}{y}=2y+c$$

using f(–1) = 1, we get

$c=1$

$$\Rightarrow \frac{x}{y}=2y+1$$

put y = 1, we get f(a) = 3

16. (a) $(x+2)\frac{dy}{dx}=x^2+4x-9 \quad x\neq -2$

$$\frac{dy}{dx}=\frac{x^2+4x-9}{x+2}$$

$$dy=\frac{x^2+4x-9}{x+2}dx$$

$$\int dy=\int\frac{x^2+4x-9}{x+2}dx$$

$$y=\int\left(x+2-\frac{13}{x+2}\right)dx$$

$$y=\int(x+2)\,dx-13\int\frac{1}{x+2}dx$$

$$y=\frac{x^2}{2}+2x-13\log|x+2|+c$$

Given that y = (0) = 0

$0=-13\log 2+c$

$$y=\frac{x^2}{2}+2x-13\log|x+2|+13\log 2$$

$y(-4)=8-8-13\log 2+13\log 2=0$

17. (c) Given differential equation is

$$\frac{dp(t)}{dt}=\frac{1}{2}p(t)-200$$

By separating the variable, we get

$$dp(t)=\left[\frac{1}{2}p(t)-200\right]dt$$

$$\Rightarrow \frac{dp(t)}{\frac{1}{2}p(t)-200}=dt$$

Integrate on both the sides,

$$\int\frac{d(p(t))}{\frac{1}{2}p(t)-200}=\int dt$$

Let $\frac{1}{2}p(t)-200=s\Rightarrow\frac{dp(t)}{2}=ds$

So, $$\int\frac{d\,p(t)}{\left(\frac{1}{2}p(t)-200\right)}=\int dt$$

$$\Rightarrow \int\frac{2ds}{s}=\int dt$$

$$\Rightarrow 2\log s=t+c$$

$$\Rightarrow 2\log\left(\frac{p(t)}{2}-200\right)=t+c$$

$$\Rightarrow \frac{p(t)}{2}-200=e^{\frac{1}{2}}k$$

Using given condition $p(t)=400-300e^{t/2}$

18. (d) Given $\frac{dy}{dx}=\frac{y}{x}+\phi\left(\frac{y}{x}\right)$ ...(1)

Let $\left(\frac{y}{x}\right)=v$ so that $y=xv$

or $\frac{dy}{dx}=x\frac{dv}{dx}+v$ ...(2)

from (1) & (2), $x\frac{dv}{dx}+\cancel{v}=\cancel{v}+\phi\left(\frac{1}{v}\right)$

or, $$\frac{dv}{\phi\left(\frac{1}{v}\right)}=\frac{dx}{x}$$

Integrating both sides, we get

$$\int \frac{dx}{x} = \int \frac{dv}{\phi\left(\frac{1}{v}\right)} \Rightarrow \ln x + c = \int \frac{dv}{\phi\left(\frac{1}{v}\right)}$$

(where c being constant of integration)

But, given $y = \frac{x}{\ln|cx|}$ is the general solution

so that $\frac{x}{y} = \frac{1}{v} = \ln|cx| = \int \frac{dv}{\phi\left(\frac{1}{v}\right)}$

Differentiating w.r.t v both sides, we get

$$\phi\left(\frac{1}{v}\right) = \frac{-1}{v^2} \Rightarrow \phi\left(\frac{x}{y}\right) = -\frac{y^2}{x^2}$$

when $\frac{x}{y} = 2$ i.e. $\phi(2) = -\left(\frac{y}{x}\right)^2 = -\left(\frac{1}{2}\right)^2 = \left(\frac{-1}{4}\right)$

19. **(c)** Given, Rate of change is $\frac{dP}{dx} = 100 - 12\sqrt{x}$

$\Rightarrow dP = (100 - 12\sqrt{x})\, dx$

By integrating

$\int dP = \int (100 - 12\sqrt{x})\, dx$

$P = 100x - 8x^{3/2} + C$

Given when $x = 0$ then $P = 2000$

$\Rightarrow C = 2000$

Now when $x = 25$ then

$P = 100 \times 25 - 8 \times (25)^{3/2} + 2000$

$= 4500 - 1000$

$\Rightarrow P = 3500$

20. **(a)** Slope $= \frac{dy}{dx} = 1 - \frac{1}{x^2}$

$$\Rightarrow \int dy = \int \left(1 - \frac{1}{x^2}\right) dx$$

$\Rightarrow y = x + \frac{1}{x} + C$, which is the equation of the curve

since curve passes through the point $\left(2, \frac{7}{2}\right)$

$$\therefore \frac{7}{2} = 2 + \frac{1}{2} + C \Rightarrow C = 1$$

$$\therefore y = x + \frac{1}{x} + 1$$

when $x = -2$, then $y = -2 + \frac{1}{-2} + 1 = \frac{-3}{2}$

21. **(d)** Given differential equation is

$$\frac{dy}{dx} = \frac{y^3}{2(xy^2 - x^2)}$$

By substituting $z = y^2$, we get diff. eqn. as

$$\frac{dz}{dx} = \frac{2z^2}{2(xz - x^2)} = \frac{z^2}{xz - x^2}$$

Now, $\frac{dx}{dz} = \frac{x}{z} - \frac{x^2}{z^2} = \frac{x}{z}\left[1 - \frac{x}{z}\right] \approx F\left(\frac{x}{z}\right)$

Hence, statement-1 is true.

Now, $y^2 e^{-y^2/x} = C$ satisfies the given diff. equation

$\therefore$ It is the solution of given diff. equation.

Thus, statement-2 is also true.

22. **(a)** Given differential equation is

$$\frac{dp(t)}{dt} = 0.5p(t) - 450$$

$$\Rightarrow \frac{dp(t)}{dt} = \frac{1}{2}p(t) - 450$$

$$\Rightarrow \frac{dp(t)}{dt} = \frac{p(t) - 900}{2}$$

$$\Rightarrow 2\frac{dp(t)}{dt} = -[900 - p(t)]$$

$$\Rightarrow 2\frac{dp(t)}{900 - p(t)} = -dt$$

Integrate both the side, we get

$$-2\int \frac{dp(t)}{900 - p(t)} = \int dt$$

Let $900 - p(t) = u$

$\Rightarrow -dp(t) = du$

$\therefore$ We have,

$$2\int \frac{du}{u} = \int dt \Rightarrow 2\ln u = t + c$$

$\Rightarrow 2\ln[900 - p(t)] = t + c$

when $t = 0$, $p(0) = 850$

$2\ln(50) = c$

$$\Rightarrow 2\left[\ln\left(\frac{900 - p(t)}{50}\right)\right] = t$$

$$\Rightarrow 900 - p(t) = 50e^{\frac{t}{2}}$$

$$\Rightarrow p(t) = 900 - 50e^{\frac{t}{2}}$$

let $p(t_1) = 0$

$0 = 900 - 50e^{\frac{t_1}{2}}$ $\quad\therefore t_1 = 2\ln 18$

23. (c) Given differential equation is

$$\frac{(2+\sin x)}{(1+y)}\cdot\frac{dy}{dx}=\cos x$$

which can be rewritten as

$$\frac{dy}{1+y}=\frac{\cos x}{2+\sin x}dx$$

Integrate both the sides, we get

$$\int\frac{dy}{1+y}=\int\frac{\cos x\,dx}{2+\sin x}$$

$\Rightarrow$ $\log(1+y)=\log(2+\sin x)+\log C$

$\Rightarrow$ $1+y=C(2+\sin x)$

Given $y(0)=2$

$\Rightarrow$ $1+2=C[2+\sin 0]\Rightarrow C=\frac{3}{2}$

Now, $y\left(\frac{\pi}{2}\right)$ can be found as

$$1+y=\frac{3}{2}\left(2+\sin\frac{\pi}{2}\right)\Rightarrow 1+y=\frac{9}{2}$$

$\Rightarrow$ $y=\frac{7}{2}$

Hence, $y\left(\frac{\pi}{2}\right)=\frac{7}{2}$

24. (b) $Y-y=\frac{dy}{dx}(X-x)$

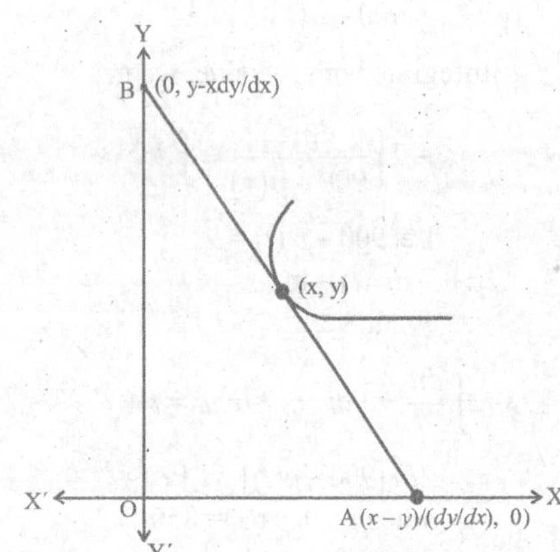

X-intercept $=x-\frac{y}{dy/dx}$

Y-intercept $=y-\frac{xdy}{dx}$

According to given statement

$$x-\frac{y}{dy}=2x \text{ and } y-\frac{xdy}{dx}=2y$$

$$\frac{-y}{\frac{dy}{dx}}=x \quad\text{and}\quad \frac{-xdy}{dx}=y$$

$$\Rightarrow \frac{dx}{x}+\frac{dy}{y}=0$$

$\ell ny=-\ell nc+\ell nc$

$y=\frac{c}{x}$

Since the above line passes through the point (2, 3).

$\therefore$ $c=6$

Hence $y=\frac{6}{x}$ is the required equation.

25. (a) $\frac{dV(t)}{dt}=-k(T-t)$

$$\Rightarrow \int dVt=-k\int(T-t)dt$$

$$V(t)=\frac{k(T-t)^2}{2}+c$$

at $t=0$, $V(t)=I\Rightarrow V(t)=I+\frac{k}{2}(t^2-2tT)$

$$V(T)=I+\frac{k}{2}(T^2-2T^2)\;=I-\frac{k}{2}T^2$$

26. (d) $\frac{dy}{dx}=y+3\Rightarrow\int\frac{dy}{y+3}=\int dx$

$\Rightarrow \ell n|y+3|=x+c$

Since $y(0)=2$, $\quad\therefore \ell n5=c$

$\Rightarrow \ell n|y+3|=x+\ell n5$

When $x=\ell n2$, then $\ell n|y+3|=\ell n2+\ell n5$

$\Rightarrow \ell n|y+3|=\ell n10$

$\therefore$ $y+3=\pm10\ \Rightarrow y=7,-13$

27. (d) $\frac{dy}{dx}=\frac{x+y}{x}=1+\frac{y}{x}$

Putting $y=vx$ and $\frac{dy}{dx}=v+x\frac{dv}{dx}$

we get

$$v+x\frac{dv}{dx}=1+v\Rightarrow\int\frac{dx}{x}=\int dv$$

$\Rightarrow v=\ln x+c\Rightarrow y=x\ln x+cx$

As $y(1)=1$

$\therefore$ $c=1$ So solution is $y=x\ln x+x$

28. (b) Equation of normal at $P(x,y)$ is

$$Y-y=-\frac{dx}{dy}(X-x)$$

Coordinate of G at X axis is $(X,0)$ (let)

$$\therefore\ 0-y=-\frac{dx}{dy}(X-x)$$

$$\Rightarrow\ y\frac{dy}{dx}=X-x$$

$\Rightarrow X = x + y\dfrac{dy}{dx}$

$\therefore$ Co-ordinate of $G\left(x + y\dfrac{dy}{dx}, 0\right)$

Given distance of G from origin = twice of the abscissa of P.

$\because$ distance cannot be –ve, therefore abscissa x should be +ve

$\therefore\ x + y\dfrac{dy}{dx} = 2x \Rightarrow y\dfrac{dy}{dx} = x$

$\Rightarrow ydy = xdx$

On Integrating, we have $\dfrac{y^2}{2} = \dfrac{x^2}{2} + c_1$

$\Rightarrow x^2 - y^2 = -2c_1$

$\therefore$ the curve is a hyperbola

29. **(c)** $\dfrac{xdy}{dx} = y(\log y - \log x + 1)$

$\dfrac{dy}{dx} = \dfrac{y}{x}\left(\log\left(\dfrac{y}{x}\right) + 1\right)$

Put $y = vx$

$\dfrac{dy}{dx} = v + \dfrac{xdv}{dx} \Rightarrow v + \dfrac{xdv}{dx} = v(\log v + 1)$

$\dfrac{xdv}{dx} = v\log v \Rightarrow \dfrac{dv}{v\log v} = \dfrac{dx}{x}$

Put $\log v = z$

$\dfrac{1}{v}dv = dz \Rightarrow \dfrac{dz}{z} = \dfrac{dx}{x}$

$\ln z = \ln x + \ln c$

$x = cx$ or $\log v = cx$ or $\log\left(\dfrac{y}{x}\right) = cx.$

30. **(b)** $\dfrac{d^2y}{dx^2} = e^{-2x}$; $\dfrac{dy}{dx} = \dfrac{e^{-2x}}{-2} + c$;

$y = \dfrac{e^{-2x}}{4} + cx + d$

31. **(b)** $y\,dx - x\,dy - 3y^2\,dy = 0$

$\Rightarrow \dfrac{dx}{dy} = \dfrac{x}{y} + 3y$

$\Rightarrow \dfrac{dx}{dy} - \dfrac{x}{y} = 3y$

if $= e^{-\int\frac{1}{y}dy} = e^{-\ln y} = \dfrac{1}{y}$

$\therefore$ solution is $\dfrac{x}{y} = \int 3y.\dfrac{1}{y}dy$

$\Rightarrow \dfrac{x}{y} = 3y + c$

which passes through (1, 1)

$\therefore\ 1 = 3 + c \Rightarrow c = -2$

$\therefore$ solution becomes

$\Rightarrow x = 3y^2 - 2y$

which also passes through $\left(-\dfrac{1}{3}, \dfrac{1}{3}\right)$

32. **(d)** $\dfrac{dy}{dx} + \dfrac{y}{2}\sec x = \dfrac{\tan x}{2y}$

$2y\dfrac{dy}{dx} + y^2\sec x = \tan x$

Put $y^2 = t \Rightarrow 2y\dfrac{dy}{dx} = \dfrac{dt}{dx}$

$\dfrac{dt}{dx} + t\sec x = \tan x$

$I.f = e^{\int\sec x dx} = e^{\ln(\sec x + \tan x)} = \sec x + \tan x$

$\dfrac{dt}{dx}(\sec x + \tan x) + t\sec x(\sec x + \tan x)$

$= \tan x(\sec x + \tan x)$

$\int d(t(\sec x + \tan x)) = \int \tan x(\sec x + \tan x)\,dx$

$t(\sec x + \tan x) = \sec x + \tan x - x$

$t = 1 - \dfrac{x}{\sec x + \tan x} \Rightarrow y^2 = 1 - \dfrac{x}{\sec x + \tan x}$

33. **(a)** Given, $\dfrac{dy}{dx} + \left(\dfrac{1}{x\log x}\right)y = 2$

I.F. $= e^{\int\frac{1}{x\log x}dx}$

$= e^{\log(\log x)} = \log x$

$y.\log x = \int 2\log x dx + c$

$y\log x = 2[x\log x - x] + c$

Put $x = 1$, $y.0 = -2 + c$

$c = 2$

Put $x = e$

$y\log e = 2e(\log e - 1) + c$

$y(e) = c = 2$

34. (c) Let $\frac{dy}{dx}+y\tan x = \sin 2x$

$\text{I.F} = e^{\int \tan x\,dx} = e^{-\log\cos x} = \sec x$

Required solution is

$y\ (\sec x) = \int \sin 2x \sec x\ dx + c$

$y\ (\sec x) = \int \frac{2\sin x\cos x}{\cos x} dx + c$

$y\ (\sec x) = 2\int \sin x\ dx + c$

$y\ (\sec x) = -2\cos x + c$ ...(1)

Given $y(0) = 1$

$\therefore$ put $x = 0$ and $y = 1$, we get

$1\ (\sec 0) = -2\cos 0 + c$

$\Rightarrow c = 1 + 2 \Rightarrow c = 3$

$\therefore$ from eqn (1), we have

$y \sec x = -2\cos x + 3$ ...(2)

To find $y\ (\pi)$, put $x = \pi$ in eqn (2), we get

$y\ (\sec\pi) = -2\cos\pi + 3$

$y = -2\ (-1)\ (-1) + 3\ (-1) = -2 - 3 = -5$

35. (d) Given, $\sin 2x\left(\frac{dy}{dx} - \sqrt{\tan x}\right) - y = 0$

or, $\frac{dy}{dx} = \frac{y}{\sin 2x} + \sqrt{\tan x}$

or, $\frac{dy}{dx} - y\,\text{cosec}\,2x = \sqrt{\tan x}$ ...(1)

Now, integrating factor (I.F) = $e^{\int -\text{cosec}\,2x}$

or, I.F = $e^{-\frac{1}{2}\log|\tan x|} = e^{\log\left(\sqrt{\tan x}\right)^{-1}}$

$= \frac{1}{\sqrt{\tan x}} = \sqrt{\cot x}$

Now, general solution of eq. (1) is written as

$y\ (\text{I. F.}) = \int Q(\text{I.F.})\,dx + c$

$\therefore\ y\sqrt{\cot x} = \int \sqrt{\tan x}.\sqrt{\cot x}\ dx + c$

$\therefore\ y\sqrt{\cot x} = \int 1.dx + c$

$\boxed{\therefore y\sqrt{\cot x} = x + c}$

36. (d) Given differential equation is

$(1+x^2)\frac{dy}{dx} + 2xy = 4x^2$

$\Rightarrow \frac{dy}{dx} + \left(\frac{2x}{1+x^2}\right)y = \frac{4x^2}{1+x^2}$

This is linear diff. equation

$\text{I.F} = e^{\int \frac{2x}{1+x^2}dx} = e^{\log(1+x^2)} = 1 + x^2$

$\therefore$ Solution is

$y(1+x^2) = \int \frac{4x^2}{1+x^2} \times 1 + x^2 + C$

$\Rightarrow y(1+x^2) = \frac{4x^3}{3} + C$

$\Rightarrow$ Required curve is

$3y\,(1+x^2) = 4x^3\ (\because\ C = 0)$

37. (b) Given differential equation is $\left(x^2-1\right)\frac{dy}{dx} + 2xy = x$

$\Rightarrow \frac{dy}{dx} + \frac{2x}{x^2-1}.y = \frac{x}{x^2-1}$

This is in linear form.

Integrating factor $= e^{\int \frac{2x}{x^2-1}dx} = e^{\int \frac{dt}{t}}$ where $t = x^2 - 1$

$= e^{\log t} = x^2 - 1$

Hence, required integrating factor $= x^2 - 1$.

38. (d) Given differential equation is

$\frac{dy}{dx} + \frac{2}{x}.y = x^2$

This is of the linear form.

$\therefore\ P = \frac{2}{x}, Q = x^2$

$\text{I.F} = e^{\int \frac{2}{x}dx} = e^{\log x^2} = x^2$

Solution is

$y.x^2 = \int x^2.x^2 dx + c = \frac{x^5}{5} + c$

$y = \frac{x^3}{5} + cx^{-2}$

39. (c) $\frac{dx}{dy} + \frac{x}{y^2} = \frac{1}{y^3}$

$\text{I.F.} = e^{\int \frac{1}{y^2}dy} = e^{-\frac{1}{y}}$

So $x.e^{-\frac{1}{y}} = \int \frac{1}{y^3} e^{-\frac{1}{y}} dy$

Let $\frac{-1}{y} = t$

$\Rightarrow \frac{1}{y^2}dy = dt$

$\Rightarrow I = -\int te^t dt = e^t - te^t = e^{-\frac{1}{y}} + \frac{1}{y}e^{-\frac{1}{y}} + c$

$$\Rightarrow \quad xe^{-\frac{1}{y}} = e^{-\frac{1}{y}} + \frac{1}{y}e^{-\frac{1}{y}} + c$$

$$\Rightarrow \quad x = 1 + \frac{1}{y} + c.e^{1/y}$$

Since $y(1) = 1$

$$\therefore \quad c = -\frac{1}{e}$$

$$\Rightarrow \quad x = 1 + \frac{1}{y} - \frac{1}{e}.e^{1/y}$$

40. **(d)** $\cos x\, dy = y(\sin x - y)\, dx$

$$\frac{dy}{dx} = y \tan x - y^2 \sec x$$

$$\frac{1}{y^2}\frac{dy}{dx} - \frac{1}{y}\tan x = -\sec x \qquad \text{...(i)}$$

Let $\frac{1}{y} = t \Rightarrow -\frac{1}{y^2}\frac{dy}{dx} = \frac{dt}{dx}$

From equation (i)

$$-\frac{dt}{dx} - t\tan x = -\sec x$$

$$\Rightarrow \frac{dt}{dx} + (\tan x)t = \sec x$$

I.F. $= e^{\int \tan x\, dx} = (e)^{\log|\sec x|} \sec x$

Solution : t(I.F) $= \int$ (I.F) $\sec x\, dx$

$$\Rightarrow \frac{1}{y}\sec x = \tan x + c$$

41. **(b)** $ydx + (x + x^2 y)dy = 0$

$$\Rightarrow \frac{dx}{dy} = -\frac{x}{y} - x^2 \Rightarrow \frac{dx}{dy} + \frac{x}{y} = -x^2,$$

It is Bernoulli form. Divide by x^2

$$x^{-2}\frac{dx}{dy} + x^{-1}\left(\frac{1}{y}\right) = -1.$$

put $x^{-1} = t, -x^{-2}\frac{dx}{dy} = \frac{dt}{dy}$

We get, $-\frac{dt}{dy} + t\left(\frac{1}{y}\right) = -1 \Rightarrow \frac{dt}{dy} - \left(\frac{1}{y}\right)t = 1$

It is linear in t.

Integrating factor $= e^{\int -\frac{1}{y}dy} = e^{-\log y} = y^{-1}$

$\therefore$ Solution is $t(y^{-1}) = \int (y^{-1})dy + C$

$$\Rightarrow \frac{1}{x}.\frac{1}{y} = \log y + C \Rightarrow \log y - \frac{1}{xy} = C$$

42. **(c)** $(1 + y^2) + (x - e^{\tan^{-1} y})\frac{dy}{dx} = 0$

$$\Rightarrow \frac{dx}{dy} + \frac{x}{(1+y^2)} = \frac{e^{\tan^{-1} y}}{(1+y^2)}$$

$$I.F = e^{\int \frac{1}{(1+y^2)}dy} = e^{\tan^{-1} y}$$

$$x(e^{\tan^{-1} y}) = \int \frac{e^{\tan^{-1} y}}{1+y^2} e^{\tan^{-1} y} dy$$

$$x(e^{\tan^{-1} y}) = \frac{e^{2\tan^{-1} y}}{2} + C$$

$$\therefore \; 2xe^{\tan^{-1} y} = e^{2\tan^{-1} y} + k$$

Vector Algebra

TOPIC-1 : Algebra of Vectors, Section Formula, Linear Dependence & Independence of Vectors, Position Vector of a Point, Modulus of a Vector, Collinearity of Three points, Coplanarity of Three Vectors & Four Points, Vector Inequality

1. Let ABC be a triangle whose circumcentre is at P. If the position vectors A, B, C and P are $\vec{a}, \vec{b}, \vec{c}$ and $\frac{\vec{a}+\vec{b}+\vec{c}}{4}$ respectively, then the position vector of the orthocentre of this triangle, is : **[Online April 10, 2016]**
   (a) $-\left(\frac{\vec{a}+\vec{b}+\vec{c}}{2}\right)$ (b) $\vec{a}+\vec{b}+\vec{c}$
   (c) $\left(\frac{\vec{a}+\vec{b}+\vec{c}}{2}\right)$ (d) $\vec{0}$

2. If the vectors $\overrightarrow{AB} = 3\hat{i} + 4\hat{k}$ and $\overrightarrow{AC} = 5\hat{i} - 2\hat{j} + 4\hat{k}$ are the sides of a triangle ABC, then the length of the median through A is **[2013]**
   (a) $\sqrt{18}$ (b) $\sqrt{72}$
   (c) $\sqrt{33}$ (d) $\sqrt{45}$

3. If $\vec{a}$ and $\vec{b}$ are non-collinear vectors, then the value of α for which the vectors $\vec{u} = (\alpha - 2)\vec{a} + \vec{b}$ and $\vec{v} = (2 + 3\alpha)\vec{a} - 3\vec{b}$ are collinear is : **[Online April 23, 2013]**
   (a) $\frac{3}{2}$ (b) $\frac{2}{3}$
   (c) $-\frac{3}{2}$ (d) $-\frac{2}{3}$

4. If $\vec{a} = \hat{i} - 2\hat{j} + 3\hat{k}$, $\vec{b} = 2\hat{i} + 3\hat{j} - \hat{k}$ and $\vec{c} = r\hat{i} + \hat{j} + (2r-1)\hat{k}$ are three vectors such that $\vec{c}$ is parallel to the plane of $\vec{a}$ and $\vec{b}$, then r is equal to **[Online May 19, 2012]**
   (a) 1 (b) -1
   (c) 0 (d) 2

5. Let $\vec{a}, \vec{b}, \vec{c}$ be three non-zero vectors which are pairwise non-collinear. If $\vec{a}+3\vec{b}$ is collinear with $\vec{c}$ and $\vec{b}+2\vec{c}$ is collinear with $\vec{a}$, then $\vec{a}+3\vec{b}+6\vec{c}$ is : **[2011RS]**
   (a) $\vec{a}$ (b) $\vec{c}$
   (c) $\vec{0}$ (d) $\vec{a}+\vec{c}$

6. If the $p\hat{i}+\hat{j}+\hat{k}, \hat{i}+q\hat{j}+\hat{k}$ and $\hat{i}+\hat{j}+r\hat{k}$ $(p \neq q \neq r \neq 1)$ vector are coplanar, then the value of $pqr-(p+q+r)$ is **[2011RS]**
   (a) 2 (b) 0
   (c) -1 (d) -2

7. The vector $\vec{a} = \alpha\hat{i} + 2\hat{j} + \beta\hat{k}$ lies in the plane of the vectors $\vec{b} = \hat{i} + \hat{j}$ and $\vec{c} = \hat{j} + \hat{k}$ and bisects the angle between $\vec{b}$ and $\vec{c}$. Then which one of the following gives possible values of α and β? **[2008]**
   (a) $\alpha = 2, \beta = 2$ (b) $\alpha = 1, \beta = 2$
   (c) $\alpha = 2, \beta = 1$ (d) $\alpha = 1, \beta = 1$

8. *ABC* is a triangle, right angled at *A*. The resultant of the forces acting along $\overline{AB}, \overline{BC}$ with magnitudes $\frac{1}{AB}$ and $\frac{1}{AC}$ respectively is the force along $\overline{AD}$, where *D* is the foot of the perpendicular from *A* onto *BC*. The magnitude of the resultant is **[2006]**
   (a) $\frac{AB^2 + AC^2}{(AB)^2(AC)^2}$ (b) $\frac{(AB)(AC)}{AB + AC}$
   (c) $\frac{1}{AB} + \frac{1}{AC}$ (d) $\frac{1}{AD}$

9. If C is the mid point of AB and P is any point outside AB, then **[2005]**
   (a) $\overrightarrow{PA} + \overrightarrow{PB} = 2\overrightarrow{PC}$
   (b) $\overrightarrow{PA} + \overrightarrow{PB} = \overrightarrow{PC}$
   (c) $\overrightarrow{PA} + \overrightarrow{PB} + 2\overrightarrow{PC} = \vec{0}$
   (d) $\overrightarrow{PA} + \overrightarrow{PB} + \overrightarrow{PC} = \vec{0}$

10. Let a, b and c be distinct non- negative numbers. If the vectors $a\hat{i}+a\hat{j}+c\hat{k}$, $\hat{i}+\hat{k}$ and $c\hat{i}+c\hat{j}+b\hat{k}$ lie in a plane, then c is **[2005]**
(a) the Geometric Mean of a and b
(b) the Arithmetic Mean of a and b
(c) equal to zero
(d) the Harmonic Mean of a and b

11. If $\vec{a}, \vec{b}, \vec{c}$ are non-coplanar vectors and λ is a real number, then the vectors $\bar{a}+2\bar{b}+3\bar{c}$, $\lambda\bar{b}+4\bar{c}$ and $(2\lambda-1)\bar{c}$ are non coplanar for **[2004]**
(a) no value of λ
(b) all except one value of λ
(c) all except two values of λ
(d) all values of λ

12. Let $\vec{a}, \vec{b}$ and $\vec{c}$ be three non-zero vectors such that no two of these are collinear. If the vector $\vec{a}+2\vec{b}$ is collinear with $\vec{c}$ and $\vec{b}+3\vec{c}$ is collinear with $\vec{a}$ (λ being some non-zero scalar) then $\vec{a}+2\vec{b}+6\vec{c}$ equals **[2004]**
(a) 0 (b) $\lambda\vec{b}$
(c) $\lambda\vec{c}$ (d) $\lambda\vec{a}$

13. Consider points A, B, C and D with position vectors $7\hat{i}-4\hat{j}+7\hat{k}, \hat{i}-6\hat{j}+10\hat{k}, -\hat{i}-3\hat{j}+4\hat{k}$ and $5\hat{i}-\hat{j}+5\hat{k}$ respectively. Then ABCD is a **[2003]**
(a) parallelogram but not a rhombus
(b) square
(c) rhombus
(d) rectangle.

14. If $\begin{vmatrix} a & a^2 & 1+a^3 \\ b & b^2 & 1+b^3 \\ c & c^2 & 1+c^3 \end{vmatrix}=0$ and vectors $(1,a,a^2)$, $(1,b,b^2)$ and $(1,c,c^2)$ are non- coplanar, then the product abc equals **[2003]**
(a) 0 (b) 2
(c) –1 (d) 1

15. The vectors $\overrightarrow{AB}=3\hat{i}+4\hat{k}$ & $\overrightarrow{AC}=5\hat{i}-2\hat{j}+4\hat{k}$ are the sides of a triangle ABC. The length of the median through A is **[2003]**
(a) $\sqrt{288}$ (b) $\sqrt{18}$
(c) $\sqrt{72}$ (d) $\sqrt{33}$

TOPIC-2 : Scalar or Dot Product of two Vectors, Projection of a Vector Along any other Vector, Component of a Vector

16. In a triangle ABC, right angled at the vertex A, if the position vectors of A, B and C are respectively $3\hat{i}+\hat{j}-\hat{k}, -\hat{i}+3\hat{j}+p\hat{k}$ and $5\hat{i}+q\hat{j}-4\hat{k}$, then the point (p, q) lies on a line : **[Online April 9, 2016]**
(a) making an obtuse angle with the positive direction of x–axis
(b) parallel to x–axis
(c) parallel to y–axis
(d) making an acute angle with the positive direction of x–axis

17. In a parallelogram ABD, $|\overrightarrow{AB}|=a, |\overrightarrow{AD}|=b$ and $|\overrightarrow{AC}|=c$, then $\overrightarrow{DA}.\overrightarrow{AB}$ has the value : **[Online April 11, 2015]**
(a) $\frac{1}{2}(a^2+b^2+c^2)$ (b) $\frac{1}{2}(a^2-b^2+c^2)$
(c) $\frac{1}{2}(a^2+b^2-c^2)$ (d) $\frac{1}{3}(b^2+c^2-a^2)$

18. If $\hat{x}, \hat{y}$ and $\hat{z}$ are three unit vectors in three-dimensional space, then the minimum value of
$|\hat{x}+\hat{y}|^2+|\hat{y}+\hat{z}|^2+|\hat{z}+\hat{x}|^2$ **[Online April 12, 2014]**
(a) $\frac{3}{2}$ (b) 3
(c) $3\sqrt{3}$ (d) 6

19. If $|\vec{a}|=2, |\vec{b}|=3$ and $|2\vec{a}-\vec{b}|=5$, then $|2\vec{a}+\vec{b}|$ equals: **[Online April 9, 2014]**
(a) 17 (b) 7
(c) 5 (d) 1

20. If $\hat{a}, \hat{b}$ and $\hat{c}$ are unit vectors satisfying $\hat{a}-\sqrt{3}\hat{b}+\hat{c}=\vec{0}$, then the angle between the vectors $\hat{a}$ and $\hat{c}$ is : **[Online April 22, 2013]**
(a) $\frac{\pi}{4}$ (b) $\frac{\pi}{3}$
(c) $\frac{\pi}{6}$ (d) $\frac{\pi}{2}$

21. Let $\vec{a}=2\hat{i}-\hat{j}+\hat{k}, \vec{b}=\hat{i}+2\hat{j}-\hat{k}$ and $\vec{c}=\hat{i}+\hat{j}-2\hat{k}$ be three vectors. A vector of the type $\vec{b}+\lambda\vec{c}$ for some scalar λ, whose projection on $\vec{a}$ is of magnitude $\sqrt{\frac{2}{3}}$ is : **[Online April 9, 2013]**

(a) $2\hat{i}+\hat{j}+5\hat{k}$ (b) $2\hat{i}+3\hat{j}-3\hat{k}$

(c) $2\hat{i}-\hat{j}+5\hat{k}$ (d) $2\hat{i}+3\hat{j}+3\hat{k}$

22. Let $ABCD$ be a parallelogram such that $\overline{AB}=\vec{q}, \overline{AD}=\vec{p}$ and $\angle BAD$ be an acute angle. If $\vec{r}$ is the vector that coincide with the altitude directed from the vertex B to the side AD, then $\vec{r}$ is given by : **[2012]**

(a) $\vec{r}=3\vec{q}-\dfrac{3(\vec{p}.\vec{q})}{(\vec{p}.\vec{p})}\vec{p}$ (b) $\vec{r}=-\vec{q}+\dfrac{(\vec{p}.\vec{q})}{(\vec{p}.\vec{p})}\vec{p}$

(c) $\vec{r}=\vec{q}-\dfrac{(\vec{p}.\vec{q})}{(\vec{p}.\vec{p})}\vec{p}$ (d) $\vec{r}=-3\vec{q}-\dfrac{3(\vec{p}.\vec{q})}{(\vec{p}.\vec{p})}\vec{p}$

23. Let $\vec{a}$ and $\vec{b}$ be two unit vectors. If the vectors $\vec{c}=\hat{a}+2\hat{b}$ and $\vec{d}=5\hat{a}-4\hat{b}$ are perpendicular to each other, then the angle between $\hat{a}$ and $\hat{b}$ is : **[2012]**

(a) $\dfrac{\pi}{6}$ (b) $\dfrac{\pi}{2}$

(c) $\dfrac{\pi}{3}$ (d) $\dfrac{\pi}{4}$

24. If $a+b+c=0$, $\left|\vec{a}\right|=3$, $\left|\vec{b}\right|=5$ and $\left|\vec{c}\right|=7$, then the angle between $\vec{a}$ and $\vec{b}$ is **[Online May 19, 2012]**

(a) $\dfrac{\pi}{3}$ (b) $\dfrac{\pi}{4}$

(c) $\dfrac{\pi}{6}$ (d) $\dfrac{\pi}{2}$

25. A unit vector which is perpendicular to the vector $2\hat{i}-\hat{j}+2\hat{k}$ and is coplanar with the vectors $\hat{i}+\hat{j}-\hat{k}$ and $2\hat{i}+2\hat{j}-\hat{k}$ is **[Online May 12, 2012]**

(a) $\dfrac{2\hat{j}+\hat{k}}{\sqrt{5}}$ (b) $\dfrac{3\hat{i}+2\hat{j}-2\hat{k}}{\sqrt{17}}$

(c) $\dfrac{3\hat{i}+2\hat{j}+2\hat{k}}{\sqrt{17}}$ (d) $\dfrac{2\hat{i}+2\hat{j}-2\hat{k}}{3}$

26. *ABCD* is parallelogram. The position vectors of *A* and *C* are respectively, $3\hat{i}+3\hat{j}+5\hat{k}$ and $\hat{i}-5\hat{j}-5\hat{k}$. If *M* is the midpoint of the diagonal *DB*, then the magnitude of the projection of $\overrightarrow{OM}$ on $\overrightarrow{OC}$, where *O* is the origin, is **[Online May 7, 2012]**

(a) $7\sqrt{51}$ (b) $\dfrac{7}{\sqrt{50}}$

(c) $7\sqrt{50}$ (d) $\dfrac{7}{\sqrt{51}}$

27. If the vectors $\vec{a}=\hat{i}-\hat{j}+2\hat{k}$, $\vec{b}=2\hat{i}+4\hat{j}+\hat{k}$ and $\vec{c}=\lambda\hat{i}+\hat{j}+\mu\hat{k}$ are mutually orthogonal, then $(\lambda,\mu)=$ **[2010]**

(a) $(2,-3)$ (b) $(-2,3)$

(c) $(3,-2)$ (d) $(-3,2)$

28. The non-zero vectors are $\vec{a}$, $\vec{b}$ and $\vec{c}$ are related by $\vec{a}=8\vec{b}$ and $\vec{c}=-7\vec{b}$. Then the angle between $\vec{a}$ and $\vec{c}$ is **[2008]**

(a) 0 (b) $\dfrac{\pi}{4}$

(c) $\dfrac{\pi}{2}$ (d) π

29. The values of a, for which points A, B, C with position vectors $2\hat{i}-\hat{j}+\hat{k}$, $\hat{i}-3\hat{j}-5\hat{k}$ and $a\hat{i}-3\hat{j}+\hat{k}$ respectively are the vertices of a right angled triangle with $C=\dfrac{\pi}{2}$ are **[2006]**

(a) 2 and 1 (b) – 2 and – 1

(c) – 2 and 1 (d) 2 and – 1

30. Let $\bar{u},\bar{v},\bar{w}$ be such that $|\bar{u}|=1, |\bar{v}|=2, |\bar{w}|=3$. If the projection $\bar{v}$ along $\bar{u}$ is equal to that of $\bar{w}$ along $\bar{u}$ and $\bar{v}$, $\bar{w}$ are perpendicular to each other then $|\bar{u}-\bar{v}+\bar{w}|$ equals **[2004]**

(a) 14 (b) $\sqrt{7}$

(c) $\sqrt{14}$ (d) 2

31. $\vec{a},\vec{b},\vec{c}$ are 3 vectors, such that $\vec{a}+\vec{b}+\vec{c}=0$, $|\vec{a}|=1$, $|\vec{b}|=2$, $|\vec{c}|=3$, then $\vec{a}.\vec{b}+\vec{b}.\vec{c}+\vec{c}.\vec{a}$ is equal to **[2003]**

(a) 1 (b) 0

(c) –7 (d) 7

32. If $|\vec{a}|=5$, $|\vec{b}|=4$, $|\vec{c}|=3$ thus what will be the value of $|\vec{a}.\vec{b}+\vec{b}.\vec{c}+\vec{c}.\vec{a}|$, given that $\vec{a}+\vec{b}+\vec{c}=0$ **[2002]**

(a) 25 (b) 50

(c) –25 (d) –50

33. If sdaa $\vec{a},\vec{b},\vec{c}$ are vectors such that $\vec{a}+\vec{b}+\vec{c}=0$ and $|\vec{a}|=7, |\vec{b}|=5, |\vec{c}|=3$ then angle between vector $\vec{b}$ and $\vec{c}$ is **[2002]**

(a) 60° (b) 30°

(c) 45° (d) 90°

TOPIC-3 : Vector or Cross Product of two vectors, Area of a Parallelogram & Triangle, Scalar & Vector Tripple Product

34. Let $\vec{a} = 2\hat{i} + \hat{j} - 2\hat{k}$ and $\vec{b} = \hat{i} + \hat{j}$. Let $\vec{c}$ be a vector such that $|\vec{c} - \vec{a}| = 3$, $\left|(\vec{a} \times \vec{b}) \times \vec{c}\right| = 3$ and the angle between $\vec{c}$ and $\vec{a} \times \vec{b}$ be 30°. Then $\vec{a}.\vec{c}$ is equal to : **[2017]**

(a) $\frac{1}{8}$ (b) $\frac{25}{8}$

(c) 2 (d) 5

35. If the vector $\vec{b} = 3\hat{j} + 4\hat{k}$ is written as the sum of a vector $\vec{b_1}$, parallel to $\vec{a} = \hat{i} + \hat{j}$ and a vector $\vec{b_2}$, perpendicular to $\vec{a}$, then $\vec{b_1} \times \vec{b_2}$ is equal to: **[Online April 9, 2017]**

(a) $-3\hat{i} + 3\hat{j} - 9\hat{k}$ (b) $6\hat{i} - 6\hat{j} + \frac{9}{2}\hat{k}$

(c) $-6\hat{i} + 6\hat{j} - \frac{9}{2}\hat{k}$ (d) $3\hat{i} - 3\hat{j} + 9\hat{k}$

36. The area (in sq. units) of the parallelogram whose diagonals are along the vectors $8\hat{i} - 6\hat{j}$ and $3\hat{i} + 4\hat{j} - 12\hat{k}$, is : **[Online April 8, 2017]**

(a) 26 (b) 65

(c) 20 (d) 52

37. Let $\vec{a}, \vec{b}$ and $\vec{c}$ be three unit vectors such that $\vec{a} \times \left(\vec{b} \times \vec{c}\right) = \frac{\sqrt{3}}{2}\left(\vec{b} + \vec{c}\right)$. If $\vec{b}$ is not parallel to $\vec{c}$, then the angle between $\vec{a}$ and $\vec{b}$ is: **[2016]**

(a) $\frac{2\pi}{3}$ (b) $\frac{5\pi}{6}$

(c) $\frac{3\pi}{4}$ (d) $\frac{\pi}{2}$

38. Let $\vec{a}, \vec{b}$ and $\vec{c}$ be three non-zero vectors such that no two of them are collinear and $(\vec{a} \times \vec{b}) \times \vec{c} = \frac{1}{3}|\vec{b}||\vec{c}|\vec{a}$. If θ is the angle between vectors $\vec{b}$ and $\vec{c}$, then a value of sin θ is : **[2015]**

(a) $\frac{2}{3}$ (b) $\frac{-2\sqrt{3}}{3}$

(c) $\frac{2\sqrt{2}}{3}$ (d) $\frac{-\sqrt{2}}{3}$

39. Let $\vec{a}$ and $\vec{b}$ be two unit vectors such that $\left|\vec{a} + \vec{b}\right| = \sqrt{3}$. If $\vec{c} = \vec{a} + 2\vec{b} + 3\left(\vec{a} \times \vec{b}\right)$, then $2\left|\vec{c}\right|$ is equal to : **[Online April 10, 2015]**

(a) $\sqrt{55}$ (b) $\sqrt{37}$

(c) $\sqrt{51}$ (d) $\sqrt{43}$

40. If $\left[\vec{a}\times\vec{b}\ \ \vec{b}\times\vec{c}\ \ \vec{c}\times\vec{a}\right] = \lambda\left[\vec{a}\,\vec{b}\,\vec{c}\right]^2$ then λ is equal to **[2014]**

(a) 0 (b) 1

(c) 2 (d) 3

41. If $\vec{x} = 3\hat{i} - 6\hat{j} - \hat{k}$, $\vec{y} = \hat{i} + 4\hat{j} - 3\hat{k}$ and $\vec{z} = 3\hat{i} - 4\hat{j} - 12\hat{k}$, then the magnitude of the projection of $\vec{x} \times \vec{y}$ on $\vec{z}$ is: **[Online April 19, 2014]**

(a) 12 (b) 15

(c) 14 (d) 13

42. If $|\vec{c}|^2 = 60$ and $\vec{c} \times \left(\hat{i} + 2\hat{j} + 5\hat{k}\right) = \vec{0}$, then a value of $\vec{c}.\left(-7\hat{i} + 2\hat{j} + 3\hat{k}\right)$ is: **[Online April 11, 2014]**

(a) $4\sqrt{2}$ (b) 12

(c) 24 (d) $12\sqrt{2}$

43. Let $\vec{a} = 2\hat{i} + \hat{j} - 2\hat{k}, \vec{b} = \hat{i} + \hat{j}$. If $\vec{c}$ is a vector such that $\vec{a} \bullet \vec{c} = |\vec{c}|, |\vec{c} - \vec{a}| = 2\sqrt{2}$ and the angle between $\vec{a} \times \vec{b}$ and $\vec{c}$ is 30°, then $|(\vec{a} \times \vec{b}) \times \vec{c}|$ equals: **[Online April 25, 2013]**

(a) $\frac{1}{2}$ (b) $\frac{3\sqrt{3}}{2}$

(c) 3 (d) $\frac{3}{2}$

44. The vector $\left(\hat{i} \times \vec{a}.\vec{b}\right)\hat{i} + \left(\hat{j} \times \vec{a}.\vec{b}\right)\hat{j} + \left(\hat{k} \times \vec{a}.\vec{b}\right)\hat{k}$ is equal to : **[Online April 9, 2013]**

(a) $\vec{b} \times \vec{a}$ (b) $\vec{a}$

(c) $\vec{a} \times \vec{b}$ (d) $\vec{b}$

45. **Statement 1:** The vectors $\vec{a}, \vec{b}$ and $\vec{c}$ lie in the same plane if and only if $\vec{a}.\left(\vec{b} \times \vec{c}\right) = 0$

Statement 2: The vectors $\vec{u}$ and $\vec{v}$ are perpendicular if and only if $\vec{u}.\vec{v} = 0$ where $\vec{u} \times \vec{v}$ is a vector perpendicular to the plane of $\vec{u}$ and $\vec{v}$. **[Online May 26, 2012]**

(a) Statement 1 is false, Statement 2 is true.

(b) Statement 1 is true, Statement 2 is true, Statement 2 is correct explanation for Statement 1.

(c) Statement 1 is true, Statement 2 is false.

(d) Statement 1 is true, Statement 2 is true, , Statement 2 is not a correct explanation for Statement 1.

46. If $\vec{u}=\hat{j}+4\hat{k}$, $\vec{v}=\hat{i}+3\hat{k}$ and $\vec{w}=\cos\theta\hat{i}+\sin\theta\hat{j}$ are vectors in 3-dimensional space, then the maximum possible value of $|\vec{u}\times\vec{v}.\vec{w}|$ is **[Online May 12, 2012]**
(a) $\sqrt{3}$ (b) 5
(c) $\sqrt{14}$ (d) 7

47. **Statement 1:** If the points (1, 2, 2), (2, 1, 2) and (2, 2, *z*) and (1, 1, 1) are coplanar, then *z* = 2.
Statement 2: If the 4 points *P*, *Q*, *R* and *S* are coplanar, then the volume of the tetrahedron *PQRS* is 0.
[Online May 12, 2012]
(a) Statement 1 is false,, Statement 2 is true.
(b) Statement 1 is true, Statement 2 is false.
(c) Statement 1 is true, Statement 2 is true, Statement 2 is a correct explanation of Statement 1.
(d) Statement 1 is true, Statement 2 is true, Statement 2 is not a correct explanation of Statement 1.

48. If $\vec{a}=\hat{i}-2\hat{j}+3\hat{k}$, $\vec{b}=2\hat{i}+3\hat{j}-\hat{k}$ and $\vec{c}=\lambda\hat{i}+\hat{j}+(2\lambda-1)\hat{k}$ are coplanar vectors, then λ is equal to **[Online May 7, 2012]**
(a) 0 (b) -1
(c) 2 (d) 1

49. The vectors $\vec{a}$ and $\vec{b}$ are not perpendicular and $\vec{c}$ and $\vec{d}$ are two vectors satisfying $\vec{b}\times\vec{c}=\vec{b}\times\vec{d}$ and $\vec{a}.\vec{d}=0$. Then the vector $\vec{d}$ is equal to **[2011]**
(a) $\vec{c}+\left(\frac{\vec{a}.\vec{c}}{\vec{a}.\vec{b}}\right)\vec{b}$ (b) $\vec{b}+\left(\frac{\vec{b}.\vec{c}}{\vec{a}.\vec{b}}\right)\vec{c}$
(c) $\vec{c}-\left(\frac{\vec{a}.\vec{c}}{\vec{a}.\vec{b}}\right)\vec{b}$ (d) $\vec{b}-\left(\frac{\vec{b}.\vec{c}}{\vec{a}.\vec{b}}\right)\vec{c}$

50. If $\vec{a}=\frac{1}{\sqrt{10}}(3\hat{i}+\hat{k})$ and $\vec{b}=\frac{1}{7}(2\hat{i}+3\hat{j}-6\hat{k})$, then the value of $(2\vec{a}-\vec{b})\left[(\vec{a}\times\vec{b})\times(\vec{a}+2\vec{b})\right]$ is **[2011]**
(a) -3 (b) 5
(c) 3 (d) -5

51. Let $\vec{a}=\hat{j}-\hat{k}$ and $\vec{c}=\hat{i}-\hat{j}-\hat{k}$. Then the vector $\vec{b}$ satisfying $\vec{a}\times\vec{b}+\vec{c}=\vec{0}$ and $\vec{a}.\vec{b}=3$ is **[2010]**
(a) $2\hat{i}-\hat{j}+2\hat{k}$ (b) $\hat{i}-\hat{j}-2\hat{k}$
(c) $\hat{i}+\hat{j}-2\hat{k}$ (d) $-\hat{i}+\hat{j}-2\hat{k}$

52. If $\vec{u},\vec{v},\vec{w}$ are non-coplanar vectors and *p*, *q* are real numbers, then the equality
$[3\vec{u}\ p\vec{v}\ p\vec{\omega}]-[p\vec{v}\ \vec{\omega}\ q\vec{u}]-[2\vec{\omega}\ q\vec{v}\ q\vec{u}]=0$
holds for : **[2009]**
(a) exactly two values of (p, q)
(b) more than two but not all values of (p, q)
(c) all values of (p, q)
(d) exactly one value of (p, q)

53. Let $\vec{a}=\hat{i}+\hat{j}+\hat{k}$, $\vec{b}=\hat{i}-\hat{j}+2\hat{k}$ and $\vec{c}=x\hat{i}+(x-2)\hat{j}-\hat{k}$. If the vector $\vec{c}$ lies in the plane of $\vec{a}$ and $\vec{b}$, then *x* equals **[2007]**
(a) -4 (b) -2
(c) 0 (d) 1.

54. If $\hat{u}$ and $\hat{v}$ are unit vectors and θ is the acute angle between them, then $2\hat{u}\times3\hat{v}$ is a unit vector for **[2007]**
(a) no value of θ
(b) exactly one value of θ
(c) exactly two values of θ
(d) more than two values of θ

55. If $(\vec{a}\times\vec{b})\times\vec{c}=\vec{a}\times(\vec{b}\times\vec{c})$ where $\vec{a},\vec{b}$ and $\vec{c}$ are any three vectors such that $\vec{a}.\vec{b}\neq0$, $\vec{b}.\vec{c}\neq0$ then $\vec{a}$ and $\vec{c}$ are **[2006]**
(a) inclined at an angle of $\frac{\pi}{3}$ between them
(b) inclined at an angle of $\frac{\pi}{6}$ between them
(c) perpendicular
(d) parallel

56. Let $\vec{a}=\hat{i}-\hat{k}$, $\vec{b}=x\hat{i}+\hat{j}+(1-x)\hat{k}$ and $\vec{c}=y\hat{i}+x\hat{j}+(1+x-y)\hat{k}$. Then $[\vec{a},\vec{b},\vec{c}]$ depends on **[2005]**
(a) only y (b) only x
(c) both x and y (d) neither x nor y

57. If $\vec{a},\vec{b},\vec{c}$ are non coplanar vectors and λ is a real number then **[2005]**
$[\lambda(\vec{a}+\vec{b})\ \lambda^2\vec{b}\ \lambda\vec{c}]=[\vec{a}\ \ \vec{b}+\vec{c}\ \ \vec{b}]$ for
(a) exactly one value of λ
(b) no value of λ
(c) exactly three values of λ
(d) exactly two values of λ

58. For any vector $\vec{a}$, the value of $(\vec{a}\times\hat{i})^2+(\vec{a}\times\hat{j})^2+(\vec{a}\times\hat{k})^2$ is equal to **[2005]**
(a) $3\vec{a}^2$ (b) $\vec{a}^2$
(c) $2\vec{a}^2$ (d) $4\vec{a}^2$

59. Let $\vec{a},\vec{b}$ and $\vec{c}$ be non-zero vectors such that $(\vec{a}\times\vec{b})\times\vec{c}=\frac{1}{3}|\vec{b}||\vec{c}|\vec{a}$. If θ is the acute angle between the vectors $\vec{b}$ and $\vec{c}$, then $\sin\theta$ equals **[2004]**

(a) $\frac{2\sqrt{2}}{3}$ (b) $\frac{\sqrt{2}}{3}$

(c) $\frac{2}{3}$ (d) $\frac{1}{3}$

60. If $\vec{u}, \vec{v}$ *and* $\vec{w}$ are three non- coplanar vectors, then $(\vec{u}+\vec{v}-\vec{w}).(\vec{u}-\vec{v})\times(\vec{v}-\vec{w})$ equals **[2003]**

(a) $3\vec{u}.\vec{v}\times\vec{w}$ (b) 0

(c) $\vec{u}.(\vec{v}\times\vec{w})$ (d) $\vec{u}.\vec{w}\times\vec{v}$.

61. A tetrahedron has vertices at O(0, 0, 0), A(1, 2, 1) B(2, 1, 3) and C(-1, 1, 2). Then the angle between the faces OAB and ABC will be **[2003]**

(a) 90° (b) $\cos^{-1}\left(\frac{19}{35}\right)$

(c) $\cos^{-1}\left(\frac{17}{31}\right)$ (d) 30°

62. Let $\vec{u}=\hat{i}+\hat{j}$, $\vec{v}=\hat{i}-\hat{j}$ and $\vec{w}=\hat{i}+2\hat{j}+3\hat{k}$. If $\hat{n}$ is a unit vector such that $\vec{u}.\hat{n}=0$ and $\vec{v}.\hat{n}=0$, then $|\vec{w}.\hat{n}|$ is equal to **[2003]**

(a) 3 (b) 0

(c) 1 (d) 2.

63. If $\vec{a}\times\vec{b}=\vec{b}\times\vec{c}=\vec{c}\times\vec{a}$ then $\vec{a}+\vec{b}+\vec{c}=$ **[2002]**

(a) abc (b) –1

(c) 0 (d) 2

64. $\vec{a}=3\hat{i}-5\hat{j}$ and $\vec{b}=6\hat{i}+3\hat{j}$ are two vectors and $\vec{c}$ is a vector such that $\vec{c}=\vec{a}\times\vec{b}$ then $|\vec{a}|:|\vec{b}|:|\vec{c}|$ **[2002]**

(a) $\sqrt{34}:\sqrt{45}:\sqrt{39}$ (b) $\sqrt{34}:\sqrt{45}:39$

(c) $34:39:45$ (d) $39:35:34$

65. If the vectors $\vec{c}$, $\vec{a}=x\hat{i}+y\hat{j}+z\hat{k}$ and $\hat{b}=\hat{j}$ are such that $\vec{a}$, $\vec{c}$ and $\vec{b}$ form a right handed system then $\vec{c}$ is: **[2002]**

(a) $z\hat{i}-x\hat{k}$ (b) $\vec{0}$

(c) $y\hat{j}$ (d) $-z\hat{i}+x\hat{k}$

66. If $\vec{a}, \vec{b}, \vec{c}$ are vectors such that $[\vec{a}\,\vec{b}\,\vec{c}]=4$ then $[\vec{a}\times\vec{b}\;\;\vec{b}\times\vec{c}\;\;\vec{c}\times\vec{a}]=$ **[2002]**

(a) 16 (b) 64

(c) 4 (d) 8

67. If $|\vec{a}|=4, |\vec{b}|=2$ and the angle between $\vec{a}$ and $\vec{b}$ is $\pi/6$ then $(\vec{a}\times\vec{b})^2$ is equal to **[2002]**

(a) 48 (b) 16

(c) $\vec{a}$ (d) none of these

TOPIC-4 : Scalar Product of Four Vectors, Reciprocal System of Vector, Application of Vectors in Mechanics

68. A particle just clears a wall of height b at a distance a and strikes the ground at a distance c from the point of projection. The angle of projection is **[2007]**

(a) $\tan^{-1}\frac{bc}{a(c-a)}$ (b) $\tan^{-1}\frac{bc}{a}$

(c) $\tan^{-1}\frac{b}{ac}$ (d) 45°.

69. A body weighing 13 kg is suspended by two strings 5m and 12m long, their other ends being fastened to the extremities of a rod 13m long. If the rod be so held that the body hangs immediately below the middle point, then tensions in the strings are **[2007]**

(a) 5 kg and 12 kg (b) 5 kg and 13 kg

(c) 12 kg and 13 kg (d) 5 kg and 5 kg

70. The resultant of two forces Pn and 3n is a force of 7n. If the direction of 3n force were reversed, the resultant would be $\sqrt{19}\,n$. The value of P is **[2007]**

(a) 3 n (b) 4 n

(c) 5 n (d) 6 n.

71. A body falling from rest under gravity passes a certain point P. It was at a distance of 400 m from P, 4s prior to passing through P. If $g=10m/s^2$, then the height above the point P from where the body began to fall is **[2006]**

(a) 720m (b) 900m

(c) 320m (d) 680m

72. A particle has two velocities of equal magnitude inclined to each other at an angle θ. If one of them is halved, the angle between the other and the original resultant velocity is bisected by the new resultant. Then θ is **[2006]**

(a) 90° (b) 120°

(c) 45° (d) 60°

73. The resultant R of two forces acting on a particle is at right angles to one of them and its magnitude is one third of the other force. The ratio of larger force to smaller one is: **[2005]**

(a) $2:1$ (b) $3:\sqrt{2}$

(c) $3:2$ (d) $3:2\sqrt{2}$

74. A and B are two like parallel forces. A couple of moment H lies in the plane of A and B and is contained with them. The resultant of A and B after combining is displaced through a distance **[2005]**

(a) $\frac{2H}{A-B}$ (b) $\frac{H}{A+B}$

(c) $\frac{H}{2(A+B)}$ (d) $\frac{H}{A-B}$

75. A particle is projected from a point O with velocity u at an angle of 60° with the horizontal. When it is moving in a direction at right angles to its direction at O, its velocity then is given by **[2005]**

(a) $\frac{u}{3}$ (b) $\frac{u}{2}$

(c) $\frac{2u}{3}$ (d) $\frac{u}{\sqrt{3}}$

76. If t_1 and t_2 are the times of flight of two particles having the same initial velocity u and range R on the horizontal, then $t_1^2 + t_2^2$ is equal to **[2004]**

(a) 1 (b) $4u^2/g^2$

(c) $u^2/2g$ (d) u^2/g

77. A velocity $\frac{1}{4}$m/s is resolved into two components along OA and OB making angles 30° and 45° respectively with the given velocity. Then the component along OB is **[2004]**

(a) $\frac{1}{8}(\sqrt{6}-\sqrt{2})$m/s (b) $\frac{1}{4}(\sqrt{3}-1)$ m/s

(c) $\frac{1}{4}$m/s (d) $\frac{1}{8}$m/s

78. A paticle moves towards east from a point A to a point B at the rate of 4 km/h and then towards north from B to C at the rate of 5km/hr. If AB = 12 km and BC = 5 km, then its average speed for its journey from A to C and resultant average velocity direct from A to C are respectively **[2004]**

(a) $\frac{13}{9}$km/h and $\frac{17}{9}$km/h

(b) $\frac{13}{4}$km/h and $\frac{17}{4}$km/h

(c) $\frac{17}{9}$km/h and $\frac{13}{9}$km/h

(d) $\frac{17}{4}$km/h and $\frac{13}{4}$km/h

79. Three forces $\vec{P}, \vec{Q}$ and $\vec{R}$ acting along IA, IB and IC, where I is the incentre of a ΔABC are in equilibrium. Then $\vec{P}:\vec{Q}:\vec{R}$ is **[2004]**

(a) $\operatorname{cosec}\frac{A}{2} : \operatorname{cosec}\frac{B}{2} : \operatorname{cosec}\frac{C}{2}$

(b) $\sin\frac{A}{2} : \sin\frac{B}{2} : \sin\frac{C}{2}$

(c) $\sec\frac{A}{2} : \sec\frac{B}{2} : \sec\frac{C}{2}$

(d) $\cos\frac{A}{2} : \cos\frac{B}{2} : \cos\frac{C}{2}$

80. In a right angle ΔABC, $\angle A = 90°$ and sides a, b, c are respectively, 5 cm, 4 cm and 3 cm. If a force $\vec{F}$ has moments 0, 9 and 16 in N cm. units respectively about vertices A, B and C, then magnitude of $\vec{F}$ is **[2004]**

(a) 9 (b) 4

(c) 5 (d) 3

81. With two forces acting at point, the maximum affect is obtained when their resultant is 4N. If they act at right angles, then their resultant is 3N. Then the forces are **[2004]**

(a) $\left(2+\frac{1}{2}\sqrt{3}\right)N$ and $\left(2-\frac{1}{2}\sqrt{3}\right)N$

(b) $\left(2+\sqrt{3}\right)N$ and $\left(2-\sqrt{3}\right)N$

(c) $\left(2+\frac{1}{2}\sqrt{2}\right)N$ and $\left(2-\frac{1}{2}\sqrt{2}\right)N$

(d) $\left(2+\sqrt{2}\right)N$ and $\left(2-\sqrt{2}\right)N$

82. A particle is acted upon by constant forces $4\hat{i}+\hat{j}-3\hat{k}$ and $3\hat{i}+\hat{j}-\hat{k}$ which displace it from a point $\hat{i}+2\hat{j}+3\hat{k}$ to the point $5\hat{i}+4\hat{j}+\hat{k}$. The work done in standard units by the forces is given by **[2004]**

(a) 15 (b) 30

(c) 25 (d) 40

83. Let R_1 and R_2 respectively be the maximum ranges up and down an inclined plane and R be the maximum range on the horizontal plane. Then R_1, R, R_2 are in **[2003]**

(a) H.P (b) A.G.P

(c) A.P (d) G.P.

84. Two particles start simultaneously from the same point and move along two straight lines, one with uniform velocity $\vec{u}$ and the other from rest with uniform acceleration $\vec{f}$. Let α be the angle between their directions of motion. The relative velocity of the second particle w.r.t. the first is least after a time **[2003]**

(a) $\frac{u\cos\alpha}{f}$ (b) $\frac{u\sin\alpha}{f}$

(c) $\frac{f\cos\alpha}{u}$ (d) $u\sin\alpha$

85. Two stones are projected from the top of a cliff h metres high, with the same speed u, so as to hit the ground at the same spot. If one of the stones is projected horizontally and the other is projected horizontally and the other is projected at an angle θ to the horizontal then $\tan\theta$ equals **[2003]**

(a) $u\sqrt{\frac{2}{gh}}$ (b) $\sqrt{\frac{2u}{gh}}$

(c) $2g\sqrt{\frac{u}{h}}$ (d) $2h\sqrt{\frac{u}{g}}$

86. A body travels a distance s in t seconds. It starts from rest and ends at rest. In the first part of the journey, it moves with constant acceleration f and in the second part with constant retardation r. The value of t is given by **[2003]**

(a) $\sqrt{2s\left(\frac{1}{f}+\frac{1}{r}\right)}$ (b) $2s\left(\frac{1}{f}+\frac{1}{r}\right)$

(c) $\frac{2s}{\frac{1}{f}+\frac{1}{r}}$ (d) $\sqrt{2s(f+r)}$

87. The resultant of forces $\vec{P}$ and $\vec{Q}$ is $\vec{R}$. If $\vec{Q}$ is doubled then $\vec{R}$ is doubled. If the direction of $\vec{Q}$ is reversed,then $\vec{R}$ is again doubled. Then $P^2 : Q^2 : R^2$ is **[2003]**

(a) 2 : 3 : 1 (b) 3 : 1 : 1
(c) 2 : 3 : 2 (d) 1 : 2 : 3.

88. A couple is of moment $\vec{G}$ and the force forming the couple is $\vec{P}$. If $\vec{P}$ is turned through a right angle the moment of the couple thus formed is $\vec{H}$. If instead, the force $\vec{P}$ are turned through an angle α, then the moment of couple becomes **[2003]**

(a) $\vec{H}\sin\alpha - \vec{G}\cos\alpha$ (b) $\vec{G}\sin\alpha - \vec{H}\cos\alpha$

(c) $\vec{H}\sin\alpha + \vec{G}\cos\alpha$ (d) $\vec{G}\sin\alpha + \vec{H}\cos\alpha$.

89. A particle acted on by constant forces $4\hat{i}+\hat{j}-3\hat{k}$ and $3\hat{i}+\hat{j}-\hat{k}$ is displaced from the point $\hat{i}+2\hat{j}-3\hat{k}$ to the point $5\hat{i}+4\hat{j}+\hat{k}$. The total work done by the forces is **[2003]**

(a) 50 units (b) 20 units
(c) 30 units (d) 40 units.

90. A bead of weight w can slide on smooth circular wire in a vertical plane. The bead is attached by a light thread to the highest point of the wire and in equilibrium, the thread is taut and make an angle θ with the vertical then tension of the thread and reaction of the wire on the bead are **[2002]**

(a) $T = w\cos\theta$ $R = w\tan\theta$
(b) $T = 2w\cos\theta$ $R = w$
(c) $T = w$ $R = w\sin\theta$
(d) $T = w\sin\theta$ $R = w\cot\theta$

91. The sum of two forces is 18 N and resultant whose direction is at right angles to the smaller force is 12 N. The magnitude of the two forces are **[2002]**

(a) 13, 5 (b) 12, 6
(c) 14, 4 (d) 11, 7

Hints & Solutions

1. **(c)** Position vector of centriod $\vec{G} = \frac{\vec{a}+\vec{b}+\vec{c}}{3}$

Position vector of circum centre $\vec{C} = \frac{\vec{a}+\vec{b}+\vec{c}}{4}$

$\vec{G} = \frac{2\vec{C}+\vec{r}}{3}$

$3\vec{G} = 2\vec{C}+\vec{r}$

$\vec{r} = 3\vec{G} - 2\vec{C} = (\vec{a}+\vec{b}+\vec{c}) - 2\left(\frac{\vec{a}+\vec{b}+\vec{c}}{4}\right)$

$= \frac{\vec{a}+\vec{b}+\vec{c}}{2}$

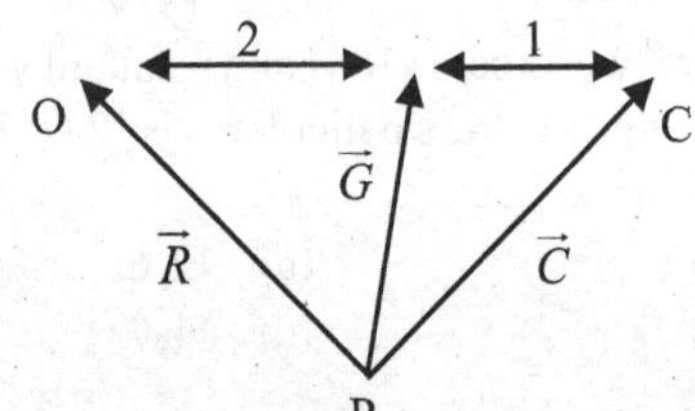

2. **(c)** We have,

$\overrightarrow{AB} + \overrightarrow{BC} + \overrightarrow{CA} = 0$

$\Rightarrow \overrightarrow{BC} = \overrightarrow{AC} - \overrightarrow{AB}$

Now, $\overrightarrow{BM} = \frac{\overrightarrow{AC} - \overrightarrow{AB}}{2} \quad \left(\because \quad \overrightarrow{BM} = \frac{\overrightarrow{BC}}{2}\right)$

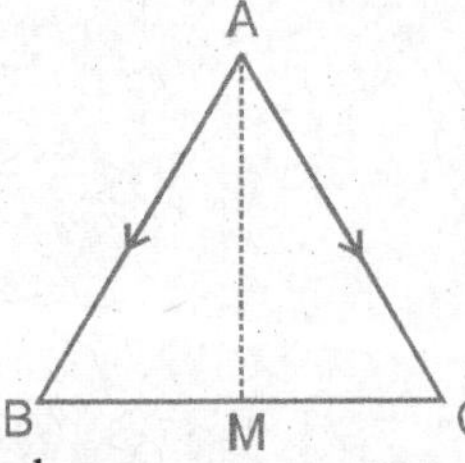

Also, we have

$\overrightarrow{AB} + \overrightarrow{BM} + \overrightarrow{MA} = 0$

$\Rightarrow \overrightarrow{AB} + \frac{\overrightarrow{AC} - \overrightarrow{AB}}{2} = \overrightarrow{AM}$

$\Rightarrow \overrightarrow{AM} = \frac{\overrightarrow{AB} + \overrightarrow{AC}}{2} = 4\hat{i} - \hat{j} + 4\hat{k}$

$\Rightarrow |\overrightarrow{AM}| = \sqrt{33}$

3. **(b)** Since, $\vec{u}$ and $\vec{v}$ are collinear, therefore $k\vec{u} + \vec{v} = 0$

$\Rightarrow [k(\alpha-2)+2+3\alpha]\,\vec{a} + (k-3)\,\vec{b} = 0$ ...(i)

Since $\vec{a}$ and $\vec{b}$ are non-collinear, then for some constant m and n,

$m\vec{a} + n\vec{b} = 0 \Rightarrow m = 0, n = 0$

Hence from equation (i)

$k - 3 = 0 \Rightarrow k = 3$

And $k(\alpha-2)+2+3\alpha = 0$

$\Rightarrow 3(\alpha-2)+2+3\alpha = 0 \Rightarrow \alpha = \frac{2}{3}$

4. **(c)** Let $\vec{a} = \hat{i} - 2\hat{j} + 3\hat{k}$, and $\vec{c} = r\hat{i} + \hat{j} + (2r-1)\hat{k}$

Since, $\vec{c}$ is parallel to the plane of $\vec{a}$ and $\vec{b}$ therefore,

$\vec{a}, \vec{b}$ and $\vec{c}$ are coplanar.

$\therefore \begin{vmatrix} 1 & -2 & 3 \\ 2 & 3 & -1 \\ r & 1 & 2r-1 \end{vmatrix} = 0$

$\Rightarrow 1\,(6r - 3 + 1) + 2\,(4r - 2 + r) + 3\,(2 - 3r) = 0$

$\Rightarrow 6r - 2 + 10r - 4 + 6 - 9r = 0$

$\Rightarrow r = 0$

5. **(c)** $\vec{a} + 3\vec{b} = \lambda\vec{c}$ ....(i)

$\vec{b} + 2\vec{c} = \mu\vec{a}$ ....(ii)

On solving equation (i) and (ii)

$(1+3\mu)\vec{a} - (\lambda+6)\vec{c} = 0$

As $\vec{a}$ and $\vec{c}$ are non collinear,

$\therefore \quad 1 + 3\mu = 0$ and $\lambda + 6 = 0$

From (i), $\vec{a} + 3\vec{b} + 6\vec{c} = \vec{0}$

6. **(d)** The given vectors are collinear if

$\begin{vmatrix} p & 1 & 1 \\ 1 & q & 1 \\ 1 & 1 & r \end{vmatrix} = 0$

$\Rightarrow \quad p(qr-1) + 1(1-r) + 1(1-q) = 0$

$\Rightarrow \quad pqr - p + 1 - r + 1 - q = 0$

$\Rightarrow \quad pqr - (p+q+r) = -2$

7. **(d)** $\because$ $\vec{a}$ lies in the plane of $\vec{b}$ and $\vec{c}$

$\therefore \quad \vec{a} = \vec{b} + \lambda\vec{c}$

$\Rightarrow \alpha\hat{i} + 2\hat{j} + \beta\hat{k} = \hat{i} + \hat{j} + \lambda(\hat{j} + \hat{k})$

$\Rightarrow \alpha = 1, 2 = 1 + \lambda, \beta = \lambda \Rightarrow \alpha = 1, \beta = 1$

ALTERNATE SOLUTION

$\because$ $\vec{a}$ bisects the angle between $\vec{b}$ and $\vec{c}$.

$\therefore$ $\vec{a} = \lambda(\hat{b} + \hat{c})$

$\Rightarrow \alpha\hat{i} + 2\hat{j} + \beta\hat{k} = \dfrac{\lambda(\hat{i} + 2\hat{j} + \hat{k})}{\sqrt{2}}$

$\Rightarrow \alpha = \dfrac{\lambda}{\sqrt{2}}, \lambda = \sqrt{2}, \beta = \dfrac{\lambda}{\sqrt{2}}$

$\Rightarrow \alpha = \beta = 1$

8. (d) If we consider unit vectors $\hat{i}$ and $\hat{j}$ in the direction AB and AC respectively, then as per quesiton, forces along AB and AC respectively are

$\left(\dfrac{1}{AB}\right)\hat{i}$ and $\left(\dfrac{1}{AC}\right)\hat{j}$

$\therefore$ Their resultant along AD

$= \left(\dfrac{1}{AB}\right)i + \left(\dfrac{1}{AC}\right)j$

$\therefore$ Magnitude of resultant is

$= \sqrt{\left(\dfrac{1}{AB}\right)^2 + \left(\dfrac{1}{AC}\right)^2} = \sqrt{\dfrac{AC^2 + AB^2}{AB^2 \times AC^2}}$

$= \dfrac{BC}{AB \times AC}$

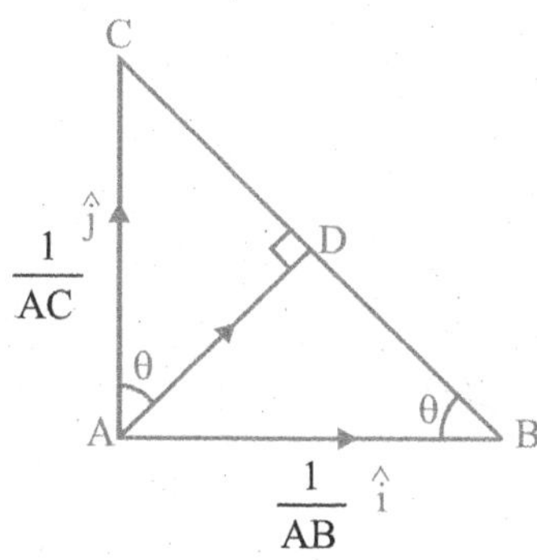

But from figure $\Delta ABC \sim \Delta DBA$

$\Rightarrow \dfrac{BC}{AB} = \dfrac{AC}{AD} \Rightarrow \dfrac{BC}{AB \times AC} = \dfrac{1}{AD}$

$\therefore$ The required magnitude of resultant becomes $\dfrac{1}{AD}$.

9. (a) $\overrightarrow{PA} + \overrightarrow{AP} = 0$ and $\overrightarrow{PC} + \overrightarrow{CP} = 0$

$\Rightarrow \quad \overrightarrow{PA} + \overrightarrow{AC} + \overrightarrow{CP} = 0$ and $\overrightarrow{PB} + \overrightarrow{BC} + \overrightarrow{CP} = 0$

Adding, we get $\overrightarrow{PA} + \overrightarrow{PB} + \overrightarrow{AC} + \overrightarrow{BC} + 2\overrightarrow{CP} = 0$.

Since $\overrightarrow{AC} = -\overrightarrow{BC}$ & $\overrightarrow{CP} = -\overrightarrow{PC}$

$\Rightarrow \quad \overrightarrow{PA} + \overrightarrow{PB} - 2\overrightarrow{PC} = 0.$

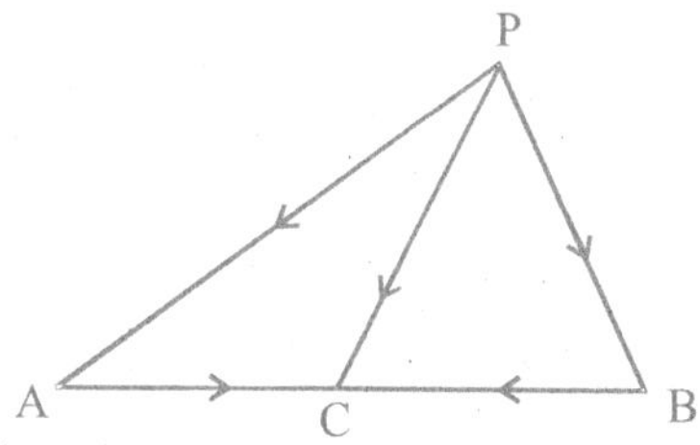

10. (a) Vector $a\vec{i} + a\vec{j} + c\vec{k}$, $\vec{i} + \vec{k}$ and $c\vec{i} + c\vec{j} + b\vec{k}$ are coplanar

$\begin{vmatrix} a & a & c \\ 1 & 0 & 1 \\ c & c & b \end{vmatrix} = 0 \Rightarrow c^2 = ab \Rightarrow c = \sqrt{ab}$

$\therefore$ c is G.M. of a and b.

11. (c) Vectors $\vec{a} + 2\vec{b} + 3\vec{c}, \lambda\vec{b} + 4\vec{c}$, and $(2\lambda - 1)\vec{c}$ are

coplanar if $\begin{vmatrix} 1 & 2 & 3 \\ 0 & \lambda & 4 \\ 0 & 0 & 2\lambda - 1 \end{vmatrix} = 0$

$\Rightarrow \lambda(2\lambda - 1) = 0 \Rightarrow \lambda = 0$ or $\dfrac{1}{2}$

$\therefore$ Forces are noncoplanar for all λ, except $\lambda = 0, \dfrac{1}{2}$

12. (c) Let $\vec{a} + 2\vec{b} = t\vec{c}$ and $\vec{b} + 3\vec{c} = s\vec{a}$, where t and s are scalars. Adding, we get

$\vec{a} + 3\vec{b} + 3\vec{c} = t\vec{c} + s\vec{a}$

$\Rightarrow \vec{a} + 2\vec{b} + 6\vec{c} = t\vec{c} + s\vec{a} - \vec{b} + 3\vec{c}$

$= t\vec{c} + (\vec{b} + 3\vec{c}) - \vec{b} + 3\vec{c} = (t + 6)\vec{c}$

$\left[\text{using } s\,\vec{a} = \vec{b} + 3\vec{c}\right]$

$= \lambda\vec{c}$, where $\lambda = t + 6$

13. (none)

$A = (7, -4, 7), B = (1, -6, 10), C = (-1, -3, 4)$ and $D = (5, -1, 5)$

$AB = \sqrt{(7-1)^2 + (-4+6)^2 + (7-10)^2}$

$= \sqrt{36 + 4 + 9} = 7$

Similarly $BC = 7$, $CD = \sqrt{41}$, $DA = \sqrt{17}$

$\therefore$ None of the options is satisfied

14. (c) $\begin{vmatrix} a & a^2 & 1+a^3 \\ b & b^2 & 1+b^3 \\ c & c^2 & 1+c^3 \end{vmatrix} = 0$

$\Rightarrow \begin{vmatrix} a & a^2 & 1 \\ b & b^2 & 1 \\ c & c^2 & 1 \end{vmatrix} + \begin{vmatrix} a & a^2 & a^3 \\ b & b^2 & b^3 \\ c & c^2 & c^3 \end{vmatrix} = 0$

$\Rightarrow (1+abc)\begin{vmatrix} 1 & a & a^2 \\ 1 & b & b^2 \\ 1 & c & c^2 \end{vmatrix} = 0$

As $\begin{vmatrix} 1 & a & a^2 \\ 1 & b & b^2 \\ 1 & c & c^2 \end{vmatrix} \neq 0$ *(given condition)*

$\therefore \quad abc = -1$

15. (d)

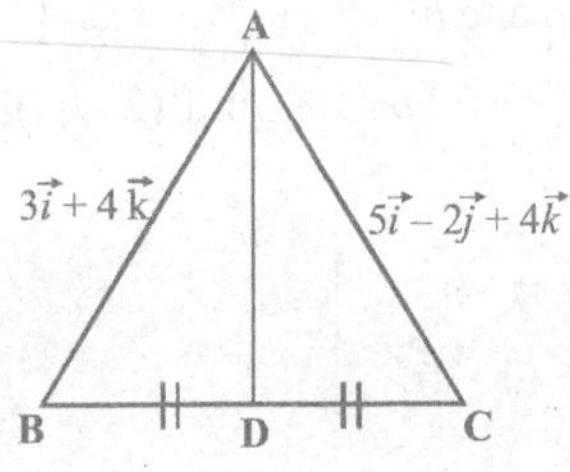

$P.V \text{ of } \overrightarrow{AD} = \dfrac{(3+5)i+(0-2)j+(4+4)k}{2}$

$= 4i - j + 4k \text{ or } |\overrightarrow{AD}| = \sqrt{16+16+1} = \sqrt{33}$

16. (d) $\overline{AB} = -4\hat{i} + 2\hat{j} + (p+1)\hat{k}$

$\overline{AC} = 2\hat{i} + (q-1)\hat{j} - 3\hat{k}$

$\overline{AB} \perp \overline{AC}$

$\Rightarrow \quad \overline{AB}.\overline{AC} = 0$

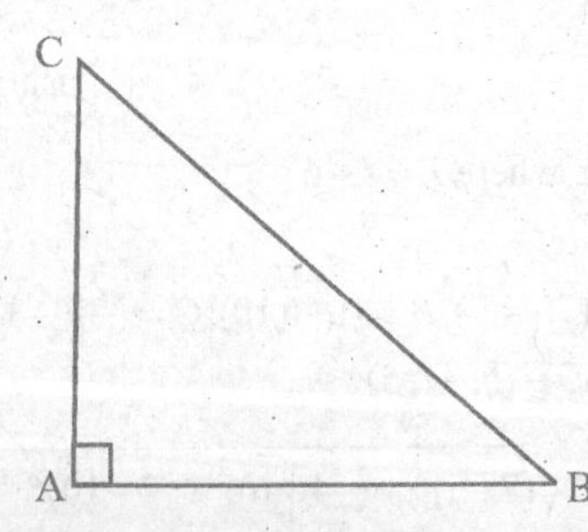

$-8 + 2(q-1) - 3(p+1) = 0$

$3p - 2q + 13 = 0$

(p, q) lies on $3x - 2y + 13 = 0$

slope $= \dfrac{3}{2}$

$\therefore$ Acute angle with x-axis

17. (c) Let $|\overrightarrow{AB}| = a$, $|\overrightarrow{AD}| = b$ and $|\overrightarrow{AC}| = c$

We have $\overrightarrow{AB} + \overrightarrow{AD} = \overrightarrow{AC}$

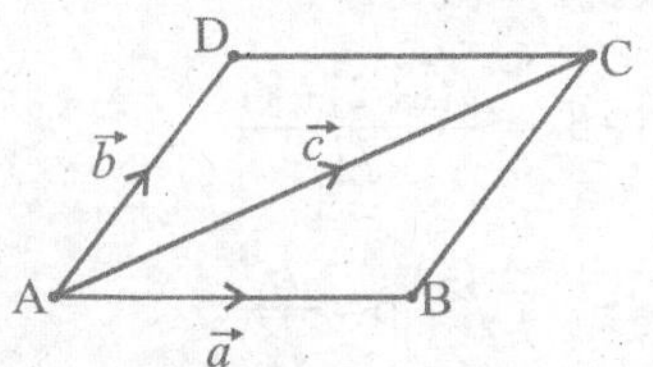

On squaring both the side, we get

$|\overrightarrow{AB}|^2 + |\overrightarrow{AD}|^2 + 2\,\overrightarrow{AB}.\overrightarrow{AD} = |\overrightarrow{AC}|^2$

$\Rightarrow a^2 + b^2 + 2\,\overrightarrow{AB}.(-\overrightarrow{DA}) = c^2$

$\Rightarrow 2\,\overrightarrow{AB}.\overrightarrow{DA} = a^2 + b^2 - c^2$

$\Rightarrow \overrightarrow{DA}.\overrightarrow{AB} = \dfrac{1}{2}(a^2 + b^2 - c^2)$

18. (b) $(\hat{x}+\hat{y}+\hat{z})^2 \geq 0$

$\Rightarrow \quad 3 + 2\Sigma\,\hat{x}.\hat{y} \geq 0$

$\Rightarrow \quad 2\Sigma\,\hat{x}.\hat{y} \geq -3$

Now, $|\hat{x}+\hat{y}|^2 + |\hat{y}+\hat{z}|^2 + |\hat{z}+\hat{x}|^2$

$= 6 + 2\Sigma\,\hat{x}.\hat{y} \geq 6 + (-3)$

$\Rightarrow \quad |\hat{x}+\hat{y}|^2 + |\hat{y}+\hat{z}|^2 + |\hat{z}+\hat{x}|^2 \geq 3$

19. (c) Given $|2\vec{a} - \vec{b}| = 5$

$\sqrt{(2|\vec{a}|)^2 + |\vec{b}|^2 - 2\times|2\vec{a}||\vec{b}|\cos\theta} = 5$

Putting values of $|\vec{a}|$ and $|\vec{b}|$, we get

$(2\times 2)^2 + (3)^2 - 24\cos\theta = 25$

$\Rightarrow \cos\theta = 0$

$\Rightarrow \theta = \dfrac{\pi}{2}$

$|2\vec{a} + \vec{b}| = \sqrt{16+9+24\cos\theta} = \sqrt{25} = 5$

20. (b) Let angle between $\hat{a}$ and $\hat{c}$ be θ.

Now, $\hat{a} - \sqrt{3}\,\hat{b} + \hat{c} = \vec{0}$

$\Rightarrow (\hat{a}+\hat{c}) = \sqrt{3}\,\hat{b}$

$\Rightarrow \quad (\hat{a}+\hat{c}).(\hat{a}+\hat{c}) = 3(\hat{b}.\hat{b})$

$\Rightarrow \quad \hat{a}.\hat{a} + \hat{a}.\hat{c} + \hat{c}.\hat{a} + \hat{c}.\hat{c} = 3\times 1$

$\Rightarrow 1 + 2\cos\theta + 1 = 3$

$\Rightarrow \cos\theta = \dfrac{1}{2} \Rightarrow \theta = \dfrac{\pi}{3}$

21. **(b)** Let $\vec{d} = \vec{b} + \lambda\vec{c}$

$\therefore\ \vec{d} = \hat{i} + 2\hat{j} - \hat{k} + \lambda(\hat{i} + \hat{j} - 2\hat{k})$

$= (1+\lambda)\hat{i} + (2+\lambda)\hat{j} - (1+2\lambda)\hat{k}$

If θ be the angle between $\vec{d}$ and $\vec{a}$, then projection of $\vec{d}$ or $(\vec{b} + \lambda\vec{c})$ on $\vec{a}$

$= |\vec{d}|\cos\theta$

$= |\vec{d}|\left(\dfrac{\vec{d}.\vec{a}}{|\vec{d}||\vec{a}|}\right) = \dfrac{\vec{d}.\vec{a}}{|\vec{a}|}$

$= \dfrac{2(\lambda+1) - (\lambda+2) - (2\lambda+1)}{\sqrt{4+1+1}} = \dfrac{-\lambda-1}{\sqrt{6}}$

But projection of $\vec{d}$ on $\vec{a} = \sqrt{\dfrac{2}{3}}$

$\therefore\ -\dfrac{\lambda+1}{\sqrt{6}} = \sqrt{\dfrac{2}{3}} \Rightarrow \dfrac{\lambda^2+2\lambda+1}{6} = \dfrac{2}{3}$

$\Rightarrow \lambda^2 + 2\lambda - 3 = 0 \Rightarrow \lambda^2 + 3\lambda - \lambda - 3 = 0$

$\Rightarrow \lambda(\lambda+3) - 1(\lambda+3) = 0, \Rightarrow \lambda = 1, -3$

when $\lambda = 1$, then $\vec{b} + \lambda\vec{c} = 2\hat{i} + 3\hat{j} - 3\hat{k}$

when $\lambda = -3$, then $\vec{b} + \lambda\vec{c} = -2\hat{i} - \hat{j} + 5\hat{k}$

22. **(b)** Let $ABCD$ be a parallelogram such that $\overline{AB} = \vec{q}$, $\overline{AD} = \vec{p}$ and ∠BAD be an acute angle.

We have

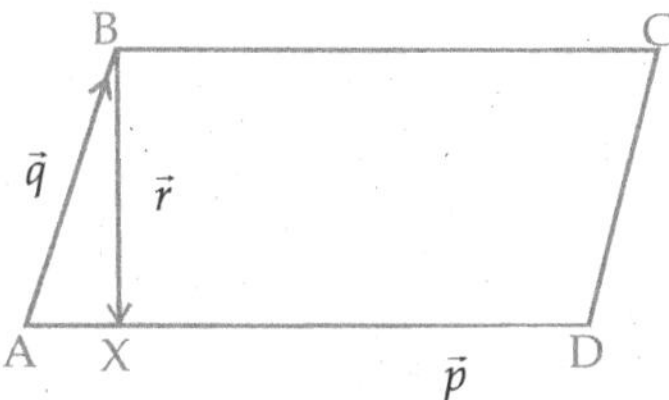

$\overline{AX} = \left(\dfrac{\vec{p}.\vec{q}}{|\vec{p}|}\right)\left(\dfrac{\vec{p}}{|\vec{p}|}\right) = \dfrac{\vec{p}.\vec{q}}{|\vec{p}|^2}\vec{p}$

Let $\vec{r} = \overline{BX} = \overline{BA} + \overline{AX} = -\vec{q} + \dfrac{\vec{p}.\vec{q}}{|\vec{p}|^2}\vec{p}$

23. **(c)** Let $\vec{c} = \hat{a} + 2\hat{b}$ and $\vec{d} = 5\hat{a} - 4\hat{b}$

Since $\vec{c}$ and $\vec{d}$ are perpendicular to each other

$\therefore\ \vec{c}.\vec{d} = 0$

$\Rightarrow\ (\hat{a} + 2\hat{b}).(5\hat{a} - 4\hat{b}) = 0$

$\Rightarrow 5 + 6\hat{a}.\hat{b} - 8 = 0 \qquad (\because \vec{a}.\vec{a} = 1)$

$\Rightarrow\ \hat{a}.\hat{b} = \dfrac{1}{2} \Rightarrow \theta = \dfrac{\pi}{3}$

24. **(a)** Let $a + b + c = 0 \Rightarrow (a+b) = -c$

$\Rightarrow\ (a+b)^2 = c^2$

$\Rightarrow\ a^2 + b^2 + 2a.b = c^2$

$\Rightarrow\ 9 + 25 + 2.3.5\cos\theta = 49$

$\left(\because |\vec{a}| = 3, |\vec{b}| = 5 \text{ and } |\vec{c}| = 7\right)$

$\therefore\ \cos\theta = \dfrac{1}{2} \Rightarrow \theta = \dfrac{\pi}{3}$

25. **(d)** Let $x\hat{i} + y\hat{j} + z\hat{k}$ be the required unit vector.

Since $\hat{a}$ is perpendicular to $(2\hat{i} - \hat{j} + 2\hat{k})$.

$\therefore\quad 2x - y + 2z = 0 \qquad$ .... (i)

Since vector $x\hat{i} + y\hat{j} + z\hat{k}$ is coplanar with the vector $\hat{i} + \hat{j} - \hat{k}$ and $2\hat{i} + 2\hat{j} - \hat{k}$.

$\therefore\quad x\hat{i} + y\hat{j} + z\hat{k} = p(\hat{i} + \hat{j} - \hat{k}) + q(2\hat{i} + 2\hat{j} - \hat{k})$,

where p and q are some scalars.

$\Rightarrow\quad x\hat{i} + y\hat{j} + z\hat{k} = (p+2q)\hat{i} + (p+2q)\hat{j} - (p+q)\hat{k}$

$\Rightarrow\quad x = p + 2q,\ y = p + 2q,\ z = -p - q$

Now from equation (i),

$2p + 4q - p - 2q - 2p - 2q = 0$

$\Rightarrow\quad -p = 0 \Rightarrow p = 0$

$\therefore\quad x = 2q,\ y = 2q,\ z = -q$

Since vector $x\hat{i} + y\hat{j} + z\hat{k}$ is a unit vector, therefore

$|x\hat{i} + y\hat{j} + z\hat{k}| = 1$

$\Rightarrow\quad \sqrt{x^2 + y^2 + z^2} = 1$

$\Rightarrow\quad x^2 + y^2 + z^2 = 1$

$\Rightarrow\quad 4q^2 + 4q^2 + q^2 = 1$

$\Rightarrow\quad 9q^2 = 1 \Rightarrow q = \pm\dfrac{1}{3}$

When $q = \dfrac{1}{3}$, then $x = \dfrac{2}{3}, y = \dfrac{2}{3}, z = -\dfrac{1}{3}$

When $q = -\dfrac{1}{3}$, then $x = -\dfrac{2}{3}, y = -\dfrac{2}{3}, z = \dfrac{1}{3}$

Here required unit vector is $\dfrac{2}{3}\hat{i} + \dfrac{2}{3}\hat{j} - \dfrac{1}{3}\hat{k}$

or $-\dfrac{2}{3}\hat{i} - \dfrac{2}{3}\hat{j} + \dfrac{1}{3}\hat{k}$.

26. (d)

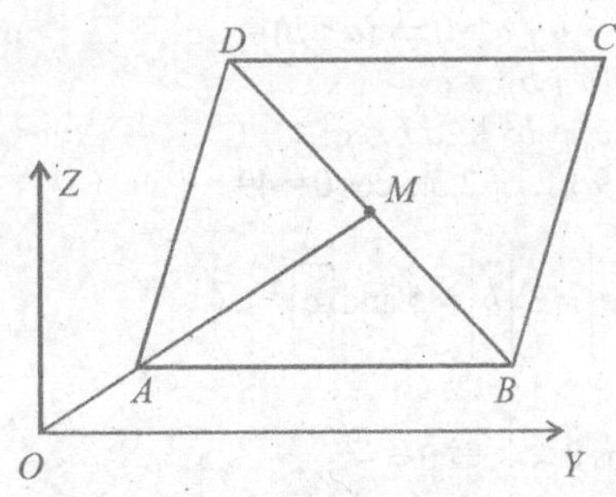

In a parallelogram, diagonals bisect each other. So, mid point of DB is also the mid-point of AC.

Mid-point of $M = 2\hat{i} - \hat{j}$

Direction ratio of $OC = (1, -5, -5)$

Direction ratio of $OM = (2, -1, 0)$

Angle θ between OM and OC is given by

$$\cos\theta = \frac{(1\times 2)+(-5)(-1)+(-5)(0)}{\sqrt{2^2+(-1)^2}\sqrt{(1)^2+(-5)^2+(-5)^2}}$$

$$= \frac{2+5}{\sqrt{5}\sqrt{51}} = \frac{7}{\sqrt{5}\sqrt{51}}$$

Projection of $\vec{OM}$ on $\vec{OC}$ is given by

$$|OM|.\cos\theta = \sqrt{5}\times\frac{7}{\sqrt{5}\times\sqrt{51}} = \frac{7}{\sqrt{51}}$$

27. (d) Since, $\vec{a}, \vec{b}$ and $\vec{c}$ are mutually orthogonal

$\therefore\ \vec{a}.\vec{b} = 0,\ \vec{b}.\vec{c} = 0,\ \vec{c}.\vec{a} = 0$

$\Rightarrow 2\lambda + 4 + \mu = 0$ ...(i)

$\lambda - 1 + 2\mu = 0$ ...(ii)

On solving (i) and (ii), we get $\lambda = -3, \mu = 2$

28. (d) Clearly $\vec{a} = -\frac{8}{7}\vec{c}$

$\Rightarrow \vec{a} \parallel \vec{c}$ and are opposite in direction

$\therefore$ Angle between $\vec{a}$ and $\vec{c}$ is π.

ALTERNATE SOLUTION

$$\cos\theta = \frac{\vec{a}.\vec{c}}{|\vec{a}||\vec{c}|} = \frac{8\vec{b}\cdot(-7\vec{b})}{8|\vec{b}|7|\vec{b}|} = -1 \Rightarrow \theta = \pi$$

29. (a) $\vec{CA} = (2-a)\hat{i} + 2\hat{j}$;

$\vec{CB} = (1-a)\hat{i} - 6\hat{k}$

$\vec{CA}.\vec{CB} = 0 \Rightarrow (2-a)(1-a) = 0$

$\Rightarrow a = 2, 1$

30. (c) Projection of $\vec{v}$ along $\vec{u}$ $= \frac{\vec{v}.\vec{u}}{|\vec{u}|} = \frac{\vec{v}.\vec{u}}{2}$

projection of $\vec{w}$ along $\vec{u}$ $= \frac{\vec{w}.\vec{u}}{|\vec{u}|} = \frac{\vec{w}\vec{u}}{2}$

Given $\frac{\vec{v}.\vec{u}}{2} = \frac{\vec{w}.\vec{u}}{2}$ ....(1)

Also, $\vec{v}.\vec{w} = 0$ ....(2)

Now $|\vec{u} - \vec{v} + \vec{w}|^2$

$= |\vec{u}|^2 + |\vec{v}|^2 + |\vec{w}|^2 - 2\vec{u}.\vec{v} - 2\vec{v}.\vec{w} + 2\vec{u}.\vec{w}$

$= 1 + 4 + 9 + 0$ [From (1) and (2)] $= 14$

$\therefore |\vec{u} - \vec{v} + \vec{w}| = \sqrt{14}$

31. (c) $\vec{a} + \vec{b} + \vec{c} = 0 \Rightarrow (\vec{a} + \vec{b} + \vec{c}).(\vec{a} + \vec{b} + \vec{c}) = 0$

$|\vec{a}|^2 + |\vec{b}|^2 + |\vec{c}|^2 + 2(\vec{a}.\vec{b} + \vec{b}.\vec{c} + \vec{c}.\vec{a}) = 0$

$\vec{a}.\vec{b} + \vec{b}.\vec{c} + \vec{c}.\vec{a} = \frac{-1-4-9}{2} = -7$

32. (a) We have, $\vec{a} + \vec{b} + \vec{c} = \vec{0}$

$\Rightarrow (\vec{a} + \vec{b} + \vec{c})^2 = 0$

$\Rightarrow |\vec{a}|^2 + |\vec{b}|^2 + |\vec{c}|^2$

$+ 2(\vec{a}\cdot\vec{b} + \vec{b}\cdot\vec{c} + \vec{c}\cdot\vec{a}) = 0$

$\Rightarrow 25 + 16 + 9 + 2(\vec{a}\cdot\vec{b} + \vec{b}\cdot\vec{c} + \vec{c}\cdot\vec{a}) = 0$

$\Rightarrow (\vec{a}\cdot\vec{b} + \vec{b}\cdot\vec{c} + \vec{c}\cdot\vec{a}) = -25$

$\therefore |\vec{a}\cdot\vec{b} + \vec{b}\cdot\vec{c} + \vec{c}\cdot\vec{a}| = 25$

33. (a) $\vec{a} + \vec{b} + \vec{c} = 0 \Rightarrow \vec{b} + \vec{c} = -\vec{a}$

$\Rightarrow (\vec{b} + \vec{c})^2 = (\vec{a})^2 = 5^2 + 3^2 + 2\vec{b}\cdot\vec{c} = 7^2$

$\Rightarrow 2|\vec{b}||\vec{c}|\cos\theta = 49 - 34 = 15$;

$\Rightarrow 2 \times 5 \times 3\cos\theta = 15$;

$\Rightarrow \cos\theta = 1/2; \Rightarrow \theta = \frac{\pi}{3} = 60°$

34. (c) Given:

$\vec{a} = 2\hat{i} + \hat{j} - 2\hat{k},\ \vec{b} = \hat{i} + \hat{j}$

$\Rightarrow |\vec{a}| = 3$

$\therefore\ \vec{a}\times\vec{b} = 2\hat{i} - 2\hat{j} + \hat{k}$

$|\vec{a}\times\vec{b}| = \sqrt{2^2 + 2^2 + 1^2} = 3$

We have $(\vec{a}\times\vec{b})\times\vec{c} = |\vec{a}\times\vec{b}||\vec{c}|\sin 30$ n

$\Rightarrow |(\vec{a}\times\vec{b})\times\vec{c}| = 3|\vec{c}|.\frac{1}{2}$

$\Rightarrow 3 = 3|\vec{c}|.\frac{1}{2}$

$\therefore\ |\vec{c}| = 2$

Now $|\vec{c}-\vec{a}| = 3$

On squaring, we get

$\Rightarrow c^2 + a^2 - 2 - \vec{c}.\vec{a} = 9$

$\Rightarrow 4 + 9 - 2 - \vec{a}.\vec{c} = 9$

$\Rightarrow \vec{a}.\vec{c} = 2 \qquad [\because \vec{c}.\vec{a} = \vec{a}.\vec{c}]$

35. (b) $\vec{b_1} = \dfrac{(\vec{b_1}.\vec{a})\hat{a}}{1}$

$$= \left\{\frac{(3\hat{j}+4\hat{k}).(\hat{i}+\hat{j})}{\sqrt{2}}\right\}\left(\frac{\hat{i}+\hat{j}}{\sqrt{2}}\right)$$

$$= \frac{3(\hat{i}+\hat{j})}{\sqrt{2}\times\sqrt{2}} = \frac{3(\hat{i}+\hat{j})}{2}$$

$\vec{b_1} + \vec{b_2} = \vec{b}$

$\Rightarrow \quad \vec{b_2} = \vec{b} - \vec{b_1}$

$$= (3\hat{j}+4\hat{k}) - \frac{3}{2}(\hat{i}+\hat{j})$$

$$\Rightarrow \boxed{\vec{b_2} = -\frac{3}{2}\hat{i} + \frac{3}{2}\hat{j} + 4\hat{k}}$$

$$\& \ \vec{b_1}\times\vec{b_2} = \begin{vmatrix} \hat{i} & \hat{j} & \hat{k} \\ \frac{3}{2} & \frac{3}{2} & 0 \\ -\frac{3}{2} & \frac{3}{2} & 4 \end{vmatrix}$$

$$\Rightarrow \quad \vec{b_1}\times\vec{b_2} = \hat{i}(6) - \hat{j}(6) + \hat{k}\left(-\frac{9}{4}+\frac{9}{4}\right) \Rightarrow 6\hat{i} - 6\hat{j} + \frac{9}{2}\hat{k}$$

36. (b) Let; $d_1 = 8\hat{i} - 6\hat{j} + 0\hat{k}$ & $d_2 = 3\hat{i} + 4\hat{j} - 12\hat{k}$

$$\therefore \quad |d_1 \times d_2| = \begin{vmatrix} \hat{i} & \hat{j} & \hat{k} \\ 8 & -6 & 0 \\ 3 & 4 & -12 \end{vmatrix}$$

$$= |72\hat{i} - (-96)\hat{j} + 50\hat{k}|$$

$$\Rightarrow \quad |d_1 \times d_2| = \sqrt{16900} = 130$$

$\therefore$ Area of parallelogram $= \dfrac{1}{2}|d_1 \times d_2| = \dfrac{1}{2}\times 130 = 65$

37. (b) $\vec{a}\times(\vec{b}\times\vec{c}) = \dfrac{\sqrt{3}}{2}(\vec{b}+\vec{c})$

$$\Rightarrow (\vec{a}\cdot\vec{c})\vec{b} - (\vec{a}\cdot\vec{b})\vec{c} = \frac{\sqrt{3}}{2}\vec{b} + \frac{\sqrt{3}}{2}\vec{c}$$

On comparing both sides

$$\vec{a}\cdot\vec{b} = -\frac{\sqrt{3}}{2} \Rightarrow \cos\theta = -\frac{\sqrt{3}}{2}$$

$[\because \vec{a}$ and $\vec{b}$ are unit vectors$]$

where θ is the angle between $\vec{a}$ and $\vec{b}$

$$\theta = \frac{5\pi}{6}$$

38. (c) $(\vec{a}\times\vec{b})\times\vec{c} = \dfrac{1}{3}|\vec{b}||\vec{c}|\vec{a}$

$$\Rightarrow \quad -\vec{c}\times(\vec{a}\times\vec{b}) = \frac{1}{3}|\vec{b}||\vec{c}|\vec{a}$$

$$\Rightarrow \quad -(\vec{c}.\vec{b})\vec{a} + (\vec{c}.\vec{a})\vec{b} = \frac{1}{3}|\vec{b}||\vec{c}|\vec{a}$$

$$\Rightarrow \quad -|\vec{b}||\vec{c}|\cos\theta\vec{a} + (\vec{c}.\vec{a})\vec{b} = \frac{1}{3}|\vec{b}||\vec{c}|\vec{a}$$

$\because \quad \vec{a}, \vec{b}, \vec{c}$ are non collinear, the above equation is possible only when

$$-\cos\theta = \frac{1}{3} \text{ and } \vec{c}.\vec{a} = 0$$

$$\Rightarrow \quad \cos\theta = -\frac{1}{3}$$

$$\Rightarrow \quad \sin\theta = \frac{2\sqrt{2}}{3}; \theta \in \text{II quad}$$

39. (a) $|\vec{a}+\vec{b}| = \sqrt{3}$

angle between $\vec{a}$ and $\vec{b}$ is 60°.

$\vec{a}\times\vec{b}$ is $\perp^r$ to plane containing $\vec{a}$ and $\vec{b}$

$\vec{c} = \vec{a} + 2\vec{b} + 3(\vec{a}\times\vec{b})$

$$\vec{c} = \sqrt{|a|^2 + 4|\vec{b}|^2 + 2.2|\vec{a}|^2\cos 60°\vec{n}_1 + 3|\vec{a}||\vec{b}|\sin 60°\vec{n}_2}$$

$$+3|\vec{a}||\vec{b}|\sin 60°.\vec{n}_2$$

$\vec{n}_1 \perp^r \vec{n}_2$

$$|\vec{c}|^2 = (1+4+2) + 9\times\frac{3}{4}$$

$$|\vec{c}|^2 = 7 + 27/4 = 55/4$$

$$2|\vec{c}| = \sqrt{55}$$

40. (b) L.H.S $= (\vec{a}\times\vec{b}).[(\vec{b}\times\vec{c})\times(\vec{c}\times\vec{a})]$

$$= (\vec{a}\times\vec{b}).[(\vec{b}\times\vec{c}.\vec{a})\vec{c} - (\vec{b}\times\vec{c}.\vec{c})\vec{a}]$$

$= (\vec{a}\times\vec{b}).[[\vec{b}\vec{c}\vec{a}]\vec{c}] \quad [\because \vec{b}\times\vec{c}.\vec{c}=0]$

$= [\vec{a}\,\vec{b}\vec{c}].(\vec{a}\times\vec{b}.\vec{c}) = [\vec{a}\vec{b}\vec{c}]^2$

$= [\vec{a}\times\vec{b}\quad \vec{b}\times\vec{c}\quad \vec{c}\times\vec{a}] = [\vec{a}\vec{b}\vec{c}]^2$

So $\lambda = 1$

41. (c) Let $\vec{x} = 3\hat{i}-6\hat{j}-\hat{k}$, $\vec{y} = \hat{i}+4\hat{j}-3\hat{k}$ and

$\vec{z} = 3\hat{i}-4\hat{j}-12\hat{k}$

Now, $\vec{x}\times\vec{y} = \begin{vmatrix}\hat{i} & \hat{j} & \hat{k}\\ 3 & -6 & -1\\ 1 & 4 & -3\end{vmatrix} = 22\hat{i}+8\hat{j}+18\hat{k}$

Projection of $\vec{x}\times\vec{y}$ on $\vec{z} = \dfrac{(\vec{x}+\vec{y}).(\vec{z})}{|\vec{z}|}$

$= \dfrac{22(3)+8(-4)+18(-12)}{\sqrt{9+16+144}} = \dfrac{-182}{13} = -14$

Now, magnitude of projection = 14.

42. (d) Let, $\vec{c} = a\hat{i}+b\hat{j}+c\hat{k}$

Given, $\vec{c}\times(\hat{i}+2\hat{j}+5\hat{k}) = \vec{0}$

$\Rightarrow \begin{vmatrix}\hat{i} & \hat{j} & \hat{k}\\ a & b & c\\ 1 & 2 & 5\end{vmatrix} = \vec{0}$

$\Rightarrow (5b-2c)\hat{i}-(5a-c)\hat{j}+(2a-b)\hat{k} = 0\hat{i}+0\hat{j}+0\hat{k}$

Comparing both sides, we get

$5b-2c=0;\ 5a-c=0;\ 2a-b=0$

or $5b=2c;\ 5a=c;\ 2a=b$

Also given $|\vec{c}|^2 = 60 \Rightarrow a^2+b^2+c^2 = 60$

Putting the value of b and c in above eqn., we get

$a^2+(2a)^2+(5a)^2 = 60$

$\Rightarrow a^2+4a^2+25a^2 = 60 \Rightarrow 30a^2 = 60$

$a^2 = 2$

$a = \pm\sqrt{2}$; $b = 2\sqrt{2}$; $c = 5\sqrt{2}$

Now, $\vec{c} = a\hat{i}+b\hat{j}+c\hat{k}$

$\therefore \vec{c} = \sqrt{2}\hat{i}+2\sqrt{2}\hat{j}+5\sqrt{2}\hat{k}$

Value of $\vec{c}.(-7\hat{i}+2\hat{j}+3\hat{k})$ is

$\left(\sqrt{2}\hat{i}+2\sqrt{2}\hat{j}+5\sqrt{2}\hat{k}\right).\left(-7\hat{i}+2\hat{j}+3\hat{k}\right)$

$= -7\sqrt{2}+4\sqrt{2}+15\sqrt{2} = 12\sqrt{2}$

43. (d) $\vec{a} = 2\hat{i}+\hat{j}-2\hat{k}$, $\vec{b} = \hat{i}+\hat{j}$

$\Rightarrow |\vec{a}| = 3$

and $\vec{a}\times\vec{b} = \begin{vmatrix}\hat{i} & \hat{j} & \hat{k}\\ 2 & 1 & -2\\ 1 & 1 & 0\end{vmatrix} = 2\hat{i}-2\hat{j}+\hat{k}$

$|\vec{a}\times\vec{b}| = \sqrt{4+4+1} = 3$

Now, $|\vec{c}-\vec{a}| = 2\sqrt{2} \Rightarrow |\vec{c}-\vec{a}|^2 = 8$

$\Rightarrow |\vec{c}-\vec{a}|.(\vec{c}-\vec{a}) = 8$

$\Rightarrow |\vec{c}|^2+|\vec{a}|^2-2\,\vec{c}.\vec{a} = 8$

$\Rightarrow |\vec{c}|^2+9-2|\vec{c}| = 8$

$\Rightarrow (|\vec{c}|-1)^2 = 0 \Rightarrow |\vec{c}| = 1$

$\therefore |(\vec{a}\times\vec{b})\times\vec{c}| = |\vec{a}\times\vec{b}||\vec{c}|\sin 30° = 3\times1\times\frac{1}{2} = \frac{3}{2}$

44. (c) $(\hat{i}\times\vec{a}\cdot\vec{b})\hat{i}+(\hat{j}\times\vec{a}\cdot\vec{b})\hat{j}+(\hat{k}\times\vec{a}\cdot\vec{b})\hat{k}$

$= (\hat{i}\cdot\vec{a}\times\vec{b})\hat{i}+(\hat{j}\cdot\vec{a}\times\vec{b})\hat{j}+(\hat{k}\cdot\vec{a}\times\vec{b})\hat{k}$

$(\because \vec{a}\times\vec{b}\cdot\vec{c} = \vec{a}\cdot\vec{b}\times\vec{c})$

$= (\vec{a}\times\vec{b})\hat{i}+(\vec{a}\times\vec{b})\hat{j}+(\vec{a}\times\vec{b})\hat{k}$

$= \vec{a}\times\vec{b}$

45. (c) Statement - 1

The vectors $\vec{a},\vec{b}$ and $\vec{c}$ lie in the same plane.

$\Rightarrow \vec{a},\vec{b}$ and $\vec{c}$ are coplanar.

We know, the necessary and sufficient conditions for three vectors to be coplanar is that $[\vec{a}\vec{b}\vec{c}] = 0$

i.e. $\vec{a}\cdot(\vec{b}\times\vec{c}) = 0$

Hence, statement-1 is true.

46. (b) Let $\vec{u} = \hat{j}+4\hat{k}$, $\vec{v} = \hat{i}-3\hat{k}$ and

$\vec{w} = \cos\theta\hat{i}+\sin\theta\hat{j}$

Now, $\vec{u}\times\vec{v} = \begin{vmatrix}\hat{i} & \hat{j} & \hat{k}\\ 0 & 1 & 4\\ 1 & 0 & -3\end{vmatrix}$

$= \hat{i}(-3)-\hat{j}(-4)+\hat{k}(-1)$

$= -3\hat{i}+4\hat{j}-\hat{k}$

Now, $\left(\vec{u}\times\vec{v}\right).\vec{w} = \left(-3\hat{i}+4\hat{j}-\hat{k}\right).\left(\cos\theta\hat{i}+\sin\theta\hat{j}\right)$

$= -3\cos\theta+4\sin\theta$

Now, maximum possible value of

$|-3\cos\theta+4\sin\theta| = \sqrt{(-3)^2+(4)^2} = \sqrt{25} = 5$

47. **(a)** **Statement - 1**

Points (1, 2, 2), (2, 1, 2), (2, 2, z) and (1, 1, 1) are coplanar then $z = 2$ which is false.

$$\because \begin{vmatrix} 1 & -1 & 0 \\ 1 & 0 & z-2 \\ 0 & -1 & -1 \end{vmatrix} = 0$$

$\Rightarrow \; 1(z-2)+1(-1)=0 \Rightarrow z=3$

Statement - 2 is the true statement.

48. **(a)** Since $\vec{a} = \hat{i} - 2\hat{j} + 3\hat{k}$, $\vec{b} = 2\hat{i} + 3\hat{j} - \hat{k}$ and

$\vec{c} = \lambda\hat{i} + \hat{j} + (2\lambda - 1)\hat{k}$ are coplanar

therefore $[\vec{a}\,\vec{b}\,\vec{c}] = 0$

i.e., $\begin{vmatrix} 1 & 2 & \lambda \\ -2 & 3 & 1 \\ 3 & -1 & 2\lambda-1 \end{vmatrix} = 0$

$\Rightarrow \; 1(6\lambda-2)-2(-4\lambda-1)+\lambda(-7)=0$

$\Rightarrow \; (6\lambda-2)+8\lambda+2+2+2\lambda-9\lambda=0$

$\Rightarrow \; 7\lambda=0 \Rightarrow \lambda=0$

49. **(c)** $\vec{a}.\vec{b} \neq 0$, $\vec{a}.\vec{d} = 0$

Now, $\vec{b} \times \vec{c} = \vec{b} \times \vec{d}$

$\Rightarrow \vec{a} \times (\vec{b} \times \vec{c}) = \vec{a} \times (\vec{b} \times \vec{d})$

$\Rightarrow (\vec{a}.\vec{c})\vec{b} - (\vec{a}.\vec{b})\vec{c} = (\vec{a}.\vec{d})\vec{b} - (\vec{a}.\vec{b})\vec{d}$

$\Rightarrow (\vec{a}.\vec{b})\vec{d} = -(\vec{a}.\vec{c})\vec{b} + (\vec{a}.\vec{b})\vec{c}$

$$\vec{d} = \vec{c} - \left(\frac{\vec{a}.\vec{c}}{\vec{a}.\vec{b}}\right)\vec{b}$$

50. **(d)** $(2\vec{a} - \vec{b}).\left((\vec{a} \times \vec{b}) \times (\vec{a} + 2\vec{b})\right)$

$= (2\vec{a} - \vec{b}).\left((\vec{a} \times \vec{b}) \times \vec{a} + 2(\vec{a} + \vec{b}) \times \vec{b}\right)$

$= (2\vec{a} - \vec{b})\begin{pmatrix}(\vec{a}.\vec{a})\vec{b} - (\vec{a}.\vec{b})\vec{a} + 2(\vec{a}.\vec{b})\vec{b} \\ -2(\vec{b}.\vec{b})\vec{a}\end{pmatrix}$

$= (2\vec{a} - \vec{b})(\vec{b} - 0 + 0 - 2\vec{a})$ [$\because \vec{a}.\vec{b} = 0$ and $\vec{b}.\vec{b} = 1$]

$= -4\vec{a}.\vec{a} - \vec{b}.\vec{b} = -5$

51. **(d)** $\vec{c} = \vec{b} \times \vec{a} \Rightarrow \vec{b}.\vec{c} = \vec{b}.(\vec{b} \times \vec{a}) \Rightarrow \vec{b}.\vec{c} = 0$

$\Rightarrow \left(b_1\hat{i} + b_2\hat{j} + b_3\hat{k}\right).\left(\hat{i} - \hat{j} - \hat{k}\right) = 0,$

where $\vec{b} = b_1\hat{i} + b_2\hat{j} + b_3\hat{k}$

$b_1 - b_2 - b_3 = 0$ ...(i)

and

$\vec{a}.\vec{b} = 3 \Rightarrow (\hat{j} - \hat{k}).(b_1\hat{i} + b_2\hat{j} + b_3\hat{k}) = 3$

$\Rightarrow b_2 - b_3 = 3$

From equation (i)

$b_1 = b_2 + b_3 = (3 + b_3) + b_3 = 3 + 2b_3$

$\vec{b} = (3 + 2b_3)\hat{i} + (3 + b_3)\hat{j} + b_3\hat{k}$

From the option given, it is clear that b_3 equal to either 2 or –2.

If $b_3 = 2$ then $\vec{b} = 7\hat{i} + 5\hat{j} + 2\hat{k}$ which is not possible

If $b_3 = -2$, then $\vec{b} = -\hat{i} + \hat{j} - 2\hat{k}$

52. **(d)** $\because$ $\vec{u}, \vec{v}, \vec{w}$ are non coplanar vectors

$\therefore [\vec{u}, \vec{v}, \vec{w}] \neq 0$

Now,

$[3\vec{u}, p\vec{v}, p\vec{w}] - [p\vec{v}, p\vec{w}, q\vec{u}] - [2\vec{w}, q\vec{v}, q\vec{u}] = 0$

$\Rightarrow \; 3p^2[\vec{u}, \vec{v}, \vec{w}] - pq[\vec{v}, \vec{w}, \vec{u}] - 2q^2[\vec{w}, \vec{v}, \vec{u}] = 0$

$\Rightarrow \; 3p^2[\vec{u}, \vec{v}, \vec{w}] - pq[\vec{u}, \vec{v}, \vec{w}] + 2q^2[\vec{u}, \vec{v}, \vec{w}]$

$\Rightarrow \; (3p^2 - pq + 2q^2)[\vec{u}, \vec{v}, \vec{w}] = 0$

$\Rightarrow \; 3p^2 - pq + 2q^2 = 0$

$\Rightarrow \; 2p^2 + p^2 - pq + \frac{q^2}{4} + \frac{7q^2}{4} = 0$

$\Rightarrow \; 2p^2 + \left(p - \frac{q}{2}\right)^2 + \frac{7}{4}q^2 = 0$

$\Rightarrow \; p = 0, q = 0, p = q/2$

This is possible only when $p = 0, q = 0$

$\therefore$ There is exactly one value of (p, q).

53. **(b)** Given $\vec{a} = \hat{i} + \hat{j} + \hat{k}$, $\vec{b} = \hat{i} - \hat{j} + 2\hat{k}$ and

$\vec{c} = x\hat{i} + (x-2)\hat{j} - \hat{k}$

If $\vec{c}$ lies in the plane of $\vec{a}$ and $\vec{b}$, then $[\vec{a}\,\vec{b}\,\vec{c}] = 0$

i.e. $\begin{vmatrix} 1 & 1 & 1 \\ 1 & -1 & 2 \\ x & (x-2) & -1 \end{vmatrix} = 0$

$\Rightarrow 1[1 - 2(x-2)] - 1[-1 - 2x] + 1[x - 2 + x] = 0$

$\Rightarrow 1 - 2x + 4 + 1 + 2x + 2x - 2 = 0$

$\Rightarrow 2x = -4 \Rightarrow x = -2$

54. **(b)** Given $|2\hat{u} \times 3\hat{v}| = 1$ and θ is acute angle between $\hat{u}$ and $\hat{v}$, $|\hat{u}| = 1, |\hat{v}| = 1$

$\Rightarrow 6|\hat{u}||\hat{v}||\sin\theta| = 1$

$\Rightarrow \; 6|\sin\theta| = 1 \Rightarrow \sin\theta = \frac{1}{6}$

Hence, there is exactly one value of θ for which $2\hat{u} \times 3\hat{v}$ is a unit vector.

55. **(d)** $(\vec{a} \times \vec{b}) \times \vec{c} = \vec{a} \times (\vec{b} \times \vec{c})$, $\vec{a}.\vec{b} \neq 0$, $\vec{b}.\vec{c} \neq 0$

$\Rightarrow \; (\vec{a}.\vec{c}).\vec{b} - (\vec{b}.\vec{c})\vec{a} = (\vec{a}.\vec{c}).\vec{b} - (\vec{a}.\vec{b}).\vec{c}$

$\Rightarrow (\vec{a}.\vec{b}).\vec{c} = (\vec{b}.\vec{c})\vec{a} \Rightarrow \vec{a} \| \vec{c}$.

56. **(d)** $\vec{a}=\hat{i}-\hat{k},\ \vec{b}=x\hat{i}+\hat{j}+(1-x)\hat{k}$ and

$\vec{c}=y\hat{i}+x\hat{j}+(1+x-y)\hat{k}$

$$[\vec{a}\ \vec{b}\ \vec{c}]=\vec{a}.\vec{b}\times\vec{c}=\begin{vmatrix}1 & 0 & -1\\ x & 1 & 1-x\\ y & x & 1+x-y\end{vmatrix}$$

$$=1\left[1+x-y-x+x^2\right]-\left[-x^2-y\right]$$

$$=1-y+x^2-x^2+y$$

$$=1$$

Hence $\left[\vec{a}\ \vec{b}\ \vec{c}\right]$ is independent of x and y both.

57. **(b)** Let us consider

$\vec{a}=a_1\hat{i}+a_2\hat{j}+a_3\hat{k}$

$\vec{b}=b_1\hat{i}+b_2\hat{j}+b_3\hat{k}$

$\vec{c}=c_1\hat{i}+c_2\hat{j}+c_3\hat{k}$

then as per question

$$\left[\lambda\left(\vec{a}+\vec{b}\right)\ \lambda^2\vec{b}\ \lambda\vec{c}\right]=\left[\vec{a}\ \vec{b}+\vec{c}\ \vec{b}\right]$$

$$\Rightarrow\begin{vmatrix}\lambda(a_1+b_1) & \lambda(a_2+b_2) & \lambda(a_3+b_3)\\ \lambda^2 b_1 & \lambda^2 b_2 & \lambda b_3\\ \lambda c_1 & \lambda c_2 & \lambda c_3\end{vmatrix}$$

$$=\begin{vmatrix}a_1 & a_2 & a_3\\ b_1+c_1 & b_2+c_2 & b_3+c_3\\ b_1 & b_2 & b_3\end{vmatrix}$$

$$\Rightarrow\lambda^4\begin{vmatrix}a_1+b_1 & a_2b_2 & a_3+b_3\\ b_1 & b_2 & b_3\\ c_1 & c_2 & c_3\end{vmatrix}$$

$$=\begin{vmatrix}a_1 & a_2 & a_3\\ b_1+c_1 & b_2+c_2 & b_3+c_3\\ b_1 & b_2 & b_3\end{vmatrix}$$

$$R_1-R_2 \qquad R_2-R_3$$

$$\Rightarrow\lambda^4\begin{vmatrix}a_1 & a_2 & a_3\\ b_1 & b_2 & b_3\\ c_1 & c_2 & c_3\end{vmatrix}=\begin{vmatrix}a_1 & a_2 & a_3\\ c_1 & c_2 & c_3\\ b_1 & b_2 & b_3\end{vmatrix}$$

$$\Rightarrow\lambda^4=-1$$

Hence λ has no real values.

58. **(c)** Let $\vec{a}=x\vec{i}+y\vec{j}+z\vec{k}$

$\vec{a}\times\vec{i}=z\vec{j}-y\vec{k}\ \Rightarrow(\vec{a}\times\vec{i})^2=y^2+z^2$

Similarly,

$(\vec{a}\times\vec{j})^2=x^2+z^2$ and $(\vec{a}\times\vec{k})^2=x^2+y^2$

$$\Rightarrow\ (\vec{a}\times\vec{i})^2+(\vec{a}\times\vec{j})^2+(\vec{a}\times\vec{k})^2$$

$$=2(x^2+y^2+z^2)=2\vec{a}^2$$

59. **(a)** Given $(\vec{a}\times\vec{b})\times\vec{c}=\frac{1}{3}|\vec{b}||\vec{c}|\vec{a}$

Clearly $\vec{a}$ and $\vec{b}$ are noncollinear

$$\Rightarrow(\vec{a}.\vec{c})\vec{b}-(\vec{b}.\vec{c})\vec{a}=\frac{1}{3}|\vec{b}||\vec{c}|\vec{a}$$

$$\therefore\ \vec{a}.\vec{c}=0 \text{ and } -\vec{b}.\vec{c}=\frac{1}{3}|\vec{b}||\vec{c}|$$

$$\Rightarrow\cos\theta=\frac{-1}{3}$$

$$\therefore\ \sin\theta=\sqrt{1-\frac{1}{9}}=\frac{2\sqrt{2}}{3}$$

[θ is acute angle between $\vec{b}$ and $\vec{c}$]

60. **(c)** $(\vec{u}+\vec{v}-\vec{w}).(\vec{u}\times\vec{v}-\vec{u}\times\vec{w}-\vec{v}\times\vec{v}+\vec{v}\times\vec{w})$

$$=(\vec{u}+\vec{v}-\vec{w}).(\vec{u}\times\vec{v}-\vec{u}\times\vec{w}+\vec{v}\times\vec{w})$$

$$=\vec{u}.(\vec{u}\times\vec{v})$$

$$-\vec{u}.(\vec{u}\times\vec{w})+\vec{u}.(\vec{v}\times\vec{w})+\vec{v}.(\vec{u}\times\vec{v})-\vec{v}.(\vec{u}\times\vec{w})$$

$$+\vec{v}.(\vec{v}\times\vec{w})-\vec{w}.(\vec{u}\times\vec{v})+\vec{w}.(\vec{u}\times\vec{w})-\vec{w}.(\vec{v}\times\vec{w})$$

$$=\vec{u}.(\vec{v}\times\vec{w})-\vec{v}.(\vec{u}\times\vec{w})-\vec{w}.(\vec{u}\times\vec{v})$$

$$=[\vec{u}\vec{v}\vec{w})]+[\vec{v}\vec{w}\vec{u})]-[\vec{w}\vec{u}\vec{v}]=\vec{u}.(\vec{v}\times\vec{w})$$

61. **(b)** Vector perpendicular to the face OAB

$$=\overrightarrow{OA}\times\overrightarrow{OB}=\begin{vmatrix}\hat{i} & \hat{j} & \hat{k}\\ 1 & 2 & 1\\ 2 & 1 & 3\end{vmatrix}=5\hat{i}-\hat{j}-3\hat{k}$$

Vector perpendicular to the face ABC

$$=\overrightarrow{AB}\times\overrightarrow{AC}=\begin{vmatrix}\hat{i} & \hat{j} & \hat{k}\\ 1 & -1 & 2\\ -2 & -1 & 1\end{vmatrix}=\hat{i}-5\hat{j}-3\hat{k}$$

Angle between the faces = angle between their normals

$$\cos\theta=\left|\frac{5+5+9}{\sqrt{35}\sqrt{35}}\right|=\frac{19}{35}\text{ or }\theta=\cos^{-1}\left(\frac{19}{35}\right)$$

62. **(a)** since $\vec{n}$ is perpendicular $\vec{u}$ *and* $\vec{v}$, $\vec{n}=\frac{\vec{u}\times\vec{v}}{|\vec{u}||\vec{v}|}$

$$\hat{n}=\frac{\begin{vmatrix}i & j & k\\ 1 & 1 & 0\\ 1 & -1 & 0\end{vmatrix}}{\sqrt{2}\times\sqrt{2}}=\frac{-2\hat{k}}{2}=-\hat{k}$$

$$|\vec{\omega}.\hat{n}|=|(i+2j+3k).(-k)|=|-3|=3$$

63. **(c)** Let $\vec{a}+\vec{b}+\vec{c}=\vec{r}$. Then

$\vec{a}\times(\vec{a}+\vec{b}+\vec{c})=\vec{a}\times\vec{r}$

$\Rightarrow 0+\vec{a}\times\vec{b}+\vec{a}\times\vec{c}=\vec{a}\times\vec{r}$

$\Rightarrow \vec{a}\times\vec{b}-\vec{c}\times\vec{a}=\vec{a}\times\vec{r}\Rightarrow\vec{a}\times\vec{r}=\vec{0}$

Similarly $\vec{b}\times\vec{r}=\vec{0}$ & $\vec{c}\times\vec{r}=\vec{0}$

Above three conditions will be satisfied for non-zero vectors if and only if $\vec{r}=\vec{0}$

64. **(b)** We have $\vec{a}\times\vec{b}=39\vec{k}=\vec{c}$

Also $|\vec{a}|=\sqrt{34}, |\vec{b}|=\sqrt{45}, |\vec{c}|=39$;

$\therefore |\vec{a}|:|\vec{b}|:|\vec{c}|=\sqrt{34}:\sqrt{45}:39$.

65. **(a)** Since $\vec{a},\vec{c},\vec{b}$ form a right handed system,

$$\therefore \quad \vec{c}=\vec{b}\times\vec{a}=\begin{vmatrix}\hat{i} & \hat{j} & \hat{k}\\ 0 & 1 & 0\\ x & y & z\end{vmatrix}=z\hat{i}-x\hat{k}$$

66. **(a)** We have, $[\vec{a}\times\vec{b}\ \ \vec{b}\times\vec{c}\ \ \vec{c}\times\vec{a}]$

$=(\vec{a}\times\vec{b}).\left\{(\vec{b}\times\vec{c})\times(\vec{c}\times\vec{a})\right\}$

$=(\vec{a}\times\vec{b}).\left\{(\vec{m}\cdot\vec{a})\vec{c}-(\vec{m}\cdot\vec{c})\vec{a}\right\}$

(where $\vec{m}=\vec{b}\times\vec{c}$)

$=\{(\vec{a}\times\vec{b}).\vec{c}\}.\{(\vec{a}\cdot(\vec{b}\times\vec{c})\}$

$=[\vec{a}\ \vec{b}\ \vec{c}]^2=4^2=16$.

67. **(b)** We have, $\vec{a}\cdot\vec{b}=|\vec{a}||\vec{b}|\cos\frac{\pi}{6}$

$=4\times2\times\frac{\sqrt{3}}{2}=4\sqrt{3}$.

Now, $(\vec{a}\times\vec{b})^2+(\vec{a}\cdot\vec{b})^2=a^2b^2$;

$\Rightarrow (\vec{a}\times\vec{b})^2+48=16\times4$

$\Rightarrow (\vec{a}\times\vec{b})^2=16$

68. **(a)** Let B be the top of the wall whose coordinates will be (a, b). Range $(R)=c$

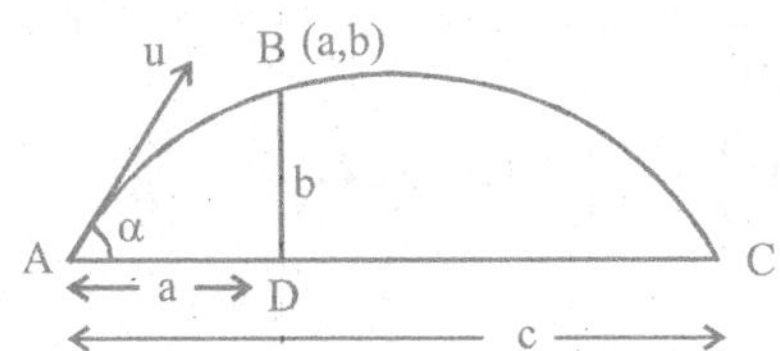

B lies on the trajectory

$$y=x\tan\alpha-\frac{1}{2}g\frac{x^2}{u^2\cos^2\alpha}$$

$$\Rightarrow b=a\tan\alpha-\frac{1}{2}g\frac{a^2}{u^2\cos^2\alpha}$$

$$\Rightarrow b=a\tan\alpha\left[1-\frac{ga}{2u^2\cos^2\alpha\tan\alpha}\right]$$

$$=a\tan\alpha\left[1-\frac{a}{\frac{2u^2}{g}\cos^2\alpha.\frac{\sin\alpha}{\cos\alpha}}\right]$$

$$=a\tan\alpha\left[1-\frac{a}{\frac{u^2.2\sin\alpha\cos\alpha}{g}}\right]$$

$$=a\tan\alpha\left[1-\frac{a}{\frac{u^2\sin2\alpha}{g}}\right]$$

$$=a\tan\alpha\left[1-\frac{a}{R}\right]\quad\left(\because R=\frac{u^2\sin^2\alpha}{g}\right)$$

$$\Rightarrow b=a\tan\alpha\left[1-\frac{a}{c}\right]\Rightarrow b=a\tan\alpha.\left(\frac{c-a}{c}\right)$$

$$\Rightarrow \tan\alpha=\frac{bc}{a(c-a)}$$

The angle of projection,

$$\alpha=\tan^{-1}\frac{bc}{a(c-a)}$$

69. **(a)**

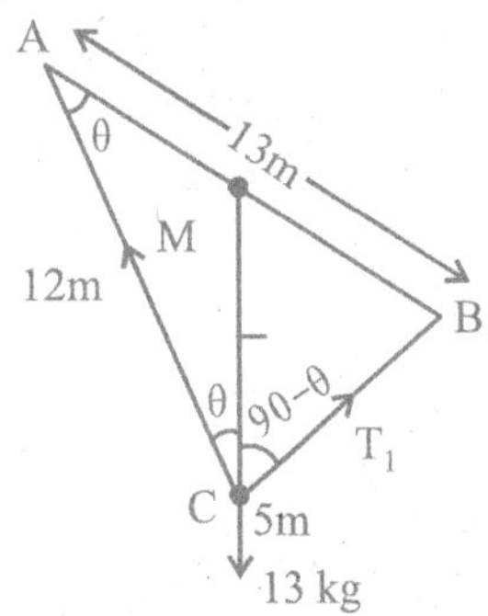

$\because 13^2=5^2+12^2\Rightarrow AB^2=AC^2+BC^2$

$\Rightarrow \angle ACB=90°$

Q m is mid point of the hypotenuse AB, therefore $MA=MB=MC$

$\Rightarrow \angle A=\angle ACM=\theta$

Applying Lami's theorem at C, we get

$$\frac{T_1}{\sin(180-\theta)}=\frac{T_2}{\sin(90+\theta)}=\frac{13kg}{\sin 90°}$$

$\Rightarrow\ T_1 = 13 \sin\theta$ and $T_2 = 13\cos\theta$

$\Rightarrow\ T_1 = 13\times\frac{5}{13}$ and $T_2 = 13\times\frac{12}{13}$

$\Rightarrow\ T_1 = 5$ kg and $T_2 = 12$ kg

70. (c) Given : Force $P = Pn$, $Q = 3n$, resultant $R = 7n$ & $P' = Pn$, $Q' = (-3)n$, $R' = \sqrt{19}\,n$

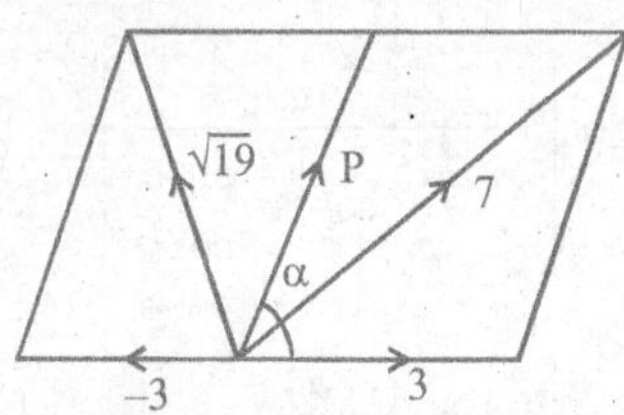

We know that $R^2 = P^2 + Q^2 + 2PQ\cos\alpha$

$\Rightarrow\ (7)^2 = P^2 + (3)^2 + 2\times P\times 3\cos\alpha$

$\Rightarrow\ 49 = P^2 + 9 + 6P\cos\alpha$

$\Rightarrow\ 40 = P^2 + 6P\cos\alpha$ .....(i)

and $\left(\sqrt{19}\right)^2 = P^2 + (-3)^2 + 2P\times -3\cos\alpha$

$\Rightarrow\ 19 = P^2 + 9 - 6P\cos\alpha$

$\Rightarrow\ 10 = P^2 - 6P\cos\alpha$ .....(ii)

Adding (i) and (ii) $50 = 2P^2$

$\Rightarrow\ P^2 = 25 \Rightarrow P = 5n.$

71. (a) Using $h = \frac{1}{2}gt^2$ and $h + 400 = \frac{1}{2}g(t+4)^2$

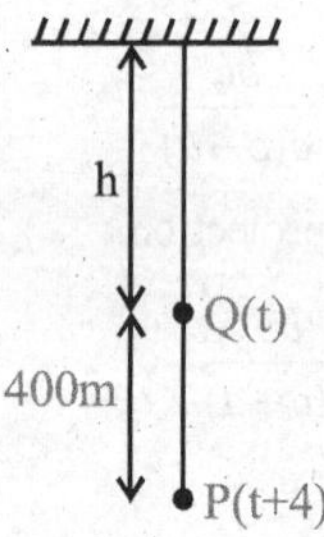

Subtracting, we get $400 = 8g + 4gt$

$\Rightarrow\ t = 8$ sec

$\therefore\ h = \frac{1}{2}\times 10\times 64 = 320m$

$\therefore$ Desired height $= 320 + 400 = 720\ m$

72. (b) For two velocities u and u at an angle θ to each other the resultant is given by

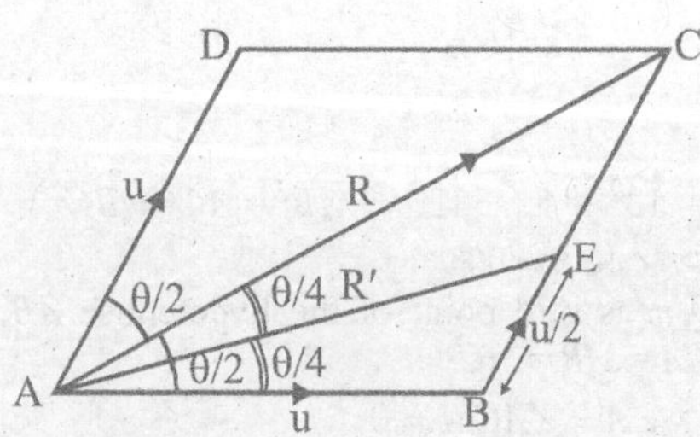

$R^2 = u^2 + u^2 + 2u^2\cos\theta = 2u^2(1+\cos\theta)$

$\Rightarrow R^2 = 4u^2\cos^2\theta/2$ or $R = 2u\cos\frac{\theta}{2}$

Now in second case, the new resultant AE (i.e., R') bisects $\angle CAB$, therefore using angle bisector theorem in ΔABC, we get

$$\frac{AB}{AC}=\frac{BE}{EC}\Rightarrow\frac{u}{R}=\frac{u/2}{u/2}\Rightarrow R=u$$

$\Rightarrow\ 2u\cos\frac{\theta}{2} = u$

$\Rightarrow\ \cos\frac{\theta}{2} = \frac{1}{2} = \cos 60° \Rightarrow \frac{\theta}{2} = 60°$

or $\theta = 120°$

ALTERNATE SOLUTION

$$\tan\frac{\theta}{4}=\frac{\frac{u}{2}\sin\theta}{u+\frac{u}{2}\cos\theta}$$

$\Rightarrow\ \sin\frac{\theta}{4}+\frac{1}{2}\sin\frac{\theta}{4}\cos\theta = \frac{1}{2}\sin\theta\cos\frac{\theta}{4}$

$\therefore\ 2\sin\frac{\theta}{4} = \sin\frac{3\theta}{4} = 3\sin\frac{\theta}{4} - 4\sin^3\frac{\theta}{4}$

$\therefore\ \sin^2\frac{\theta}{4} = \frac{1}{4} \Rightarrow \frac{\theta}{4} = 30°$ or $\theta = 120°$

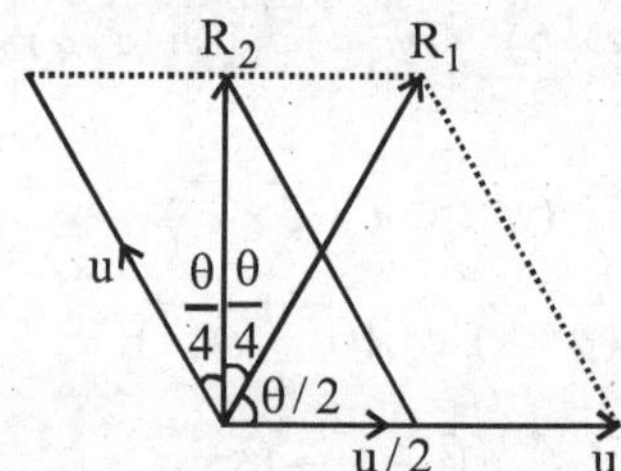

73. (d) $F' = 3F\cos\theta$ and $F = 3F\sin\theta$

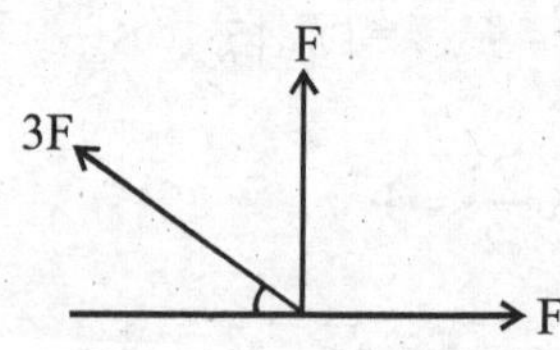

$\Rightarrow F' = 2\sqrt{2}\,F \Rightarrow F : F' :: 3 : 2\sqrt{2}.$

74. (b) Let A and B be displaced by a distance x then Change in moment of $(A+B)$ = applied moments

$$\Rightarrow (A+B)\times x = H \Rightarrow x = \frac{H}{A+B}$$

75. (d) $u\cos 60° = v\cos 30°$

(as horizontal component of velocity remains the same)

$\Rightarrow u\cdot\frac{1}{2} = v\cdot\frac{\sqrt{3}}{2}$ or $v = \frac{1}{\sqrt{3}}u$

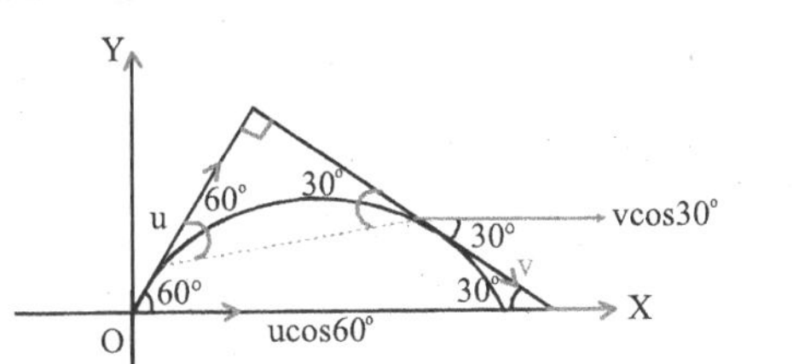

76. **(b)** For same horizontal range the angles of projection must be α and $\frac{\pi}{2}-\alpha$

$\therefore t_1 = \frac{2u\sin\alpha}{g}$ and

$$t_2 = \frac{2u\sin\left(\frac{\pi}{2}-\alpha\right)}{g} = \frac{2u\cos\alpha}{g}$$

$$\therefore t_1^2 + t_2^2 = \frac{4u^2}{g^2}$$

77. **(a)** If $v = \frac{1}{4}$, component along OB

$$= \frac{v\sin 30°}{\sin(45°+30°)} = \frac{\frac{1}{4}\times\frac{1}{2}}{\frac{\sqrt{3}+1}{2\sqrt{2}}} = \frac{\sqrt{6}-\sqrt{2}}{8}$$

78. **(d)** Time taken by the particle in complete journey

$$T = \frac{12}{4}+\frac{5}{5} = 4\ hr.$$

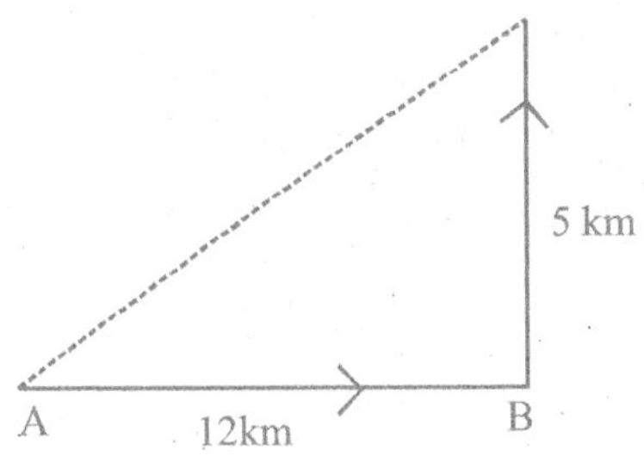

$\therefore$ Average speed $= \frac{12+5}{4} = \frac{17}{4}$

Average velocity $= \sqrt{\frac{12^2+5^2}{4}} = \frac{13}{4}$

[using vector addition]

79. **(d)** IA, IB, IC are bisectors of the angles A, B and C as I is incentre of ΔABC.

Now $\angle BIC = 180 - \frac{B}{2} - \frac{C}{2} = 90° + \frac{A}{2}$ *etc.*

Applying Lami's theorem at I

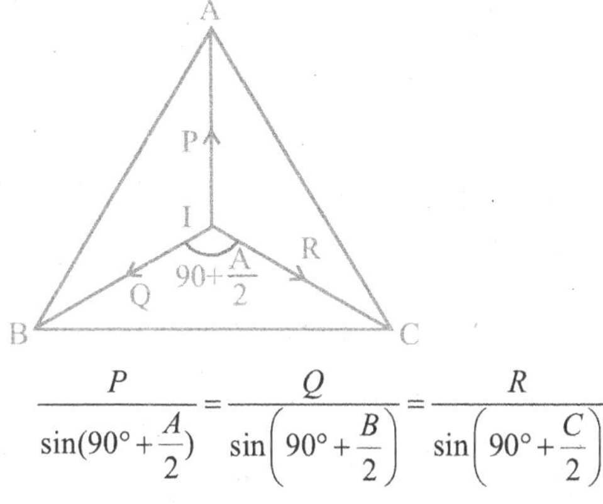

$$\frac{P}{\sin(90°+\frac{A}{2})} = \frac{Q}{\sin\left(90°+\frac{B}{2}\right)} = \frac{R}{\sin\left(90°+\frac{C}{2}\right)}$$

$$\Rightarrow \quad P:Q:R = \cos\frac{A}{2} : \cos\frac{B}{2} : \cos\frac{C}{2}$$

80. **(c)** Since, the moment about A is zero, hence $\vec{F}$ passes through A. Taking A as origin. Let the line of action of force $\vec{F}$ be $y = mx$. (see figure)

Moment about $B = \frac{3m}{\sqrt{1+m^2}}|\vec{F}| = 9$ ....(1)

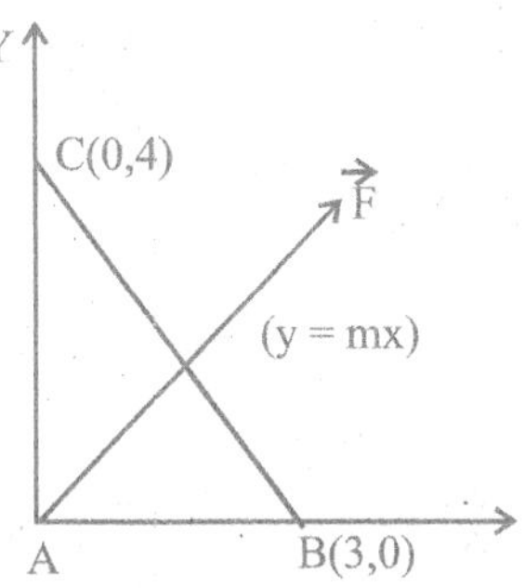

Moment about $C = \frac{4}{\sqrt{1+m^2}}|\vec{F}| = 16$ ....(2)

Dividing (1) by (2), we get

$m = \frac{3}{4} \Rightarrow |\vec{F}| = 5N.$

81. **(c)** Let forces be P and Q. then $P+Q=4$ ....(1)

and $P^2+Q^2=3^2$ ....(2)

Solving we get the forces

$$\left(2+\frac{\sqrt{2}}{2}\right)N \text{ and } \left(2-\frac{\sqrt{2}}{2}\right)N$$

82. **(d)** Resultant of forces $\vec{F} = 7\hat{i}+2\hat{j}-4\hat{k}$

Displacement $\vec{d} = 4\hat{i}+2\hat{j}-2\hat{k}$

$\therefore$ Work done $= \vec{F}.\vec{d} = 28+4+8 = 40$

83. **(a)** Let β be the inclination of the plane to the horizontal and u be the velocity of projection of the projectile

$$R_1 = \frac{u^2}{g(1+\sin\beta)} \text{ and } R_2 = \frac{u^2}{g(1-\sin\beta)}$$

$$\frac{1}{R_1}+\frac{1}{R_2}=\frac{2g}{u^2} \text{ or } \frac{1}{R_1}+\frac{1}{R_2}=\frac{2}{R}\left[\because R=\frac{u^2}{g}\right]$$

$\therefore R_1, R, R_2$ are in H.P.

84. **(a)** We can consider the two velocities as $\vec{v}_1 = u\hat{i}$ and $\vec{v}_2 = (ft\cos\alpha)\hat{i} + (ft\sin\alpha)\hat{j}$

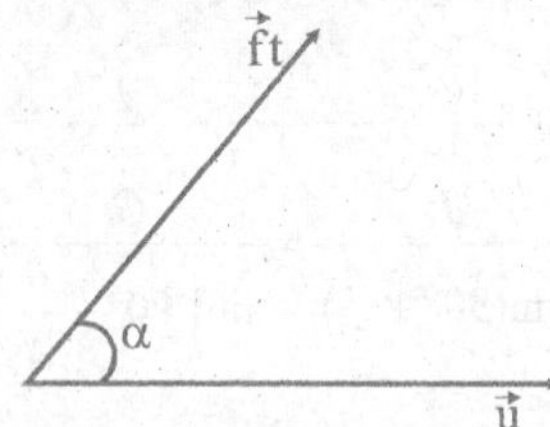

$\therefore$ Relative velocity of second with respect to first

$$\vec{v} = \vec{v}_2 - \vec{v}_1 = (ft\cos\alpha - u)\hat{i} + ft\sin\alpha\,\hat{j}$$

$$\Rightarrow |\vec{v}|^2 = (ft\cos\alpha - u)^2 + (ft\sin\alpha)^2$$

$$= f^2t^2 + u^2 - 2uft\cos\alpha$$

For $|\vec{v}|$ to be min we should have

$$\frac{d|v|^2}{dt} = 0 \Rightarrow 2f^2t - 2uf\cos\alpha = 0$$

$$\Rightarrow t = \frac{u\cos\alpha}{f}$$

Also $\frac{d^2|v|^2}{dt^2} = 2f^2 = +ve$

$\therefore |v|^2$ and hence $|v|$ is least at the time $\frac{u\cos\alpha}{f}$

85. **(a)** For the stone projected horizontally, for horizontal motion, using distance = speed × time $\Rightarrow R = ut$

and for vertical motion

$$h = 0\times t + \frac{1}{2}gt^2$$

$$\Rightarrow t = \sqrt{\frac{2h}{g}}$$

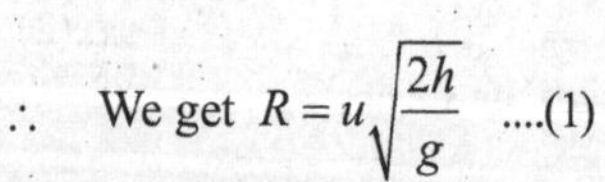

$\therefore$ We get $R = u\sqrt{\frac{2h}{g}}$ ....(1)

For the stone projected at an angle θ, for horizontal and vertical motions, we have

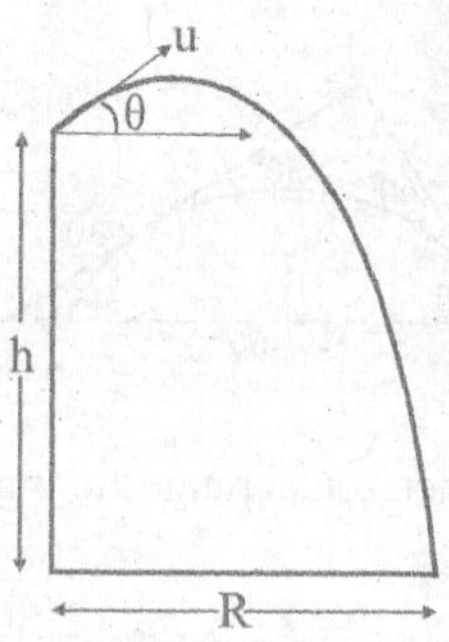

$R = u\cos\theta \times t$ ....(2)

and $h = -u\sin\theta \times t + \frac{1}{2}gt^2$ ....(3)

From (1) and (2) we get

$$u\sqrt{\frac{2h}{g}} = u\cos\theta \times t$$

$$\Rightarrow t = \frac{1}{\cos\theta}\sqrt{\frac{2h}{g}}$$

Substituting this value of t in eq (3) we get

$$h = -\frac{u\sin\theta}{\cos\theta}\sqrt{\frac{2h}{g}} + \frac{1}{2}g\left[\frac{2h}{g\cos^2\theta}\right]$$

$$h = -u\sqrt{\frac{2h}{g}}\tan\theta + h\sec^2\theta$$

$$h = -u\sqrt{\frac{2h}{g}}\tan\theta + h\tan^2\theta + h$$

$$\tan^2\theta - u\sqrt{\frac{2}{hg}}\tan\theta = 0; \therefore \tan\theta = u\sqrt{\frac{2}{hg}}$$

86. **(a)** Let the body travels from A to B with constant acceleration t and from B to C with constant retardation r.

A —x— B —y— C (t_1, t_2)

If $AB = x$, $BC = y$, time taken from A to $B = t_1$ and time taken from B to $C = t_2$, then $s = x + y$ and $t = t_1 + t_2$

For the motion from A to B

$$v^2 = u^2 + 2fs \Rightarrow v^2 = 2fx \;(\because u = 0)$$

$$\Rightarrow x = \frac{v^2}{2f} \qquad ....(1)$$

and $v = u + ft \Rightarrow v = ft_1$

$$\Rightarrow t_1 = \frac{v}{f} \qquad ...(2)$$

For the motion from B to C

$$v^2 = u^2 + 2fs$$

$$\Rightarrow 0 = v^2 - 2ry$$

$\Rightarrow \ y=\frac{v^2}{2r}$ ...(3)

and $v=u+ft \Rightarrow 0=v-rt_2$

$\Rightarrow \ t_2=\frac{v}{r}$

Adding equations (1) and (3), we get

$$x+y=\frac{v^2}{2}\left[\frac{1}{f}+\frac{1}{r}\right]=s$$

Adding equations (2) and (4), we get

$$t_1+t_2=v\left[\frac{1}{f}+\frac{1}{r}\right]=t$$

$$\therefore \ \frac{t^2}{2s}=\frac{v^2\left[\frac{1}{f}+\frac{1}{r}\right]^2}{2\times\frac{v^2}{2}\left(\frac{1}{f}+\frac{1}{r}\right)}=\frac{1}{f}+\frac{1}{r}$$

$$\Rightarrow \ t=\sqrt{2s\left(\frac{1}{f}+\frac{1}{r}\right)}$$

87. (c) $R^2=P^2+Q^2+2PQ\cos\theta$ ....(1)

$4R^2=P^2+4Q^2+4PQ\cos\theta$ ....(2)

$4R^2=P^2+Q^2-2PQ\cos\theta$ ....(3)

On $(1)+(3)$, $5R^2=2P^2+2Q^2$ ....(4)

On $(3)\times 2+(2)$, $12R^2=3P^2+6Q^2$ .....(5)

$2P^2+2Q^2-5R^2=0$ .....(6)

$3P^2+6Q^2-12R^2=0$ .....(7)

$$\frac{P^2}{-24+30}=\frac{Q^2}{24-15}=\frac{R^2}{12-6}$$

$$\frac{P^2}{6}=\frac{Q^2}{9}=\frac{R^2}{6} \text{ or } P^2:Q^2:R^2=2:3:2$$

88. (c) $\vec{G}=\vec{r}\times\vec{p}$; $\quad |\vec{G}|=rp\sin\theta$

$|\vec{H}|=rp\cos\theta \left[\because \sin(90^o+\theta)=\cos\theta\right]$

$G=rp\sin\theta$.......(1) $\quad H=rp\cos\theta$........(2)

$x=rp\sin(\theta+\alpha)$......(3)

From (1), (2) & (3), $\quad x=\vec{G}\cos\alpha+\vec{H}\sin\alpha$.

89. (d) $\vec{F}+\vec{F}_1+\vec{F}_2=7i+2j-4k$

$\vec{d}=P.V\ of\ \vec{B}-P.V\ of\ \vec{A}=4i+2j-2k$

$W=\vec{F}.\vec{d}=28+4+8=40\ unit$

90. (b) $\angle TQW=180-\theta$; $\angle RQW=2\theta$;
$\angle RQT=180-\theta$

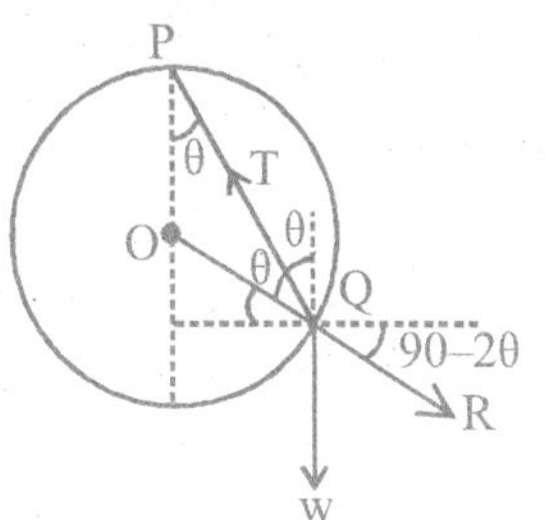

Applying Lami's theorem at Q.

$$\frac{T}{\sin 2\theta}=\frac{R}{\sin(180-\theta)}=\frac{W}{\sin(180-\theta)}$$

$\Rightarrow \ R=W$ and $T=2W\cos\theta$

91. (a) Given $P+Q=18$ ....(1)
$P^2+Q^2+2PQ\cos\alpha=144$ ......(2)

$$\tan 90^\circ=\frac{Q\sin\alpha}{P+Q\cos\alpha}$$

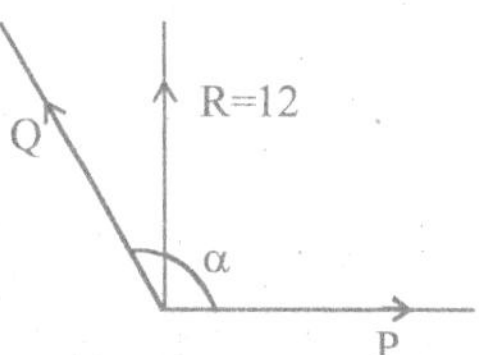

$\Rightarrow \ P+Q\cos\alpha=0$ ......(3)

From (2) and (3),

$Q^2-P^2=144 \Rightarrow (Q-P)(Q+P)=144$

$\therefore \ Q-P=\frac{144}{18}=8$

From (1), On solving, we get $Q=13, P=5$

Chapter 26

Three Dimensional Geometry

TOPIC-1 : Direction Ratios & Direction cosines of a Line, Angle between two lines in terms of dc's and dr's, Condition of Parallelism & Perpendicularity of two Lines, Projection of a Point on a Line, Projection of a Line Segment Joining two Points

1. ABC is triangle in a plane with vertices A (2, 3, 5), B (–1, 3, 2) and C (λ, 5, μ). If the median through A is equally inclined to the coordinate axes, then the value of $(\lambda^3 + \mu^3 + 5)$ is : **[Online April 10, 2016]**

(a) 1130 (b) 1348
(c) 1077 (d) 676

2. The angle between the lines whose direction cosines satisfy the equations $l+m+n=0$ and $l^2+m^2+n^2$ is **[2014]**

(a) $\frac{\pi}{6}$ (b) $\frac{\pi}{2}$
(c) $\frac{\pi}{3}$ (d) $\frac{\pi}{4}$

3. Let A (2, 3, 5), B (– 1, 3, 2) and C (λ, 5, μ) be the vertices of a ΔABC. If the median through A is equally inclined to the coordinate axes, then: **[Online April 11, 2014]**

(a) $5\lambda-8\mu=0$ (b) $8\lambda-5\mu=0$
(c) $10\lambda-7\mu=0$ (d) $7\lambda-10\mu=0$

4. A line in the 3-dimensional space makes an angle θ $\left(0<\theta\leq\frac{\pi}{2}\right)$ with both the x and y axes. Then the set of all values of θ is the interval: **[Online April 9, 2014]**

(a) $\left(0,\frac{\pi}{4}\right]$ (b) $\left[\frac{\pi}{6},\frac{\pi}{3}\right]$
(c) $\left[\frac{\pi}{4},\frac{\pi}{2}\right]$ (d) $\left(\frac{\pi}{3},\frac{\pi}{2}\right]$

5. Let ABC be a triangle with vertices at points A (2, 3, 5), B (–1, 3, 2) and C (λ, 5, μ) in three dimensional space. If the median through A is equally inclined with the axes, then (λ, μ) is equal to : **[Online April 25, 2013]**

(a) (10, 7) (b) (7, 5)
(c) (7, 10) (d) (5, 7)

6. If the projections of a line segment on the x, y and z-axes in 3-dimensional space are 2, 3 and 6 respectively, then the length of the line segment is : **[Online April 23, 2013]**

(a) 12 (b) 7
(c) 9 (d) 6

7. The acute angle between two lines such that the direction cosines l, m, n, of each of them satisfy the equations $l+m+n=0$ and $l^2+m^2-n^2=0$ is :**[Online April 22, 2013]**

(a) 15° (b) 30°
(c) 60° (d) 45°

8. A line AB in three-dimensional space makes angles 45° and 120° with the positive x-axis and the positive y-axis respectively. If AB makes an acute angle θ with the positive z-axis, then θ equals **[2010]**

(a) 45° (b) 60°
(c) 75° (d) 30°

9. The projections of a vector on the three coordinate axis are 6, –3, 2 respectively. The direction cosines of the vector are : **[2009]**

(a) $\frac{6}{5},\frac{-3}{5},\frac{2}{5}$ (b) $\frac{6}{7},\frac{-3}{7},\frac{2}{7}$
(c) $\frac{-6}{7},\frac{-3}{7},\frac{2}{7}$ (d) $6,-3,2$

10. If a line makes an angle of $\pi/4$ with the positive directions of each of x- axis and y- axis, then the angle that the line makes with the positive direction of the z-axis is **[2007]**

(a) $\frac{\pi}{4}$ (b) $\frac{\pi}{2}$
(c) $\frac{\pi}{6}$ (d) $\frac{\pi}{3}$

11. A line makes the same angle θ, with each of the x and z axis. If the angle β, which it makes with y-axis, is such that $\sin^2\beta=3\sin^2\theta$, then $\cos^2\theta$ equals **[2004]**

(a) $\frac{2}{5}$ (b) $\frac{1}{5}$
(c) $\frac{3}{5}$ (d) $\frac{2}{3}$

TOPIC-2 : Equation of a Straight Line in Cartesian and Vector Form, Angle Between two Lines, Condition for Coplanarity of two Lines Perpendicular Distance of a Point from a Line, Shortest Distance between two Skew Lines, Distance Between two Parallel Lines.

12. The number of distinct real values of λ for which the lines $\frac{x-1}{1}=\frac{y-2}{2}=\frac{z+3}{\lambda^2}$ and $\frac{x-3}{1}=\frac{y-2}{\lambda^2}=\frac{z-1}{2}$ are coplanar is : **[Online April 10, 2016]**
(a) 2 (b) 4
(c) 3 (d) 1

13. The shortest distance between the lines $\frac{x}{2}=\frac{y}{2}=\frac{z}{1}$ and $\frac{x+2}{-1}=\frac{y-4}{8}=\frac{z-5}{4}$ lies in the interval : **[Online April 9, 2016]**
(a) $(3,4]$ (b) $(2,3]$
(c) $[1,2)$ (d) $[0,1)$

14. Equation of the line of the shortest distance between the lines $\frac{x}{1}=\frac{y}{-1}=\frac{z}{1}$ and $\frac{x-1}{0}=\frac{y+1}{-2}=\frac{z}{1}$ is: **[Online April 19, 2014]**
(a) $\frac{x}{1}=\frac{y}{-1}=\frac{z}{-2}$ (b) $\frac{x-1}{1}=\frac{y+1}{-1}=\frac{z}{-2}$
(c) $\frac{x-1}{1}=\frac{y+1}{-1}=\frac{z}{1}$ (d) $\frac{x}{-2}=\frac{y}{1}=\frac{z}{2}$

15. If the lines $\frac{x-2}{1}=\frac{y-3}{1}=\frac{z-4}{-k}$ and $\frac{x-1}{k}=\frac{y-4}{2}=\frac{z-5}{1}$ are coplanar, then k can have **[2013]**
(a) any value (b) exactly one value
(c) exactly two values (d) exactly three values

16. If two lines L_1 and L_2 in space, are defined by
$L_1=\left\{x=\sqrt{\lambda}y+\left(\sqrt{\lambda}-1\right),\ z=\left(\sqrt{\lambda}-1\right)y+\sqrt{\lambda}\right\}$ and
$L_2=\left\{x=\sqrt{\mu}y+\left(1-\sqrt{\mu}\right),\ z=\left(1-\sqrt{\mu}\right)y+\sqrt{\mu}\right\}$
then L_1 is perpendicular to L_2, for all non-negative reals λ and μ, such that : **[Online April 23, 2013]**
(a) $\sqrt{\lambda}+\sqrt{\mu}=1$ (b) $\lambda\neq\mu$
(c) $\lambda+\mu=0$ (d) $\lambda=\mu$

17. If the lines $\frac{x+1}{2}=\frac{y-1}{1}=\frac{z+1}{3}$ and $\frac{x+2}{2}=\frac{y-k}{3}=\frac{z}{4}$ are coplanar, then the value of k is : **[Online April 9, 2013]**
(a) $\frac{11}{2}$ (b) $-\frac{11}{2}$
(c) $\frac{9}{2}$ (d) $-\frac{9}{2}$

18. If the line $\frac{x-1}{2}=\frac{y+1}{3}=\frac{z-1}{4}$ and $\frac{x-3}{1}=\frac{y-k}{2}=\frac{z}{1}$ intersect, then k is equal to: **[2012]**
(a) -1 (b) $\frac{2}{9}$
(c) $\frac{9}{2}$ (d) 0

19. The distance of the point $-\hat{i}+2\hat{j}+6\hat{k}$ from the straight line that passes through the point $2\hat{i}+3\hat{j}-4\hat{k}$ and is parallel to the vector $6\hat{i}+3\hat{j}-4\hat{k}$ is **[Online May 26, 2012]**
(a) 9 (b) 8
(c) 7 (d) 10

20. **Statement 1:** The shortest distance between the lines $\frac{x}{2}=\frac{y}{-1}=\frac{z}{2}$ and $\frac{x-1}{4}=\frac{y-1}{-2}=\frac{z-1}{4}$ is $\sqrt{2}$.
Statement 2: The shortest distance between two parallel lines is the perpendicular distance from any point on one of the lines to the other line. **[Online May 19, 2012]**
(a) Statement 1 is true, Statement 2 is false.
(b) Statement 1 is true, Statement 2 is true, Statement 2 is a correct explanation for Statement 1.
(c) Statement 1 is false, Statement 2 is true.
(d) Statement 1 is true, Statement 2 is true, , Statement 2 is not a correct explanation for Statement 1

21. The coordinates of the foot of perpendicular from the point $(1, 0, 0)$ to the line $\frac{x-1}{2}=\frac{y+1}{-3}=\frac{z+10}{8}$ are **[Online May 12, 2012]**
(a) $(2,-3,8)$ (b) $(1,-1,-10)$
(c) $(5,-8,-4)$ (d) $(3,-4,-2)$

22. The length of the perpendicular drawn from the point $(3,-1,11)$ to the line $\frac{x}{2}=\frac{y-2}{3}=\frac{z-3}{4}$ is : **[2011RS]**
(a) $\sqrt{29}$ (b) $\sqrt{33}$
(c) $\sqrt{53}$ (d) $\sqrt{66}$

23. **Statement-1:** The point $A(1, 0, 7))$ is the mirror image of the point $B(1, 6, 3)$ in the line : $\frac{x}{1}=\frac{y-1}{2}=\frac{z-2}{3}$

Statement-2: The line $\frac{x}{1}=\frac{y-1}{2}=\frac{z-2}{3}$ bisects the line segment joining $A(1, 0, 7)$ and $B(1, 6, 3)$. **[2011]**

(a) Statement-1 is true, Statement-2 is true; Statement-2 is **not a** correct explanation for Statement-1.
(b) Statement-1 is true, Statement-2 is false.
(c) Statement-1 is false, Statement-2 is true.
(d) Statement-1 is true, Statement-2 is true; Statement-2 is a correct explanation for Statement-1.

24. The line L given by $\frac{x}{5}+\frac{y}{b}=1$ passes through the point (13, 32). The line K is parallel to L and has the equation $\frac{x}{c}+\frac{y}{3}=1$. Then the distance between L and K is **[2010]**

(a) $\sqrt{17}$ (b) $\frac{17}{\sqrt{15}}$

(c) $\frac{23}{\sqrt{17}}$ (d) $\frac{23}{\sqrt{15}}$

25. If the straight lines $\frac{x-1}{k}=\frac{y-2}{2}=\frac{z-3}{3}$ and $\frac{x-2}{3}=\frac{y-3}{k}=\frac{z-1}{2}$ intersect at a point, then the integer k is equal to **[2008]**

(a) –5 (b) 5
(c) 2 (d) –2

26. If non zero numbers a, b, c are in H.P., then the straight line $\frac{x}{a}+\frac{y}{b}+\frac{1}{c}=0$ always passes through a fixed point. That point is **[2005]**

(a) $(-1, 2)$ (b) $(-1,-2)$

(c) $(1,-2)$ (d) $\left(1,-\frac{1}{2}\right)$

27. The angle between the lines 2x = 3y = – z and 6x = – y = – 4z is **[2005]**

(a) 0° (b) 90°
(c) 45° (d) 30°

28. If the straight lines **[2004]**

$x=1+s, y=-3-\lambda s, z=1+\lambda s$

and $x=\frac{t}{2}, y=1+t, z=2-t,$ with parameters s and t respectively, are co-planar, then λ equals.

(a) 0 (b) –1

(c) $-\frac{1}{2}$ (d) –2

29. A line with direction cosines proportional to 2, 1, 2 meets each of the lines $x=y+a=z$ and $x+a=2y=2z$. The co-ordinates of each of the points of intersection are given by **[2004]**

(a) $(2a,3a,3a),(2a,a,a)$ (b) $(3a,2a,3a),(a,a,a)$

(c) $(3a,2a,3a),(a,a,2a)$ (d) $(3a,3a,3a),(a,a,a)$

30. The lines $\frac{x-2}{1}=\frac{y-3}{1}=\frac{z-4}{-k}$ **[2003]**

and $\frac{x-1}{k}=\frac{y-4}{1}=\frac{z-5}{1}$ are coplanar if

(a) k = 3 or –2 (b) k = 0 or –1
(c) k = 1 or –1 (d) k = 0 or –3.

31. The two lines $x = ay + b, z = cy + d$ and $x = a'y + b', z = c'y + d'$ will be perpendicular, if and only if **[2003]**

(a) $aa' + cc' + 1 = 0$
(b) $aa' + bb' + cc' + 1 = 0$
(c) $aa' + bb' + cc' = 0$
(d) $(a+a')(b+b')+(c+c')=0.$

TOPIC-3 : Equation of a Plane in Different Forms, Equation of a Plane Passing Through the Intersection of two Given Planes, Plane Containing two Lines, Angle Between two Planes, Angle Between a Plane and a Line, Distance Between two Parallel Planes, Position of Point and Line wrt a Plane, Projection of a Line on a Plane

32. If the image of the point P(1, –2, 3) in the plane, $2x + 3y - 4z + 22 = 0$ measured parallel to line, $\frac{x}{1}=\frac{y}{4}=\frac{z}{5}$ is Q, then PQ is equal to : **[2017]**

(a) $6\sqrt{5}$ (b) $3\sqrt{5}$

(c) $2\sqrt{42}$ (d) $\sqrt{42}$

33. The distance of the point (1, 3, –7) from the plane passing through the point (1, –1, –1), having normal perpendicular to both the lines **[2017]**

$\frac{x-1}{1}=\frac{y+2}{-2}=\frac{z-4}{3}$ and $\frac{x-2}{2}=\frac{y+1}{-1}=\frac{z+7}{-1}$, is :

(a) $\frac{10}{\sqrt{74}}$ (b) $\frac{20}{\sqrt{74}}$

(c) $\frac{10}{\sqrt{83}}$ (d) $\frac{5}{\sqrt{83}}$

34. If $x = a, y = b, z = c$ is a solution of the system of linear equations **[Online April 9, 2017]**

$x + 8y + 7z = 0$
$9x + 2y + 3z = 0$
$x + y + z = 0$

such that the point (a, b, c) lies on the plane $x + 2y + z = 6$, then $2a + b + c$ equals :

(a) –1 (b) 0
(c) 1 (d) 2

35. If a variable plane, at a distance of 3 units from the origin, intersects the coordinate axes at A, B and C, then the locus of the centroid of ΔABC is : **[Online April 9, 2017]**

(a) $\frac{1}{x^2}+\frac{1}{y^2}+\frac{1}{z^2}=1$

(b) $\frac{1}{x^2}+\frac{1}{y^2}+\frac{1}{z^2}=3$

(c) $\frac{1}{x^2}+\frac{1}{y^2}+\frac{1}{z^2}=\frac{1}{9}$

(d) $\frac{1}{x^2}+\frac{1}{y^2}+\frac{1}{z^2}=9$

36. If the line, $\frac{x-3}{1}=\frac{y+2}{-1}=\frac{z+\lambda}{-2}$ lies in the plane, $2x - 4y + 3z = 2$, then the shortest distance between this line and the line, $\frac{x-1}{12}=\frac{y}{9}=\frac{z}{4}$ is: **[Online April 9, 2017]**

(a) 2 (b) 1
(c) 0 (d) 3

37. The coordinates of the foot of the perpendicular from the point (1, –2, 1) on the plane containing the lines,

$\frac{x+1}{6}=\frac{y-1}{7}=\frac{z-3}{8}$ and

$\frac{x-1}{3}=\frac{y-2}{5}=\frac{z-3}{7}$, is: **[Online April 8, 2017]**

(a) (2, –4, 2) (b) (–1, 2, –1)
(c) (0, 0, 0) (d) (1, 1, 1)

38. The line of intersection of the planes

$\vec{r}.(3\hat{i}-\hat{j}+\hat{k}) = 1$ and

$\vec{r}.(\hat{i}+4\hat{j}-2\hat{k}) = 2$, is: **[Online April 8, 2017]**

(a) $\frac{x-\frac{4}{7}}{-2}=\frac{y}{7}=\frac{z-\frac{5}{7}}{13}$

(b) $\frac{x-\frac{4}{7}}{2}=\frac{y}{-7}=\frac{z+\frac{5}{7}}{13}$

(c) $\frac{x-\frac{6}{13}}{2}=\frac{y-\frac{5}{13}}{-7}=\frac{z}{-13}$

(d) $\frac{x-\frac{6}{13}}{2}=\frac{y-\frac{5}{13}}{7}=\frac{z}{-13}$

39. If the line, $\frac{x-3}{2}=\frac{y+2}{-1}=\frac{z+4}{3}$ lies in the plane, $lx + my - z = 9$, then $l^2 + m^2$ is equal to : **[2016]**

(a) 5 (b) 2
(c) 26 (d) 18

40. The distance of the point (1, –5, 9) from the plane $x - y + z = 5$ measured along the line $x = y = z$ is : **[2016]**

(a) $\frac{10}{\sqrt{3}}$ (b) $\frac{20}{3}$

(c) $3\sqrt{10}$ (d) $10\sqrt{3}$

41. The distance of the point (1, –2, 4) from the plane passing through the point (1, 2, 2) and perpendicular to the planes $x - y + 2z = 3$ and $2x - 2y + z + 12 = 0$, is : **[Online April 9, 2016]**

(a) 2 (b) $\sqrt{2}$

(c) $2\sqrt{2}$ (d) $\frac{1}{\sqrt{2}}$

42. The equation of the plane containing the line $2x - 5y + z = 3$; $x + y + 4z = 5$, and parallel to the plane, $x + 3y + 6z = 1$, is : **[2015]**

(a) $x + 3y + 6z = 7$ (b) $2x + 6y + 12z = -13$
(c) $2x + 6y + 12z = 13$ (d) $x + 3y + 6z = -7$

43. The distance of the point (1, 0, 2) from the point of intersection of the line $\frac{x-2}{3}=\frac{y+1}{4}=\frac{z-2}{12}$ and the plane $x - y + z = 16$, is **[2015]**

(a) $3\sqrt{21}$ (b) 13
(c) $2\sqrt{14}$ (d) 8

44. The shortest distance between the z–axis and the line $x + y + 2z - 3 = 0 = 2x + 3y + 4z - 4$, is **[Online April 11, 2015]**

(a) 1 (b) 2
(c) 4 (d) 3

45. A plane containing the point (3, 2, 0) and the line $\frac{x-1}{1}=\frac{y-2}{5}=\frac{z-3}{4}$ also contains the point : **[Online April 11, 2015]**

(a) (0, 3, 1) (b) (0, 7, –10)
(c) (0, –3, 1) (d) 0, 7, 10

46. If the points (1, 1, λ) and (–3, 0, 1) are equidistant from the plane, $3x + 4y - 12z + 13 = 0$, then λ satisfies the equation : **[Online April 10, 2015]**

(a) $3x^2 + 10x - 13 = 0$ (b) $3x^2 - 10x + 21 = 0$
(c) $3x^2 - 10x + 7 = 0$ (d) $3x^2 + 10x - 7 = 0$

47. If the shortest distance between the lines

$\frac{x-1}{\alpha} = \frac{y+1}{-1} = \frac{z}{1}, (\alpha \neq -1)$ and $x + y + z + 1 = 0$

$= 2x - y + z + 3$ is $\frac{1}{\sqrt{3}}$, then a value α is : **[Online April 10, 2015]**

(a) $-\frac{16}{19}$ (b) $\frac{19}{16}$

(c) $\frac{32}{19}$ (d) $\frac{19}{32}$

48. The image of the line $\frac{x-1}{3} = \frac{y-3}{1} = \frac{z-4}{-5}$ in the plane $2x - y + z + 3 = 0$ is the line: **[2014]**

(a) $\frac{x-3}{3} = \frac{y+5}{1} = \frac{z-2}{-5}$

(b) $\frac{x-3}{-3} = \frac{y+5}{-1} = \frac{z-2}{5}$

(c) $\frac{x+3}{3} = \frac{y-5}{1} = \frac{z-2}{-5}$

(d) $\frac{x+3}{-3} = \frac{y-5}{-1} = \frac{z+2}{5}$

49. If the angle between the line $2(x + 1) = y = z + 4$ and the plane $2x - y + \sqrt{\lambda}\, z + 4 = 0$ is $\frac{\pi}{6}$, then the value of λ is: **[Online April 19, 2014]**

(a) $\frac{135}{7}$ (b) $\frac{45}{11}$

(c) $\frac{45}{7}$ (d) $\frac{135}{11}$

50. If the distance between planes, $4x - 2y - 4z + 1 = 0$ and $4x - 2y - 4z + d = 0$ is 7, then d is: **[Online April 12, 2014]**

(a) 41 or –42 (b) 42 or – 43
(c) – 41 or 43 (d) – 42 or 44

51. A symmetrical form of the line of intersection of the planes $x = ay + b$ and $z = cy + d$ is **[Online April 12, 2014]**

(a) $\frac{x-b}{a} = \frac{y-1}{1} = \frac{z-d}{c}$

(b) $\frac{x-b-a}{a} = \frac{y-1}{1} = \frac{z-d-c}{c}$

(c) $\frac{x-a}{b} = \frac{y-0}{1} = \frac{z-c}{d}$

(d) $\frac{x-b-a}{b} = \frac{y-1}{0} = \frac{z-d-c}{d}$

52. The plane containing the line $\frac{x-1}{1} = \frac{y-2}{2} = \frac{z-3}{3}$ and parallel to the line $\frac{x}{1} = \frac{y}{1} = \frac{z}{4}$ passes through the point: **[Online April 11, 2014]**

(a) $(1, -2, 5)$ (b) $(1, 0, 5)$
(c) $(0, 3, -5)$ (d) $(-1, -3, 0)$

53. Equation of the plane which passes through the point of intersection of lines

$\frac{x-1}{3} = \frac{y-2}{1} = \frac{z-3}{2}$ and

$\frac{x-3}{1} = \frac{y-1}{2} = \frac{z-2}{3}$

and has the largest distance from the origin is: **[Online April 9, 2014]**

(a) $7x + 2y + 4z = 54$ (b) $3x + 4y + 5z = 49$
(c) $4x + 3y + 5z = 50$ (d) $5x + 4y + 3z = 57$

54. Distance between two parallel planes $2x + y + 2z = 8$ and $4x + 2y + 4z + 5 = 0$ is **[2013]**

(a) $\frac{3}{2}$ (b) $\frac{5}{2}$

(c) $\frac{7}{2}$ (d) $\frac{9}{2}$

55. The equation of a plane through the line of intersection of the planes $x + 2y = 3$, $y - 2z + 1 = 0$, and perpendicular to the first plane is : **[Online April 25, 2013]**

(a) $2x - y - 10z = 9$ (b) $2x - y + 7z = 11$
(c) $2x - y + 10z = 11$ (d) $2x - y - 9z = 10$

56. Let Q be the foot of perpendicular from the origin to the plane $4x - 3y + z + 13 = 0$ and R be a point $(-1, -6)$ on the plane. Then length QR is : **[Online April 22, 2013]**

(a) $\sqrt{14}$ (b) $\sqrt{\frac{19}{2}}$

(c) $3\sqrt{\frac{7}{2}}$ (d) $\frac{3}{\sqrt{2}}$

57. A vector $\vec{n}$ is inclined to x-axis at 45°, to y-axis at 60° and at an acute angle to z-axis. If $\vec{n}$ is a normal to a plane passing through the point $(\sqrt{2}, -1, 1)$ then the equation of the plane is : **[Online April 9, 2013]**

(a) $4\sqrt{2}x + 7y + z - 2$ (b) $2x + y + 2z = 2\sqrt{2} + 1$
(c) $3\sqrt{2}x - 4y - 3z = 7$ (d) $\sqrt{2}x - y - z = 2$

58. A equation of a plane parallel to the plane $x-2y+2z-5=0$ and at a unit distance from the origin is : **[2012]**

(a) $x-2y+2z-3=0$ (b) $x-2y+2z+1=0$
(c) $x-2y+2z-1=0$ (d) $x-2y+2z+5=0$

59. The equation of a plane containing the line $\frac{x+1}{-3}=\frac{y-3}{2}=\frac{z+2}{1}$ and the point (0, 7, – 7) is **[Online May 26, 2012]**

(a) $x+y+z=0$
(b) $x+2y+z=21$
(c) $3x-2y+5z+35=0$
(d) $3x+2y+5z+21=0$

60. Consider the following planes
$P: x+y-2z+7=0$
$Q: x+y+2z+2=0$
$R: 3x+3y-6z-11=0$ **[Online May 26, 2012]**

(a) P and R are perpendicular
(b) Q and R are perpendicular
(c) P and Q are parallel
(d) P and R are parallel

61. If the three planes $x = 5$, $2x - 5ay + 3z - 2 = 0$ and $3bx + y - 3z = 0$ contain a common line, then(a, b) is equal to **[Online May 19, 2012]**

(a) $\left(\frac{8}{15},-\frac{1}{5}\right)$ (b) $\left(\frac{1}{5},-\frac{8}{15}\right)$

(c) $\left(-\frac{8}{15},\frac{1}{5}\right)$ (d) $\left(-\frac{1}{5},\frac{8}{15}\right)$

62. A line with positive direction cosines passes through the point $P(2,-1,2)$ and makes equal angles with the coordinate axes. If the line meets the plane $2x+y+z=9$ at point Q, then the length PQ equals **[Online May 7, 2012]**

(a) $\sqrt{2}$ (b) 2
(c) $\sqrt{3}$ (d) 1

63. The values of a for which the two points (1, a, 1) and (– 3, 0, a) lie on the opposite sides of the plane $3x+4y-12z+13=0$, satisfy **[Online May 7, 2012]**

(a) $0<a<\frac{1}{3}$ (b) $-1<a<0$

(c) $a<-1$ or $a<\frac{1}{3}$ (d) $a=0$

64. The distance of the point (1, – 5, 9) from the plane $x-y+z=5$ measured along a straight $x=y=z$ is **[2011RS]**

(a) $10\sqrt{3}$ (b) $5\sqrt{3}$
(c) $3\sqrt{10}$ (d) $3\sqrt{5}$

65. If the angle between the line $x=\frac{y-1}{2}=\frac{z-3}{\lambda}$ and the plane $x+2y+3z=4$ is $\cos^{-1}\left(\sqrt{\frac{5}{14}}\right)$, then λ equals **[2011]**

(a) $\frac{3}{2}$ (b) $\frac{2}{5}$

(c) $\frac{5}{3}$ (d) $\frac{2}{3}$

66. **Statement -1 :** The point A(3, 1, 6) is the mirror image of the point B(1, 3, 4) in the plane $x-y+z=5$.
Statement -2: The plane $x-y+z=5$ bisects the line segment joining A(3, 1, 6) and B(1, 3, 4). **[2010]**

(a) Statement -1 is true, Statement -2 is true ; Statement -2 is **not** a correct explanation for Statement -1.
(b) Statement -1 is true, Statement -2 is false.
(c) Statement -1 is false, Statement -2 is true .
(d) Statement - 1 is true, Statement 2 is true ; Statement -2 is a correct explanation for Statement -1.

67. Let the line $\frac{x-2}{3}=\frac{y-1}{-5}=\frac{z+2}{2}$ lie in the plane $x+3y-\alpha z+\beta=0$. Then (α, β) equals **[2009]**

(a) (–6, 7) (b) (5, –15)
(c) (–5, 5) (d) (6, –17)

68. The line passing through the points (5, 1, a) and (3, b, 1) crosses the yz-plane at the point $\left(0,\frac{17}{2},\frac{-13}{2}\right)$. Then **[2008]**

(a) $a=2, b=8$ (b) $a=4, b=6$
(c) $a=6, b=4$ (d) $a=8, b=2$

69. Let L be the line of intersection of the planes $2x+3y+z=1$ and $x+3y+2z=2$. If L makes an angle α with the positive x-axis, then cos α equals **[2007]**

(a) 1 (b) $\frac{1}{\sqrt{2}}$

(c) $\frac{1}{\sqrt{3}}$ (d) $\frac{1}{2}$.

70. The image of the point (–1, 3, 4) in the plane $x-2y=0$ is **[2006]**

(a) $\left(-\frac{17}{3},-\frac{19}{3},4\right)$ (b) (15,11,4)

(c) $\left(-\frac{17}{3},-\frac{19}{3},1\right)$ (d) None of these

71. The distance between the line $\vec{r} = 2\hat{i} - 2\hat{j} + 3\hat{k} + \lambda(i - j + 4k)$ and the plane $\vec{r}.(\hat{i} + 5\hat{j} + \hat{k}) = 5$ is **[2005]**

(a) $\frac{10}{9}$ (b) $\frac{10}{3\sqrt{3}}$

(c) $\frac{3}{10}$ (d) $\frac{10}{3}$

72. If the angle θ between the line $\frac{x+1}{1} = \frac{y-1}{2} = \frac{z-2}{2}$ and the plane $2x - y + \sqrt{\lambda}\, z + 4 = 0$ is such that $\sin\theta = \frac{1}{3}$ then the value of λ is **[2005]**

(a) $\frac{5}{3}$ (b) $\frac{-3}{5}$

(c) $\frac{3}{4}$ (d) $\frac{-4}{3}$

73. Distance between two parallel planes $2x+y+2z=8$ and $4x+2y+4z+5=0$ is **[2004]**

(a) $\frac{9}{2}$ (b) $\frac{5}{2}$

(c) $\frac{7}{2}$ (d) $\frac{3}{2}$

74. Two system of rectangular axes have the same origin. If a plane cuts them at distances a, b, c and a', b', c' from the origin then **[2003]**

(a) $\frac{1}{a^2}+\frac{1}{b^2}+\frac{1}{c^2}-\frac{1}{a'^2}-\frac{1}{b'^2}-\frac{1}{c'^2}=0$

(b) $\frac{1}{a^2}+\frac{1}{b^2}+\frac{1}{c^2}+\frac{1}{a'^2}+\frac{1}{b'^2}+\frac{1}{c'^2}=0$

(c) $\frac{1}{a^2}+\frac{1}{b^2}-\frac{1}{c^2}+\frac{1}{a'^2}+\frac{1}{b'^2}-\frac{1}{c'^2}=0$

(d) $\frac{1}{a^2}-\frac{1}{b^2}-\frac{1}{c^2}+\frac{1}{a'^2}-\frac{1}{b'^2}-\frac{1}{c'^2}=0$.

75. The d.r. of normal to the plane through (1, 0, 0), (0, 1, 0) which makes an angle $\pi/4$ with plane $x+y=3$ are **[2002]**

(a) $1, \sqrt{2}, 1$ (b) $1, 1, \sqrt{2}$

(c) $1, 1, 2$ (d) $\sqrt{2}, 1, 1$

76. A plane which passes through the point (3, 2, 0) and the line $\frac{x-4}{1} = \frac{y-7}{5} = \frac{z-4}{4}$ is **[2002]**

(a) $x-y+z=1$ (b) $x+y+z=5$

(c) $x+2y-z=1$ (d) $2x-y+z=5$

TOPIC-4 : Sphere and Miscellaneous Problems on Sphere

77. If (2, 3, 5) is one end of a diameter of the sphere $x^2+y^2+z^2-6x-12y-2z+20=0$, then the cooordinates of the other end of the diameter are **[2007]**

(a) (4, 3, 5) (b) (4, 3, – 3)

(c) (4, 9, – 3) (d) (4, –3, 3).

78. The plane $x+2y-z=4$ cuts the sphere $x^2+y^2+z^2-x+z-2=0$ in a circle of radius **[2005]**

(a) 3 (b) 1

(c) 2 (d) $\sqrt{2}$

79. If the plane $2ax - 3ay + 4az + 6 = 0$ passes through the midpoint of the line joining the centres of the spheres $x^2+y^2+z^2+6x-8y-2z=13$ and $x^2+y^2+z^2-10x+4y-2z=8$ then a equals **[2005]**

(a) – 1 (b) 1

(c) – 2 (d) 2

80. The intersection of the spheres $x^2+y^2+z^2+7x-2y-z=13$ and $x^2+y^2+z^2-3x+3y+4z=8$ is the same as the intersection of one of the sphere and the plane **[2004]**

(a) $2x-y-z=1$ (b) $x-2y-z=1$

(c) $x-y-2z=1$ (d) $x-y-z=1$

81. The radius of the circle in which the sphere $x^2+y^2+z^2+2x-2y-4z-19=0$ is cut by the plane $x+2y+2z+7=0$ is **[2003]**

(a) 4 (b) 1

(c) 2 (d) 3

82. The shortest distance from the plane $12x+4y+3z=327$ to the sphere $x^2+y^2+z^2+4x-2y-6z=155$ is **[2003]**

(a) 39 (b) 26

(c) $11\frac{4}{13}$ (d) 13.

Hints & Solutions

1. (b) DR's of AD are $\frac{\lambda-1}{2}-2, 4-3, \frac{\mu+2}{2}-5$

i.e. $\frac{\lambda-5}{2}, 1, \frac{\mu-8}{2}$

∵ This median is making equal angles with coordinate axes, therefore,

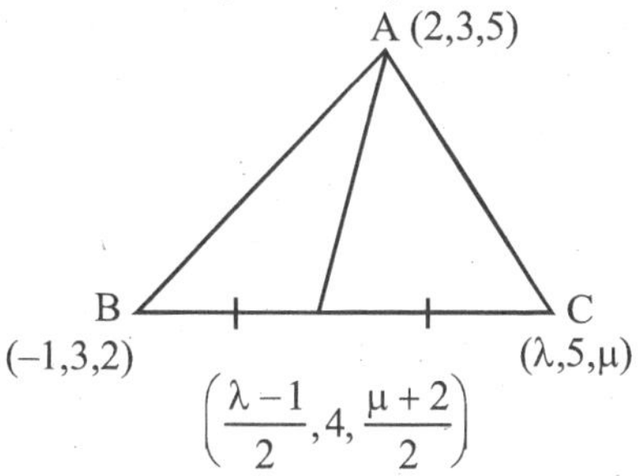

$\frac{\lambda-5}{2}=1=\frac{\mu-8}{2}$

$\Rightarrow \lambda=7 \;\&\; \mu=10$

$\therefore \lambda^3+\mu^3=5=1348$

2. (c) Given, $l+m+n=0$ and $l^2=m^2+n^2$

Now, $(-m-n)^2=m^2+n^2$

$\Rightarrow mn=0 \Rightarrow m=0$ or $n=0$

If $m=0$ then $l=-n$

We know $l^2+m^2+n^2=1 \Rightarrow n=\pm\frac{1}{\sqrt{2}}$

i.e. $(l_1, m_1, n_1)=\left(-\frac{1}{\sqrt{2}}, 0, \frac{1}{\sqrt{2}}\right)$

If $n=0$ then $l=-m$

$l^2+m^2+n^2=1 \Rightarrow 2m^2=1$

$\Rightarrow m=\pm\frac{1}{\sqrt{2}}$

Let $m=\frac{1}{\sqrt{2}} \Rightarrow l=-\frac{1}{\sqrt{2}}$ and $n=0$

$(l_2, m_2, n_2)=\left(-\frac{1}{\sqrt{2}}, \frac{1}{\sqrt{2}}, 0\right)$

$\therefore \cos\theta=\frac{1}{2} \Rightarrow \theta=\frac{\pi}{3}$

3. (c) If D be the mid-point of BC, then

$D=\left(\frac{\lambda-1}{2}, 4, \frac{\mu+2}{2}\right)$

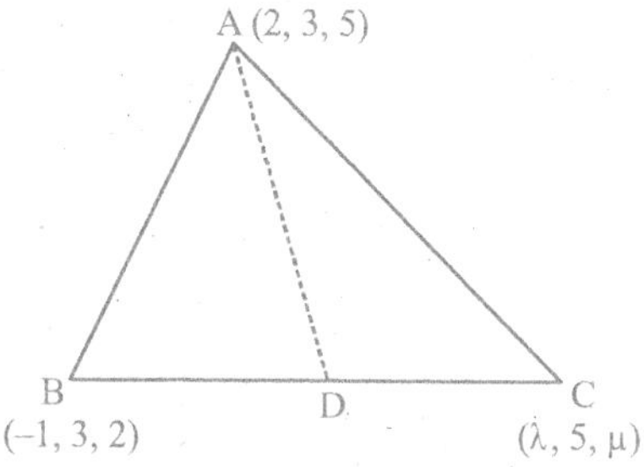

Direction ratios of AD are $\frac{\lambda-5}{2}, 1, \frac{\mu-8}{2}$

Since median AD is equally inclined with coordinate axes, therefore direction ratios of AD will be equal, i.e,

$$\frac{\left(\frac{\lambda-5}{2}\right)^2}{\left(\frac{\lambda-5}{2}\right)^2+1+\left(\frac{\mu-8}{2}\right)^2}=\frac{1}{\left(\frac{\lambda-5}{2}\right)^2+1+\left(\frac{\mu-8}{2}\right)^2}$$

$$=\frac{\left(\frac{\mu-8}{2}\right)^2}{\left(\frac{\lambda-5}{2}\right)^2+1+\left(\frac{\mu-8}{2}\right)^2}$$

$\Rightarrow \left(\frac{\lambda-5}{2}\right)^2=1=\left(\frac{\mu-8}{2}\right)^2$

$\Rightarrow \lambda=7, 3$ and $\mu=10, 6$

If $\lambda=7$ and $\mu=10$

Then $\frac{\lambda}{\mu}=\frac{7}{10} \Rightarrow 10\lambda-7\mu=0$

4. (c) It makes θ with x and y-axes.

$l=\cos\theta,\ m=\cos\theta,\ n=\cos(\pi-2\theta)$

we have $l^2+m^2+n^2=1$

$\Rightarrow \cos^2\theta+\cos^2\theta+\cos^2(\pi-2\theta)=1$

$\Rightarrow 2\cos^2\theta+(-\cos 2\theta)^2=1$

$\Rightarrow 2\cos^2\theta-1+\cos^2 2\theta=0$

$\Rightarrow \cos 2\theta-[1+\cos 2\theta]=0$

$\Rightarrow \cos 2\theta=0$ or $\cos 2\theta=-1$

$\Rightarrow 2\theta=\pi/2$ or $2\theta=\pi$

$\Rightarrow \theta=\pi/4$ or $\theta=\frac{\pi}{2}$

$\Rightarrow \theta=\left[\frac{\pi}{4}, \frac{\pi}{2}\right]$

5. (c) Since AD is the median

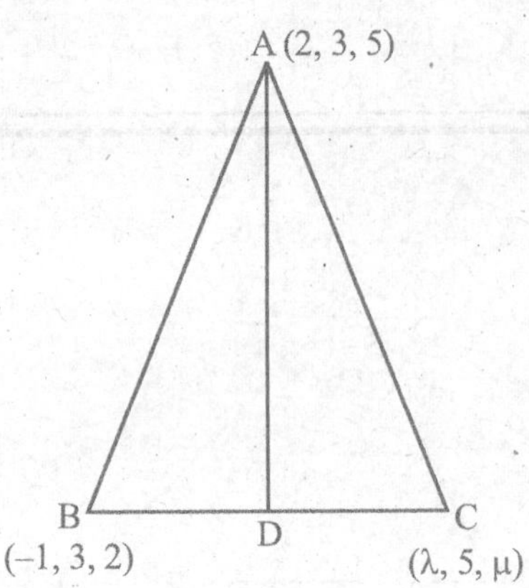

$\therefore\ D = \left(\frac{\lambda-1}{2}, 4, \frac{\mu+2}{2}\right)$

Now, dR's of AD is

$a = \left(\frac{\lambda-1}{2} - 2\right) = \frac{\lambda-5}{2}$

$b = 4 - 3 = 1,\ c = \frac{\mu+2}{2} - 5 = \frac{\mu-8}{2}$

Also, a, b, c are dR's

$\therefore\ a = kl, b = km, c = kn$ where $l = m = n$

and $l^2 + m^2 + n^2 = 1$

$\Rightarrow l = m = n = \frac{1}{\sqrt{3}}$

Now, $a = 1, b = 1$ and $c = 1$

$\Rightarrow \lambda = 7$ and $\mu = 10$

6. (b) Length of the line segment

$= \sqrt{(2)^2 + (3)^2 + (6)^2} = 7$

7. (c) Let l_1, m_1, n_1 and l_2, m_2, n_2 be the d.c of line 1 and 2 respectively, then as given

$l_1 + m_1 + n_1 = 0$

and $l_2 + m_2 + n_2 = 0$

and $l_1^2 + m_1^2 - n_1^2 = 0$ and

$l_2^2 + m_2^2 - n_2^2 = 0$

$(\because\ l + m + n = 0$ and $l^2 + m^2 - n^2 = 0)$

Angle between lines, θ is

$\cos\theta = l_1l_2 + m_1m_2 + n_1n_2$ ...(1)

As given $l^2 + m^2 = n^2$ and $l + m = -n$

$\Rightarrow (-n)^2 - 2lm = n^2 \Rightarrow 2lm = 0$ or $lm = 0$

So $l_1m_1 = 0, l_2m_2 = 0$

If $l_1 = 0, m_1 \neq 0$ then $l_1m_2 = 0$.

If $m_1 = 0, l_1 \neq 0$ then $l_2m_1 = 0$

If $l_2 = 0, m_2 \neq 0$ then $l_2m_1 = 0$

If $m_2 = 0, l_2 \neq 0$ then $l_1m_2 = 0$

Also $l_1l_2 = 0$ and $m_1m_2 = 0$

$l^2 + m^2 - n^2 = l^2 + m^2 + n^2 - 2n^2 = 0$

$\Rightarrow 1 - 2n^2 = 0 \Rightarrow n = \pm\frac{1}{\sqrt{2}}$

$\therefore\ n_1 = \pm\frac{1}{\sqrt{2}}, n_2 = \pm\frac{1}{\sqrt{2}}$

$\therefore\ \cos\theta = \frac{1}{2}\ \theta = 60°$ (acute angle)

8. (b) Direction cosines of the line :

$\ell = \cos 45° = \frac{1}{\sqrt{2}},\ m = \cos 120° = \frac{-1}{2},\ n = \cos\theta$

where θ is the angle, which line makes with positive z-axis.

Now $\ell^2 + m^2 + n^2 = 1$

$\Rightarrow \frac{1}{2} + \frac{1}{4} + \cos^2\theta = 1$

$\cos^2\theta = \frac{1}{4}$

$\Rightarrow \cos\theta = \frac{1}{2}$ (θ being acute)

$\Rightarrow \theta = \frac{\pi}{3}$

9. (b) Let $P(x_1, y_1, z_1)$ and $Q(x_2, y_2, z_2)$ be the initial and final points of the vector whose projections on the three coordinate axes are 6, – 3, 2 then

$x_2 - x_1, = 6;\ y_2 - y_1 = -3;\ z_2 - z_1 = 2$

So that direction ratios of $\overrightarrow{PQ}$ are 6, – 3, 2

$\therefore$ Direction cosines of $\overrightarrow{PQ}$ are

$\frac{6}{\sqrt{6^2 + (-3)^2 + 2^2}}, \frac{-3}{\sqrt{6^2 + (-3)^2 + 2^2}},$

$\frac{2}{\sqrt{6^2 + (-3)^2 + 2^2}} = \frac{6}{7}, \frac{-3}{7}, \frac{2}{7}$

10. (b) Let the angle of line makes with the positive direction of z-axis is α direction cosines of line with the +ve directions of x-axis, y-axis, and z-axis is l, m, n respectively.

$\therefore\ l = \cos\frac{\pi}{4}, m = \cos\frac{\pi}{4}, n = \cos\alpha$

as we know that, $l^2 + m^2 + n^2 = 1$

$\therefore\ \cos^2\frac{\pi}{4} + \cos^2\frac{\pi}{4} + \cos^2\alpha = 1$

$\Rightarrow \frac{1}{2} + \frac{1}{2} + \cos^2\alpha = 1$

$\Rightarrow \cos^2\alpha = 0 \Rightarrow \alpha = \frac{\pi}{2}$

Hence, angle with positive direction of the z-axis is $\frac{\pi}{2}$.

11. **(c)** The direction cosines of the line are $\cos\theta, \cos\beta, \cos\theta$

$\therefore \cos^2\theta + \cos^2\beta + \cos^2\theta = 1$

$\Rightarrow 2\cos^2\theta = \sin^2\beta = 3\sin^2\theta$ (given)

$\Rightarrow 2\cos^2\theta = 3 - 3\cos^2\theta$

$\therefore \cos^2\theta = \frac{3}{5}$

12. (c) Lines are coplanar

$$\begin{vmatrix} 3-1 & 2-2 & 1-(-3) \\ 1 & 2 & \lambda^2 \\ 1 & \lambda^2 & 2 \end{vmatrix} = 0$$

$$\Rightarrow \begin{vmatrix} 2 & 0 & 4 \\ 1 & 2 & \lambda^2 \\ 1 & \lambda^2 & 2 \end{vmatrix} = 0$$

$\Rightarrow 2(4-\lambda^4) + 4(\lambda^2 - 2) = 0$

$\Rightarrow 4 - \lambda^4 + 2\lambda^2 - 4 = 0$

$\Rightarrow \lambda^2(\lambda^2 - 2) = 0$

$\Rightarrow \lambda = 0, \sqrt{2}, -\sqrt{2}$

13. **(b)** Shortest distance between two lines

$\frac{x-x_1}{a_1} = \frac{y-y_1}{b_1} = \frac{z-z_1}{c_1}$ and

$\frac{x-x_2}{a_2} = \frac{y-y_2}{b_2} = \frac{z-z_2}{c_2}$ is given by,

$$\left| \frac{\begin{vmatrix} x_2-x_1 & y_2-y_1 & z_2-z_1 \\ a_1 & b_1 & c_1 \\ a_2 & b_2 & c_2 \end{vmatrix}}{\sqrt{(b_1c_2-b_2c_1)^2 + (c_1a_2-c_2a_1)^2 + (a_1b_2-a_2b_1)^2}} \right|$$

$\therefore$ The shortest distance between given lines are

$$\left| \frac{\begin{vmatrix} -2 & 4 & 5 \\ 2 & 2 & 1 \\ -1 & 8 & 4 \end{vmatrix}}{\sqrt{(8-8)^2 + (-1-8)^2 + (16+2)^2}} \right|$$

$$= \left| \frac{0-36+90}{\sqrt{405}} \right| = \frac{54}{20.1} = 2.68$$

14. **(b)** Let equation of the required line be

$\frac{x-x_1}{a} = \frac{y-y_1}{b} = \frac{z-z_1}{c}$ ...(i)

Given two lines

$\frac{x}{1} = \frac{y}{-1} = \frac{z}{1}$ ...(ii)

and $\frac{x-1}{0} = \frac{y+1}{0} = \frac{z}{1}$ ...(iii)

Since the line (i) is perpendicular to both the lines (ii) and (iii), therefore

$a - b + c = 0$ ...(iv)

$-2b + c = 0$ ...(v)

From (iv) and (v) $c = 2b$ and $a + b = 0$, which are not satisfy by options (c) and (d). Hence options (c) and (d) are rejected.

Thus point (x_1, y_1, z_1) on the required line will be either (0, 0, 0) or (1, –1, 0).

Now foot of the perpendicular from point (0, 0, 0) to the line (iii)

$= (1, -2r - 1, r)$

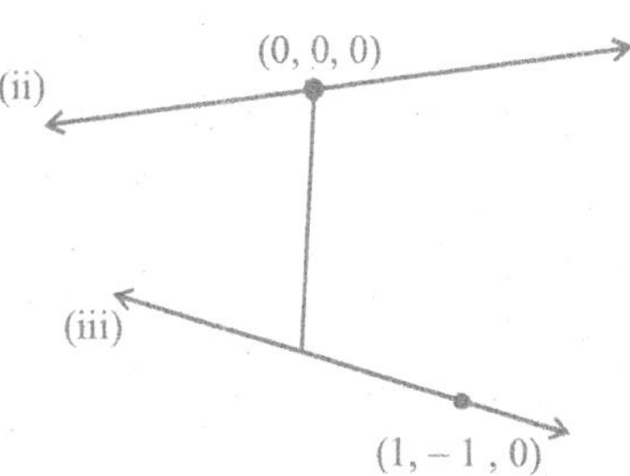

The direction ratios of the line joining the points (0, 0, 0) and $(1, -2r-1, r)$ are $1, -2r-1, r$

Since sum of the x and y-coordinate of direction ratio of the required line is 0.

$\therefore 1 - 2r - 1 = 0, \Rightarrow r = 0$

Hence direction ratio are 1, – 1, 0

But the z-direction ratio of the required line is twice the y-direction ratio of the required line

i.e. $0 = 2(-1)$, which is not true.

Hence the shortest line does not pass through the point (0, 0, 0). Therefore option (a) is also rejected.

15. **(c)** Given lines will be coplanar

If $\begin{vmatrix} -1 & 1 & 1 \\ 1 & 1 & -k \\ k & 2 & \end{vmatrix} = 0$

$\Rightarrow -1(1+2k) - (1+k^2) + 1(2-k) = 0$

$\Rightarrow k = 0, -3$

16. (d) For L_1,

$$x=\sqrt{\lambda}y+(\sqrt{\lambda}-1) \Rightarrow y=\frac{x-(\sqrt{\lambda}-1)}{\sqrt{\lambda}} \quad ...(i)$$

$$z=(\sqrt{\lambda}-1)y+\sqrt{\lambda} \Rightarrow y=\frac{z-\sqrt{\lambda}}{\sqrt{\lambda}-1} \quad ...(ii)$$

From (i) and (ii)

$$\frac{x-(\sqrt{\lambda}-1)}{\sqrt{\lambda}}=\frac{y-0}{1}=\frac{z-\sqrt{\lambda}}{\sqrt{\lambda}-1} \quad ...(A)$$

The equation (A) is the equation of line L_1.
Similarly equation of line L_2 is

$$\frac{x-(1-\sqrt{\mu})}{\sqrt{\mu}}=\frac{y-0}{1}=\frac{z-\sqrt{\mu}}{1-\sqrt{\mu}} \quad ...(B)$$

Since $L_1 \perp L_2$, therefore

$$\sqrt{\lambda}\sqrt{\mu}+1\times1+(\sqrt{\lambda}-1)(1-\sqrt{\mu})=0$$

$$\Rightarrow \sqrt{\lambda}+\sqrt{\mu}=0 \Rightarrow \sqrt{\lambda}=-\sqrt{\mu}$$

$$\Rightarrow \lambda=\mu$$

17. (a) Two given planes are coplanar, if

$$\begin{vmatrix} -2-(-1) & k-1 & 0-(-1) \\ 2 & 1 & 3 \\ 2 & 3 & 4 \end{vmatrix}=0$$

$$\Rightarrow \begin{vmatrix} -1 & k-1 & 1 \\ 2 & 1 & 3 \\ 2 & 3 & 4 \end{vmatrix}=0$$

$$\Rightarrow(-1)(4-9)-(k-1)(8-6)+6-2=0$$

$$\Rightarrow k=\frac{11}{2}$$

18. (c) Given lines are $\frac{x-1}{2}=\frac{y+1}{3}=\frac{z-1}{4}$

and $\frac{x-3}{1}=\frac{y-k}{2}=\frac{z}{1}$

Thus, $\vec{a}$, $\vec{b}$, $\vec{c}$ and $\vec{d}$ are given as

$\vec{a}(1,-1,1)$, $\vec{b}(2,3,4)$, $\vec{c}(3,k,0)$; and $\vec{d}(1,2,1)$

These lines will intersect if lines are coplanar

i.e., $\vec{a}-\vec{c}, \vec{b}$ & $\vec{d}$ are coplanar

$$\therefore \quad [\vec{a}-\vec{c}, \vec{b}, \vec{d}]=0$$

Now, $\vec{a}-\vec{c}=(3-1, k+1, 0-1)$
$=(2, k+1, -1)$

$$\Rightarrow \begin{vmatrix} 2 & k+1 & -1 \\ 2 & 3 & 4 \\ 1 & 2 & 1 \end{vmatrix}=0$$

$$\Rightarrow 2(3-8)-k+1(2-4)-1(4-3)=0$$

$$\Rightarrow 2(-5)-(k+1)(-2)-1(1)=0$$

$$\Rightarrow -10+2k+2-1=0 \Rightarrow k=\frac{9}{2}$$

19. (c) Point is (–1, 2, 6)
Line passes through the point (2, 3, –4) parallel to vector whose direction ratios is 6, 3, – 4.

Equation is $\frac{x-2}{6}=\frac{y-3}{3}=\frac{z+4}{-4}=\lambda$

Any point on this line is given by $x = 6\lambda + 2$, $y = 3\lambda + 3$, $z = -4\lambda - 4$
Now, d.Rs of line passing through (–1, 2, 6) and $\perp$ to this line is
$\{(x + 1), (y - 2), (z - 6)\}$
So, $6(x + 1) + 3(y - 2) - 4(z - 6) = 0$
$\Rightarrow 6x + 3y - 4z + 24 = 0$
Now, $6(6\lambda + 2) + 3(3\lambda + 3) + 4(4\lambda + 4) + 24 = 0$
$\Rightarrow 61\lambda + 61 = 0 \Rightarrow \lambda = -1$
So, $x = -4$, $y = 0$, $z = 0$
Now, distance between (–1, 2, 6) and (– 4, 0, 0) is
$\sqrt{9+4+36}=\sqrt{49}=7$

20. (c) On solving we will get shortest distance $\neq \sqrt{2}$

21. (d) Let the equation of AB is

$$\frac{x-1}{2}=\frac{y-(-1)}{-3}=\frac{z-(-10)}{8}=k$$

Let L be the foot of the perpendicular drawn from $P(1, 0, 0)$.

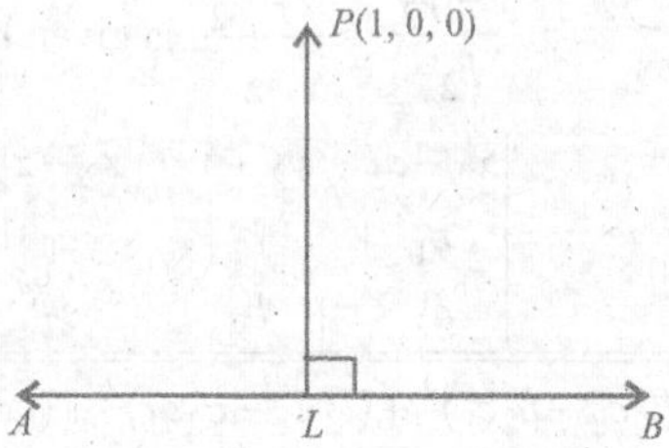

$\therefore \quad L=(2k+1, -3k-1, 8k-10)$.
Now, direction ratio of $PL=(2k, -3k-1, 8k-10)$ and direction ratio of $AB=(2, -3, 8)$
Since, PL is perpendicular to AB
$\therefore \quad 2(2k)-3(-3k-1)+8(8k-10)=0$

$$\text{Now, } k=\frac{2(1-1)+(-3)(0+1)+8(0+10)}{(2)^2+(-3)^2+(8)^2}$$

$$=\frac{0-3+80}{4+9+64}=\frac{77}{77}=1$$

$\therefore$ Required co-ordinate
$=L=(2+1, -3-1, 8-10)=(3, -4, -2)$.

22. (c) Let feet of perpendicular is

$(2\alpha, 3\alpha+2, 4\alpha+3)$

$\Rightarrow$ Direction ratio of the $\perp$ line is

$2\alpha-3, 3\alpha+3, 4\alpha-8$. and

Direction ratio of the line 2, 3, 4 are

$\Rightarrow\ 2(2\alpha-3)+3(3\alpha+3)+4(4\alpha-8)=0$

$\Rightarrow\ 29\alpha-29=0$

$\Rightarrow\ \alpha=1$

$\Rightarrow$ Feet of $\perp$ is (2, 5, 7)

$\Rightarrow$ Length $\perp$ is $\sqrt{1^2+6^2+4^2}=\sqrt{53}$

23. (a) The direction ratio of the line segment joining points A(1, 0, 7) and B(1, 6, 3) is 0, 6, –4.
The direction ratio of the given line is 1, 2, 3.
Clearly $1\times0+2\times6+3\times(-4)=0$
So, the given line is perpendicular to line AB.
Also, the mid point of A and B is (1, 3, 5) which lies on the given line.
So, the image of B in the given line is A, because the given line is the perpendicular bisector of line segment joining points A and B.

24. (c) Slope of line L $=-\dfrac{b}{5}$

Slope of line K $=-\dfrac{3}{c}$.

Line L is parallel to line k.

$\Rightarrow \dfrac{b}{5}=\dfrac{3}{c} \Rightarrow bc=15$

(13, 32) is a point on L.

$\therefore\ \dfrac{13}{5}+\dfrac{32}{b}=1 \Rightarrow \dfrac{32}{b}=-\dfrac{8}{5}$

$\Rightarrow b=-20 \Rightarrow c=-\dfrac{3}{4}$

Equation of K :

$y-4x=3 \Rightarrow 4x-y+3=0$

Distance between L and K

$=\dfrac{|52-32+3|}{\sqrt{17}}=\dfrac{23}{\sqrt{17}}$

25. (a) The two lines intersect if shortest distance between them is zero i.e.

$$\frac{(\vec{a}_2-\vec{a}_1)\cdot\vec{b}_1\times\vec{b}_2}{|\vec{b}_1\times\vec{b}_2|}=0 \Rightarrow (\vec{a}_2-\vec{a}_1)\cdot\vec{b}_1\times\vec{b}_2=0$$

where $\vec{a}_1=\hat{i}+2\hat{j}+3\hat{k}$, $\vec{b}_1=k\hat{i}+2\hat{j}+3\hat{k}$

$\vec{a}_2=2\hat{i}+3\hat{j}+\hat{k}$, $\hat{b}_2=3\hat{i}+k\hat{j}+2\hat{k}$

$$\Rightarrow \begin{vmatrix}1 & 1 & -2\\ k & 2 & 3\\ 3 & k & 2\end{vmatrix}=0$$

$\Rightarrow 1(4-3k)-1(2k-9)-2(k^2-6)=0$

$\Rightarrow -2k^2-5k+25=0 \Rightarrow k=-5$ or $\dfrac{5}{2}$

$\because$ k is an integer, therefore $k=-5$

26. (c) a, b, c are in H.P. $\Rightarrow \dfrac{1}{a},\dfrac{1}{b},\dfrac{1}{c}$ are in A.P.

$\Rightarrow \dfrac{2}{b}=\dfrac{1}{a}+\dfrac{1}{c} \Rightarrow \dfrac{1}{a}-\dfrac{2}{b}+\dfrac{1}{c}=0$

$\therefore\ \dfrac{x}{a}+\dfrac{y}{a}+\dfrac{1}{c}=0$ passes through (1, –2)

27. (b) The given lines are $2x=3y=-z$

or $\dfrac{x}{3}=\dfrac{y}{2}=\dfrac{z}{-6}$ [Dividing by 6]

and $6x=-y=-4z$

or $\dfrac{x}{2}=\dfrac{y}{-12}=\dfrac{z}{-3}$ [Dividing by 12]

$\therefore$ Angle between two lines is

$$\cos\theta=\frac{3.2+2.(-12)+(-6).(-3)}{\sqrt{3^2+2^2+(-6)^2}\ \sqrt{2^2+(-12)^2+(-3)^2}}$$

$$=\frac{6-24+18}{\sqrt{49}\ \sqrt{157}}=0 \Rightarrow \theta=90^\circ$$

28. (d) The given lines are

$x-1=\dfrac{y+3}{-\lambda}=\dfrac{z-1}{\lambda}=s$ ....(1)

and $2x=y-1=\dfrac{z-2}{-1}=t$ ....(2)

The lines are coplanar, if

$$\begin{vmatrix}0-(-1) & -1-3 & -2-(-1)\\ 1 & -\lambda & \lambda\\ \frac{1}{2} & 1 & -1\end{vmatrix}=0$$

$$c_2\to c_2+c_3;\ \begin{vmatrix}1 & -5 & -1\\ 1 & 0 & \lambda\\ \frac{1}{2} & 0 & -1\end{vmatrix}=0$$

$\Rightarrow 5(-1-\dfrac{\lambda}{2})=0 \Rightarrow \lambda=-2$

29. **(b)** Let a point on the line $x = y + a = z$ is $(\lambda, \lambda - a, \lambda)$ and a point on the line $x + a = 2y = 2z$ is $\left(\mu - a, \frac{\mu}{2}, \frac{\mu}{2}\right)$, then direction ratio of the line

joining these points are $\lambda - \mu + a,\ \lambda - a - \frac{\mu}{2},\ \lambda - \frac{\mu}{2}$

If it respresents the required line, then

$$\frac{\lambda - \mu + a}{2} = \frac{\lambda - a - \frac{\mu}{2}}{1} = \frac{\lambda - \frac{\mu}{2}}{2}$$

on solving we get $\lambda = 3a, \mu = 2a$

$\therefore$ The required points of intersection are

$(3a, 3a\text{-}a, 3a)$ and $\left(2a - a, \frac{2a}{2}, \frac{2a}{2}\right)$

or $(3a, 2a, 3a)$ and (a, a, a)

30. **(d)** $\begin{vmatrix} x_2 - x_1 & y_2 - y_1 & z_2 - z_1 \\ l_1 & m_1 & n_1 \\ l_2 & m_2 & n_2 \end{vmatrix} = 0$

$$\begin{vmatrix} 1 & -1 & -1 \\ 1 & 1 & -k \\ k & 2 & 1 \end{vmatrix} = 0 \Rightarrow \begin{vmatrix} 0 & 0 & -1 \\ 2 & 1+k & -k \\ k+2 & 1 & 1 \end{vmatrix} = 0$$

$k^2 + 3k = 0 \Rightarrow k(k+3) = 0 \ or \ k = 0 \, or - 3$

31. **(a)** $\frac{x-b}{a} = \frac{y}{1} = \frac{z-d}{c}; \frac{x-b'}{a'} = \frac{y}{1} = \frac{z-d'}{c'}.$

For perpendicularity of lines

$aa' + 1 + cc' = 0$

32. **(c)** Equation of line PQ is $\frac{x-1}{1} = \frac{y+2}{4} = \frac{z-3}{5}$

Let F be $(\lambda + 1, 4\lambda - 2, 5\lambda + 3)$

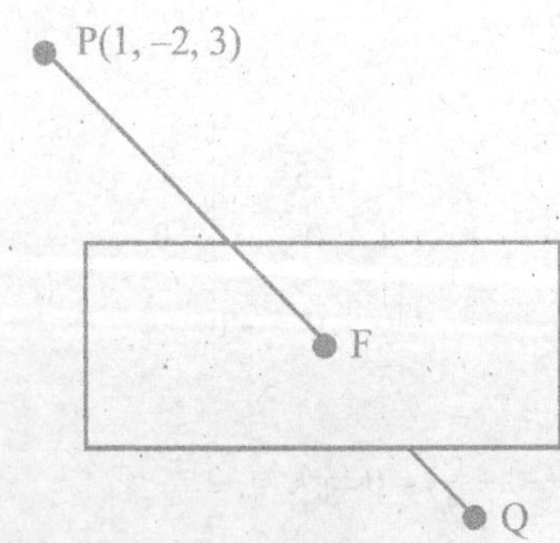

Since F lies on the plane

$\therefore 2(\lambda+1) + 3(4\lambda - 2) - 4(5\lambda + 3) + 22 = 0$

$2\lambda + 2 + 12\lambda - 6 - 20\lambda - 12 + 22 = 0$

$\Rightarrow -6\lambda + 6 = 0 \Rightarrow \lambda = 1$

$\therefore$ F is (2, 2, 8)

$PQ = 2\,PF = 2\sqrt{1^2 + 4^2 + 5^2} = 2\sqrt{42}$

33. **(c)** Let the plane be

$a(x-1) + b(y+1) + c(z+1) = 0$

Normal vector

$$\begin{vmatrix} \hat{i} & \hat{j} & \hat{k} \\ 1 & -2 & 3 \\ 2 & -1 & -1 \end{vmatrix} = 5\hat{i} + 7\hat{j} + 3\hat{k}$$

So plane is $5(x-1) + 7(y+1) + 3(z+1) = 0$

$\Rightarrow 5x + 7y + 3z + 5 = 0$

Distance of point (1, 3, –7) from the plane is

$$\frac{5 + 21 - 21 + 5}{\sqrt{25 + 49 + 9}} = \frac{10}{\sqrt{83}}$$

34. **(c)** $x + 8y + 7z = 0$

$9x + 2y + 3z = 0$

$x + y + z = 0$

$x = \lambda \quad y = 6\lambda \quad z = -7\lambda$

$x = \lambda \quad y = 6\lambda \quad z = -7\lambda$

Now, $\lambda + 12\lambda - 7\lambda = 6$; $6\lambda = 6$; $\lambda = 1$ | $\therefore\ 2\lambda + 6\lambda - 7\lambda = \lambda = 1$

35. **(a)** Suppose centroid be (h, k, ℓ)

$\therefore$ x – intp = $3h$, y – intp = $3k$, z – intp = 3ℓ

Equation $\frac{x}{3h} + \frac{y}{3k} + \frac{z}{3\ell} = 1$

$\therefore$ Distance from (0, 0, 0)

$$\left| \frac{-1}{\sqrt{\frac{1}{9h^2} + \frac{1}{9k^2} + \frac{1}{9\ell^2}}} \right| = 3$$

$$\Rightarrow \boxed{\frac{1}{x^2} + \frac{1}{y^2} + \frac{1}{z^2} = 1}$$

36. **(c)** Point $(3, -2, -\lambda)$ on p line $2x - 4y + 3z - 2 = 0$

$= 6 + 8 - 3\lambda - 2 = 0$

$= 3\lambda = 12$

$\boxed{\lambda = 4}$

Now,

$\frac{x-3}{1} = \frac{y+2}{-1} = \frac{z+4}{-2} = k_1$ ...(i)

$\frac{x-1}{12} = \frac{y}{9} = \frac{z}{4} = k_2$ ...(ii)

Point on equation (i) P $(k_1+3, -k_1-2, -2k_1-4)$
Point on equation (ii) Q $(12k_2+1, 9k_2, 4k_2)$
$k_1+3=12k_2+1 \mid -k_1-2=9k_2 \mid -2k_1-4=4k_2$
$k_2=0$
$k_1=-2$
p (1, 0, 0) lie on equation of a line 1
gives shortest distance = 0

37. (c) $\vec{n}=\vec{n_1}\times\vec{n_2}=\begin{vmatrix}\hat{i} & \hat{j} & \hat{k}\\ 6 & 7 & 8\\ 3 & 5 & 7\end{vmatrix}$

$=(9,-18,9)$
$=(1,-2,1)$

$\therefore$ Equation of plane is
$1(x+1)-2(y-1)+(z-3)=0$

$\Rightarrow$ $x-2y+z=0$

foot to z

$$\frac{x-1}{1}=\frac{y+2}{-2}=\frac{z-1}{1}=-\frac{[1+4+1]}{6}$$

$$\boxed{x=0, y=0, z=0}$$

38. (c) $\vec{n}=\vec{n_1}\times\vec{n_2}$

$$\Rightarrow \begin{vmatrix}\hat{i} & \hat{j} & \hat{k}\\ 3 & -1 & 1\\ 1 & 4 & -2\end{vmatrix}=\hat{i}(-2)-\hat{j}(-7)+\hat{k}(13)$$

$\Rightarrow$ $\vec{n}=-2\hat{i}+7\hat{j}+13\hat{k}$

Now,
$3x-y+z=1$
$x+4y-2z=2$

but $z=0$ & solving the given
$x=6/13$ & $y=5/13$

$\therefore$ required equation of a line is

$$\frac{x-6/13}{2}=\frac{y-5/13}{-7}=\frac{z}{-13}$$

39. (b) Line lies in the plane $\Rightarrow(3,-2,-4)$ lie in the plane
$\Rightarrow 3\ell-2m+4=9$ or $3\ell-2m=5$ ..... (1)
Also, ℓ, m, –1 are dr's of line perpendicular to plane and 2, –1, 3 are dr's of line lying in the plane
$\Rightarrow 2\ell-m-3=0$ or $2\ell-m=3$ .....(2)
Solving (1) and (2) we get $\ell=1$ and m = –1
$\Rightarrow \ell^2+m^2=2.$

40. (d)

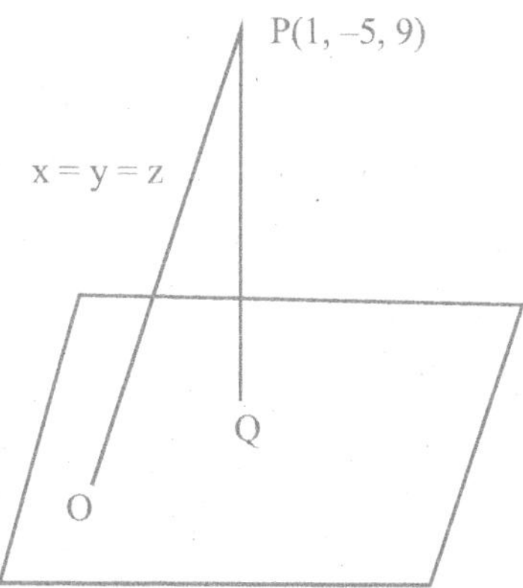

eq^n of PO : $\frac{x-1}{1}=\frac{y+5}{1}=\frac{z-9}{1}=\lambda$

$\Rightarrow x=\lambda+1;\ y=\lambda-5; z=\lambda+9.$

Putting these in eq^n of plane :-

$\lambda+1-\lambda+5+\lambda+9=5$

$\Rightarrow \lambda=-10$

$\Rightarrow$ O is $(-9,-15,-1)$

$\Rightarrow$ distance OP = $10\sqrt{3}$

41. (c) Let equation of plane be
$a(x-1)+b(y-2)+c(z-2)=0$ .....(1)
(1) is perpendicular to given planes then
$a-b+2c=0$
$2a-2b+c=0$
Solving above equation $c=0$ and $a=b$
equation of plane (1) can be
$x+y-3=0$
distance from $(1,-2,4)$ will be

$$D=\frac{|1-2-3|}{\sqrt{1+1}}=\frac{4}{\sqrt{2}}=2\sqrt{2}$$

42. (a) Equation of the plane containing the lines
$2x-5y+z=3$ and $x+y+4z=5$ is

$2x-5y+z-3+\lambda(x+y+4z-5)=0$

$\Rightarrow(2+\lambda)x+(-5+\lambda)y+(1+4\lambda)z+(-3-5\lambda)=0$ ...(i)

Since the plane (i) parallel to the given plane $x+3y+6z=1$

$$\therefore \frac{2+\lambda}{1}=\frac{-5+\lambda}{3}=\frac{1+4\lambda}{6}$$

$$\Rightarrow \lambda=-\frac{11}{2}$$

Hence equation of the required plane is

$$\left(2-\frac{11}{2}\right)x+\left(-5-\frac{11}{2}\right)y+\left(1-\frac{44}{2}\right)z+\left(-3+\frac{55}{2}\right)=0$$

$\Rightarrow (4-11)x+(-10-11)y+(2-44)z+(-6+55)=0$

$\Rightarrow -7x-21y-42z+49=0$

$\Rightarrow x+3y+6z-7=0$

$\Rightarrow x+3y+6z=7$

43. (b) General point on given line $\equiv P(3r+2, 4r-1, 12r+2)$

Point P must satisfy equation of plane

$(3r+2)-(4r-1)+(12r+2)=16$

$11r+5=16$

$r=1$

$P(3\times 1+2, 4\times 1-1, 12\times 1+2)=P(5, 3, 14)$

distance between P and (1, 0, 2)

$$D=\sqrt{(5-1)^2+3^2+(14-2)^2}=13$$

44. (b) The equation of any plane passing through given line is

$(x+y+2z-3)+\lambda(2x+3y+4z-4)=0$

$\Rightarrow (1+2\lambda)x+(1+3\lambda)y+(2+4\lambda)z-(3+4\lambda)=0$

If this plane is parallel to z–axis then normal to the plane will be perpendicular to z–axis.

$\therefore (1+2\lambda)(0)+(1+3\lambda)(0)+(2+4\lambda)(1)=0$

$\lambda=-\frac{1}{2}$

Thus, Required plane is

$(x+y+2z-3)-\frac{1}{2}(2x+3y+4z-4)=0\Rightarrow y+2=0$

$\therefore \text{S.D}=\frac{2}{\sqrt{(1)^2}}=2$

45. (c) Equation of the plane containing the given line $\frac{x-1}{1}=\frac{y-2}{5}=\frac{z-3}{4}$ is

$A(x-1)+B(y-2)+C(z-3)=0$ ...(i)

where $A+5B+4C=0$ ...(ii)

Since the point (3, 2, 0) contains in the plane (i), therefore

$2A+0.B-3C=0$ ...(iii)

From equations (ii) and (iii),

$$\frac{A}{-15-0}=\frac{B}{6+3}=\frac{C}{0-10}=k \text{ (let)}$$

$\Rightarrow A=-15k, B=9k$ and $C=-10k$

Putting the value of A, B and C in equation (i), we get

$-15(x-1)+9(y-2)-10(z-3)=0$...(iv)

Now the coordinates of the point (0, –3, 1) satisfy the equation of the plane (iv) as

$-15(0-1)+9(-3-2)-10(1-3)$

$=15-45+20=0$

Hence the point (0, –3, 1) contains in the plane.

46. (c) $|3+4-12\lambda+13|=|-9+0-12+13|$

$\Rightarrow |-12\lambda+20|=|8|$

$\Rightarrow |3\lambda-5|=2$

$\Rightarrow 9\lambda^2+25-30\lambda=4$

$\Rightarrow 9\lambda^2-30\lambda+21=0$

$\Rightarrow 3\lambda^2-10\lambda+7=0$

47. (c) Plane passing through $x+y+z+1=0$ and $2x-y+z+3=0$ is $x+y+z+1+\lambda(2x-y+z+3)=0$

$\Rightarrow (2\lambda+1)x+(1-\lambda)y+(1+\lambda)z+3\lambda+1=0$

Parallel to the given line if

$\alpha(2\lambda+1)-1(1-\lambda)+1(1+\lambda)=0$

$\Rightarrow \alpha=\frac{-2\lambda}{2\lambda+1}$ ...(i)

Also, $\left|\frac{2\lambda+1-(1-\lambda)+0+3\lambda+1}{\sqrt{(2\lambda+1)^2+(1-\lambda)^2+(1+\lambda)^2}}\right|=\frac{1}{\sqrt{3}}$

$\Rightarrow \lambda=0, \frac{-32}{102}; \alpha=0 \text{ or } \alpha=\frac{32}{19}$

48. (c) $\frac{a-1}{2}=\frac{b-3}{-1}=\frac{c-4}{1}=\lambda$(let)

$\Rightarrow a=2\lambda+1$

$b=3-\lambda$

$c=4+\lambda$

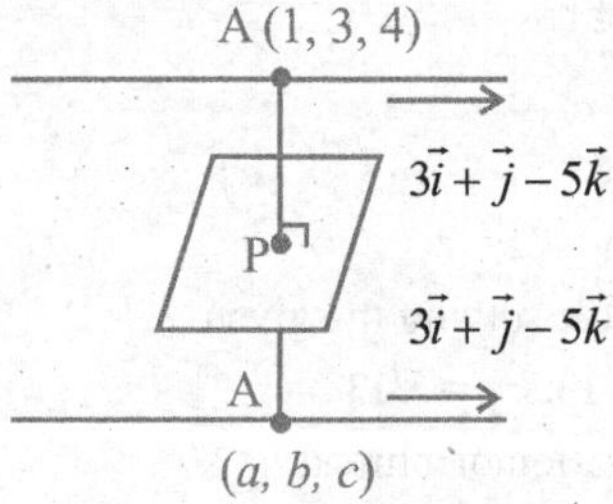

$$P=\left(\frac{a+1}{2},\frac{b+3}{2},\frac{c+4}{2}\right)=\left(\lambda+1,\frac{6-\lambda}{2},\frac{\lambda+8}{2}\right)$$

$\therefore 2(\lambda+1)-\frac{6-\lambda}{2}+\frac{\lambda+8}{2}+3=0$

$3\lambda+6=0\Rightarrow\lambda=-2$

$a=-3, b=5, c=2$

Required line is $\frac{x+3}{3}=\frac{y-5}{1}=\frac{z-2}{-5}$

49. (c) Given equation of line can be written as

$$\frac{x+1}{1}=\frac{y}{2}=\frac{z+4}{2}$$

Eqn of plane is $2x-y+\sqrt{\lambda}z+4=0$

Since, angle between the line and the plane is $\frac{\pi}{6}$

therefore

$$\sin\frac{\pi}{6}=\frac{2(1)+2(-1)+2(\sqrt{\lambda})}{\sqrt{1+4+4}\sqrt{4+1+\lambda}}$$

$$\frac{1}{2}=\frac{2-2+2\sqrt{\lambda}}{\sqrt{9}\sqrt{5+\lambda}}$$

$$\Rightarrow \frac{\sqrt{\lambda}}{\sqrt{5+\lambda}}=\frac{3}{4}\Rightarrow\frac{\lambda}{5+\lambda}=\frac{9}{16}$$

$$\Rightarrow 7\lambda=45\Rightarrow\lambda=\frac{45}{7}$$

50. (c) Given planes are

$4x-2y-4z+1=0$

and $4x-2y-4z+d=0$

They are parallel.

Distance between them is $\pm 7=\frac{d-1}{\sqrt{16+4+16}}$

$$\Rightarrow \frac{d-1}{6}=\pm 7\Rightarrow d=42+1$$

or $-42+1$ i.e. $d=-41$ or 43.

51. (b) Given two planes :

$x-ay-b=0$ and $cy-z+d=0$

Let, l, m, n be the direction ratio of the required line.

Since the required line is perpendicular to normal of both the plane, therefore $l-am=0$ and $cm-n=0$

$\Rightarrow l-am+0.n=0$ and $0.l+cm-n=0$

$$\therefore \frac{l}{a-0}=\frac{m}{0+1}=\frac{n}{c-0}$$

Hence, d.R of the required line are a, 1, c.

Hence, options (c) and (d) are rejected.

Now, the point $(a+b, 1, c+d)$ satisfy the equation of the two given planes.

$\therefore$ Option (b) is correct.

52. (b) Equation of the plane containing the line

$$\frac{x-1}{1}=\frac{y-2}{2}=\frac{z-3}{3}\text{ is}$$

$a(x-1)+b(y-2)+c(z-3)=0$ .... (i)

where $a.1+b.2+c.3=0$

i.e., $a+2b+3c=0$ .... (ii)

Since the plane (i) parallel to the line

$$\frac{x}{1}=\frac{y}{1}=\frac{z}{4}$$

$\therefore$ $a.1+b.1+c.4=0$

i.e., $a+b+4c=0$ .... (iii)

From (ii) and (iii),

$$\frac{a}{8-3}=\frac{b}{3-4}=\frac{c}{1-2}=k\text{ (let)}$$

$\therefore$ $a=5k,\ b=-k,\ c=-k$

On putting the value of a, b and c in equation (i),

$5(x-1)-(y-2)-(z-3)=0$

$\Rightarrow$ $5x-y-z=0$ .... (iv)

when $x=1$, $y=0$ and $z=5$; then

L.H.S. of equation (iv) $=5x-y-2$

$=5\times 1-0-5$

$=0$

$=$ R.H.S. of equation (iv)

Hence coordinates of the point (1, 0, 5) satisfy the equation plane represented by equations (iv),

Therefore the plane passes through the point (1,0,5)

53. (c) Given equation of lines are

$$\frac{x-1}{3}=\frac{y-2}{1}=\frac{z-3}{2}\quad ...(1)$$

$$\text{and}\quad\frac{x-3}{1}=\frac{y-1}{2}=\frac{z-2}{3}\quad ...(2)$$

Any point on line (1) is P $(3\lambda+1, \lambda+2, 2\lambda+3)$ and on line (2) is Q $(\mu+3, 2\mu+1, 3\mu+2)$.

On solving $3\lambda+1=\mu+3$ and $\lambda+2=2\mu+1$

we get $\lambda=1$, $\mu=1$

$\therefore$ Point of intersection of two lines is R (4, 3, 5)

So, equation of plane $\perp$ to OR where O is (0, 0, 0) and passing through R is

$4x+3y+5z=50$

54. (c) $2x+y+2z-8=0$ ...(Plane 1)

$2x+y+2z+\frac{5}{2}=0$ ...(Plane 2)

Distance between Plane 1 and 2

$$=\left|\frac{-8-\frac{5}{2}}{\sqrt{2^2+1^2+2^2}}\right|=\left|\frac{-21}{6}\right|=\frac{7}{2}$$

55. (c) Equation of a plane through the line of intersection of the planes

$x+2y=3, y-2z+1=0$ is

$(x+2y-3)+\lambda(y-2z+1)=0$

$\Rightarrow x+(2+\lambda)y-2\lambda(z)-3+\lambda=0$ (i)

Now, plane (i) is $\perp$ to $x+2y=3$

$\therefore$ Their dot product is zero

i.e. $1+2(2+\lambda)=0\Rightarrow\lambda=-\frac{5}{2}$

Thus, required plane is

$$x+\left(2-\frac{5}{2}\right)y-2\times\frac{-5}{2}(z)-3-\frac{5}{2}=0$$

$$\Rightarrow x-\frac{y}{2}+5z-\frac{11}{2}=0$$

$$\Rightarrow 2x-y+10z-11=0$$

56. (c) Let P be the image of O in the given plane.

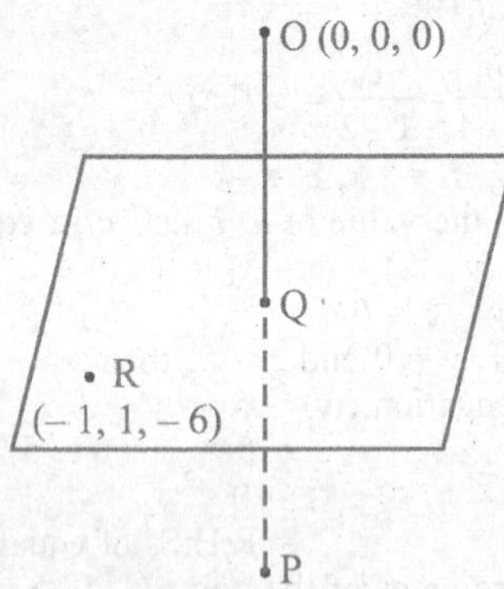

Equation of the plane, $4x-3y+z+13=0$

OP is normal to the plane, therefore direction ratio of OP are proportional to 4, – 3, 1

Since OP passes through (0, 0, 0) and has direction ratio proportional to 4, –3, 1. Therefore equation of OP is

$$\frac{x-0}{4}=\frac{y-0}{-3}=\frac{z-0}{1}=r \text{ (let)}$$

$\therefore x=4r, y=-3r, z=r$

Let the coordinate of P be $(4r, -3r, r)$

Since Q be the mid point of OP

$$\therefore Q=\left(2r,-\frac{3}{2}r,\frac{r}{2}\right)$$

Since Q lies in the given plane

$4x-3y+z+13=0$

$$\therefore 8r+\frac{9}{2}r+\frac{r}{2}+13=0$$

$$\Rightarrow r=\frac{-13}{8+\frac{9}{2}+\frac{1}{2}}=\frac{-26}{26}=-1$$

$$\therefore Q=\left(-2,\frac{3}{2},-\frac{1}{2}\right)$$

$$QR=\sqrt{(-1+2)^2+\left(1-\frac{3}{2}\right)^2+\left(-6+\frac{1}{2}\right)^2}$$

$$=\sqrt{1+\frac{1}{4}+\frac{121}{4}}=3\sqrt{\frac{7}{2}}$$

57. (b) Direction cosines of $\vec{n}$ are $\frac{1}{2},\frac{1}{4},\frac{1}{2}$.

Equation of the plane,

$$\frac{1}{2}(x-\sqrt{2})+\frac{1}{4}(y+1)+\frac{1}{2}(z-1)=0$$

$$\Rightarrow 2(x-\sqrt{2})+(y+1)+2(z-1)=0$$

$$\Rightarrow 2x+y+2z=2\sqrt{2}-1+2$$

$$\Rightarrow 2x+y+2z=2\sqrt{2}+1$$

58. (a) Given equation of a plane is $x-2y+2z-5=0$

So, Equation of parallel plane is given by $x-2y+2z+d=0$

Now, it is given that distance from origin to the parallel plane is 1.

$$\therefore \left|\frac{d}{\sqrt{1^2+2^2+2^2}}\right|=1 \Rightarrow d=\pm 3$$

So equation of required plane

$$x-2y+2z\pm 3=0$$

59. (a) The equation of the plane containing the line $\frac{x+1}{-3}=\frac{y-3}{2}=\frac{z+2}{1}$ is a $(x + 1) + b\ (y - 3) + c\ (z + 2) = 0$ where

$-3a+2b+c=0$ ...(A)

This passes through (0, 7, – 7)

$\therefore a\ (0+1)+b\ (7-3)+c\ (-7+2)=0$

$\Rightarrow a+4b-5c=0$ ...(B)

On solving equation (A) and (B) we get

$a=1, b=1, c=1$

$\therefore$ Required plane is

$x+1+y-3+z+2=0$

$\Rightarrow x+y+z=0$

60. (d) Given planes are

$P: x+y-2z+7=0$

$Q: x+y+2z+2=0$

and $R: 3x+3y-6z-11=0$

Consider Plane P and R.

Here $a_1=1, b_1=1, c_1=-2$

and $a_2=3, b_2=3, c_2=-6$

Since, $\frac{a_1}{a_2}=\frac{b_1}{b_2}=\frac{c_1}{c_2}=\frac{1}{3}$

therefore P and R are parallel.

61. (b) Let the direction ratios of the common line be l, m and n.

$\therefore\ l\times 1+m\times 0+n\times 0=0 \Rightarrow l=0$ ....(1)

$2l-5ma+3n=0 \Rightarrow 5ma-3n=0$ ....(2)

$3lb+m-3n=0 \Rightarrow m-3n=0$ ....(3)

Subtracting (3) from (1), we get

$m(5a-1)=0$

Now, value of m can not be zero because if $m=0$ then $n=0$

$\Rightarrow l=m=n=0$ which is not possible.

Hence, $5a-1=0 \Rightarrow a=\frac{1}{5}$

Thus, option (b) is correct.

62. **(c)** Point P is $(2, -1, 2)$

Let this line meet at $Q(h, k, w)$

Direction ratio of this line is

$(h-2, k+1, w-2)$

Since, dc_s are equal & dr_s are also equal,

So, $h-2 = k+1+w-2$

$\Rightarrow k = h-3$ and $w = h$

This line meets the plane

$2x+y+z=9$ at Q, so,

$2h+k+w=9$ or $2h+h-3+h=9$

$\Rightarrow 4h-3=9 \Rightarrow h=3$

and $k=0$ and $w=3$

Distance

$$PQ = \sqrt{(3-2)^2+(0-(-1))^2+(3-2)^2}$$

$$= \sqrt{1^2+1^2+1^2} = \sqrt{3}$$

63. **(d)** Given equation of plane is

$3x+4y-12z+13=0$

$(1, a, 1)$ and $(-3, 0, a)$ satisfy the equation of plane.

$\therefore$ We have

$3+4(a)-12+13=0$ and $3(-3)-12(a)+13=0$

$\Rightarrow 4+4a=0$ and $4-12a=0$

$\Rightarrow a=-1$ and $a=\frac{1}{3}$

Since, $(1, a, 1)$ and $(-3, 0, a)$ lie on the opposite sides of the plane $\therefore a=0$

64. **(a)** Equation of line through $P(1,-5,9)$ and parallel to the plane $x=y=z$ is

$$\frac{x-1}{1}=\frac{y+5}{1}=\frac{z-9}{1}=\lambda(say)$$

$Q=(x=1+\lambda, y=-5+\lambda, z=9+\lambda)$

Given plane $x-y+z=5$

$\therefore 1+\lambda+5-\lambda+9+\lambda=5$

$\Rightarrow \lambda=-10$

$\therefore Q=(-9,-15,-1)$

$$\therefore PQ=\sqrt{(1+9)^2+(15-5)^2+(9+1)^2}$$

$$=\sqrt{300}=10\sqrt{3}$$

65. **(d)** If θ be the angle between the given line and plane, then

$$\sin\theta = \frac{1\times1+2\times2+\lambda\times3}{\sqrt{1^2+2^2+\lambda^2}.\sqrt{1^2+2^2+3^2}}$$

$$=\frac{5+3\lambda}{\sqrt{14}.\sqrt{5+\lambda^2}}$$

$$\Rightarrow \cos\theta = \sqrt{1-\frac{(5+3\lambda)^2}{14(5+\lambda^2)}}$$

$$\therefore \theta = \cos^{-1}\sqrt{1-\frac{(5+3\lambda)^2}{14(5+\lambda^2)}}$$

But it is given that $\theta = \cos^{-1}\sqrt{\frac{5}{14}}$

$$\therefore \sqrt{1-\frac{(5+3\lambda)^2}{14(5+\lambda^2}} = \sqrt{\frac{5}{14}}$$

$$\Rightarrow \lambda = \frac{2}{3}$$

66. **(a)** A(3, 1, 6); B = (1, 3, 4)

Mid-point of AB = (2, 2, 5) lies on the plane.

and d.r's of AB = (2, –2, 2)

d.r's of normal to plane = (1, –1, 1).

Direction ratio of AB and normal to the plane are proportional therefore,

AB is perpendicular to the plane

$\therefore$ A is image of B

Statement-2 is correct but it is not correct explanation.

67. **(a)** $\because$ The line $\frac{x-2}{3}=\frac{y-1}{-5}=\frac{z+2}{2}$ lie in the plane

$x+3y-\alpha z+\beta=0$

$\therefore Pt\,(2, 1, -2)$ lies on the plane

i.e. $2+3+2\alpha+\beta=0$

or $2\alpha+\beta+5=0$ ....(i)

Also normal to plane will be perpendicular to line,

$\therefore 3\times1-5\times3+2\times(-\alpha)=0$

$\Rightarrow \alpha=-6$

From equation (i) then, $\beta=7$

$\therefore (\alpha, \beta)=(-6, 7)$

68. **(c)** Equation of line through $(5, 1, a)$ and $(3, b, 1)$ is $\frac{x-5}{-2}=\frac{y-1}{b-1}=\frac{z-a}{1-a}=\lambda$

$\therefore$ Any point on this line is a

$[-2\lambda+5, (b-1)\lambda+1, (1-a)\lambda+a]$

It crosses yz plane where $-2\lambda+5=0$

$$\lambda=\frac{5}{2}$$

$$\therefore \left(0,(b-1)\frac{5}{2}+1,(1-a)\frac{5}{2}+a\right)=\left(0,\frac{17}{2},\frac{-13}{2}\right)$$

$$\Rightarrow (b-1)\frac{5}{2}+1=\frac{17}{2} \text{ and } (1-a)\frac{5}{2}+a=-\frac{13}{2}$$

$\Rightarrow b=4$ and $a=6$

69. **(c)** Let the direction cosines of line L be l, m, n, then

$2l+3m+n=0$ ....(i)

and $l+3m+2n=0$ ....(ii)

on solving equation (i) and (ii), we get

$$\frac{l}{6-3}=\frac{m}{1-4}=\frac{n}{6-3} \Rightarrow \frac{l}{3}=\frac{m}{-3}=\frac{n}{3}$$

$$\text{Now } \frac{l}{3}=\frac{m}{-3}=\frac{n}{3}=\frac{\sqrt{l^2+m^2+n^2}}{\sqrt{3^2+(-3)^2+3^2}}$$

$\because l^2+m^2+n^2=1$

$\therefore \frac{l}{3}=\frac{m}{-3}=\frac{n}{3}=\frac{1}{\sqrt{27}}$

$\Rightarrow l=\frac{3}{\sqrt{27}}=\frac{1}{\sqrt{3}}, m=-\frac{1}{\sqrt{3}}, n=\frac{1}{\sqrt{3}}$

Line L, makes an angle α with +ve x-axis

$\therefore l=\cos\alpha \Rightarrow \cos\alpha=\frac{1}{\sqrt{3}}$

70. (d) If (α, β, γ) be the image, then mid point of (α, β, γ) and $(-1, 3, 4)$ must lie on $x-2y=0$

$\therefore \frac{\alpha-1}{2}-2\left(\frac{\beta+3}{2}\right)=0$

$\therefore \alpha-1-2\beta-6=0 \Rightarrow \alpha-2\beta=7 \ldots(1)$

Also line joining (α, β, γ) and $(-1, 3, 4)$ should be parallel to the normal of the plane $x-2y=0$

$\therefore \frac{\alpha+1}{1}=\frac{\beta-3}{-2}=\frac{\gamma-4}{0}=\lambda$

$\Rightarrow \alpha=\lambda-1, \beta=-2\lambda+3, \gamma=4 \ldots(2)$

From (1) and (2)

$\alpha=\frac{9}{5}, \ \beta=-\frac{13}{5}, \gamma=4$

None of the option matches.

71. (b) The given line is $\vec{r}=2\vec{i}-2\vec{j}+3\vec{k}+\lambda(\vec{i}-\vec{j}+4\vec{k})$

and the plane is $\vec{r}\cdot(\vec{i}+5\vec{j}+\vec{k})=5$

or $x+5y+z=5$

Required distance $=\left|\frac{2-10-2+3-5}{\sqrt{1+25+1}}\right|=\frac{10}{3\sqrt{3}}$

72. (a) If θ is the angle between line and plane then $\left(\frac{\pi}{2}-\theta\right)$ is the angle between line and normal to plane given by

$$\cos\left(\frac{\pi}{2}-\theta\right)=\frac{(\hat{i}+2\hat{j}+2\hat{k}).(2\hat{i}-\hat{j}+\sqrt{\lambda}\hat{k})}{3\sqrt{4+1+\lambda}}$$

$$\cos\left(\frac{\pi}{2}-\theta\right)=\frac{2-2+2\sqrt{\lambda}}{3\times\sqrt{5+\lambda}}$$

$$\Rightarrow \sin\theta=\frac{2\sqrt{\lambda}}{3\sqrt{5+\lambda}}=\frac{1}{3}\Rightarrow 4\lambda=5+\lambda$$

$$\Rightarrow \lambda=\frac{5}{3}.$$

73. (c) The planes are $2x+y+2z-8=0$. ...(1)

and $4x+2y+4z+5=0$

or $2x+y+2z+\frac{5}{2}=0$ ...(2)

$\therefore$ Distance between (1) and (2)

$$=\left|\frac{\frac{5}{2}+8}{\sqrt{2^2+1^2+2^2}}\right|=\left|\frac{21}{2\sqrt{9}}\right|=\frac{7}{2}$$

74. (a) Eq. of planes be $\frac{x}{a}+\frac{y}{b}+\frac{z}{c}=1$ & $\frac{x}{a'}+\frac{y}{b'}+\frac{z}{c'}=1$

($\perp r$ distance on plane from origin is same.)

$$\left|\frac{-1}{\sqrt{\frac{1}{a^2}+\frac{1}{b^2}+\frac{1}{c^2}}}\right|=\left|\frac{-1}{\sqrt{\frac{1}{a'^2}+\frac{1}{b'^2}+\frac{1}{c'^2}}}\right|$$

$$\frac{1}{a^2}+\frac{1}{b^2}+\frac{1}{c^2}-\frac{1}{a'^2}-\frac{1}{b'^2}-\frac{1}{c'^2}=0$$

75. (b) Equation of plane through (1, 0, 0) is

$a(x-1)+by+cz=0$ ...(i)

(i) passes through (0, 1, 0).

$-a+b=0 \Rightarrow b=a$; Also,

$\cos 45°=\frac{a+a}{\sqrt{2(2a^2+c^2)}} \Rightarrow 2a=\sqrt{2a^2+c^2}$

$\Rightarrow 2a^2=c^2 \quad \Rightarrow c=\sqrt{2}a$.

So d.r of normal are a, a $\sqrt{2}a$ i.e. 1, 1, $\sqrt{2}$.

76. (a) As the point (3, 2, 0) lies on the given line

$\frac{x-4}{1}=\frac{y-7}{5}=\frac{z-4}{4}$

$\therefore$ There can be infinite many planes passing through this line. But here out of the four options only first option is satisfied by the coordinates of both the points (3, 2, 0) and (4, 7, 4)

$\therefore x-y+z=1$ is the required plane.

77. (c) We know that equation of sphere is

$x^2+y^2+z^2+2ux+2vy+2wz+d=0$

where centre is $(-u, -v, -w)$

given $x^2+y^2+z^2-6x-12y-2z+20=0$

$\therefore$ centre $\equiv(3, 6, 1)$

Coordinates of one end of diameter of the sphere are (2, 3, 5). Let the coordinates of the other end of diameter are (α, β, γ)

$\therefore \frac{\alpha+2}{2}=3, \frac{\beta+3}{2}=6, \frac{\gamma+5}{2}=1$

$\Rightarrow \alpha=4, \beta=9$ and $\gamma=-3$

$\therefore$ Coordinate of other end of diameter are (4, 9, –3)

78. (b)

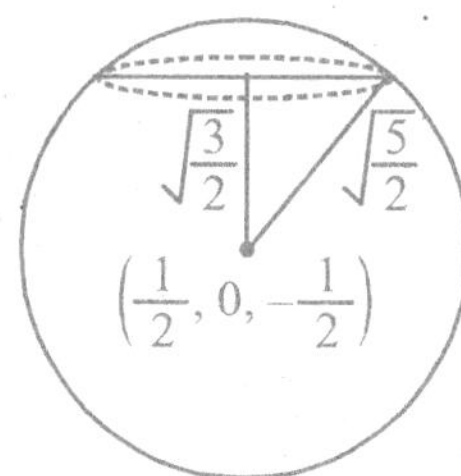

Perpendicular distance of centre $\left(\frac{1}{2}, 0, -\frac{1}{2}\right)$ from $x + 2y - 2 = 4$ is given by

$$\frac{\left|\frac{1}{2} + \frac{1}{2} - 4\right|}{\sqrt{6}} = \sqrt{\frac{3}{2}}$$

radius of sphere $= \sqrt{\frac{1}{4} + \frac{1}{4} + 2} = \sqrt{\frac{5}{2}}$

$\therefore$ radius of circle $= \sqrt{\frac{5}{2} - \frac{3}{2}} = 1$.

79. (c) Plane $2ax - 3ay + 4az + 6 = 0$ passes through the mid point of the centre of spheres

$x^2 + y^2 + z^2 + 6x - 8y - 2z = 13$ and

$x^2 + y^2 + z^2 - 10x + 4y - 2z = 8$ respectively centre of spheres are $(-3, 4, 1)$ and $(5, -2, 1)$. Mid point of centres is $(1, 1, 1)$.

Satisfying this in the equation of plane, we get

$2a - 3a + 4a + 6 = 0$

$\Rightarrow a = -2$.

80. (a) The equations of spheres are

$S_1 : x^2 + y^2 + z^2 + 7x - 2y - z - 13 = 0$ *and*

$S_2 : x^2 + y^2 + z^2 - 3x + 3y + 4z - 8 = 0$

Their plane of intersection is

$S_1 - S_2 = 0 \Rightarrow 10x - 5y - 5z - 5 = 0$

$\Rightarrow 2x - y - z = 1$

81. (d)

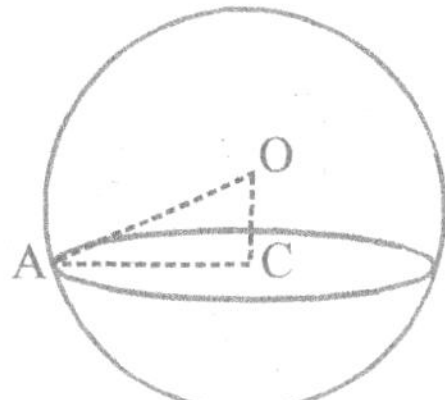

centre of sphere = (-1, 1, 2)

Radius of sphere $\sqrt{1+1+4+19} = 5$

Perpendicular distance from centre to the plane

$$OC = d = \left|\frac{-1+2+4+7}{\sqrt{1+4+4}}\right| = \frac{12}{3} = 4.$$

$AC^2 = AO^2 - OC^2 = 5^2 - 4^2 = 9$

$\Rightarrow AC = 3$

82. (d) Shortest distance = perpendicular distance between the plane and sphere = distance of plane from centre of sphere – radius

$$= \left|\frac{-2\times12 + 4\times1 + 3\times3 - 327}{\sqrt{144+9+16}}\right| - \sqrt{4+1+9+155}$$

$= 26 - 13 = 13$

Chapter 27

Probability

TOPIC-1 : Multiplication Theorem on Probability, Independent events, Conditional Probability, Baye's Theorem

1. If two different numbers are taken from the set (0, 1, 2, 3, ..., 10), then the probability that their sum as well as absolute difference are both multiple of 4, is : **[2017]**

(a) $\frac{7}{55}$ (b) $\frac{6}{55}$

(c) $\frac{12}{55}$ (d) $\frac{14}{55}$

2. Let E and F be two independent events. The probability that both E and F happen is $\frac{1}{12}$ and the probability that neither E nor F happens is $\frac{1}{2}$, then a value of $\frac{P(E)}{P(F)}$ is : **[Online April 9, 2017]**

(a) $\frac{4}{3}$ (b) $\frac{3}{2}$

(c) $\frac{1}{3}$ (d) $\frac{5}{12}$

3. Three persons P, Q and R independently try to hit a target. If the probabilities of their hitting the target are $\frac{3}{4}, \frac{1}{2}$ and $\frac{5}{8}$ respectively, then the probability that the target is hit by P or Q but not by R is : **[Online April 8, 2017]**

(a) $\frac{21}{64}$ (b) $\frac{9}{64}$

(c) $\frac{15}{64}$ (d) $\frac{39}{64}$

4. An unbiased coin is tossed eight times. The probability of obtaining at least one head and at least one tail is : **[Online April 8, 2017]**

(a) $\frac{255}{256}$ (b) $\frac{127}{128}$

(c) $\frac{63}{64}$ (d) $\frac{1}{2}$

5. Let two fair six-faced dice A and B be thrown simultaneously. If E_1 is the event that die A shows up four, E_2 is the event that die B shows up two and E_3 is the event that the sum of numbers on both dice is odd, then which of the following statements is NOT true ? **[2016]**

(a) E_1 and E_3 are independent.
(b) E_1, E_2 and E_3 are independent.
(c) E_1 and E_2 are independent.
(d) E_2 and E_3 are independent.

6. If A and B are any two events such that $P(A)=\frac{2}{5}$ and $P(A \cap B)=\frac{3}{20}$, then the conditional probability, $P(A \mid A' \cup B'))$, where A' denotes the complement of A, is equal to : **[Online April 9, 2016]**

(a) $11/20$ (b) $5/17$

(c) $8/17$ (d) $1/4$

7. Let X be a set containing 10 elements and P(X) be its power set. If A and B are picked up at random from P(X), with replacement, then the probability that A and B have equal number elements, is : **[Online April 10, 2015]**

(a) $\frac{\left(2^{10}-1\right)}{2^{10}}$ (b) $\frac{{}^{20}C_{10}}{2^{10}}$

(c) $\frac{\left(2^{10}-1\right)}{2^{20}}$ (d) $\frac{{}^{20}C_{10}}{2^{20}}$

8. Let A and B be two events such that $P\left(\overline{A \cup B}\right)=\frac{1}{6}$, $P\left(\overline{A \cap B}\right)=\frac{1}{4}$ and $P\left(\overline{A}\right)=\frac{1}{4}$, where $\overline{A}$ stands for the complement of the event A. Then the events A and B are **[2014]**
(a) independent but not equally likely.
(b) independent and equally likely.
(c) mutually exclusive and independent.
(d) equally likely but not independent.

9. Let A and E be any two events with positive probabilities:
Statement - 1: $P(E/A) \geq P(A/E)\,P(E)$
Statement - 2: $P(A/E) \geq P(A \cap E)$
[Online April 19, 2014]
(a) Both the statements are true
(b) Both the statements are false
(c) Statement-1 is true, Statement-2 is false
(d) Statement-1 is false, Statement-2 is true

10. A, B, C try to hit a target simultaneously but independently. Their respective probabilities of hitting the targets are $\frac{3}{4}, \frac{1}{2}, \frac{5}{8}$. The probability that the target is hit by A or B but not by C is : **[Online April 23, 2013]**
(a) 21/64 (b) 7/8
(c) 7/32 (d) 9/64

11. Given two independent events, if the probability that exactly one of them occurs is $\frac{26}{49}$ and the probability that none of them occurs is $\frac{15}{49}$, then the probability of more probable of the two events is : **[Online April 22, 2013]**
(a) 4/7 (b) 6/7
(c) 3/7 (d) 5/7

12. The probability of a man hitting a target is $\frac{2}{5}$. He fires at the target k times (k, a given number). Then the minimum k, so that the probability of hitting the target at least once is more than $\frac{7}{10}$, is : **[Online April 9, 2013]**
(a) 3 (b) 5
(c) 2 (d) 4

13. Three numbers are chosen at random without replacement from {1,2,3,..8}. The probability that their minimum is 3, given that their maximum is 6, is : **[2012]**
(a) $\frac{3}{8}$ (b) $\frac{1}{5}$
(c) $\frac{1}{4}$ (d) $\frac{2}{5}$

14. Let A, B, C, be pairwise independent events with $P(C) > 0$ and $P(A \cap B \cap C) = 0$. Then $P\left(A^c \cap B^c / C\right)$. **[2011RS]**
(a) $P\left(B^c\right) - P(B)$ (b) $P\left(A^c\right) + P\left(B^c\right)$
(c) $P\left(A^c\right) - P\left(B^c\right)$ (d) $P\left(A^c\right) - P(B)$

15. If C and D are two events such that $C \subset D$ and $P(D) \neq 0$, then the correct statement among the following is **[2011]**
(a) $P(C \mid D) \geq P(C)$ (b) $P(C \mid D) < P(C)$
(c) $P(C \mid D) = \frac{P(D)}{P(C)}$ (d) $P(C \mid D) = P(C)$

16. One ticket is selected at random from 50 tickets numbered 00,01,02,...,49. Then the probability that the sum of the digits on the selected ticket is 8, given that the product of these digits is zero, equals: **[2009]**
(a) $\frac{1}{7}$ (b) $\frac{5}{14}$
(c) $\frac{1}{50}$ (d) $\frac{1}{14}$

17. It is given that the events A and B are such that $P(A) = \frac{1}{4}, P(A \mid B) = \frac{1}{2}$ and $P(B \mid A) = \frac{2}{3}$. Then $P(B)$ is **[2008]**
(a) $\frac{1}{6}$ (b) $\frac{1}{3}$
(c) $\frac{2}{3}$ (d) $\frac{1}{2}$

18. Two aeroplanes I and II bomb a target in succession. The probabilities of I and II scoring a hit correctly are 0.3 and 0.2, respectively. The second plane will bomb only if the first misses the target. The probability that the target is hit by the second plane is **[2007]**
(a) 0.2 (b) 0.7
(c) 0.06 (d) 0.14.

19. Three houses are available in a locality. Three persons apply for the houses. Each applies for one house without consulting others. The probability that all the three apply for the same house is **[2005]**

(a) $\frac{2}{9}$ (b) $\frac{1}{9}$

(c) $\frac{8}{9}$ (d) $\frac{7}{9}$

20. Let A and B be two events such that $P(\overline{A \cup B}) = \frac{1}{6}$, $P(A \cap B) = \frac{1}{4}$ and $P(\bar{A}) = \frac{1}{4}$, where $\bar{A}$ stands for complement of event A. Then events A and B are **[2005]**

(a) equally likely and mutually exclusive
(b) equally likely but not independent
(c) independent but not equally likely
(d) mutually exclusive and independent

21. The probability that A speaks truth is $\frac{4}{5}$, while the probability for B is $\frac{3}{4}$. The probability that they contradict each other when asked to speak on a fact is **[2004]**

(a) $\frac{4}{5}$ (b) $\frac{1}{5}$

(c) $\frac{7}{20}$ (d) $\frac{3}{20}$

22. A problem in mathematics is given to three students A, B, C and their respective probability of solving the problem is $\frac{1}{2}, \frac{1}{3}$ and $\frac{1}{4}$. Probability that the problem is solved is **[2002]**

(a) $\frac{3}{4}$ (b) $\frac{1}{2}$

(c) $\frac{2}{3}$ (d) $\frac{1}{3}$

TOPIC-2 : Random Variables, Probability Distribution, Bernoulli Trails, Binomial Distribution, Poisson Distribution

23. A box contains 15 green and 10 yellow balls. If 10 balls are randomly drawn, one-by-one, with replacement, then the variance of the number of green balls drawn is : **[2017]**

(a) $\frac{6}{25}$ (b) $\frac{12}{5}$

(c) 6 (d) 4

24. An experiment succeeds twice as often as it fails. The probability of at least 5 successes in the six trials of this experiment is : **[Online April 10, 2016]**

(a) $\frac{496}{729}$ (b) $\frac{192}{729}$

(c) $\frac{240}{729}$ (d) $\frac{256}{729}$

25. If the mean and the variance of a binomial variate X are 2 and 1 respectively, then the probability that X takes a value greater than or equal to one is : **[Online April 11, 2015]**

(a) $\frac{9}{16}$ (b) $\frac{3}{4}$

(c) $\frac{1}{16}$ (d) $\frac{15}{16}$

26. If X has a binomial distribution, B(n, p) with parameters n and p such that $P(X = 2) = P(X = 3)$, then E(X), the mean of variable X, is **[Online April 11, 2014]**

(a) $2 - p$ (b) $3 - p$

(c) $\frac{p}{2}$ (d) $\frac{p}{3}$

27. A multiple choice examination has 5 questions. Each question has three alternative answers of which exactly one is correct. The probability that a student will get 4 or more correct answers just by guessing is: **[2013]**

(a) $\frac{17}{3^5}$ (b) $\frac{13}{3^5}$

(c) $\frac{11}{3^5}$ (d) $\frac{10}{3^5}$

28. Consider 5 independent Bernoulli's trials each with probability of success p. If the probability of at least one failure is greater than or equal to $\frac{31}{32}$, then p lies in the interval **[2011]**

(a) $\left(\frac{3}{4}, \frac{11}{12}\right]$ (b) $\left[0, \frac{1}{2}\right]$

(c) $\left(\frac{11}{12}, 1\right]$ (d) $\left(\frac{1}{2}, \frac{3}{4}\right]$

29. In a binomial distribution $B\left(n, p=\frac{1}{4}\right)$, if the probability of at least one success is greater than or equal to $\frac{9}{10}$, then n is greater than: **[2009]**

(a) $\frac{1}{\log_{10} 4+\log_{10} 3}$ (b) $\frac{9}{\log_{10} 4-\log_{10} 3}$

(c) $\frac{4}{\log_{10} 4-\log_{10} 3}$ (d) $\frac{1}{\log_{10} 4-\log_{10} 3}$

30. A pair of fair dice is thrown independently three times. The probability of getting a score of exactly 9 twice is **[2007]**

(a) 8/729 (b) 8/243

(c) 1/729 (d) 8/9.

31. At a telephone enquiry system the number of phone calls regarding relevant enquiry follow Poisson distribution with an average of 5 phone calls during 10 minute time intervals. The probability that there is at the most one phone call during a 10-minute time period is **[2006]**

(a) $\frac{6}{5^e}$ (b) $\frac{5}{6}$

(c) $\frac{6}{55}$ (d) $\frac{6}{e^5}$

32. A random variable X has Poisson distribution with mean 2. Then $P(X > 1.5)$ equals **[2005]**

(a) $\frac{2}{e^2}$ (b) 0

(c) $1-\frac{3}{e^2}$ (d) $\frac{3}{e^2}$

33. The mean and the variance of a binomial distribution are 4 and 2 respectively. Then the probability of 2 successes is **[2004]**

(a) $\frac{28}{256}$ (b) $\frac{219}{256}$

(c) $\frac{128}{256}$ (d) $\frac{37}{256}$

34. A random variable X has the probability distribution:

X:	1	2	3	4	5	6	7	8
p(X):	0.2	0.2	0.1	0.1	0.2	0.1	0.1	0.1

For the events $E = \{X \text{ is a prime number}\}$ and $F = \{X < 4\}$, the $P(E \cup F)$ is **[2004]**

(a) 0.50 (b) 0.77

(c) 0.35 (d) 0.87

35. The mean and variance of a random variable X having binomial distribution are 4 and 2 respectively, then $P(X=1)$ is **[2003]**

(a) $\frac{1}{4}$ (b) $\frac{1}{32}$

(c) $\frac{1}{16}$ (d) $\frac{1}{8}$

36. A dice is tossed 5 times. Getting an odd number is considered a success. Then the variance of distribution of success is **[2002]**

(a) 8/3 (b) 3/8

(c) 4/5 (d) 5/4

Hints & Solutions

1. (b) Let $A \equiv \{0, 1, 2, 3, 4, ..., 10\}$

$n(S) = {}^{11}C_2 = 55$ where 'S' denotes sample space

Let E be the given event

$\therefore E \equiv \{(0,4), (0,8), (2,6), (2,10), (4,8), (6,10)\}$

$\Rightarrow n(E) = 6$

$\therefore P(E) = \frac{n(E)}{n(S)} = \frac{6}{55}$

2. (a) $P(E \cap F) = P(E).P(F) = \frac{1}{12}$

$P(\bar{E} \cap \bar{F}) = P(\bar{E}).P(\bar{F}) = \frac{1}{2}$

$\Rightarrow (1 - P(E))(1 - P(F)) = \frac{1}{2}$

Let $P(E) = x$

$P(F) = y$

$\Rightarrow 1 - x - y + xy = \frac{1}{2}$

$\Rightarrow 1 - x - y = \frac{1}{2} - \frac{1}{12} = \frac{5}{12}$

$\Rightarrow \boxed{x + y = \frac{7}{12}}$

$\Rightarrow x + \frac{1}{12x} = \frac{7}{12} \quad \left[\because x.y = \frac{1}{12}\right]$

$\Rightarrow 12x^2 - 7x + 1 = 0$

$\Rightarrow 12x^2 - 4x - 3x + 1 = 0$

$\Rightarrow (4x - 1)(3x - 1) = 0$

$\Rightarrow x = \frac{1}{3}, x = \frac{1}{4}$

and $y = \frac{1}{4}, y = \frac{1}{3}$

$\therefore \frac{x}{y} = \frac{1/3}{1/4} = \frac{4}{3}$ *or* $\frac{1/4}{1/3} = \frac{3}{4}$

3. (a) Required probability =

$\left(\frac{3}{4}\right)\left(\frac{1}{2}\right)\left(\frac{3}{8}\right) + \left(\frac{1}{4}\right)\left(\frac{1}{2}\right)\left(\frac{3}{8}\right) + \left(\frac{3}{4}\right)\left(\frac{1}{2}\right)\left(\frac{3}{8}\right)$

$= \frac{12+9}{64} = \frac{21}{64}$

4. (b) Required probability $= 1 - \{P(\text{All Head}) + P(\text{All Tail})\}$

$= 1 - \left\{\frac{1}{2^8} + \frac{1}{2^8}\right\}$

$= 1 - \left\{\frac{1}{2^7}\right\}$

$= 1 - \left\{\frac{1}{128}\right\} = \frac{127}{128}$

5. (b) $P(E_1) = \frac{1}{6};\ P(E_2) = \frac{1}{6};\ P(E_3) = \frac{1}{2}$

$P(E_1 \cap E_2) = \frac{1}{36}, P(E_2 \cap E_3) = \frac{1}{12}, P(E_1 \cap E_3) = \frac{1}{12}$

And $P(E_1 \cap E_2 \cap E_3) = 0 \neq P(E_1).P(E_2).P(E_3)$

$\Rightarrow E_1, E_2, E_3$ are not independent.

6. (b) $P(A) = \frac{2}{5} = \frac{8}{20}$; $P(A \cap B) = \frac{3}{20}$

$P(\overline{A \cap B}) = 1 - \frac{3}{20}$

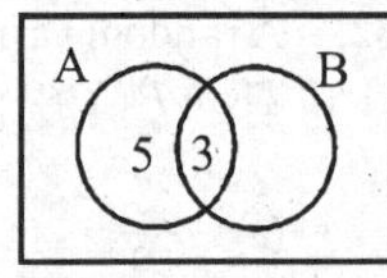

$\Rightarrow P(\bar{A} \cup \bar{B}) = \frac{17}{20}$

$A \cap (A' \cup B')$

$= A - (A \cap B)$

$\therefore P(A - (A \cap B)) = \frac{5}{20}$

$\therefore P(A / (A' \cap B')) = \frac{P(A - (A \cap B))}{P(\bar{A} \cup \bar{B})} = \frac{5}{17}$

7. (d) Required probability is

$$\frac{\left({}^{10}C_0\right)^2 + \left({}^{10}C_1\right)^2 + \left({}^{10}C_2\right)^2 + ... + \left({}^{10}C_{10}\right)^2}{2^{10}}$$

$$= \frac{{}^{20}C_{10}}{2^{20}}$$

8. (a) Given,

$P(\overline{A \cup B}) = \frac{1}{6} \Rightarrow P(A \cup B) = 1 - \frac{1}{6} = \frac{5}{6}$

$P(\bar{A}) = \frac{1}{4} \Rightarrow P(A) = 1 - \frac{1}{4} = \frac{3}{4}$

We know,

$P(A \cup B) = P(A) + P(B) - P(A \cap B)$

$\Rightarrow \quad \frac{5}{6} = \frac{3}{4} + P(B) - \frac{1}{4} \qquad \left(\because P(A \cap B) = \frac{1}{4}\right)$

$\Rightarrow \quad P(B) = \frac{1}{3}$

$\because \; P(A) \neq P(B)$ so they are not equally likely.

Also $P(A) \times P(B) = \frac{3}{4} \times \frac{1}{3} = \frac{1}{4}$

$= P(A \cap B)$

So A & B are independent.

9. (a) Let A and E be any two events with positive probabilities.

Consider statement-1 :

$P(E/A) \geq P(A/E)P(E)$

LHS : $P(E/A) = \frac{P(E \cap A)}{P(A)}$ ...(1)

RHS : $P(A/E).\,P(E) = \frac{P(E \cap A)}{P(E)}.P(E)$

$= P(A \cap E)$ ...(2)

Clearly, from (1) and (2),

we have

$P(E/A) \geq P(A \cap E)$

Thus, statement - 1 is true.

Similarly, statement-2 is also true.

10. (a) $P(\text{A or B but not by C}) = P((A \cup B) \cap \bar{C})$

$= P(A \cup B) \times P(\bar{C})$

$= [P(A) + P(B) - P(A \cap B)] \times P(\bar{C})$

$= \left[\frac{3}{4} + \frac{1}{2} - \frac{3}{4} \times \frac{1}{2}\right] \times \frac{3}{8} = \left(\frac{6+4-3}{8}\right) \times \frac{3}{8} = \frac{21}{64}$

11. (a) Let the probability of occurrence of first event A, be 'a'

i..e., P(A) = a

$\therefore$ P(not A) = $1 - a$

And also suppose that probability of occurrence of second event B, P(B) = b,

$\therefore$ P(not B) = $1 - b$

Now, P(A and not B) + P(not A and B) = $\frac{26}{49}$

$\Rightarrow P(A) \times P(\text{not } B) + P(\text{not } A) \times P(B) = \frac{26}{49}$

$\Rightarrow a \times (1 - b) + (1 - a)\, b = \frac{26}{49}$

$\Rightarrow a + b - 2ab = \frac{26}{49}$ ...(i)

And P(not A and not B) = $\frac{15}{49}$

$\Rightarrow P(\text{not } A) \times P(\text{not } B) = \frac{15}{49}$

$\Rightarrow (1 - a) \times (1 - b) = \frac{15}{49}$

$\Rightarrow 1 - b - a + ab = \frac{15}{49}$

$\Rightarrow a + b - ab = \frac{34}{49}$ ...(ii)

From (i) and (ii),

$a + b = \frac{42}{49}$ ...(iii)

and $ab = \frac{8}{49}$

$(a - b)^2 = (a + b)^2 - 4ab = \frac{42}{49} \times \frac{42}{49} - \frac{4 \times 8}{49} = \frac{196}{2401}$

$\therefore \quad a - b = \frac{14}{49}$ ...(iv)

From (iii) and (iv),

$a = \frac{4}{7}, b = \frac{2}{7}$

Hence probability of more probable of the two events

$= \frac{4}{7}$

12. (a) $\frac{2}{5} + \frac{3}{5} \times \frac{2}{5} + \left(\frac{3}{5}\right)^2 \times \frac{2}{5} + \ldots\ldots + \left(\frac{3}{5}\right)^k . \frac{2}{5} > \frac{7}{10}$

$\Rightarrow \quad \frac{2}{5}\left[1 + \frac{3}{5} + \left(\frac{3}{5}\right)^2 + \ldots\ldots + \left(\frac{3}{5}\right)^k\right] > \frac{7}{10}$

$\Rightarrow \quad \frac{2}{5} \times \frac{1 - \left(\frac{3}{5}\right)^k}{1 - \frac{3}{5}} > \frac{7}{10} \quad \Rightarrow \quad 1 - \left(\frac{3}{5}\right)^k > \frac{7}{10}$

$\Rightarrow \quad \left(\frac{3}{5}\right)^k < \frac{3}{10} \quad \Rightarrow \quad k \geq 3$

Hence minimum value of $k = 3$

13. (b) Given sample space $= \{1,2,3,.....,8\}$
Let Event
A : Maximum of three numbers is 6.
B : Minimum of three numbers is 3.
This is the case of conditional probability
We have to find P (minimum) is 3 when it is given that P (maximum) is 6.

$$\therefore P\left(\frac{B}{A}\right)=\frac{P(B\cap A)}{P(A)}=\frac{{}^2C_1}{{}^5C_2}$$

$$=\frac{2}{10}=\frac{1}{5}$$

14. (d) $P(A^c \cap B^c/C) =$

$$\frac{P\left(\left(A^c\cap B^c\right)\cap C\right)}{P(C)}=\frac{P\left(\left(A\cup B\right)^c\cap C\right)}{P(C)}$$

$$=\frac{P((1-A\cup B)\cap C)}{P(C)}$$

$$=\frac{P((1-A-B+A\cap B)\cap C)}{P(C)}$$

$$=\frac{P(C)-P(A\cap C)-P(B\cap C)+P(A\cap B\cap C)}{P(C)}$$

$$=\frac{P(C)-P(A).P(C)-P(B)P(C)+0}{P(C)}$$

$$=1-P(A)-P(B)$$
$$=P\left(A^c\right)-P(B)$$

15. (a) In this case

$$P\left(\frac{C}{D}\right)=\frac{P(C\cap D)}{P(D)}=\frac{P(C)}{P(D)}$$

Where, $0 \le P(D) \le 1$, hence

$$P\left(\frac{C}{D}\right)\ge P(C)$$

16. (d) Let $A \equiv$ Sum of the digits is 8
$B \equiv$ Product of the digits is 0
Then A= {08, 17, 26, 35, 44}
B= {00, 01, 02, 03, 04, 05, 06, 07, 08, 09, 10, 20, 30, 40,}
$A \cap B = \{08\}$

$$\therefore \quad P(A/B)=\frac{P(A\cap B)}{P(B)}=\frac{1/50}{14/50}=\frac{1}{14}$$

17. (b) $P(A) = 1/4, P(A/B) = \frac{1}{2}, P(B/A) = 2/3$

By conditional probability,
$P(A \cap B) = P(A)P(B/A) = P(B)P(A/B)$

$$\Rightarrow \frac{1}{4}\times\frac{2}{3}=P(B)\times\frac{1}{2}\Rightarrow P(B)=\frac{1}{3}$$

18. (d) Given : Probability of aeroplane I, scoring a target correctly i.e., $P(I) = 0.3$ probability of scoring a target correctly by aeroplane II, i.e. $P(II) = 0.2$

$\therefore P(\overline{I}) = 1 - 0.3 = 0.7$

$\therefore$ The required probability

$= P(\overline{I} \cap II) = P(\overline{I}).P(II) = 0.7 \times 0.2$

19. (b) For a particular house being selected

$$\text{Probability}=\frac{1}{3}$$

P (all the persons apply for the same house)

$$=\left(\frac{1}{3}\times\frac{1}{3}\times\frac{1}{3}\right)3=\frac{1}{9}.$$

20. (c) $P(\overline{A\cup B})=\frac{1}{6}, P(A\cap B)=\frac{1}{4}$ and $P(\overline{A})=\frac{1}{4}$

$$\Rightarrow P(A\cup B)=\frac{5}{6},\ P(A)=\frac{3}{4}$$

Also $\Rightarrow P(A \cup B) = P(A) + P(B) - P(A \cap B)$

$$\Rightarrow P(B)=\frac{5}{6}-\frac{3}{4}+\frac{1}{4}=\frac{1}{3}$$

$$\Rightarrow P(A)\ P(B)=\frac{3}{4}\cdot\frac{1}{3}=\frac{1}{4}=P(A\cap B)$$

Hence A and B are independent but not equally likely.

21. (c) A and B will contradict each other if one speaks truth and other false . So , the required

$$\text{Probability}=\frac{4}{5}\left(1-\frac{3}{4}\right)+\left(1-\frac{4}{5}\right)\frac{3}{4}$$

$$=\frac{4}{5}\times\frac{1}{4}+\frac{1}{5}\times\frac{3}{4}=\frac{7}{20}$$

22. (a) $P(E_1)=\frac{1}{2}, P(E_2)=\frac{1}{3}$ and $P(E_3)=\frac{1}{4}$;

$$P(E_1UE_2UE_3)=1-P(\bar{E}_1)P(\bar{E}_2)P(\bar{E}_3)$$

$$=1-\left(1-\frac{1}{2}\right)\left(1-\frac{1}{3}\right)\left(1-\frac{1}{4}\right)$$

$$=1-\frac{1}{2}\times\frac{2}{3}\times\frac{3}{4}=\frac{3}{4}$$

23. (b) We can apply binomial probability distribution

We have n = 10

$p = \text{Probability of drawing a green ball} = \frac{15}{25} = \frac{3}{5}$

Also $q = 1 - \frac{3}{5} = \frac{2}{5}$

Variance = npq

$= 10 \times \frac{3}{5} \times \frac{2}{5} = \frac{12}{5}$

24. (d) Let $p(F) = p \Rightarrow p(S) = 2p$

$\because \quad p + 2p = 1 \Rightarrow p = \frac{1}{3}$

$p(x \geq 5) = p(x = 5) + p(x = 6)$

$= {}^6C_5\left(\frac{2}{3}\right)^5\left(\frac{1}{3}\right)^1 + {}^6C_5\left(\frac{2}{3}\right)^6\left(\frac{1}{3}\right)^0$

$= \left(\frac{2}{3}\right)^5\left(6 \times \frac{1}{3} + \frac{2}{3}\right) = \frac{256}{729}$

25. (d) Let mean = np = 2 ...(1)

and variance = npq = 1 ...(2)

On solving eqn (1) and (2), we get

$q = \frac{1}{2}$ and $p = \frac{1}{2}$

From eqn (1), we have

n = 4

$P(x \geq 1) = {}^4C_1p^1q^3 + {}^4C_2p^2q^2 + {}^4C_3p^3q + {}^4C_4p^4$

$= 1 - {}^4C_0p^0q^4 = 1 - \left(\frac{1}{2}\right)^4 = 1 - \frac{1}{16} = \frac{15}{16}$

26. (b) Since X has a binomial distribution, B (n, p)

$\therefore$ P $(X = 2) = {}^nC_2\,(p)^2\,(1 - p)^{n-2}$

and P $(X = 3) = {}^nC_3\,(p)^3\,(1 - p)^{n-3}$

Given P $(X = 2)$ = P $(X = 3)$

$\Rightarrow {}^nC_2\,p^2\,(1 - p)^{n-2} = {}^nC_3\,(p)^3\,(1 - p)^{n-3}$

$\Rightarrow \frac{n!}{2!(n-2)!}\cdot\frac{p^2(1-p)^n}{(1-p)^2} = \frac{n!}{3!(n-3)!}\cdot\frac{p^3(1-p)^n}{(1-p)^3}$

$\Rightarrow \frac{1}{n-2} = \frac{1}{3}\cdot\frac{p}{1-p}$

$\Rightarrow 3\,(1 - p) = p\,(n - 2)$

$\Rightarrow 3 - 3p = np - 2p$

$\Rightarrow np = 3 - p$

$\Rightarrow$ E(X) = mean = $3 - p$

($\because$ mean of B $(n, p) = np$)

27. (c) $p = p$ (correct answer), $q = p$ (wrong answer)

$\Rightarrow \pi = \frac{1}{3}, q = \frac{2}{3}, n = 5$

By using Binomial distribution

Required probability

$= {}^5C_4\left(\frac{1}{3}\right)^4\cdot\frac{2}{3} + {}^5C_5\left(\frac{1}{3}\right)^5$

$= 5\cdot\frac{2}{3^5} + \frac{1}{3^5} = \frac{11}{3^5}$

28. (b) p (at least one failure) $\geq \frac{31}{32}$

$\Rightarrow 1 - p\text{ (no failure)} \geq \frac{31}{32}$

$\Rightarrow 1 - p^5 \geq \frac{31}{32}$

$\Rightarrow p^5 \leq \frac{1}{32}$

$\Rightarrow p \leq \frac{1}{2}$

But $p \geq 0$

Hence p lies in the interval $\left[0, \frac{1}{2}\right]$.

29. (d) We have

$P(x \geq 1) \geq \frac{9}{10}$

$\Rightarrow 1 - P(x = 0) \geq \frac{9}{10}$

$\Rightarrow 1 - {}^nC_0\left(\frac{1}{4}\right)^0\left(\frac{3}{4}\right)^n \geq \frac{9}{10}$

$\Rightarrow 1 - \frac{9}{10} \geq \left(\frac{3}{4}\right)^n$

$\Rightarrow \left(\frac{3}{4}\right)^n \leq \left(\frac{1}{10}\right)$

Taking log to the base 3/4, on both sides, we get

$n\log_{3/4}\left(\frac{3}{4}\right) \geq \log_{3/4}\left(\frac{1}{10}\right)$

$\Rightarrow \quad n \geq -\log_{3/4} 10 = \frac{-\log_{10} 10}{\log_{10}\left(\frac{3}{4}\right)}$

$= \dfrac{-1}{\log_{10} 3 - \log_{10} 4}$

$\Rightarrow n \geq \dfrac{1}{\log_{10} 4 - \log_{10} 3}$

$= 0.14$

30. **(b)** A pair of fair dice is thrown, the sample space $S = (1, 1), (1, 2)(1, 3) .... = 36$.
Possibility of getting 9 are (5, 4), (4, 5), (6, 3), (3,6)
∴ Possibility of getting score 9 in a single throw

$= \dfrac{4}{36} = \dfrac{1}{9}$

∴ Probability of getting score 9 exactly twice

$= {}^3C_2 \times \left(\dfrac{1}{9}\right)^2 . \left(1 - \dfrac{1}{9}\right) = \dfrac{3!}{2!} \times \dfrac{1}{9} \times \dfrac{1}{9} \times \dfrac{8}{9}$

$= \dfrac{3.2!}{2!} \times \dfrac{1}{9} \times \dfrac{1}{9} \times \dfrac{8}{9} = \dfrac{8}{243}$

31. **(d)** $P(X = r) = \dfrac{e^{-m} m^r}{r!}$

P (at most 1 phone call)

$= P(X \leq 1) = P(X = 0) + P(X = 1)$

$= e^{-5} + 5 \times e^{-5} = \dfrac{6}{e^5}$

32. **(c)** According to Poission distribution, prob. of getting k successes is

$P(x = k) = e^{-\lambda} \dfrac{\lambda^k}{k!}$

$P(x \geq 2) = 1 - P(x = 0) - P(x = 1)$

$= 1 - e^{-\lambda} - e^{-\lambda} \left(\dfrac{\lambda}{1!}\right) = 1 - \dfrac{3}{e^2}$.

33. **(a)** mean $= np = 4$ and variance $= npq = 2$

$\therefore p = q = \dfrac{1}{2}$ and $n = 8$

$\therefore P(2 \text{ success}) = {}^8C_2 \left(\dfrac{1}{2}\right)^6 \left(\dfrac{1}{2}\right)^2$

$= \dfrac{28}{2^8} = \dfrac{28}{256}$

34. **(b)** $P(E) = P(2 \text{ or } 3 \text{ or } 5 \text{ or } 7)$

$= 0.23 + 0.12 + 0.20 + 0.07 = 0.62$

$P(F) = P(1 \text{ or } 2 \text{ or } 3) = 0.15 + 0.23 + 0.12 = 0.50$

$P(E \cap F) = P(2 \text{ or } 3)$

$= 0.23 + 0.12 = 0.35$

$\therefore P(EUF) = P(E) + P(F) - P(E \cap F)$

$= 0.62 + 0.50 - 0.35 = 0.77$

35. **(b)** $\left.\begin{matrix} np = 4 \\ npq = 2 \end{matrix}\right\} \Rightarrow q = \dfrac{1}{2}, p = \dfrac{1}{2}, n = 8$

$P(X = 1) = {}^8C_1 \left(\dfrac{1}{2}\right)\left(\dfrac{1}{2}\right)^7$

$= 8 . \dfrac{1}{2^8} = \dfrac{1}{2^5} = \dfrac{1}{32}$

36. **(d)** The event follows binomial distribution with $n = 5, p = 3/6 = 1/2$.
$q = 1 - p = 1/2$.; ∴ Variance $= npq = 5/4$.

Properties of Triangles

TOPIC-1 : Properties of Triangle, Solutions of Triangles, Inscribed & Enscribed Circles, Regular Polygons

1. In a ΔABC, $\frac{a}{b} = 2 + \sqrt{3}$ and $\angle C = 60°$. Then the ordered pair ($\angle A$, $\angle B$) is equal to : **[Online April 10, 2015]**
(a) $(45°, 75°)$ (b) $(105°, 15°)$
(c) $(15°, 105°)$ (d) $(75°, 45°)$

2. ABCD is a trapezium such that AB and CD are parallel and $BC \perp CD$. If $\angle ADB = \theta$, $BC = p$ and $CD = q$, then AB is equal to : **[2013]**
(a) $\frac{(p^2+q^2)\sin\theta}{p\cos\theta + q\sin\theta}$ (b) $\frac{p^2+q^2\cos\theta}{p\cos\theta + q\sin\theta}$
(c) $\frac{p^2+q^2}{p^2\cos\theta + q^2\sin\theta}$ (d) $\frac{(p^2+q^2)\sin\theta}{(p\cos\theta + q\sin\theta)^2}$

3. If in a triangle ABC, $\frac{b+c}{11} = \frac{c+a}{12} = \frac{a+b}{13}$, then cosA is equal to **[2012]**
(a) 5/7 (b) 1/5
(c) 35/19 (d) 19/35

4. In a ΔPQR, If $3\sin P + 4\cos Q = 6$ and $4\sin Q + 3\cos P = 1$, then the angle R is equal to : **[2012]**
(a) $\frac{5\pi}{6}$ (b) $\frac{\pi}{6}$
(c) $\frac{\pi}{4}$ (d) $\frac{3\pi}{4}$

5. For a regular polygon, let r and R be the radii of the inscribed and the circumscribed circles. A ***false*** statement among the following is **[2010]**
(a) There is a regular polygon with $\frac{r}{R} = \frac{1}{\sqrt{2}}$
(b) There is a regular polygon with $\frac{r}{R} = \frac{2}{3}$
(c) There is a regular polygon with $\frac{r}{R} = \frac{\sqrt{3}}{2}$
(d) There is a regular polygon with $\frac{r}{R} = \frac{1}{2}$

6. If in a ΔABC, the altitudes from the vertices A, B, C on opposite sides are in H.P, then $\sin A$, $\sin B$, $\sin C$ are in **[2005]**
(a) G.P. (b) A. P.
(c) A.P-G.P. (d) H. P

7. In a triangle ABC, let $\angle C = \frac{\pi}{2}$. If r is the inradius and R is the circumradius of the triangle ABC, then $2(r+R)$ equals **[2005]**
(a) $b+c$ (b) $a+b$
(c) $a+b+c$ (d) $c+a$

8. The sides of a triangle are $\sin\alpha, \cos\alpha$ and $\sqrt{1+\sin\alpha\cos\alpha}$ for some $0 < \alpha < \frac{\pi}{2}$. Then the greatest angle of the triangle is **[2004]**
(a) 150° (b) 90°
(c) 120° (d) 60°

9. If in a ΔABC $a\cos^2\left(\frac{C}{2}\right) + c\cos^2\left(\frac{A}{2}\right) = \frac{3b}{2}$, then the sides a, b and c **[2003]**
(a) satisfy $a+b=c$ (b) are in A.P
(c) are in G.P (d) are in H.P.

10. In a triangle ABC, medians AD and BE are drawn. If AD = 4, $\angle DAB = \frac{\pi}{6}$ and $\angle ABE = \frac{\pi}{3}$, then the area of the ΔABC is **[2003]**
(a) $\frac{64}{3}$ (b) $\frac{8}{3}$
(c) $\frac{16}{3}$ (d) $\frac{32}{3\sqrt{3}}$

11. The sum of the radii of inscribed and circumscribed circles for an n sided regular polygon of side a , is **[2003]**

(a) $\frac{a}{4}\cot\left(\frac{\pi}{2n}\right)$ (b) $a\cot\left(\frac{\pi}{n}\right)$

(c) $\frac{a}{2}\cot\left(\frac{\pi}{2n}\right)$ (d) $a\cot\left(\frac{\pi}{2n}\right)$.

12. In a triangle with sides $a, b, c, r_1 > r_2 > r_3$ (which are the ex-radii) then **[2002]**

(a) $a > b > c$ (b) $a < b < c$

(c) $a > b$ and $b < c$ (d) $a < b$ and $b > c$

13. The sides of a triangle are $3x+4y$, $4x+3y$ and $5x+5y$ where $x, y > 0$ then the triangle is **[2002]**

(a) right angled (b) obtuse angled

(c) equilateral (d) none of these

TOPIC-2 : Heights & Distances

14. Let a vertical tower AB have its end A on the level ground. Let C be the mid-point of AB and P be a point on the ground such that AP = 2AB. If $\angle BPC = \beta$, then $\tan\beta$ is equal to : **[2017]**

(a) $\frac{4}{9}$ (b) $\frac{6}{7}$

(c) $\frac{1}{4}$ (d) $\frac{2}{9}$

15. A man is walking towards a vertical pillar in a straight path, at a uniform speed. At a certain point A on the path, he observes that the angle of elevation of the top of the pillar is 30°. After walking for 10 minutes from A in the same direction, at a point B, he observes that the angle of elevation of the top of the pillar is 60°. Then the time taken (in minutes) by him, from B to reach the pillar, is: **[2016]**

(a) 20 (b) 5

(c) 6 (d) 10

16. The angle of elevation of the top of a vertical tower from a point A, due east of it is 45°. The angle of elevation of the top of the same tower from a point B, due south of A is 30°. If the distance between A and B is $54\sqrt{2}$ m, then the height of the tower (in metres), is : **[Online April 10, 2016]**

(a) 108 (b) $36\sqrt{3}$

(c) $54\sqrt{3}$ (d) 54

17. If the angles of elevation of the top of a tower from three collinear points A, B and C, on a line leading to the foot of the tower, are 30°, 45° and 60° respectively, then the ratio, AB : BC, is : **[2015]**

(a) $1:\sqrt{3}$ (b) $2:3$

(c) $\sqrt{3}:1$ (d) $\sqrt{3}:\sqrt{2}$

18. Let 10 vertical poles standing at equal distances on a straight line, subtend the same angle of elevation at a point O on this line and all the poles are on the same side of O. If the height of the longest pole is 'h' and the distance of the foot of the smallest pole from O is 'a'; then the distance between two consecutive poles, is : **[Online April 11, 2015]**

(a) $\frac{h\cos\alpha - a\sin\alpha}{9\sin\alpha}$ (b) $\frac{h\sin\alpha + a\cos\alpha}{9\sin\alpha}$

(c) $\frac{h\cos\alpha - a\sin\alpha}{9\cos\alpha}$ (d) $\frac{h\sin\alpha - a\cos\alpha}{9\cos\alpha}$

19. A bird is sitting on the top of a vertical pole 20 m high and its elevation from a point O on the ground is $45°$. It flies off horizontally straight away from the point O. After one second, the elevation of the bird from O is reduced to $30°$. Then the speed (in m/s) of the bird is **[2014]**

(a) $20\sqrt{2}$ (b) $20\left(\sqrt{3}-1\right)$

(c) $40\left(\sqrt{2}-1\right)$ (d) $40\left(\sqrt{3}-\sqrt{2}\right)$

20. The angle of elevation of the top of a vertical tower from a point P on the horizontal ground was observed to be α. After moving a distance 2 metres from P towards the foot of the tower, the angle of elevation changes to β. Then the height (in metres) of the tower is: **[Online April 11, 2014]**

(a) $\frac{2\sin\alpha\sin\beta}{\sin(\beta-\alpha)}$ (b) $\frac{\sin\alpha\sin\beta}{\cos(\beta-\alpha)}$

(c) $\frac{2\sin(\beta-\alpha)}{\sin\alpha\sin\beta}$ (d) $\frac{\cos(\beta-\alpha)}{\sin\alpha\sin\beta}$

21. AB is a vertical pole with B at the ground level and A at the top. A man finds that the angle of elevation of the point A from a certain point C on the ground is 60°. He moves away from the pole along the line BC to a point D such that CD = 7 m. From D the angle of elevation of the point A is 45°. Then the height of the pole is **[2008]**

(a) $\frac{7\sqrt{3}}{2}\frac{1}{\sqrt{3}-1}m$ (b) $\frac{7\sqrt{3}}{2}(\sqrt{3}+1)m$

(c) $\frac{7\sqrt{3}}{2}(\sqrt{3}-1)m$ (d) $\frac{7\sqrt{3}}{2}\frac{1}{\sqrt{3}+1}m$

22. A tower stands at the centre of a circular park. A and B are two points on the boundary of the park such that $AB\ (= a)$ subtends an angle of $60°$ at the foot of the tower, and the angle of elevation of the top of the tower from A and B is $30°$. The height of the tower is **[2007]**

(a) $a/\sqrt{3}$ (b) $a\sqrt{3}$

(c) $2a/\sqrt{3}$ (d) $2a\sqrt{3}$

23. A person standing on the bank of a river observes that the angle of elevation of the top of a tree on the opposite bank of the river is $60°$ and when he retires 40 meters away from the tree the angle of elevation becomes $30°$. The breadth of the river is **[2004]**

(a) 60m (b) 30 m

(c) 40m (d) 20 m

24. The upper $\frac{3}{4}$ th portion of a vertical pole subtends an angle $\tan^{-1}\frac{3}{5}$ at a point in the horizontal plane through its foot and at a distance 40 m from the foot. A possible height of the vertical pole is **[2003]**

(a) $80\,m$ (b) $20\,m$

(c) $40\,m$ (d) $60\,m$.

Hints & Solutions

1. (b) $\frac{\sin A}{\sin B} = 2+\sqrt{3}$

$\frac{\sin(105°)}{\sin(15°)} = 2+\sqrt{3} \quad \frac{\cos 15°}{\sin 15°} = 2+\sqrt{3}$

2. (a) From Sine Rule

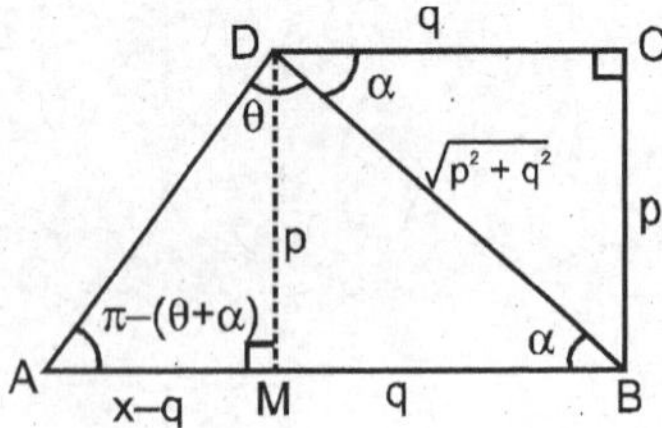

$\frac{AB}{\sin\theta} = \frac{\sqrt{p^2+q^2}}{\sin(\pi-(\theta+\alpha))}$

$AB = \frac{\sqrt{p^2+q^2}\,\sin\theta}{\sin\theta\cos\alpha + \cos\theta\sin\alpha}$

$= \frac{(p^2+q^2)\sin\theta}{q\sin\theta + p\cos\theta}$

$\left(\because \cos\alpha = \frac{q}{\sqrt{p^2+q^2}} \text{ and } \sin\alpha = \frac{p}{\sqrt{p^2+q^2}}\right)$

3. (b) Let $\frac{b+c}{11} = \frac{c+a}{12} = \frac{a+b}{13} = K$ in a triangle ABC.

$\Rightarrow b+c = 11K, c+a = 12K, a+b = 13K$

On solving these, we get

$a = 7K, b = 6K, c = 5K$

Now we know,

$\cos A = \frac{b^2+c^2-a^2}{2bc}$

$= \frac{36K^2+25K^2-49K^2}{2(6K)(5K)} = \frac{1}{5}$

4. (b) Given $3\sin P + 4\cos Q = 6$ ...(i)

$4\sin Q + 3\cos P = 1$ ...(ii)

Squaring and adding (i) & (ii) we get

$9\sin^2 P + 16\cos^2 Q + 24\sin P\cos Q$

$+ 16\sin^2 Q + 9\cos^2 P + 24\sin Q\cos P$

$= 36+1 = 37$

$\Rightarrow 9(\sin^2 P + \cos^2 P) + 16(\sin^2 Q + \cos^2 Q)$

$+ 24(\sin P\cos Q + \cos P\sin Q) = 37$

$\Rightarrow 9 + 16 + 24\sin(P+Q) = 37$

$[\because \sin^2\theta + \cos^2\theta = 1$ and $\sin A\cos B + \cos A\sin B = \sin(A+B)]$

$\Rightarrow \sin(P+Q) = \frac{1}{2}$

$\Rightarrow P+Q = \frac{\pi}{6}$ or $\frac{5\pi}{6}$

$\Rightarrow R = \frac{5\pi}{6}$ or $\frac{5\pi}{6}$ $\quad (\because P+Q+R = \pi)$

If $R = \frac{5\pi}{6}$ then $0 < P, Q < \frac{\pi}{6}$

$\Rightarrow \cos Q < 1$ and $\sin P < \frac{1}{2}$

$\Rightarrow 3\sin P + 4\cos Q < \frac{11}{2}$

So, $R = \frac{\pi}{6}$

5. (b) If O is centre of polygon and AB is one of the side, then by figure

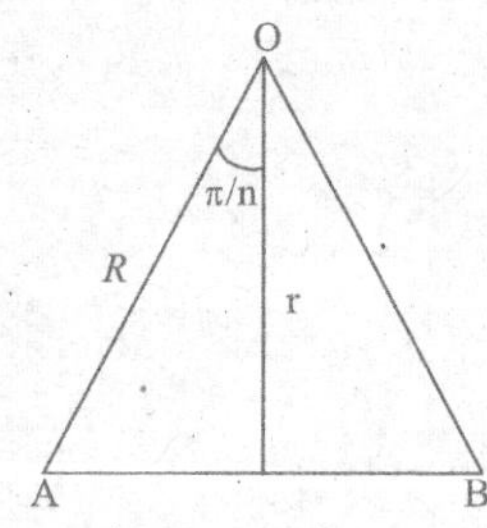

$\cos\frac{\pi}{n} = \frac{r}{R}$

$\Rightarrow \frac{r}{R} = \frac{1}{2}, \frac{1}{\sqrt{2}}, \frac{\sqrt{3}}{2}$ for $n = 3, 4, 6$ respectively.

6. (b) $\Delta = \frac{1}{2}p_1 a = \frac{1}{2}p_2 b = \frac{1}{2}p_3 b$

p_1, p_2, p_3, are in H.P.

$\Rightarrow \frac{2\Delta}{a}, \frac{2\Delta}{b}, \frac{2\Delta}{c}$ are in H.P.

$\Rightarrow \frac{1}{a}, \frac{1}{b}, \frac{1}{c}$ are in H.P.

$\Rightarrow$ a, b, c are in A.P.

$\Rightarrow KsinA, K\sin B, K\sin C$ are in AP

$\Rightarrow$ $\sin A, \sin B, \sin C$ are in A.P.

7. (b) We know that for the circle circumscribing a right triangle, hypotenutse is the diameter As $\angle C = 90°$

$$\therefore 2R = c \Rightarrow R = \frac{c}{2}$$

also $r = \dfrac{\Delta}{s} = \dfrac{\frac{1}{2}\times a\times b}{\frac{a+b+c}{2}}$

$\Rightarrow r = \dfrac{ab}{a+b+c}$ $\quad\therefore\ 2r + 2R = \dfrac{2ab}{a+b+c} + c$

$$= \frac{2ab+ac+bc+c^2}{a+b+c} = \frac{2ab+ac+bc+a^2b^2}{a+b+c}$$

$$\left(\because c^2 = a^2 + b^2\right)$$

$$= \frac{(a+b)^2 + (a+b)c}{a+b+c} = (a+b)$$

8. (c) Let $a = \sin\alpha, b = \cos\alpha$ and $c = \sqrt{1+\sin\alpha\cos\alpha}$

Clearly a and $b < 1$ but $c > 1$ as $\sin\alpha > 0$ and $\cos\alpha > 0$

$\therefore c$ is the greatest side and greatest angle is C

$$\therefore \cos C = \frac{a^2+b^2-c^2}{2ab}$$

$$= \frac{\sin^2\alpha + \cos^2\alpha - 1 - \sin\alpha\cos\alpha}{2\sin\alpha\cos\alpha} = -\frac{1}{2}$$

$\therefore C = 120°$

9. (b) If $a\cos^2\left(\dfrac{C}{2}\right) + c\cos^2\left(\dfrac{A}{2}\right) = \dfrac{3b}{2}$

$a[\cos C + 1] + c[\cos A + 1] = 3b$

$(a+c) + (a\cos C + c\cos B) = 3b$

$a + c + b = 3b$ or $a + c = 2b$

or a, b, c are in $A.P.$

10. (d)

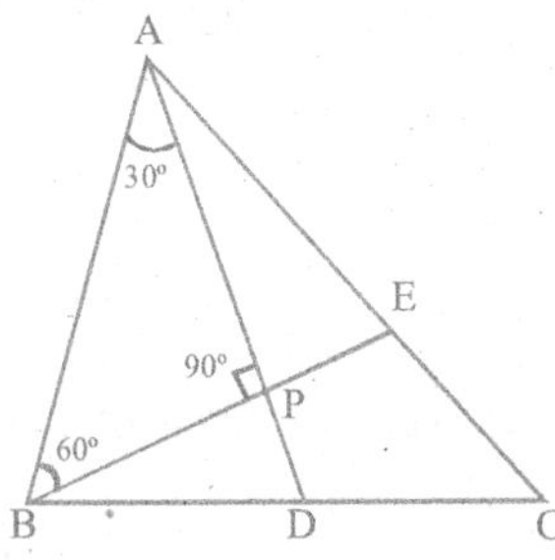

$AP = \dfrac{2}{3}AD = \dfrac{8}{3}$; $\quad PD = \dfrac{4}{3}$; $\quad$ Let $PB = x$

$\tan 60^o = \dfrac{8/3}{x}$ or $x = \dfrac{8}{3\sqrt{3}}$

Area of $\Delta ABD = \dfrac{1}{2}\times 4\times\dfrac{8}{3\sqrt{3}} = \dfrac{16}{3\sqrt{3}}$

$\therefore$ Area of $\Delta ABC = 2\times\dfrac{16}{3\sqrt{3}} = \dfrac{32}{3\sqrt{3}}$

[$\because$ Median of a Δ divides it into two Δ's of equal area.]

11. (c) $\tan\left(\dfrac{\pi}{n}\right) = \dfrac{a}{2r}$; $\sin\left(\dfrac{\pi}{n}\right) = \dfrac{a}{2R}$

$$r + R = \frac{a}{2}\left[\cot\frac{\pi}{n} + \operatorname{cosec}\frac{\pi}{n}\right]$$

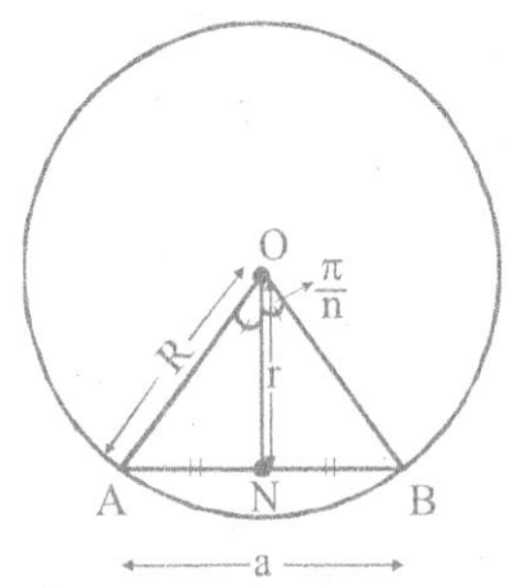

$$= \frac{a}{2}\left[\frac{\cos\frac{\pi}{n}+1}{\sin\frac{\pi}{n}}\right] = \frac{a}{2}\left[\frac{2\cos^2\frac{\pi}{2n}}{2\sin\frac{\pi}{2n}\cos\frac{\pi}{2n}}\right]$$

$$= \frac{a}{2}\cot\frac{\pi}{2\pi}$$

12. (a) $r_1 > r_2 > r_3 \Rightarrow \dfrac{\Delta}{s-a} > \dfrac{\Delta}{s-b} > \dfrac{\Delta}{s-c}$;

$\Rightarrow s-a < s-b < s-c \Rightarrow -a < -b < -c \Rightarrow a > b > c$

13. (b) Let $a = 3x + 4y$, $b = 4x + 3y$ and $c = 5x + 5y$

as $x, y > 0$, $c = 5x + 5y$ is the largest side

$\therefore$ C is the largest angle. Now

$$\cos C = \frac{(3x+4y)^2 + (4x+3y)^3 - (5x+5y)^2}{2(3x+4y)(4x+3y)}$$

$$= \frac{-2xy}{2(3x+4y)(4x+3y)} < 0$$

$\therefore$ C is obtuse angle $\Rightarrow \Delta$ABC is obtuse angled

14. (d) Since AP = 2AB $\Rightarrow \dfrac{AB}{AP} = \dfrac{1}{2}$ ...(1)

Let $\angle$APC = α

$\tan\alpha = \dfrac{AC}{AP} = \dfrac{1}{2}\dfrac{AB}{AP} = \dfrac{1}{4}$ $\quad$ ($\because$ C is the mid point $\therefore$ AC = $\dfrac{1}{2}$AB)

$\Rightarrow \tan\alpha = \dfrac{1}{4}$

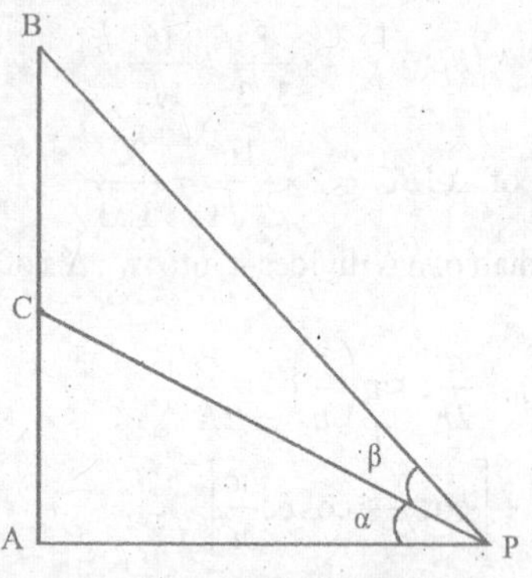

As $\tan(\alpha+\beta) = \frac{\tan\alpha + \tan\beta}{1-\tan\alpha\tan\beta}$

$$\Rightarrow \frac{\tan\alpha+\tan\beta}{1-\tan\alpha\tan\beta} = \frac{1}{2} \left[\begin{array}{l} \because \tan(\alpha+\beta) = \frac{AB}{AP} \\ \tan(\alpha+\beta) = \frac{1}{2} \ [\text{From(1)}] \end{array}\right]$$

$$\Rightarrow \frac{\frac{1}{4}+\tan\beta}{1-\frac{1}{4}\tan\beta} = \frac{1}{2}$$

$\therefore \tan\beta = \frac{2}{9}$

15. (b) $\tan 30° = \frac{h}{x+a}$

$\Rightarrow \frac{1}{\sqrt{3}} = \frac{h}{x+a} \Rightarrow \sqrt{3}h = x+a$ ...(1)

$\tan 60° = \frac{h}{a} \Rightarrow \sqrt{3} = \frac{h}{a}$

$\Rightarrow h = \sqrt{3}a$ ...(2)

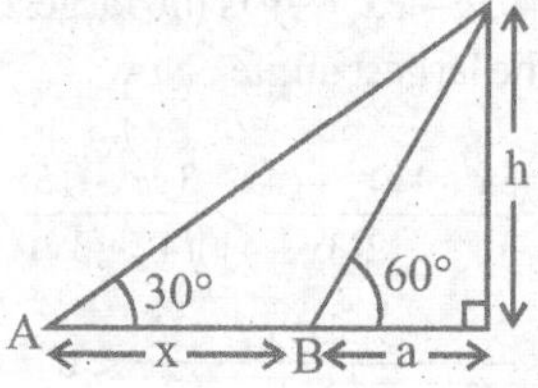

From (1) and (2)

$3a = x + a \Rightarrow x = 2a$

Here, the speed is uniform

So, time taken to cover x = 2 (time taken to cover a)

$\therefore$ Time taken to cover $a = \frac{10}{2}$ minutes = 5 minutes

16. (d) Let $AP = x$

$BP = y$

$\tan 45° = \frac{H}{x} \Rightarrow H = x$

$\tan 30° = \frac{H}{y} \Rightarrow y = \sqrt{3}H$

$x^2 + (54\sqrt{2})^2 = y^2$

$H^2 + (54\sqrt{2})^2 = 3H^2$

$(54\sqrt{2})^2 = 2H^2$

$54\sqrt{2} = \sqrt{2}H$

$54 = H$

17. (c)

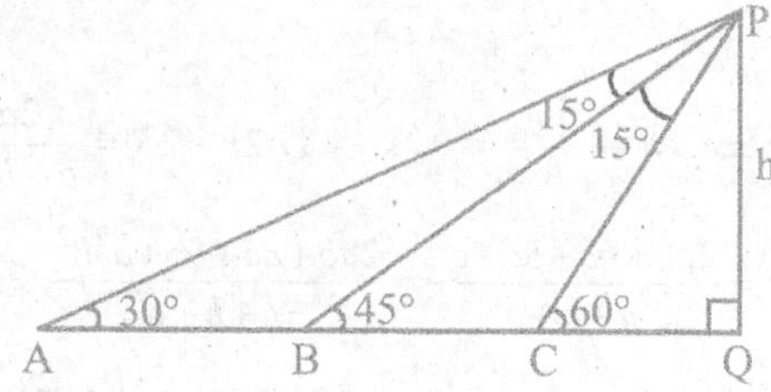

$\because$ PB bisects $\angle APC$, therefore

$AB : BC = PA : PC$

Also in ΔAPQ, $\sin 30° = \frac{h}{PA} \Rightarrow PA = 2h$

and in ΔCPQ, $\sin 60° = \frac{h}{PC} \Rightarrow PC = \frac{2h}{\sqrt{3}}$

$\therefore$ $AB : BC = 2h : \frac{2h}{\sqrt{3}} = \sqrt{3} : 1$

18. (a)

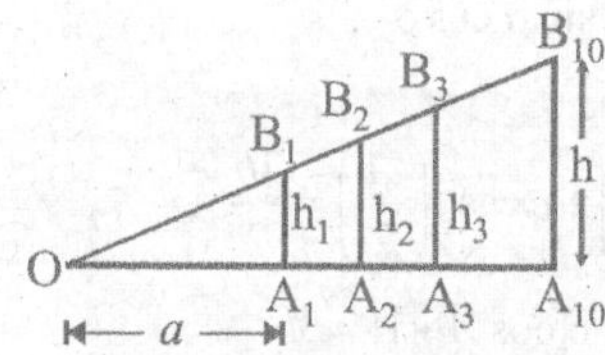

$\Delta OA_1B_1, \Delta OA_2B_2, \Delta OA_3B_3, \ldots\ldots, \Delta OA_{10}B_{10}$ all are similar triangles.

$\Rightarrow \frac{h_1}{a_1} = \frac{h_2}{a_2} = \frac{h_3}{a_3} = \ldots\ldots = \frac{h_{10}}{a_{10}} = \tan\alpha$.

Since, $h_{10} = h = a_{10}\tan\alpha$ ...(1)

and $a_1 = a \Rightarrow h_1 = a\tan\alpha$ ...(2)

$\Rightarrow h = (a+9d)\tan\alpha$ where d is distance between poles $(\because a_{10} = a + 9d)$

$\Rightarrow h = a\tan\alpha + 9d\tan\alpha$

$$\Rightarrow \frac{h - a\tan\alpha}{9\tan\alpha} = d \Rightarrow \frac{h - \frac{a\sin\alpha}{\cos\alpha}}{9\frac{\sin\alpha}{\cos\alpha}} = d$$

$$\Rightarrow d = \frac{h\cos\alpha - a\sin\alpha}{9\sin\alpha}$$

19. (b) Let the speed be y m/sec.

Let AC be the vertical pole of height 20 m.

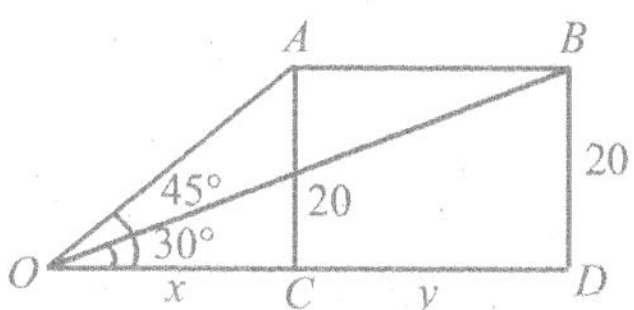

Let O be the point on the ground such that $\angle AOC = 45°$

Let $OC = x$

Time $t = 1$ s

From ΔAOC,

$$\tan 45° = \frac{20}{x} \quad \text{...(i)}$$

and from ΔBOD,

$$\tan 30° = \frac{20}{x+y} \quad \text{...(ii)}$$

From (i) and (ii), we have $x = 20$ and $\frac{1}{\sqrt{3}} = \frac{20}{x+y}$

$$\Rightarrow \frac{1}{\sqrt{3}} = \frac{20}{20+y} \Rightarrow 20 + y = 20\sqrt{3}$$

So, $y = 20(\sqrt{3}-1)$

i.e., speed $= 20(\sqrt{3}-1)$ m/s

20. (a) Let AB be the tower of height 'h'.

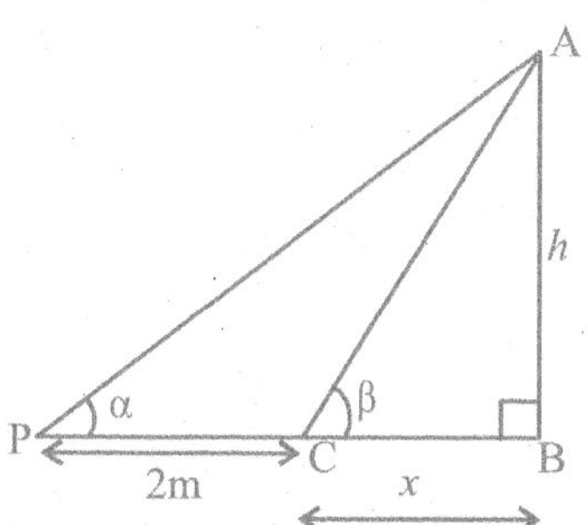

Given : In ΔABP

$$\tan\alpha = \frac{AB}{PB}$$

or $\frac{\sin\alpha}{\cos\alpha} = \frac{h}{x+2}$

$\Rightarrow (x + 2)\sin\alpha = h\cos\alpha$

$$\Rightarrow h = \frac{x\sin\alpha + 2\sin\alpha}{\cos\alpha} \quad \text{...(1)}$$

Now, In ΔABC, $\tan\beta = \frac{AB}{BC}$

$$\Rightarrow \frac{\sin\beta}{\cos\beta} = \frac{h}{x} \Rightarrow x = \frac{h\cos\beta}{\sin\beta} \quad \text{...(2)}$$

Putting the value of x in eq. (2) to eq. (1), we get

$$h = \frac{\frac{h\cos\beta\sin\alpha}{\sin\beta} + \frac{2\sin\alpha}{1}}{\cos\alpha}$$

$$\Rightarrow h = \frac{h\cos\beta.\sin\alpha + 2\sin\alpha\sin\beta}{\sin\beta.\cos\alpha}$$

$\Rightarrow h(\sin\beta.\cos\alpha - \cos\beta.\sin\alpha) = 2\sin\alpha.\sin\beta$

$\Rightarrow h[\sin(\beta - \alpha)] = 2\sin\alpha.\sin\beta$

$$\Rightarrow h = \frac{2\sin\alpha.\sin\beta}{\sin(\beta-\alpha)}$$

21. (b) In ΔABC $\frac{h}{x} = \tan 60° = \sqrt{3}$

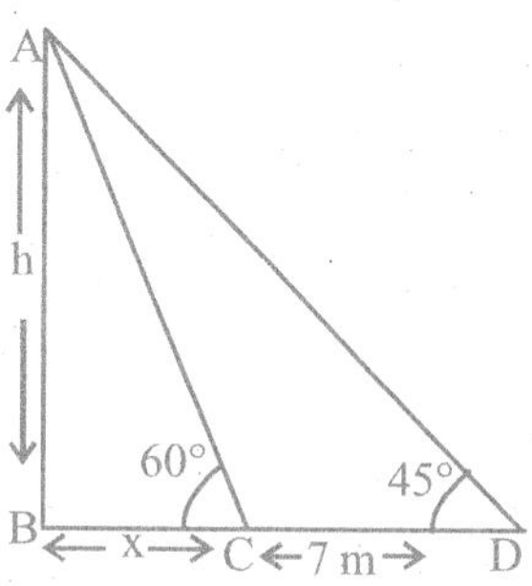

$$\Rightarrow x = \frac{h}{\sqrt{3}}$$

In ΔABD

$$\frac{h}{x+7} = \tan 45° = 1$$

$$\Rightarrow h = x + 7 \Rightarrow h - \frac{h}{\sqrt{3}} = 7$$

$$\Rightarrow h = \frac{7\sqrt{3}}{\sqrt{3}-1} \times \frac{\sqrt{3}+1}{\sqrt{3}+1}$$

$$\Rightarrow h = \frac{7\sqrt{3}}{2}\left(\sqrt{3}+1\right)m$$

22. (a) In the ΔAOB, $\angle AOB = 60°$, and $\angle OBA = \angle OAB$ (since $OA = OB = AB$ radius of same circle). $\therefore$ ΔAOB is a equilateral triangle. Let the height of tower is h

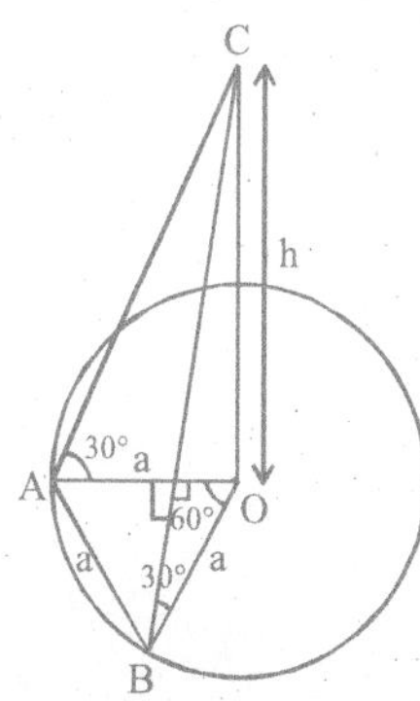

m. Given distance between two points A & B lie on boundary of circular park, subtends an angle of 60° at the foot of the tower is AB i.e. $AB = a$. A tower OC

stands at the centre of a circular park. Angle of elevation of the top of the tower from A and B is 30°. In

$\Delta OAC,\ \tan 30° = \frac{h}{a} \Rightarrow \frac{1}{\sqrt{3}} = \frac{h}{a}$

$\Rightarrow h = \frac{a}{\sqrt{3}}$

23. (d)

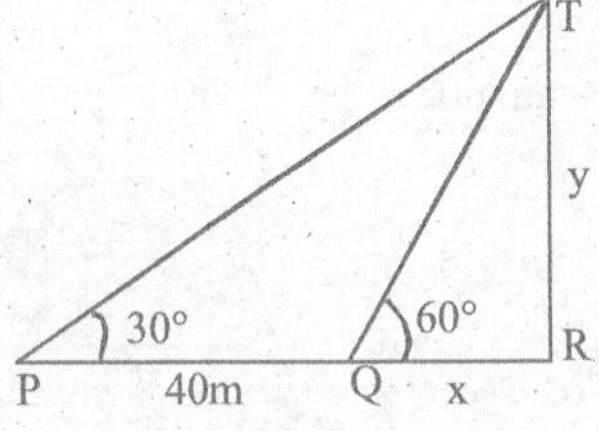

From the figure

$\tan 60° = \frac{y}{x} \Rightarrow y = \sqrt{3}x$ ....(1)

$\tan 30° = \frac{y}{x+40} \Rightarrow y = \frac{x+40}{\sqrt{3}}$ ....(2)

From (1) and (2), $\sqrt{3}x = \frac{x+40}{\sqrt{3}} \Rightarrow x = 20m$

24. (c)

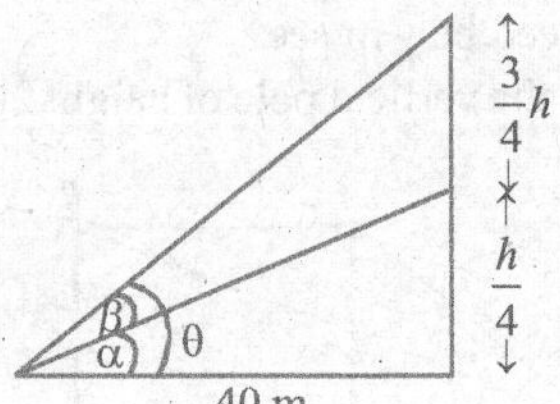

$\theta = \alpha + \beta, \beta = \tan^{-1}\left(\frac{3}{5}\right)$

or $\beta = \theta - \alpha$

$\Rightarrow \tan\beta = \frac{\tan\theta - \tan\alpha}{1 + \tan\theta . \tan\alpha}$

or $\frac{3}{5} = \frac{\frac{h}{40} - \frac{h}{160}}{1 + \frac{h}{40} . \frac{h}{160}}$

$h^2 - 200h + 6400 = 0$

$\Rightarrow h = 40$ or 160 metre

$\therefore$ possible height $= 40$ metre